Deborah Tomlinson
Nancy E. Kline
(Eds.)

Pediatric Oncology Nursing

Advanced Clinical Handbook

With 43 Figures and 203 Tables

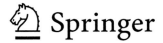 Springer

Library of Congress
Control Number 2004101947
ISBN 3-540-40851-7
Springer Berlin Heidelberg New York
ISSN 1613-53

Deborah Tomlinson MN, RSCN, RGN,
Dip. Cancer Nursing
Macmillan Lecturer/Project Leader
School of Nursing Studies
University of Edinburgh
31 Buccleuch Place
Edinburgh, EH8 9JT
Scotland, UK

Nancy E. Kline PhD, RN, CPNP, FAAN,
Director
Center for Innovation and Clinical Scholarship
Children's Hospital Boston
Wolbach 201
300 Longwood Avenue
Boston, MA 02115
USA

Springer is a part of Springer Science + Business Media

springeronline.com

© Springer-Verlag Berlin Heidelberg 2005
Printed in Germany

Medical Editor: Dr. Julia Heidelmann, Heidelberg, Germany
Desk Editor: Meike Stoeck, Heidelberg, Germany
Cover design: Erich Kirchner, Heidelberg, Germany
Layout: Bernd Wieland, Heidelberg, Germany
Production: Pro Edit GmbH, Heidelberg, Germany
Reproduction and typesetting: AM-productions GmbH, Wiesloch, Germany

21/3150 – 5 4 3 2 1 0
Printed on acid-free paper

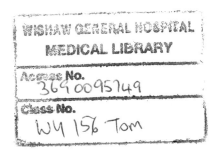

Dedication

To the nurses, and others,
who use the information in this book,
and to the children they serve,
we dedicate this work.

To my husband Chris and our children,
Vivian, Sam and Suzanne –
to the moon and back.
Deborah Tomlinson

To my parents, and Michael.
I am forever grateful for your love and support.
Nancy E. Kline

Preface

"Pediatric Oncology Nursing: Advanced Clinical Handbook" is a joint effort between nurses in Canada, the UK, and the USA. This is a first-time collaboration between pediatric hematology and oncology nurses from two continents and represents a blending of knowledge from these experts. The book is designed to be a comprehensive clinical handbook for nurses in advanced practice working with pediatric hematology / oncology patients. Specific issues related to young children and adolescents with cancer and hematologic disorders are discussed.

Twenty-two contributors and two editors participated in the writing of this text. Nurses in advanced practice and academic roles – nurse practitioners, clinical nurse specialists, clinical instructors, lecturers, and educators – were involved. One of the most appealing features of this text is the varied experience represented by nurses from different countries and different educational backgrounds.

The book is divided into five sections: pediatric cancers, hematologic disorders, treatment of childhood cancer, side effects of treatment and disease, and supportive and palliative care. Many tables and illustrations are included for quick reference in the clinical setting. Future perspectives and opportunities for new treatment options and research are discussed.

Part One focuses on pediatric cancers: the leukemias and solid tumors. The most common pediatric tumors, as well as some rare tumors, are discussed with regard to epidemiology, etiology, molecular genetics, symptoms and clinical signs, diagnostic and laboratory testing, staging and classification, treatment, prognosis, and follow-up care.

Part Two focuses on pediatric hematology. The anemias, bleeding disorders, neutropenia, and thrombocytopenia are discussed in detail. Epidemiology, etiology, symptoms and clinical signs, diagnostic and laboratory procedures, treatment, prognosis, and follow up care are included for each of the disorders.

Part Three covers cancer treatment, including chemotherapy, radiation therapy, peripheral stem cell transplantation, surgery, gene therapy, and complementary and alternative medicine. The principles and description of treatment, method of treatment delivery, potential side effects, and special considerations for each type of treatment are discussed.

Part Four focuses on the side effects of cancer treatment in relation to metabolic processes and the gastrointestinal, hematologic, respiratory, urinary, cardiovascular, neurologic, musculoskeletal, integumentary, and endocrine systems. The incidence, etiology, treatment, prevention, and prognosis are included for each side effect reviewed.

Part Five includes essential information regarding supportive and palliative care of pediatric cancer patients. Nutrition, hydration, pain, transfusion therapy, growth factors, and care of the dying child are covered. The principles of treatment for these conditions, method of delivery, and special considerations for certain conditions are included.

As the editors of "Pediatric Oncology Nursing: Advanced Clinical Handbook" we want to recognize and thank everyone who participated in the development of this text. We are profoundly aware of the personal time and commitment that was devoted to make this an outstanding resource, and we are grateful. It is our hope that nurses in advanced clinical practice will find this publication useful and that it will enrich knowledge and improve care for young people with cancer and hematologic disorders.

Deborah Tomlinson, Nancy E. Kline

Contributors

Sharon Beardsmore SRN, RSCN, Dip Palliative Care
Paediatric Macmillan Nurse,
Birmingham's Children's Hospital NHS Trust,
Birmingham, UK

Jane Belmore RSCN, RGN, Dip Palliative Care
Macmillan Clinical Nurse Specialist, Schiehallion
Day Care Unit, Royal Hospital for Sick Children,
Yorkhill NHS Trust, Glasgow, G3 8SJ, Scotland, UK

Rosalind Bryant MN, RN, PNP
Instructor of Pediatrics,
Pediatric Nurse Practitioner,
Texas Children's Cancer Center
and Hematology Service, 6621 Fannin MC1-3320,
Houston, TX 77030, USA

Christine Chordas MSN, RN, CPNP
Pediatric Nurse Practitioner, Jimmy Fund Clinic,
Dana Farber Cancer Institute, 44 Binney Street,
D306, Boston, MA 02115, USA

Sandra Doyle MN, RN
Clinical Nurse Specialist, Hospital For Sick Children,
Division of Hematology Oncology,
555 University Avenue, Toronto, Ontario M5G 1X8,
Canada

Angela M. Ethier MSN, RN, CNS, CPN
Clinical Instructor and Fellow,
UTSHC School of Nursing, 4223 University Blvd.,
Houston, TX 77005, USA

Nicki Fitzmaurice RGN, RSCN, Dip N, BSc
Paediatric Macmillan Nurse, Birmingham's
Children's Hospital NHS Trust, Birmingham, UK

Ali Hall RSCN, RGN, BA, M.Phil,
Ad Dip Child Development
Paediatric Oncology Outreach Nurse Specialist,
Schiehallion Day Care Unit, Yorkhill NHS Trust,
Glasgow, G3 8SJ, Scotland, UK

Eleanor Hendershot RN, BScN, MN
Clinical Nurse Specialist/Acute Care Nurse
Practitioner, Hospital For Sick Children,
Division of Hematology Oncology –
Solid Tumor Program, 555 University Avenue,
Toronto, Ontario, M5G 1X8, Canada

Kathleen E. Houlahan MS, RN
Nurse Manager, Hematology/Oncology/
Stem Cell Transplant, Children's Hospital Boston,
300 Longwood Avenue, Boston, MA 02115, USA

Elizabeth Kassner MSN, RN, CPNP
Instructor of Pediatrics, Pediatric Nurse
Practitioner, Texas Children's Cancer Center
and Hematology Service, 3000 Bissonnet Street,
#2304, Houston, TX 77005, USA

Mark W. Kieran MD, PhD
Director, Pediatric Medical Neuro-Oncology,
Assistant Professor of Pediatrics,
Harvard Medical School,
Dana-Farber Cancer Institute, Boston, MA, USA

Nancy E. Kline PhD, RN, CPNP, FAAN
Children's Hospital Boston, Wolbach 201,
300 Longwood Avenue, Boston, MA 02115, USA

Nan D. McIntosh RSCN, RGN, BSc (Hons),
NP Diploma
Haematology Advanced Nurse Practitioner,
Schiehallion Day Care Unit, Yorkhill NHS Trust,
Glasgow, G3 8SJ, Scotland, UK

Anne-Marie Maloney RN, BSc, MSc
CNS/NP, The Hospital for Sick Children,
555 University Avenue, Toronto, Ontario M5G 1X8,
Canada

Ethel McNeill RSCN, RGN, BSc
Endocrine Nurse Specialist, Department
of Child Health, Yorkhill NHS Trust,
Glasgow, G3 8SJ, Scotland, UK

Colleen Nixon RN, BSN, CPON
Patient Educator, Inpatient Oncology, Children's
Hospital Boston, 300 Longwood Avenue, Boston,
MA 02115, USA

Robbie Norville MSN, RN, CNS
Bone Marrow Transplant/Cell and Gene Therapy,
Clinical Nurse Specialist, Texas Children's Cancer
Center and Hematology Service,
6621 Fannin MC1-3320, Houston, TX 77030, USA

Joan M. O'Brien RN, BSN, CPON
Hematology/Oncology Clinical Educator,
Children's Hospital Boston, 300 Longwood Avenue,
Boston, MA 02115, USA

Jill Brace O'Neill MS, RN-CS, PNP
David B. Perini Quality of Life Clinic,
Dana-Farber Cancer Institute,
D-321, 44 Binney Street,
Boston, MA 02115, USA

Margaret Parr RGN, RSCN, ENB240
Paediatric Oncology Nurse Specialist,
Children's Services, E Floor, East Block,
Queen's Medical Centre, Derby Road,
Nottingham, NG7 2UH, UK

Fiona Reid RSCN, RGN
Staff Nurse
Raigmore Hospital, Old Perth Road, Inverness,
1V2 3UJ, Scotland, UK

Debbie Rembert MSN, RN, CNS
Clinical Instructor and Fellow,
UTSHC School of Nursing, 4201 Ruskin,
Houston, TX 77005, USA

Chris M. Senter RGN, RSCN, ONC
Macmillan Clinical Nurse Specialist,
Royal Orthopaedic Hospital, Orthopaedic Oncology
Service, Bristol Road South, Northfield,
Birmingham, B31 2AP, UK

Nicole M. Sevier MSN, RN, CPNP
Instructor of Pediatrics, Pediatric Nurse
Practitioner, Texas Children's Cancer Center
and Hematology Service, 6621 Fannin MC1-3320,
Houston, TX 77030, USA

Cara Simon MSN, RN, CPNP
Instructor of Pediatrics, Pediatric Nurse
Practitioner, Texas Children's Cancer Center
and Hematology Service, 6621 Fannin MC1-3320,
Houston, TX 77030, USA

Deborah Tomlinson MN, RSCN, RGN,
Dip. Cancer Nursing
Macmillan Lecturer/Project Leader,
School of Nursing Studies,
University of Edinburgh,
31 Buccleuch Place, Edinburgh, EH8 9JT,
Scotland, UK

Contents

3   **Common Central Nervous System Tumours**

Nicki Fitzmaurice · Sharon Beardsmore

9   Radiation Therapy
Joan M. O'Brien · Deborah Tomlinson

10   Hematopoietic Stem Cell Transplantation
      Robbie Norville

11   Surgical Approaches to Childhood Cancer
      Jill Brace O'Neill

12   Gene Therapy
      Kathleen E. Houlahan · Mark W. Kieran

13   Complementary and Alternative Therapy
      Nancy E. Kline

PART IV

14   Metabolic System
      Deborah Tomlinson

15 Gastrointestinal Tract
Anne-Marie Maloney

19   Cardiovascular System
     Ali Hall

20   Central Nervous System
     Jane Belmore · Deborah Tomlinson

29   Growth Factors
Nancy E. Kline

30   Care of the Dying Child
       and the Family
Angela M. Ethier

PART I

Leukemia

Deborah Tomlinson

Contents

Leukemia is the most common malignancy that affects children, accounting for approximately a third of cancer diagnoses. It may be defined as a neoplastic disease that involves the blood-forming tissues of the bone marrow, lymph nodes, and spleen.

Normal hematopoiesis occurs in these blood-forming tissues; the development of blood cells is shown in Fig. 1.1. A range of extracellular protein factors regulates the growth and differentiation of pathways of developing cells. This ensures that the mature blood cell types are produced in appropriate proportions. Leukemia is a clonal disease that is due to genetic mutations and transformation of a single early progenitor myeloid or lymphoid cell during hematopoiesis. The type of leukemia that results is therefore dependent on the cell lineage that is affected by the mutation. Table 1.1 shows the blood cells that can be affected from either stem cell lineage. In leukemia, there is an overproduction of immature white blood cells that cannot function effectively. These immature white blood cells, such as the myeloblasts, lymphoblasts, and monoblasts, are commonly called "blasts." An abnormal population of immature white blood cells decreases the space available for the production of other healthy blood cells produced by the bone marrow. The blast cells may then enter the blood and may also infiltrate the central nervous system (CNS).

The two broad classifications of leukemia are acute and chronic. The most common types of leukemia are

- Acute lymphoblastic leukemia (ALL), which accounts for 75–80% of childhood leukemia

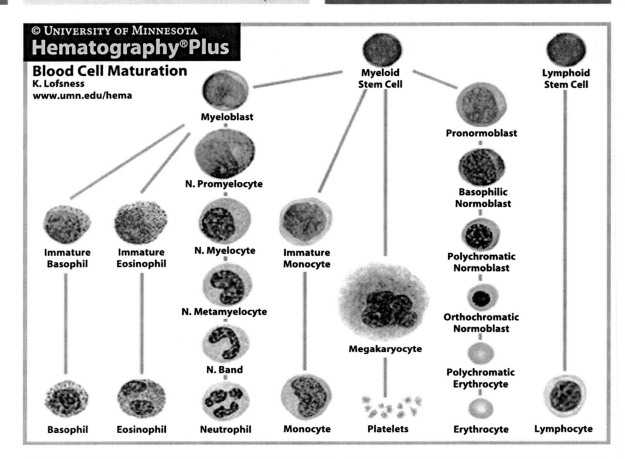

© UNIVERSITY OF MINNESOTA
Hematography®Plus

Blood Cell Maturation
K. Lofsness
www.umn.edu/hema

Figure 1.1

Hemopoiesis: The lymphoid stem cell differentiates into T-lymphocytes and B-lymphocytes. Natural Killer (NK) cells are also thought to derive from the lymphocyte stem cell. Image credit: K. Lofsness, University of Minnesota

— Acute myeloid leukemia (AML), also known as acute nonlymphoblastic leukemia (ANLL), which accounts for 20–25% of childhood leukemia
The most common type of chronic leukemia is

— Chronic myeloid (or myelocytic) leukemia (CML), which accounts for less than 5% of childhood leukemia

1.1 Acute Lymphoblastic Leukemia

1.1.1 Epidemiology

ALL affects slightly more males than females (1.2:1) and peaks between the ages of 2 and 6 years. In infants there is a higher number of females affected.

Globally, the highest incidence of ALL appears to be in Europe and North America, with about 5 cases in 100,000 of 0–14-year-old children. The lowest incidence, of about 0.9 in 100,000, is in Kuwait and Bombay. There may be a lack of clarity regarding some

Table 1.1. Lineage and function of major types of blood cells

Blood cell	Lineage	Function	Half-life
Red blood cells (erythrocytes)	Myeloid stem cells	Transport oxygen from lungs to tissue Transport some carbon dioxide from tissues to lungs	About 120 days
Platelets (thrombocytes)	Myeloid stem cells	Repair blood vessels and participate in clotting mechanism	7–10 days
White blood cells (leucocytes)		Crucial in immunity	
Monocytes	Myeloid stem cells	Can differentiate into macrophages; phagocytosis; antigen presentation; immune regulation	1–3 days in blood 3 months in tissues
Granulocytes			
– Neutrophils	Myeloid stem cells	Phagocytosis, killing bacteria	6–12 hours in blood
– Eosinophils	Myeloid stem cells	Detoxify products from allergic response; phagocytosis	2–3 days in tissues
– Basophils	Myeloid stem cells	Involved in allergic response; source of immune inhibitors (e.g., histamine)	Minutes to hours in blood, then in tissue for about 12 days
– Monocytes	Myeloid stem cells	Contain enzymes that kill foreign bacteria	Undetermined
Lymphocytes	Lymphoid stem cells	Role in immunity	Undetermined; cells can move between blood and lymphoid tissues
– T lymphocytes		Attack invaders directly	
– B lymphocytes		Produce antibodies	
– Others: null cells, natural killer cells, lymphokine-activated killer cells, tumor-infiltrating lymphocytes			

incidence figures due to the lack of true population-based registration of cancer. However, ALL generally has a higher incidence in affluent industrialized nations within white populations. The incidence tends to be lower among the black populations of the same nations.

In a study in the United States, Pan et al. (2002) compared the incidence of leukemia in Asian-Americans and their descendents and in Caucasians. This study reported a lower incidence of leukemia in Asian-Americans irrespective of birthplace. In 1991, Stiller et al. reported that children of Asian and West Indian ethnic origin had patterns of ALL incidence that were similar to those of Caucasians. Interestingly, other later studies of ALL incidence in areas of the United Kingdom have reported an increased risk, although not significantly so, of ALL among South Asian children compared with non-Asian children (McKinney et al. 2003; Powell et al. 1994). However, these increases may be due to socioeconomic status, which has been linked to childhood cancers.

Table 1.2. Syndromes with a predisposition to leukemia

Genetic bone marrow failure syndromes predisposed
to leukemia:
  Fanconi's anemia
  Diamond-Blackfan anemia
  Shwachman-Diamond syndrome
  Congenital dyskeratosis
  Kostmann's infantile genetic agranulocytosis

Genetic syndromes predisposed to leukemia
as one of the illnesses:
  Chromosomal abnormality:
  Down's syndrome (trisomy 21)
  Chromosome 8 trisomy syndrome

DNA repair/tumor suppressor deficiency:
  Ataxia telangiectasia
  Li-Fraumeni syndrome
  Neurofibromatosis type 1
  Bloom syndrome
  Nijmegen/Berlin breakage syndrome
  Retinoblastoma:
  RB1 gene is important in the histiogenesis of ALL

(Table compiled from Mizutani 1998)

1.1.2 Etiology

The factors involved in the cause of childhood cancers are unclear. Many different etiologies have been
suggested and investigated, but few are well established. It would be misleading to associate the cause
of any childhood malignancy wholly to genetic or environmental factors, but the study of various factors
can improve the understanding of events that may
lead to leukemia in children.

1.1.2.1 Genetic Factors

Syndromes that have a component of hereditary or
genetic predisposition to leukemia have been identified and are listed in Table 1.2. A study by Mellemkjaer et al. in 2000 has shown that children of parents
with autoimmune disease are slightly more susceptible to leukemia.

1.1.2.2 Environmental Factors

It is accepted that ionizing radiation is a causal factor
in leukemia. Following the atomic bombs in Japan,
children who were exposed acquired an increased
risk of developing leukemia. Individuals exposed in
utero, however, showed no increase in incidence of
leukemia. This finding is in contrast to the suggested
results of various studies that showed an increased
risk of leukemia and other cancers (by about 40%) to
children exposed in utero to diagnostic radiography
(Doll and Wakeford 1997). There is no doubt that ionizing radiation is a causal factor in leukemia; however, there are uncertainties regarding various aspects
of its effect on leukemogenesis.

A significant change in thought surrounds the
clusters of reported childhood ALL around nuclear
installations. The suspicion that background radiation was the cause of these clusters has moved towards Kinlen's theory (1995) that population mixing,
herd immunity, and abnormal response to infection
of unusually susceptible children increases the risk of
ALL. This "delayed infection" or "hygiene" hypothesis
suggests that ALL in children is caused by a lack of
exposure to infection in infancy, with an abnormal
response to a later common infection incurred after
mixing with other children in playgroups or schools.
Therefore, circumstances that alter the pattern of infections in infants may contribute to the etiology of
ALL.

Table 1.3 highlights studies that have been undertaken to investigate various possible factors in the
etiology of childhood leukemia and other cancers. All
theories surrounding the causes of ALL, or indeed the
majority of childhood cancers, leave much unexplained, and further studies are necessary to confirm
or reject the conclusions of those available.

Because of the public interest that surrounds the
majority of these potential risk factors, parents will
continue to form theories regarding their children's
illnesses (Ruccione et al. 1994). Nurses have a role in
eliciting parents' causal explanations so that the content of these concerns can be related to the parents'
adjustment and management of their experience of
childhood cancer.

Table 1.3. Reported environmental links to childhood leukemia and current conclusions

Possible environmental link	Current conclusions
Parental use of tobacco	Paternal smoking before pregnancy may be a potential risk factor for the generality of childhood cancers. Studies do not provide significant evidence (Pang et al. 2003; Sorahan et al. 2001)
Vitamin K prophylaxis in infants	Inconsistent associations reported. However, confirmed benefits of vitamin K outweigh the hypothetical association with any childhood cancer (Parker et al. 1998; Passmore et al. 1998; Roman et al. 2002; Ross and Davies 2000).
Living near landfill sites	No excess risk of any cancer reported (Jarup et al. 2002)
Proximity to railways	No association reported between risk of childhood leukemia and railway proximity (Dickinson et al. 2003). Small association with railway density assumed consequence of population mixing and proximity of railways in deprived urban areas
Children born after in-vitro fertilization	No increased risk of childhood cancer reported in studies published (Bergh et al. 1999; Klip et al. 2001)
Prenatal ultrasound	No association with childhood leukemia found (Naumburg et al. 2000)
Supplementary oxygen	Resuscitation with 100% oxygen immediately postpartum is associated with childhood ALL; further studies warranted (Naumburg et al. 2002a)
Breastfeeding	Contradicting reports of association with a reduced risk of acute leukemia (Lancashire and Sorahan 2003; UK Childhood Cancer Study Investigators 2001; Shu et al. 1999)
Pet (healthy or sick) ownership	No relationship (Swensen et al. 2001)
Family cancer history	May be a risk factor for childhood acute leukemia (Perrillat et al. 2001)
Electromagnetic fields (EMF)/ power lines	Do not support hypothesis of an association (Skinner et al. 2002; Steinbuch et al. 1999)
Natural radionucleotides in drinking water, including uranium	Results do not indicate increased risk of leukemia (Auvinen et al. 2002)
In utero exposure to metronidazole	No reported increased risk (Thapa et al. 1998)
Allergies or family history of allergies	Reduced risk of ALL; no such pattern seen with AML (Schuz et al. 2003)
Exposure to pesticides	May increase risk (Ma et al. 2002); further studies needed
Perinatal exposure to infection	Some association reported between maternal lower genitourinary tract infection in utero and risk of childhood leukemia (Naumburg et al. 2002b). This supports hypothesis that an infectious agent is involved in etiology of ALL (Kinlen 1995)
Population mixing	Increased risk of ALL in children 1–6 years old in high tertile of population mixing (Alexander et al. 1999; Boutou et al. 2002). Further support for infectious agents possessing direct or indirect cause

1.1.3 Molecular Genetics

Clonal chromosomal abnormalities (originating in a single cell) are detectable in around 90% of childhood ALL cases. The leukemia then evolves by the accrual of mutations within a clone. The abnormalities are responsible for a loss of controlled cell growth, division, and differentiation.

To review the biology of chromosomes:

- Genes carry instructions to make proteins essential for cell growth, division, and differentiation.
- A deoxyribonucleic acid (DNA) molecule carries the genetic information in coded form.
- DNA is a nucleic acid made of chains of nucleotides.
- Nucleotides have three components – a phosphate group, a pentose sugar, and a base.
- In DNA the sugar is deoxyribose, and the bases are adenine, guanine, thymine, and cytosine.
- DNA consists of two chains of nucleotides linked across their bases by weak hydrogen ions. These two complementary strands of nucleotides are linked in a double helix formation.
- The bases have specific affinities with each other, so that thymine pairs only with adenine, and cytosine pairs only with guanine.
- The base sequence is the key to the control of the cell and is referred to as the genetic code.
- The length of DNA in cells is so great that there is a significant risk of entanglement and breakage. During mitosis, proteins called histones bind to DNA and wrap it into 46 compact manageable chromosomes (23 pairs).
- The complete chromosome complement of a cell is referred to as the karyotype.

Some genes are associated with the transformation of a normal cell to a malignant cell. These are known as oncogenes (or proto-oncogenes) and tumor suppressor genes. Mutations in the DNA of these genes may cause them to produce an abnormal product or disrupt their control so that they are expressed inappropriately, making products in excessive amounts or at the wrong time. Some oncogenes may cause extra production of growth factors, which are chemicals that stimulate cell growth. Other oncogenes may cause changes in a surface receptor, causing it to send signals as though it were being activated by a growth factor.

The exact number of mutations required to transform a normal cell into a malignant cell is unknown, but research indicates that two or more mutations, or "hits," are involved. The first hit is thought to occur in the womb, which in ALL is likely to be a developmental accident affecting a chromosome. This would then suggest that a second hit after birth is necessary before ALL develops. This theory has arisen mainly from observed high concordance rates of leukemia in infant monozygotic twins (that is, if one twin has leukemia, so will the other) and the study of neonatal blood spots or Guthrie cards. In twins, it is considered that the leukemogenic event arises in one twin, and the cells from the abnormal clone then spread to the other via shared placental anastomosis. Polymerase chain reaction (PCR) has been used to identify the same fusion gene sequence in neonatal blood spots as is in patients' leukemic cells at diagnosis. In all cases of infant leukemia, there are fusions of the MLL gene; in many cases of childhood ALL, there are fusions of the TEL-AML 1 gene. These gene fusions would indicate the first hit or mutation. Table 1.4 shows the classification of types of mutation that can occur. In childhood ALL, reciprocal translocations account for approximately 25% of the chromosomal abnormalities. The translocations involve exchanges of tracks of DNA between chromosomes, resulting in the generation of chimeric or fusion genes. There may also be changes in chromosome number (ploidy), gene deletions, or single nucleotide base changes in genes. (The chromosome number is also measurable as the DNA index, in which 46 chromosomes equals a DNA index of 1).

As discussed earlier, the process by which a normal cell transforms into a leukemic cell is unclear. However, improved molecular analysis techniques have assisted in identifying mechanisms regulating cell growth and differentiation. These include the following:

- Polymerase chain reaction (PCR)
- Fluorescence in situ hybridization (FISH)
- Flow cytometry for immunophenotyping

Table 1.4. Types of mutation to genetic code

Mutation	Description	Presentations
Point mutation	Change in DNA sequence Can occur in base substitution, deletion, or addition May result in wrong amino acid being inserted into protein	Mis-sense mutation, usually a decrease in function
Chromosomal mutation	Alteration in the gross structure of chromosomes Results from cell breakage and reunion of chromosomal material during the cell cycle	Translocation Rearrangement
Genomic mutation	Change in number of chromosomes in the genome	Amplification Aneuploidy (loss or gain of single chromosome

- Digitized karyotype imaging/multicolor spectral karyotyping
- Microarray profiling
- Southern blotting
- Western blotting

Molecular analysis has proved indispensable for identifying prognostic factors and therapeutically important genetic subtypes of childhood ALL. The ranges of subtypes are based on gene expression, antigens that delineate cell type, and chromosomal and molecular abnormalities. There is currently a relatively sophisticated understanding of the genetic basis of ALL, which will be discussed further in the following sections.

1.1.4 Symptoms and Clinical Signs

ALL usually presents as an acute illness of short onset, but symptoms are occasionally slow and insidious. Symptoms relate to the infiltration of the bone marrow and other affected organs by the proliferation of lymphoblastic cells. The presenting features often appear like many childhood illnesses. Parents or children may describe the following:

- irritability
- night sweats
- fatigue
- bone pain, which may present as limping
- loss of appetite

Initially, symptoms may fluctuate daily, with the child feeling exhausted one day and fine the next. The child may have suffered from repeated ear or other infections that have been frequently resistant to treatment. This is often associated with a history of frequent visits to the family general practitioner.

Physical findings may include the following:

- pallor and lethargy
- pain at the sites of disease infiltration, especially in long bones
- petechiae
- bruising or unusual bleeding (including nose bleeds)
- enlarged liver or spleen, causing the abdomen to protrude
- enlarged lymph nodes and fever

In less than 10 % of cases the disease has spread to the CNS at diagnosis. This may cause related symptoms of

- headache
- poor school performance
- weakness
- vomiting
- blurred vision
- seizures
- difficulty maintaining balance

In 60–70 % of children with the T-cell type of ALL, there is involvement of the thymus. Enlargement of the thymus caused by an accumulation of white blood cells can give rise to an anterior mediastinal mass that can cause pressure on the trachea, causing coughing, shortness of breath, pain, and dysphagia. In some cases the pressure may also compress the superior vena cava and cause swelling of the head and arms.

In rare circumstances acute leukemia may present with extremely high blast cell counts, known as hyperleukocytosis. This state of the disease can cause respiratory failure, intracranial bleeding, and severe metabolic abnormalities, conditions that are the main causes of high early mortality. The process that leads to these complications has become known as leukostasis. It had been thought that leukostasis was caused by overcrowding of leukemic blasts. However, it is now evident that leukostasis results from adhesive interactions between blasts and the vascular endothelium. Damage to the endothelium is likely due to cytokines that are released. The adhesion molecules displayed by the blasts and their response to the environment are probably more important factors in leukostasis formation than numbers of cells. Leukopheresis is routinely used to reduce the leukocyte count in the initial phase when there is hyperleukocytosis. It remains unclear whether this is the most efficient method of treating leukostasis. However, further research should indicate the most appropriate use of this procedure.

1.1.5 Diagnostics

If ALL is suspected following the history and physical examination of the child, initial investigations include a complete blood count, urea and electrolyte counts, and a chest x-ray. The blood count may point to a diagnosis of leukemia with blast cells present or an elevated white blood cell count. Figure 1.2a shows a normal blood film, and Fig. 1.2b is a blood film from a child with ALL. However, the necessary diagnostic investigation is a bone marrow examination. The bone marrow is usually taken from the iliac bone at the iliac crest. Despite the new technologies available, ALL is still usually diagnosed by an experienced pediatric oncologist and/or pathologist examining a Romanowsky-stained bone marrow smear with a high-powered microscope. More than a 25% blast cell count in the marrow confirms a diagnosis of leukemia. A portion of the bone marrow aspirate and the chloroma biopsy/trephine are then analyzed to detect other features of the leukemic cells to help determine what type of leukemia is present. Other techniques are used to extend the diagnosis.

A lumbar puncture is performed to determine any CNS involvement; a sample of cerebrospinal fluid (CSF) is examined for blast cells.

These procedures are most often performed using sedation or anesthetic. Therefore, because of the potential anesthetic difficulties that could develop, a chest x-ray is vital to assist in diagnosing infection or detecting a mediastinal mass.

1.1.6 Staging and Classification

1.1.6.1 Risk Classification

Once a diagnosis of ALL has been confirmed, cell morphology, cytogenetics, and immunophenotyping are determined to elicit more defined prognostic factors. Treatment can then focus on "risk-directed" protocols developed through well-designed clinical trials. This strategy uses the child's likelihood of relapse or resistance to treatment to intensify or reduce the treatment to ensure adequate cell kill within acceptable levels of toxicity. The significance of various reported risk factors has led to some debate. Difficulty also arises when comparing results between different countries and centers using locally-assigned risk categories. However, over the past few decades several features have been determined to be more favorable prognostic factors. In 1993, following a previous initiative in Rome, collaborative groups met to establish those features that would indicate "standard risk" ALL. These are known as the Rome/NCI (National Cancer Institute) criteria:

- WBC <50,000/mm^3
- Female
- 1–9 years of age
- non-T/non-B

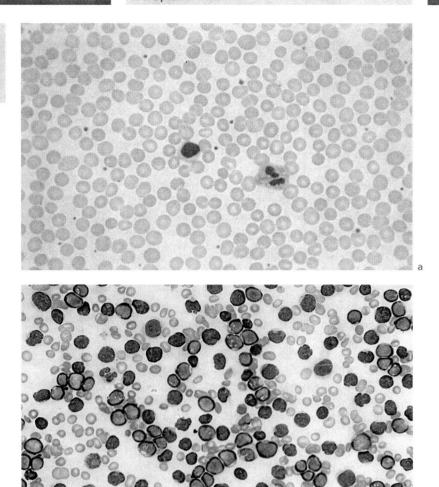

All other patients are "high risk."

Other factors are used to determine risk classification, but the number and array of factors used to classify ALL make it difficult to establish any one system. Consequently, there is a lack of precision within most risk classification systems. Varying conclusions have been reported with regard to the prognostic significance of other characteristics, including the presence of Down's syndrome; liver and spleen size; the presence of an anterior mediastinal mass; French-American-British subtype; body mass index; and CNS involvement, hemoglobin level, platelet count, and number of blast cells in the CSF at diagnosis. However, subgroups of patients with different outcomes can be predicted by blast karyotype, molecular abnormalities, and early response to treatment, with response to treatment proving to be increasingly more important. The persistence of lymphoblasts in bone marrow following a week of induction therapy is associated with a poor prognosis, with less than 30 % survival at 5 years no matter what subsequent therapy is given (Hann 2001).

Table 1.5. French-American-British Classification of acute lymphoblastic leukemia

Category	Definition	Features	% of patients
L1	Small cells with scant cytoplasm	Associated with good treatment response	90%
L2	Large cells with abundant cytoplasm	Indicates more refractory to therapy if 10–20% L2 cells are present	9%
L3	Large cells with prominent nucleoli	Mature B-cell phenotype; frequently presents as lymphoma; poor prognosis	1%

Interestingly, a study by Gajjar and colleagues in 2000 found that traumatic lumbar puncture at diagnosis of childhood ALL indicated adverse outcomes and was an indication to intensify intrathecal (IT) therapy.

1.1.6.2 Cell Morphology

Despite other ways of looking at cells, a morphological classification that is still widely applied is the French-American-British (FAB) system. This classification is based on the morphology (appearance, structure, and cytochemistry) and number of cells, and it defines three categories (Table 1.5). This system is limited due to very unevenly divided numbers of patients in each category and to a morphological feature that correlates with responsiveness to conventional therapy – the presence of cytoplasmic vacuoles – not included in the FAB system. Vacuoles are present in 25–30% of patients and are associated with a lower presenting white cell count and the "common" ALL immunophenotype.

1.1.6.3 Cytochemistry

Several biochemical markers have been identified to assist in the classification of leukemia. However, little is added to the morphology of ALL, with the exception of

- Periodic-acid Schiff positivity, seen in around 15% of cases correlating with common ALL
- Acid phosphatase positivity in T-ALL

Table 1.6. Categories of acute lymphoblastic leukemia

Category of ALL	Percentage (approximately)
Common or pre-B	80%
T-cell	10%
Mature B	7%
Null (early B-precursor)	3%

All forms other than T-cell are considered as B-precursor cell ALL

1.1.6.4 Immunophenotyping

ALL is probably best classified on the basis of immunophenotyping. Antigens on the surface of normal hematopoietic cells express changes as the cells mature in the bone marrow. Technology has produced monoclonal antibodies to many of these cell cluster-of-differentiation (CD) antigen groups. These are each given a classification number prefixed with CD. Some CD antigen groups relate to lymphocyte sublineage (CDs 1–8 mark various stages of T-cell lineage; CDs 19–22, 24, and 79a mark B cells) and some to myeloid lineage, whereas others mark more primitive features (CD10 and CD34). Other useful immunologically defined cell characteristics include the following:

- Cytoplasmic immunoglobulins found in pre-B-cell ALL
- Surface immunoglobulins found in mature B-ALL
- Terminal deoxynucleotidyl transferase (TdT) found in immature lymphoid cells

Using these markers enables the classification of ALL into major categories (Table 1.6).

Table 1.7. Outcome prediction associated with ploidy status of acute lymphoblastic leukemia

Ploidy status	Number of chromosomes per malignant cell	Percentage of childhood ALL cases	Predicted response to treatment
Hyperdiploidy	>50	25–30%	Favorable
Hypodiploidy	<50	5–10%	Poor
Near-haploidy	<30	<1%	Very poor

ALL cells occasionally express cell antigens more usually associated with myeloid lineage. Opinion is divided as to whether this is clinically significant.

1.1.6.5 Cytogenetics

Cytogenetic abnormalities are detectable in most cases of childhood ALL. They can be categorized either by the number of chromosomes (ploidy) or by the structural changes and rearrangements based on detailed analysis of the karyotype. The assessment of ploidy status is clinically useful in predicting prognosis (Table 1.7).

With regard to structural changes, the identification of translocations and marker chromosomes and the delineation of complex chromosome aberrations have been possible with multicolor spectral karyotyping. The most significant chromosome (Ch') translocations identified in childhood ALL include the following:

- Ch'12 and Ch'22; i.e., t(12;22), resulting in the ETV6/AML1 fusion gene
- the Philadelphia chromosome, which is translocation t(9;22) and gives rise to the BCR/ABL fusion gene in ALL that indicates a poor prognosis
- t(1;19), giving rise to E2A/PBX1 which is a translocation of pre-B ALL
- t(12;21), giving rise to TEL/AML1 (also termed ETV6/CBFA2 fusion gene), which has been commonly reported as indicating a good prognosis
- t(4;11), giving rise to MLL/AF4, which is a typical translocation occurring in infant leukemia

Other significant abnormalities include

- rearrangements of the MLL gene
- rearrangements of the MYC gene with immunoglobulin genes
- rearrangements of T-cell receptor genes
- mutations of p16 (a tumor suppressor gene)
- mutations of p53 gene (although uncommon in childhood ALL, these mutations are associated with relapse or refractory leukemia)

The effects of these genetic alterations in leukemia help to explain adverse clinical outcomes. For example, the Philadelphia chromosome results in the production of an active kinase enzyme that drives cell proliferation independently of normal requirements for growth factor and blocks apoptosis (programmed cell death). Therefore, drug responsiveness pathways may be blocked. Normal p53 protein is required to induce cell death following anoxia or DNA damage from exposure to drugs or irradiation. Mutations in the p53, common in relapse of leukemia, may explain drug resistance in more advanced disease.

Although the risk criteria features must be considered important predictors of outcome, it would appear that they are most beneficial in predicting risk groups in B-cell lineage but not consistently in T-cell disease (Eden et al. 2000). Overall, 30–40% of children with T-lineage ALL relapse within the first 18 months after diagnosis, and approximately 20% of children with "standard risk" ALL relapse. Some groups of patients require further intensification of therapy. Consequently, more sophisticated approaches to risk classification that incorporate the molecular genetic findings and minimal residual disease measurement have the potential for identifying higher-risk children.

1.1.7 Treatment

Therapy for ALL has improved to such a degree that about 80% of childhood ALL is curable. The cytotoxic drugs used have been available for over 20 years, but better understanding of the pharmacology of these drugs has led to more effective protocols being devised that also attempt to avoid long-term adverse effects. Improvements have also been made in supportive care to reduce morbidity and mortality. The aim of treatment for ALL is to effectively halt the production of abnormal cells and eradicate the disease. Treatment protocols for ALL are constantly attempting to improve in terms of efficacy and long-term toxicity. Protocols for ALL generally include the following features:

1. Induction
2. Intensification/consolidation
3. CNS-directed therapy
4. Maintenance/continuing treatment

The drugs normally administered during the treatment for ALL are shown in Table 1.8. (Part 3 will detail cytotoxic drugs further). Treatment for ALL continues for a period of 2 or 3 years. However, infant ALL remains a challenge to treat. Most investigators treat infants as a unique subgroup, giving multiple drugs at high doses. Intensive systemic and IT treatments seem to provide adequate therapy for the CNS, even in infants with CNS involvement at diagnosis, thus avoiding cranial irradiation in these infants.

1.1.7.1 Induction

The drugs used initially to induce a remission are vincristine, steroids, and a third drug – L-asparaginase or an anthracycline – given over a 4-week period. This three-drug induction usually produces remission in about 95% of children. CNS prophylaxis/treatment is also started immediately with IT methotrexate. In the past, protocols included daunorubicin during induction. This was later omitted due to treatment-related mortality and potential late cardiotoxicity. However, research suggests that early treatment with daunorubicin could achieve a reduced relapse risk if it is not replaced by alternative intensification strategies (Chessells et al. 2002).

When treatment begins, the lysis of leukemic cells causes an increase in uric acid levels in the blood. Therefore, a uricolytic agent (uric acid depletor) is routinely prescribed. This is usually allopurinol, but investigations continue to seek a more effective agent, such as nonrecombinant urate oxidase.

The steroid of choice is normally prednisolone, but research continues to establish the efficacy of dexamethasone.

L-asparaginase can be derived from several sources, including

- Polyethylene-glycol (PEG) L-asparaginase
- *Escherichia coli (E. coli)* asparaginase
- *Erwinia* asparaginase (derived from *Erwinia carotovora* or *Erwinia chrysanthemi*).

Each of these L-asparaginase preparations has different pharmacokinetic properties and different toxic tendencies. PEG L-asparaginase has a longer half-life than *E. coli* asparaginase, which in turn has a longer half-life than *Erwinia* asparaginase. Given in equivalent doses, the one with a longer half-life should be more effective but is also more toxic. Reports comparing the efficacy of different preparations have debated the clinical significance of the results. Due to the sources of the preparations, they can all display immunogenicity and cause allergic side effects. However, the presence of antibodies does not necessarily cause an allergic reaction. Other toxicities, including coagulation disorders, liver toxicity, and acute pancreatitis, are related to the inhibition of protein synthesis. Few studies have compared the effect of the various asparaginase preparations on the coagulation proteins. *Erwinia* asparaginase has been reported as having a less pronounced effect on coagulation than *E. coli* asparaginase does. This may be argued to be dose-related rather than preparation-related. Fresh frozen plasma (FFP) was often transfused prior to L-asparaginase if coagulation screening showed a decrease in any coagulation proteins, but this is now thought to be of no clinical benefit. Protocols for the treatment of ALL usually specify one particular preparation of L-asparaginase. However, allergic reactions usually require the discontinuation of thera-

Table 1.8. Drugs commonly used in the treatment of acute lymphoblastic leukemia

Drugs	Route of administration	Induction	Intensification	CNS prophylaxis	Maintenance
Vincristine	Intravenous	*	*		*
L-asparaginase	Subcutaneous/ intramuscular	*			
Prednisolone/ dexamethasone	Oral	*	*		*
Co-trimoxazole	Oral				*
Methotrexate	Oral				*
Methotrexate	Intrathecal	*	*	*	*
Methotrexate (with folinic acid rescue)	Intravenous			*	
Daunorubicin	Intravenous	*possibly	*		
Etoposide or cyclophosphamide	Intravenous		*		
Cytarabine	Intravenous		*		
Thioguanine (may be replaced with mercaptopurine)	Oral		*		
Mercaptopurine	Oral				*

py and subsequent substitution with a different preparation. This substitution is necessary, but it is generally thought that the different preparations are not therapeutically interchangeable, although there is probably no adverse prognostic impact of allergy to asparaginase.

Because of the risk of *Pneumocystis jiroveci* pneumonia (PCP) in immunocompromised patients, sulfamethoxazole/trimethoprim (SMX/TMP) or co-trimoxazole is given as effective prophylaxis. This is normally administered as an oral preparation (usually two or three times per week) but may be given intravenously if the patient's condition requires it. On occasion, due to adverse reactions including prolonged periods of neutropenia, a secondary alternative may be necessary. These alternatives include aerosolized/nebulized pentamidine, oral dapsone, and oral atovaquone. Pentamidine can be given intravenously, but systemic toxicities may be higher with this method of administration.

1.1.7.2 Intensification/Consolidation

This block of treatment is given following induction and again about 4 months later (depending on the protocol). Clinical trials have also investigated the introduction of a third block, which seemed to compensate for the omission of anthracyclines in induction but with possibly little other benefit.

1.1.7.3 CNS-directed Therapy

Prophylactic CNS therapy is based on the premise that the CNS provides a sanctuary site for leukemic cells that are undetectable at diagnosis and that can be protected from systemic therapy by the blood-brain barrier. If preventative therapy were not given to children with ALL, over 50% would develop CNS disease. Regular (usually every 12 weeks) lumbar punctures are performed in order to administer IT methotrexate. Additionally, high-dose methotrexate is given intravenously, usually at 4-weekly intervals between intensification blocks. High-dose methotrexate infusions were introduced to protocols to replace cranial irradiation because of its associated adverse side effects, and the benefits are still under investigation. Cranial radiotherapy may be reserved for children thought to be at especially high risk of CNS involvement (T-cell with high white count at diagnosis) or for those with CNS infiltration at diagnosis. Triple IT therapy (including the addition of cytarabine and hydrocortisone) is also under investigation in some protocols.

> Note: It is vital that the IT methotrexate NEVER be confused with the intravenous vincristine that is normally given on the same day. This would result in fatality.

1.1.7.4 Maintenance/Continuing Treatment

Oral methotrexate administered weekly and oral 6-mercaptopurine administered daily are the mainstay of most continuation regimens. Administering these drugs in the evening appears to give a better clinical outcome. This result may be mainly due to issues surrounding compliance; it may be easier for parents or adolescents to remember drugs at this time of day. Studies have indicated the need to give continuation therapy to the limits of tolerance by titrating doses against myelosuppression and reiterating the importance of compliance. This may result in periods of discontinuing therapy during this phase, but this is thought to be a positive event if it is related to neutropenia. Therapy is not usually discontinued if there is an episode of elevated liver enzymes. Maintenance therapy also includes continuing intravenous (IV) vincristine, PCP prophylaxis, and CNS-directed therapy every 4 weeks.

The progression of each stage of the protocol relies on a degree of return of normal bone marrow function, where the blood component levels are within normal limits. Periods of neutropenia are associated with any ALL treatment protocol during which the child/adolescent becomes immunocompromised. Procedures regarding supportive care are adhered to and are as important as the cytotoxic therapy with regard to ensuring the best outcomes for these children and adolescents.

1.1.7.5 Allogeneic Stem Cell Transplant

Some high-risk leukemias may indicate the need for transplantation from the time of diagnosis, such as Philadelphia-chromosome-positive ALL. However, as transplantation and chemotherapy are improving, these patients are continually subject to review. Stem cell transplantation has not been shown to improve outcomes for infant ALL or other very-high-risk ALL.

1.1.8 Prognosis

The prognosis of ALL is one of the highest of childhood malignancies, with a survival rate of around 80%. Studies have investigated the influence on survival of ethnicity and socioeconomic status. Increasing levels of deprivation were associated with poorer survival from all cancers, including leukemia, but only before other prognostic factors were taken into consideration (McKinney et al. 1999). However, despite continuing improved protocols, the rate of relapse has decreased only slightly over the last decade. The main improvements in survival rates have been due to improved management of relapse, especially for those relapsing off treatment. Relapse of ALL is most commonly treated with marrow ablative chemotherapy and allogeneic stem cell transplant following the achievement of a second remission. Late bone marrow relapse of several years may be treated by intense chemotherapy alone, leaving the possibility of transplant in third remission if necessary. Allografts from unrelated donors are an option that has provided encouraging results when there is a lack of suitable related donors. Transplant with umbilical cord blood stem cells is another option.

The survival rate of 80% is the mean that disguises rates that range from 10–90%. The failure of improved rates of survival has been most notable in high-risk groups. However, the relapse that occurs in standard risk groups must also be explained. Reasons may be pharmacological in cases of noncompliance or drug resistance. Drug sensitivity testing and greater vigilance may help to identify those at risk and allow for intervention. Other reasons for treatment failure may be due to intrinsically resistant disease or to recurrence from residual disease. Testicular relapse of ALL can occur, possibly because this area is a sanctuary site. However, this is a rare event, affecting approximately 1% of boys with ALL, and is normally treated with local radiation therapy and chemotherapy. Approximately 10–13% of pediatric ALL cases have T-lineage phenotype, and 30–40% of these still relapse during treatment. More sophisticated approaches to risk classification and measurement of minimal residual disease to capture patients who would benefit from more intense treatment may go some way to increase overall event-free survival rates (survival free from relapse).

1.1.9 Follow-up

Following the completion of therapy for ALL, it is crucial to monitor these children and adolescents for two reasons:

1. Blood counts will be carried out to ensure that signs of relapse can be detected, but with decreasing frequency over a number of years. Follow-up may also include bone marrow aspiration yearly initially for the same reason.
2. As therapy becomes more successful, late side effects are of increasing concern.

Long-term effects of antileukemic treatment include the following:

- Chronic cardiotoxicity induced by anthracyclines (daunorubicin), which can manifest as sudden onset irreversible heart failure. The severity of cardiac dysfunction is related to the cumulative dose of anthracycline.
- Hypothalamic-pituitary axis and gonadal damage induced by radiation. Growth problems may cause short stature and obesity later in life, and girls may undergo precocious puberty. Growth hormone therapy may be required. It is less clear if chemotherapy alone can impair growth. Testicular radiotherapy renders males sterile, and most will require androgen replacement throughout puberty. Chemotherapy may lead to subfertility, which can improve over time. Ovaries are less sensitive to chemotherapy, but if they are irradiated, estrogen replacement will be necessary. Alkylating agents are also likely to cause gonadal damage.

- Secondary malignancies induced by epipodophyllotoxins (etoposide), radiation, or alkylating agents. Exposure to epipodophyllotoxins has produced an increase in secondary acute myeloid leukemia. There is a marked excess of brain tumors among children who received cranial irradiation before the age of 5.
- Osteonecrosis caused by glucocorticoids (prednisolone, dexamethasone). This is most often seen in adolescents.
- Altered bone density induced by glucocorticoids, which increases susceptibility to fractures.
- Some potential impairment of intellectual development, which is measurable by a fall in IQ of 10–20 points.
- Psychosocial sequelae of a diagnosis of and treatment for leukemia, which are significant. There may be problems regarding relationships, career, insurance, and mortgage application, and emotional issues such as depression, anger, and confusion. Many studies have highlighted the need to include excellent psychosocial care throughout the disease trajectory and beyond.

Approaches to minimize adverse effects without affecting treatment outcome have included the development of new drugs, such as the liposomal formulation of daunorubicin; the use of cardioprotective agents; alternative administration schedules, such as continuous infusions/prolonged infusion times (the advantages of which are debatable); and the monitoring of minimal residual disease, which allows for reduction or optimization of drug doses.

1.1.10 Future Perspectives

The lack of specificity of most prognostic factors, as previously discussed, has led to the search for more relevant features of disease. Minimal residual disease (MRD) – that is, submicroscopic leukemia – can be detected at defined time points by identifying clone-specific T-cell receptors using PCR or immunoglobulin gene rearrangements using flow cytometry. This highly sensitive and highly specific prognostic information allows for definition of new risk groups. Treatment may possibly be reduced in children and adolescents with fast clearance of leukemic cells. Persistent disease could require treatment modification and intensification.

Levels of MRD may be defined as

- Negative – nothing detectable with two markers
- Indeterminate – no result or low positive (1×10^{-5}–1×10^{-4} nucleated bone marrow cells)
- Positive – more than one nucleated bone marrow cell in 10,000 ($>1\times10^{-4}$).

Bone marrow samples from diagnosis and a later defined time point, such as the end of induction therapy, are compared. Treatment can then be assigned according to the clinical trial in place. Sequential monitoring of MRD can also elicit further risk assessment. For example, the persistence of MRD beyond 4 months is associated with an increased risk of relapse.

Remarkable advances have been made by defining molecular abnormalities involved in leukemogenesis and drug resistance. This has led to the development of promising new therapeutic strategies. Recognition of inherited differences in the metabolism of antileukemic drugs has enabled the selection of optimal drug dosages and scheduling. This could be useful to increase antileukemic effects and to reduce late effects. Future strategies will incorporate more specific risk-directed therapy and greater international collaboration. Ultimately, progress made should result in improved clinical management and increased cure rates for childhood ALL.

1.2 Acute Myeloid Leukemia

1.2.1 Epidemiology

Acute myeloid leukemia (AML) is most often seen in adults over age 40, but the annual incidence of childhood AML is approximately 4.7 per 100,000 and is constant from birth to 10 years of age. Incidence peaks slightly in adolescence, and AML is the more common leukemia found in neonates. Boys and girls appear to be affected equally. It is generally reported that AML is equally distributed among ethnic groups, but a study by McKinney et al. (2003) indicated a significantly higher incidence of AML among South Asians in an urban English city.

Children with Down's syndrome have an increased risk of AML, with an estimated 10–15-fold increase in incidence compared with that of the general childhood population (Hasle et al. 2000). These children's risk of ALL is also increased but not to the same degree. The reasons for their predisposition to leukemia are unclear. Presence of the extra chromosome 21 may disrupt the genetic balance, which in turn increases susceptibility to further trauma. However, individuals with Down's syndrome do not appear to have a higher risk of other malignancies. Hypotheses for this may include an increased susceptibility for apoptosis (programmed cell death) in Down's syndrome, causing cell death rather than malignant transformation after cell injuries (Hasle 2001).

1.2.2 Etiology

1.2.2.1 Genetic Factors

The various conditions that have a predisposition to AML are akin to those of any acute leukemia (Table 1.2), with the addition of myelodysplastic syndrome (monosomy 7).

1.2.2.2 Environmental Factors

Similarly, the causal risk factors associated with AML are the same as for ALL (see Table 3). Interestingly, allergy or a family history of allergy (including hay fever, neurodermatitis, asthma, and, to a lesser degree, eczema) have been associated with a decreased risk of ALL but not of AML (Schuz 2003).

Until recently, a Vietnam-era herbicide, Agent Orange (dioxin), was reported to be a parental exposure link to childhood AML. However, subsequent studies have ruled out any increased risk (Ahmad 2002).

1.2.3 Molecular Genetics

The defect that occurs in AML appears to be an arrest in the differentiation pathway of myeloid progenitors or precursors. Fusion genes generated by translocations of chromosomes block cell differentiation. These genes can be detected by PCR, and clonal chromosomal abnormalities of dividing bone marrow cells have been identified in more than 70% of children diagnosed with AML. The most common fusion genes detected in AML are

- AML1/ETO from t(8,21), most often seen in acute myeloblastic leukemia
- MLL/AF10 from t(10,11)
- Inversion of ch16, creating CRFB/SMMHC
- Trisomy 8
- Monosomy 7
- PML/RARA from t(15,17), most common in acute promyelocytic leukemia

Fusions of the MLL gene occur in about 50% of cases of AML. These fusions are thought to be fetal in origin, as this fusion is often detected on the Guthrie card or neonatal blood spot of those children who subsequently develop AML. This is possibly the initiating event in childhood AML that requires additional secondary genetic alterations to cause leukemia.

1.2.4 Symptoms and Clinical Signs

AML can have a similar presentation to that of ALL, with symptoms appearing 1–6 weeks before diagnosis. The presenting signs and symptoms include the following:

- Pallor
- Fatigue, weakness
- Petechiae
- Fever, infection
- Sore throat
- Lymphadenopathy
- Skin lesions
- Gastrointestinal symptoms, including pain, nausea, and vomiting
- Gingival changes or infiltrates

The presenting lesions or infiltrates result from chloromas (or granulocytic sarcomas or myeloblastomas), which are localized collections of leukemic blast cells. Presentation with bleeding can be due to disseminated intravascular coagulation (DIC) and may be indicative of acute promyelocytic leukemia. DIC can occur as a result of the release of procoagulants from abnormal promyelocytic granules (see Chapter 16). Complaints of presenting bone pain are

less common in AML, and hepatosplenomegaly is more marked in infants with AML.

CNS involvement of AML, occurring in 5–15% of cases, can cause symptoms similar to those of CNS involvement in ALL:

- Headache
- Poor school performance
- Weakness
- Vomiting
- Blurred vision
- Seizures
- Difficulty maintaining balance

Hyperleukocytosis can be present at diagnosis of childhood AML and may or may nor require leukopheresis therapy. Approximately 15–20% of children present with leukocyte counts $>100\times10^9$g/l, which may lead to leukostasis. Testicular infiltrates are uncommon in AML.

1.2.5 Diagnostics

If the history and physical examination suggest leukemia, examination of peripheral blood and bone marrow samples is required, as with the diagnosis of ALL. Bone marrow findings include a hypercellular trephine/biopsy sample and an aspirate sample showing more than 30% blast cells. To confirm a diagnosis of AML, the same procedures as for diagnosing ALL are applied.

1.2.6 Staging and Classification

There is presently no therapeutically or prognostically meaningful staging system for AML. Cytochemical staining of bone marrow smears using Sudan black stain produces a positive result in AML, and esterase stains distinguish further subgroups. Immunophenotyping also assists in determining the originating cell line. Cluster-of-differentiation antigen groups related to myeloid lineage include CD11, CD13–15, and CD33.

If the myeloid cell line is involved and a diagnosis of AML is confirmed, the French-American-British classification system for AML is applied. There are eight different classifications or types of AML (M0 to

M7), based on appearance of the diseased cells under the microscope (Table 1.9). Each subtype refers to the particular myeloid lineage affected and the degree of

Table 1.9. French-American-British (FAB) classification of acute myeloid leukemia

FAB group	Cell morphology
M0	Myeloid leukemia with minimal differentiation
M1	Myeloblastic leukemia
M2	Myeloblastic leukemia – undifferentiated
M3	Promyelocytic leukemia with 15;17 translocation
M4	Myelomonocytic leukemia
M5	Monocytic leukemia: M5a – without differentiation M5b – with differentiation
M6	Erythroblastic leukemia
M7	Megakaryoblastic leukemia

blast cell differentiation. This standardization began in 1976, but with improvements in treatment outcome, this approach to classification has limited clinical relevance. Approximately 80% of children less than 2 years of age have either M4 or M5 FAB subtypes. M7 is most common in children under 3 years, particularly in those with Down's syndrome.

Myelodysplastic syndrome (MDS) is a preleukemic syndrome that has a relationship with some types of AML (MDS-related AML or MDR-AML). Approximately half of the cases of AML follow MDS, and these patients generally have a very poor prognosis. The other main group consists of those cases unrelated to MDS, with a suggested name of true de novo AML (TDN-AML). This led to subclassification of AML based on its relationship with MDS. The World Health Organization (WHO) attempted to refine the FAB classification by incorporating the AML/MDS relationship. This classification, shown in Table 1.10, has been a cause for debate over the past few years. However, the WHO classification incorporates subcategories of AML with recurring translocations, AML related to MDS, and subsets of treatment-relat-

Table 1.10. World Health Organization classification of acute myeloid leukemia

Group	Subgroups
Acute myeloid leukemia with recurrent genetic abnormalities	Acute myeloid leukemia with t(8;21) Acute myeloid leukemia with abnormal bone marrow eosinophils inv(16) or t(16;16) Acute promyelocytic leukemia (AML with t(15;17) and variants Acute myeloid leukemia with MLL abnormalities
Acute myeloid leukemia with multilineage dysplasia	Following an MDS or MDS/myeloproliferative disorder Without antecedent myelodysplastic syndrome
Acute myeloid leukemia and MDS, therapy-related	Alkylating agent-related Topoisomerase type II inhibitor-related Other types
Acute myeloid leukemia not otherwise specified	Acute myeloid leukemia minimally differentiated Acute myeloid leukemia without maturation Acute myeloid leukemia with maturation Acute myelomonocytic leukemia Acute monoblastic and monocytic leukemia Acute erythroid leukemia Acute megakaryoblastic leukemia Acute basophilic leukemia Acute panmyelosis with myelofibrosis Myeloid sarcoma

Adapted from Head 2002

ed AML based on their relation to the first two groups. Therefore, this system may assist clinical decisions and be useful in analyzing biologic studies in AML. It is of note that MDS-AML is more prominent in the elderly, with only 15% of cases in children and young adults (Head 2002). The TDN-AML group, related to a set of recurring cytogenetic translocations and inversions, has a median age approximating the median age of the population (Head 2002).

1.2.7 Treatment

The most dramatic outcomes for children with AML have resulted from intensive therapy over a brief period of time. Treatment usually includes a protocol with an induction anthracycline (usually daunorubicin) and cytarabine. An important component of post-remission therapy appears to be several courses of high-dose cytarabine. The addition of mitoxantrone is possibly also beneficial. Intensive therapy usually induces remission in about 90% of children. The challenge then is to prolong the remission. In over 60% of these children, an allogeneic stem cell transplant is the chosen treatment option once first remission has been achieved. However, if cytogenetics are favorable, such as t(15;17), t(8;21) or inv16, intensive chemotherapy consolidation may be the treatment of choice even if a matched sibling donor is available (Sung et al. 2003). These patients would be transplanted after relapse. There is no evidence to suggest that autologous transplant is of any benefit in pediatric acute leukemia. (Part 3 will cover stem cell transplants in detail.) The use of some form of CNS treatment is included. Children with M4 and M5 have the highest incidence of CNS disease.

Acute promyelocytic leukemia (APM) (i.e., FAB subtype M3) can often be treated with all-trans retinoic acid and chemotherapy, which achieves a remission and cure in most children with AML of this type. This outcome is possible due to the translocation t(15;17) involving a breakpoint that includes the retinoid acid receptor. Fatal hemorrhagic complications can occur before or during induction in this subtype. There is a low incidence of CNS disease in children with APM. A lumbar puncture is not performed, and IT chemotherapy is not required.

Down's syndrome patients have a markedly increased responsiveness to therapy. However, this causes an increased treatment-related morbidity and mortality, which has meant that AML protocols have been tailored specifically for this population of children. Stem cell transplant is rarely indicated in these circumstances. Of note are cases when infants with Down's syndrome, usually under 2 months of age, are diagnosed with AML or transient leukemia and achieve complete spontaneous remission.

1.2.8 Prognosis

Despite significant improvements in the outcomes of children with AML, the cure rate is only approximately 50%. About 45% of children with AML relapse, and there remains little information about the best treatment for this group of children.

In 2002 (a), Rubnitz and colleagues reported that the only independent factors indicating a favorable prognosis were

- a presenting leukocyte count of $<50 \times 10^9/l$
- the genetic factor of translocation t(9;11)

Another favorable prognostic factor, as mentioned previously, is the constitutional trisomy 21 (Down's syndrome), despite the increased risk for developing AML. These children also have a decreased risk of relapse that is unrelated to having the favorable abnormalities of t(15;17), inv16, or t(8;21).

It is worth noting that results of another study by Rubnitz et al. (2002b) debate the favorable outcome of t(8;21) that was previously reported.

1.2.9 Follow-up

Children and adolescents need appropriate and sensitive follow-up, similar to that following ALL treatment. The specific features of follow-up for AML concern the increased incidence of relapse and the increased number of children and adolescents who receive transplant as a standard modality of treatment.

1.2.10 Future Perspectives

The progress in therapy for AML lags behind that for ALL. Allogeneic bone marrow transplant from a matched family donor appears to remain the best option for most patients. Drug resistance is an apparent factor in AML and is being investigated by studying leukemic blast cells or minimal residual disease.

In adult patients with AML, the expression of the multidrug resistance gene (MRD1) defines a poor prognostic group. This is not a similar finding in children with AML (Steinbach et al. 2003). A study by Steinbach et al. (2003) investigated the expression of five of the genes encoding the multidrug resistance-associated proteins (MRP) in children with AML and their response to chemotherapy. Expression of MRP3 was found to be involved in drug resistance, producing a poorer prognosis, and the expression of MRP2 was, to a lesser extent, also associated with poor prognosis. Expression of high levels of both these genes indicated a particularly poor prognosis. This study suggests that these proteins, MRP3 and possibly MRP2, could provide markers for risk-adapted therapy and possible targets for the development of drugs that would overcome multidrug resistance in childhood AML.

Alternative approaches to therapy may include risk-directed therapy based on different prognostic criteria, differentiation therapy with all-trans-retinoic acid, immunotherapy with monoclonal antibodies, or tumor vaccines.

1.3 Chronic Myeloid Leukemia

1.3.1 Epidemiology and Etiology

An increase in the incidence of adult chronic myeloid leukemia (CML) has been seen in three populations:

- The Japanese exposed to radiation released from atomic bombs in Nagasaki and Hiroshima
- Patients with ankylosing spondylitis treated with spine irradiation
- Women with uterine cervical carcinoma who received radiation treatment (Freedman 1994)

Despite this obvious relationship between radiation and CML, only 5–7% of adult cases of CML have documented exposure to excessive radiation, and previous exposure is infrequent in children with CML (Freedman 1994). In patients younger than 20 years of age, the incidence is less than 1 in 100,000, with 80% of these cases being over the age of 4 years.

1.3.2 Molecular Genetics

CML is normally a hematological disease of the elderly, characterized by the BCR/ABL oncogene caused by a translocation between the ABL gene on Ch'9 and the BCR gene on Ch'22. The resulting chromosome 22, with a shortening of the long arm, is known as the Philadelphia (Ph') chromosome. The BCR/ABL gene fusion product is thought to be causative in CML and has multiple effects on diverse cell functions, such as growth, differentiation, adhesion, and apoptosis.

1.3.3 Symptoms and Clinical Signs

The "chronic phase" of leukemia that results then evolves into a more rapidly progressive phase known as the "accelerated phase" and ultimately "blast crisis." The chronic phase lasts about 3 years but can range from a few months to 20 years. The accelerated phase generally occurs over a 3–6-month period. The final phase is generally resistant to current treatment and is therefore fatal.

The signs and symptoms of CML can vary depending on the phase the disease has reached:

- The *chronic phase* has a nonspecific onset over weeks to months, with complaints of fatigue, anorexia, weight loss, and excessive sweating. Physical presentation includes pallor, bruising, low-grade fever, sternal bone pain, and splenomegaly that is sometimes accompanied by hepatomegaly.
- Signs and symptoms of the *accelerated phase* present over a few months and are similar to those of the chronic phase but with more episodes of unexplained fever, lymphadenopathy, and bruising and petechiae caused by thrombocytopenia.

— The *blastic phase* presents with symptoms identical to those of acute leukemia

1.3.4 Diagnostics

CML is characterized by the presence of large numbers of granulocytes in the blood, with mild anemia and thrombocytosis. The numbers of basophils and eosinophils are increased. A characteristic laboratory feature is a marked reduction or absence of leukocyte alkaline phosphatase (LAP) activity, which results from a decrease in monocytes that normally secrete a factor that induces LAP activity (Freedman 1994).

Cytogenetic analysis of the marrow cells will display the Philadelphia chromosome in over 90% of new patients with CML. Absence of cytogenetic or molecular abnormalities in chromosome 22 would rule out a diagnosis of CML.

1.3.5 Treatment

In children with CML, allogeneic bone marrow transplant is normally the treatment of choice. This treatment is providing promising survival rates even in the event of advanced disease and histoincompatibility with donor marrow (Sharathkumar et al. 2002). Another treatment that has produced encouraging results, reported by Millot et al. (2002), uses a combination of interferon and cytarabine for children with Philadelphia-chromosome-positive CML. This may offer an alternative to transplantation in children and adolescents in the chronic phase of CML.

1.3.6 Prognosis

For children with the adult form of CML, the importance of prognostic factors is difficult to define due to the low incidence of disease. Remissions can be induced, but relapse is common and long-term survivors are rare.

1.3.7 Future Perspectives

For children with CML, current efforts should aim to reduce transplant-related deaths. Cytogenetic studies to identify further risk factors will assist in the understanding of the cell biology of this disease.

1.4 Juvenile Myelomonocytic Leukemia

A subgroup of CML is juvenile myelomonocytic leukemia (JMML), formerly called juvenile chronic myeloid leukemia (JCML). This subgroup represents less than 1% of cases of childhood leukemia. Controversy surrounds the classification of this subgroup, and it may be termed as chronic myelomonocytic leukemia (CMML). Most patients are less than 2 years of age, with 95% younger than 4 years (Freedman 1994).

Children frequently present with complaints of malaise, bleeding, or fever, often with localized infection. Less common presentations include pulmonary symptoms (cough, wheezing, tachypnea), abdominal distension and discomfort, weight loss, and occasionally bone pain. On examination, splenomegaly is a frequent feature; pallor and hepatomegaly may also be present. Skin manifestations may be seen, with an eczematous rash that is unresponsive to topical treatment. Xanthoma and café-au-lait spots are often associated with JMML. These skins findings are also common in neurofibromatosis, and an interrelationship between neurofibromatosis and JMML has been established (Freedman 1994).

Peripheral blood samples show an increasing number of circulating monocytes in all cases. Immature granulocytes, anemia, and thrombocytopenia are also frequently present. The cells in JMML do not contain the Philadelphia chromosome, although other chromosomal abnormalities are present.

This disease is more progressive and less responsive to treatment than Ph'-chromosome-positive CML. Prognosis is poor, and a bone marrow transplant is required as early as possible for these children, particularly when a matched relative donor is available.

Table 1.11. Common Symptoms of Histiocytosis

System	Symptom
Gastrointestinal	Abdominal pain, vomiting, diarrhea, jaundice, weight loss, esophageal bleeding
Bone	Bone pain, headaches (skull lesions), limp (leg lesions)
CNS (brain)	Diabetes insipidus, mental deterioration, headaches, dizziness, seizures, increased intracranial pressure
CNS (pituitary gland)	Polydipsia, polyuria, dehydration, short stature, delayed puberty
Pulmonary	Feeding problems (infants), chest pain, dyspnea, cough, hemoptysis
Oral	Facial swelling and pain, loss of teeth, swollen and bleeding gingiva, swollen lymph nodes
Skin	Scaly rash
Ear	Inflamed, draining ear canal, rash behind ears

1.5 Langerhans Cell Histiocytosis

Histiocytosis is not defined as a malignancy, but it is treated with cancer therapies (e. g., chemotherapy, radiotherapy) and pediatric oncology nurses may be involved in the care of a child with Langerhan's cell histiocytosis.

A histiocyte is a normal cell in the immune system found in the bone marrow, blood, skin, liver, lungs, lymph glands and spleen. Histiocytosis identifies a group of disorders that have proliferation of cells of the mononuclear phagocyte and dendritic cell systems. In Langerhans cell histiocytosis (LCH), the histiocytes move into tissues where they are not normally found and cause damage to those tissues. The cause of LCH is unknown. Suggested hypotheses include the possibility of clonal abnormalities; cytokine or chemokine abnormality causing abnormal expression of Langerhan's cells; a combination of oncogenesis and immune dysregulation (Egeler et al., 2004); and lesional Langerhans cells that control the persistance and progression themselves (Annels et al., 2003).

The Histiocyte Society, an international body, was formed in 1987 and has outlined morphology, immnohistiochemistry and clinial criteria required for LCH. The symptoms of LCH are dependent on the body system involved and are listed in Table 1.11. Tests to diagnose LCH may include radiographs, CT studies, complete blood count and blood chemistries, and tissue or skin biopsy.

Single-system (localised) LCH usually disappears on its own without any treatment. Although treated with chemotherapy there has been no specific research trial for the use of cytotoxic therapy in LCH. This may occur following a biopsy. In a small number of children, treatment will be needed and low-dose radiotherapy, surgery and steroids may be used. Multi-system (disseminated) disease is usually treated with chemotherapy and steroids. The combination and duration of therapy will vary depending on the severity of the illness. Eighty percent of children who develop LCH will recover from it.

A small number of children may develop side effects many years later, because of the treatment they have received. This is more likely to happen when treatments have been intensive. Possible late side effects include reduced growth, infertility, pulmonary and cardiac abnormalities, and second malignancy.

References

Ahmad K (2002) Agent Orange no longer linked to childhood AML. The Lancet Oncology 3(4):199

Alexander FE, Boyle P, Carli PM, Coebergh JW, Ekbom A, Levi F, McKinney PA, McWhirter W, Michaelis J, Peris-Bonet R, Petridou E, Pompe-Kirn V, Plesko I, Pukkala E, Rahu M, Stiller CA, Storm H, Terracini B, Vatten L, Wray N (1999) Population density and childhood leukaemia: results of the EUROCLUS Study. European Journal of Cancer 35(3):439–444

Annels NE, Da Costa CE, Prins FA, Willemze A, Hogendoorn, Egeler RM (2003) Aberrant chemokine receptor expression and chemokine production by Langerhans cells underlies the pathogenesis of Langerhans cell histiocytosis. Journal of Experimental Medicine 197(10): 1385–1390.

Auvinen A, Kurttio P, Pekkanen J, Pukkala E, Ilus T, Salonen L (2002) Uranium and other natural radionuclides in drinking water and risk of leukemia: a case-cohort study in Finland. Cancer Causes and Control 13(9):825–829

Bergh T, Ericson A, Hillensjo T, Nygren KG, Wennerholm UB (1999) Deliveries and children born after in-vitro fertilisation in Sweden 1982–1995: a retrospective cohort study. Lancet 354(9190):1579–1585

Boutou O, Guizard AV, Slama R, Pottier D, Spira A (2002) Population mixing and leukaemia in young people around the la Hague nuclear waste reprocessing plant. British Journal of Cancer 87(7):740–745

Chessells JM, Harrison G, Richards SM, Gibson BE, Bailey CC, Hill FG, Hann IM (2002) Failure of a new protocol to improve treatment results in paediatric lymphoblastic leukaemia: lessons from the UK Medical Research Council trials UKALL X and UKALL XI. British Journal of Haematology 118(2):445–55

Dickinson HO, Hammal DM, Dummer TJB, Parker L, Bithell JF (2003) Childhood leukaemia and non-Hodgkin's lymphoma in relation to proximity to railways. British Journal of Cancer 88(5):695–698

Doll R, Wakeford R (1997) Risk of childhood cancer from fetal irradiation. The British Journal of Radiology 70: 130–139

Eden OB, Harrison G, Richards S, Lilleyman JS, Bailey CC, Chessells JM, Hann IM, Hill FG, Gibson BE (2000) Long-term follow-up of the United Kingdom Medical Research Council protocols for childhood acute lymphoblastic leukaemia, 1980–1997. Medical Research Council Childhood Leukaemia Working Party. Leukaemia 14(12):2307–2320

Egeler RM, Annels NE, Hogendoorn PC (2004) Langherhans cell histiocytosis: A pathological combination of oncogenesis and immune dysregulation. Pediatric Blood Cancer 42(5): 401–403.

Freedman MH (1994) Chronic myelocytic leukemia in infancy and childhood. In: Pochedly C (ed) Neoplastic Diseases of Childhood Volume 1. Harwood Academic Publishers, Switzerland

Gajjar A, Harrison PL, Sandlund JT, Rivera GK, Ribeiro RC, Rubnitz JE, Razzouk B, Relling MV, Evans WE, Boyett JM, Pui CH (2000) Traumatic lumbar puncture at diagnosis adversely affects outcome in childhood acute lymphoblastic leukemia. Blood 96(10):3381–3384

Hann I, Vora A, Harrison G, Harrison C, Eden O, Hill F, Gibson B and Richards S (2001) Determinants of outcome after intensified therapy of childhood lymphoblastic leukaemia: results from Medical Research Council United Kingdom acute lymphoblastic leukaemia XI protocol. British Journal of Haematology 113(1):103–114

Hasle H (2001) Pattern of malignant disorders in individuals with Down's syndrome. The Lancet Oncology 2(7):429–436

Hasle H, Clemmensen IH, Mikelsen M (2000) Risks of leukemia and solid tumours in individuals with Down's syndrome. Lancet 355(9199):165–169

Head DR (2002) Proposed changes in the definitions of acute myeloid leukemia and myelodysplastic syndrome: are they helpful? Current Opinion in Oncology 14(1):19–23

Jarup L, Briggs D, de Hoogh C, Morris S, Hurt C, Lewin A, Maitland I, Richardson S, Wakefield J, Elliott P (2002) Cancer risks in population living near landfill sites in Great Britain. British Journal of Cancer 86(11):1732–1736

Kinlen LJ (1995) Epidemiological evidence for an infective basis in childhood leukaemia. British Journal of Cancer 71(1):1–5

Klip H, Burger CW, de Kraker J, van Leeuwen FE, OMEGA-project group (2001) Risk of cancer in the offspring of women who underwent ovarian stimulation for IVF. Human Reproduction16(11):2451–2458

Lancashire RJ, Sorahan T; OSCC (2003) Breastfeeding and childhood cancer risks: OSCC data. British Journal of Cancer 88(7):1035–1037

Ma X, Buffler PA, Gunier RB, Dahl G, Smith MT, Reinier K, Reynolds P. (2002) Critical windows of exposure to household pesticides and risk of childhood leukemia. Environmental Health Perspective 110(9):955–960

McKinney PA, Feltbower RG, Parslow RC, Lewis IJ, Glaser AW, Kinsey SE (2003) Patterns of childhood cancer by ethnic group in Bradford, UK 1974–1997. European Journal of Cancer 39(1):92–7

McKinney PA, Feltbower RG, Parslow RC, Lewis IJ, Picton S, Kinsey SE, Bailey CC (1999) Survival from childhood cancer in Yorkshire, UK: Effect of ethnicity and socio-economic status. European Journal of Cancer 35(13):1816–1823

Mellemkjaer L, Alexander F, Olsen JH. (2000) Cancer among children of parents with autoimmune diseases. British Journal of Cancer 82(7):1353–7

Millot F, Brice P, Phillipe N, Thyss A, Demeoq F, Wetterwald M, Boccara JM, Vilque J-P, Guyotat D, Guilhot J, Guilhot F (2002) α-Interferon in combination with cytarabine in children with Philadelphia chromosome-positive chronic myeloid leukemia. Journal of Pediatric Hematology/Oncology 24(1):18–22

Naumburg E, Bellocco R, Cnattinigius S, Jonzon A, Ekbom A (2000) Prenatal ultrasound examinations and risk of childhood leukaemia: case-control study. British Medical Journal 320(7230):282–283

Naumburg E, Bellocco R, Cnattinigius S, Jonzon A, Ekbom A (2002a) Supplementary oxygen and risk of childhood lymphatic leukaemia. Acta Paediatrica 91(12):1328–1333

Naumburg E, Bellocco R, Cnattinigius S, Jonzon A, Ekbom A (2002b) Perinatal exposure to infection and risk to childhood leukemia. Medical and Pediatric Oncology 38(6):391–397

Pan JW, Cook LS, Schwartz SM, Weis NS (2002) Incidence of leukemia in Asian migrants to the United States and their descendants. Cancer Causes and Control 13(9):791–795

Pang D, McNally R, Birch JM on behalf of the UK Childhood Cancer Study Investigators (2003) Parental smoking and childhood cancer: results from the United Kingdom Childhood Cancer Study. British Journal of Cancer 88(3):373–381

Parker L, Cole M, Craft AW, Hey EN (1998) Neonatal vitamin K administration and childhood cancer in the north of England: retrospective case-control study. British Medical Journal 316(7126):189–193

Passmore SJ, Draper G, Brownbill P, Kroll M (1998) Case-control studies of relation between childhood cancer and neonatal vitamin K administration. British Medical Journal 316(7126):178–184

Perrillat F, Clavel J, Jaussent I, Baruchel A, Leverger G, Nelkn B, Phillippe N, Schaison, Sommelet D, Vilmer E, Bonaiti-Pellie C, Hemon D (2001) Family cancer history and risk of childhood acute leukemia (France). Cancer Causes and Control 12(10):935–941

Powell JE, Parkes SE, Cameron AH, Mann JR (1994) Is the risk of cancer increased in Asians living in the UK? Archives of Disease in Childhood 71(5):398–403

Roman E, Fear NT, Ansell P, Bull D, Draper G, McKinney P, Michaelis J, Passmore SJ, von Kries R (2002)Vitamin K and childhood cancer: analysis of individual patient data from six case-control studies. British Journal of Cancer 86(1):63–9

Ross JA, Davies SM (2000) Vitamin K prophylaxis and childhood cancer. Medical and Pediatric Oncology 34(6):434–437

Rubnitz JE, Raimondi SC, Halbert AR, Tong X, Srivastava DK, Razzouk BI, Downing JR, Pui CH, Ribeiro RC, Behm FG (2002b) Characteristics and outcome of t(8;21)-positive childhood acute myeloid leukemia: a single institution's experience. Leukemia 16(10):2072–2077

Rubnitz JE, Raimondi SC, Tong X, Srivastava DK, Razzouk BI, Shurtleff SA, Downing JR, Pui CH, Ribeiro RC, Behm FG (2002a) Favourable impact of the t(9;11) in childhood acute myeloid leukemia. Journal of Clinical Oncology 20(9):2302–2309

Ruccione KS, Waskerwitz M, Buckley J, Perin G, Hammond GD (1994) What caused my child's cancer? Parents' responses to an epidemiology study of childhood cancer. Journal of Pediatric Oncology Nursing 11(2):71–84

Schuz J, Morgan G, Bohler E, Kaatsch P, Michaelis J (2003) Atopic disease and childhood acute lymphoblastic leukemia. International Journal of Cancer 105(2):255–260

Sharathkumar A, Thornley I, Saunders EF, Calderwood S, Freedman MH, Doyle J (2002) Allogenic bone marrow transplantation in children with chronic myelogenous leukemia. Journal of Pediatric Hematology/Oncology 24(3):215–219

Shu XO, Linet MS, Steinbuch M, Wen WQ, Buckley JD, Neglia JP, Potter JD, Reaman GH, Robison LL (1999) Breast feeding and risk of childhood acute leukemia Journal of the National Cancer Institute 91(20): 1765–1772

Skinner J, Mee TJ, Blackwell RP, Maslanyj MP, Simpson J, Allen SG, Day NE, Cheng KK, Gilman E, Williams D, Cartwright R, Craft A, Birch JM, Eden OB, McKinney PA, Deacon J, Peto J, Beral V, Roman E, Elwood P, Alexander FE, Mott M, Chilvers CE, Muir K, Doll R, Taylor CM, Greaves M, Goodhead D, Fry FA, Adams G, Law G (2002) Exposure to power frequency electric fields and the risk of childhood cancer in the UK. British Journal of Cancer 87(11):1257–1266

Sorahan T, McKinney PA, Mann JR, Lancashire RJ, Stiller CA, Birch JM, Dodd HE, Cartwright RA (2001) Childhood cancer and parental use of tobacco: findings from the interregional epidemiological study of childhood cancer (IRESCC). British Journal of Cancer 84(1):141–146

Steinbach D, Lengemann J, Voigt A, Hermann J, Zintl F, Sauerbrey A (2003) Response to chemotherapy and expression of the genes encoding the multidrug resistance-associated proteins MRP2, MRP3, MRP4, MRP5, and SMRP in childhood acute myeloid leukemia. Clinical Cancer Research 9(3):1083–1086

Steinbuch M, Weinberg CR, Buckley JD, Robison LL, Sandler DP (1999) Indoor residential radon exposure and risk of childhood acute myeloid leukaemia. British Journal of Cancer 81(5):900–906

Stiller CA, McKinney PA, Bunch KJ, Bailey CC, Lewis IJ (1991) Childhood cancer and ethnic group in Britain: a United Kingdom children's Cancer Study Group (UKCCSG) study. British Journal of Cancer 64(3):543–548

Sung L, Buckstein R, Doyle JJ, Crump M, Detsky AS (2003) Treatment options for patients with acute myeloid leukemia with a matched sibling donor: a decision analysis. Cancer 97(3):592–600

Swensen AR, Ross JA, Shu XO, Reaman GH, Steinbuch M, Robison LL (2001) Pet ownership and childhood acute leukemia (USA and Canada). Cancer Causes Control 12(4):301–303

Thapa PB, Whitlock JA, Brockman Worrell KG, Gideon P, Mitchel EF Jr., Roberson P, Pais R, Ray WA (1998) Prenatal exposure to metronidazole and risk of childhood cancer: a retrospective cohort study of children younger than 5 years. Cancer 83(7):1461–1468

UK Childhood Cancer Study Investigators (2001) Breastfeeding and childhood cancer. British Journal of Cancer 85(11):1685–1694

Solid Tumors

Eleanor Hendershot

Contents

Solid tumors account for 30% of all pediatric malignancies. Pediatric tumors are most often classified by histology rather than anatomic location, as is done in adult tumors. The most commonly occurring pediatric solid neoplasms are brain tumors, neuroblastoma, and Wilms' tumor. Other malignancies that affect the pediatric population include Hodgkin's lymphoma, non-Hodgkin's lymphoma, Ewing's sarcoma, osteosarcoma, hepatoblastoma, retinoblastoma, and rhabdomyosarcoma. These and other less commonly occurring tumors will be reviewed in this chapter.

2.1 Hodgkin's Disease

Hodgkin's disease (HD) is a malignant disease of the reticuloendothelial and lymphatic systems. It has a predictable pattern of spread through contiguous nodes. It does occur, although rarely, in extralymphatic organs.

2.1.1 Epidemiology

HD comprises 5% of all pediatric malignancies. The overall incidence of HD each year is approximately 6.6 per million children under the age of 15, with a peak in incidence in 14-year-olds of 23.1 per million. (Gurney et al., 1999). There tends to be a male predominance in children less than 15, at which point the incidence becomes more equal between males and females. There is a characteristic bimodal distribution of age of onset that differs geographically. In industrialized nations, there is a peak incidence around the age of 20, followed by a second peak that occurs in the 50s. In developing countries, however, the first peak occurs earlier into childhood. HD is rare in children less than 5 years of age.

2.1.2 Etiology

In general, HD tends to be diagnosed most frequently in patients with abnormal immune systems. There has been a strong association noted between the development of HD and previous Epstein-Barr virus (EBV) infection, especially early and prolonged exposure. The virus has been noted in the Reed-Sternberg cells in 50% of HD patients (Hudson and Donaldson, 2002); HD is characterized by the presence of Reed-Sternberg cells (see section 2.1.5). EBV has been associated with HD to varying degrees based on ethnicity and is found in 93% of Asians, 86% of Hispanics, 46% of whites, and 17% of African-American children who are affected (Hudson and Donaldson, 2002).

The role of HHV6 in disease development is also being investigated. HD has been noted with greater frequency in patients with a family history of HD, ataxia telangiectasia, or immunodeficiency syndromes such as human immunodeficiency virus (HIV).

2.1.3 Molecular Genetics

Cytogenetic abnormalities, often characteristic in other tumors, are not diagnostic in HD.

2.1.4 Symptoms and Clinical Signs

HD usually presents with painless lymphadenopathy. On physical examination the lymph node is usually described as firm and rubbery, and it may be sensitive or painful if it has enlarged quickly. Eighty percent of individuals present with disease in the cervical area, and 60% of those affected have some degree of mediastinal disease. Systemic symptoms are present in 25–30% of children and include

- fever >38°C for more than 3 days
- drenching night sweats
- weight loss comprising 10% of body weight over a period of 6 months (Chauvenet et al., 2000)

Respiratory symptoms of cough or chest pain may be obvious if significant mediastinal disease is present. Superior vena cava syndrome can also occur due to a mediastinal mass. Other systemic symptoms include pruritus, urticaria, and fatigue. Splenic enlargement may be observed with abdominal involvement, and splenic disease is present in one-third of patients. Idiopathic thrombocytopenia purpura occurs in 1–2% of children with HD and is often associated with autoimmune hemolytic anemia (Hudson and Donaldson, 2002).

HD typically spreads via lymphatics rather than hematogenous routes. Extralymphatic organs such as the bone and bone marrow may be involved in advanced disease. Parenchymal lung lesions are also sometimes present.

2.1.5 Diagnostics

Physical examination will demonstrate the presence of any significant lymphadenopathy. Although a chest x-ray can be performed quickly to determine the presence of a mediastinal mass, computerized tomography (CT) of the neck, chest, abdomen, and pelvis is necessary to evaluate the extent of disease. Nuclear imaging such as a gallium scan and, more recently, positron emission tomography (PET) scanning provides additional information on the extent of disease and the response to treatment. Gallium positivity is found in 70% of patients (Chauvenet et al., 2000). Gallium is taken up by underlying pathology, predominantly malignancy; however, it can be taken up by infection and thrombosis as well. Bone scan should be done if clinically warranted; i.e., bone pain, elevated alkaline phosphatase, or metastatic disease. Bilateral bone marrow aspirate and biopsies are necessary to rule out bone marrow involvement. A staging surgical laparotomy is no longer routinely performed in pediatric patients.

A biopsy of the affected node is required for diagnosis. An excisional biopsy is preferred because it preserves the architecture of the node and because the sample must be large enough to locate the presence of Reed-Sternberg cells. HD is characterized by the presence of Reed-Sternberg cells, which are giant multinucleated cells with abundant cytoplasm, the nucleolus having a characteristic "owl's eye" appearance. In most cases the Reed Sternberg cells are B-cells, and in 10–20% of cases, T-cells (Hudson and

Table 2.1. Ann Arbor staging classification for Hodgkin's lymphoma (adapted from Pinkerton et al., 1999)

Stage	Characteristics
I	Involvement of a single lymph node region or a single extralymphatic organ or site
II	Involvement of two or more lymph node regions on the same side of the diaphragm or solitary involvement of an extralymphatic organ or site and of one or more lymph node regions on the same side of the diaphragm
III	Involvement of lymph node regions on both sides of the diaphragm, which may be accompanied by localized involvement of extralymphatic organ or site or by involvement of the spleen, or both
IV	Diffuse or disseminated involvement of one or more extralymphatic organs or tissues with or without associated lymph node enlargement

"B" staging includes subjective symptoms such as fever, night sweats, and weight loss (10% of body weight in previous 6 months) Pinkerton et al., 1999

Donaldson, 2002). Malignant cells comprise less than 1% of tumor cells, with the remainder being inflammatory infiltrates. Histopathological studies carried out on Hodgkin's tumors consist of hematoxylin, eosin, and special immunohistochemical staining for surface markers, including CD15, CD20, and CD30. Immunophenotyping of RS cells indicates expression of certain activation antigens, including the IL2 receptor, Ki-1, the transferrin receptor, and HLA-DR (Hudson and Donaldson, 2002).

Blood work should include a complete/full blood count (CBC) and differential; cytopenias may be seen with bone marrow disease. Liver and renal function tests including alkaline phosphatase, should be done. Elevations of the erythrocyte sedimentation rate (ESR), copper, and ferritin are often seen because of increased activity of the reticuloendothelial system.

2.1.6 Staging and Classification

HD includes four major subtypes: nodular sclerosing, mixed cellularity, lymphocyte-predominant, and lymphocyte-depleted. Nodular sclerosing (NS) is the most common subtype, occurring in 60% of patients; disease is often found in the lower cervical, supraclavicular, and mediastinal lymph nodes. Mixed cellularity occurs in 30% of patients, often in children less than 10 years of age, those with advanced disease, and those with extranodal involvement. Lymphocyte-predominant HD occurs in 10–15% of patients, is more common in males and younger children, and

presents as localized disease. Lymphocyte-depleted HD occurs very rarely in children and is more common in HIV infection; it frequently presents as advanced disease involving bone or bone marrow (Hudson and Donaldson, 2002).

The Ann Arbor Staging Classification System is generally used to stage disease (Table 2.1).

2.1.7 Treatment

The goal of treatment for children with HD has become increasingly focused on response-based therapy and on minimizing late effects. Chemotherapy and radiation therapy are the cornerstones of treatment in HD. Surgery is not used in HD treatment; its only role is to obtain tissue biopsy. Children are at an increased risk for late secondary malignancies resulting from having both chemotherapy and radiotherapy at a time when they are still growing. For this reason, attempts to minimize treatment for those children who already do well based on stage and histology are being trialed.

Chemotherapy is an important part of the treatment for HD. Nitrogen mustard was one of the first drugs to be used for treating this disease, but due to subsequently recognized significant toxicities, specifically a relatively high incidence of secondary malignancies (predominantly acute myeloid leukemia) and infertility, it is no longer commonly used. Currently treatment is being modified and efforts made to avoid the use of alkylators and other drugs with significant long-term sequelae. Drugs that are pre-dominantly used in the treatment of HD include mechlorethamine (M), vincristine (O), prednisone (P), procarbazine (P), adriamycin (A), methotrexate (MT) bleomycin (B), vinblastine (V), etoposide (E), dacarbazine (D), and cyclophosphamide (C). Drug combinations that have and are currently being used in the treatment of HD are MOPP-ABV; ABVD, COPP-ABV, ABVE-PC, VEPA, BEACOPP, and VAMP.

Radiation therapy also plays a vital role in treating HD. Involved field radiation therapy includes the areas that are clinically involved as well as the surrounding lymph nodes. This approach is being used more commonly now in efforts to decrease the radiation field, thereby decreasing late effects. Mantle radiation, involving a larger field (submandibular, submental, cervical, supraclavicular, infraclavicular, axillary, mediastinal, and pulmonary hilar nodes), was typically used in previous protocols. In some instances of mantle radiation, the tumor volume may be enlarged to include the cardiac silhouette or lung fields as well. When pelvic radiation is needed, surgical repositioning of the ovaries to a central midline position is possible, enabling a midline pelvic block to protect ovaries and minimize toxicity.

Tailored therapy considers and evaluates early response to therapy for the purpose of limiting the cumulative chemotherapy doses while maintaining efficacy. Early responders continue to have improved outcomes compared with slow responders. Schwartz (2003) describes a protocol using VEPA (vincristine, etoposide, prednisone, adriamycin) that does not include any alkylators, which has been shown to be effective for low-stage disease without radiation therapy. Donaldson et al. (2002) also studied low-risk children and adolescents with stage I, stage IIa, and IIb without bulky mediastinal disease or peripheral nodal disease. These patients were treated with four cycles of VAMP (vincristine, adriamycin, methotrexate and prednisone) followed by low-dose involved field radiation. Those who had a complete response after two cycles of VAMP were treated with 15 Gy of involved field radiation therapy, and those who had only a partial response to two cycles of VAMP received 22.5 Gy of radiation therapy. The mean follow-up for these patients has been 5–10 years, and the

5 year overall survival is 99%, event-free survival is 93%, and there have been no toxicity concerns. Schwartz describes a North American Pediatric Oncology Group (POG) trial for advanced disease (POG 9425) in which the early responder received three courses of ABVE-PC versus five courses for the slow responders or partial responders, followed by radiation therapy. The results show that the overall 2 year event-free survival is 88.2%, with 90.8% for early responders, which comprised 61% of the children, and 87.7% for slow responders, which represented 38% of the children. Progressive disease was found in 1% of children. These results suggest that tailoring therapy has good outcomes in both cohorts of early and late responders but, by reducing treatment, may avoid late effects in those who respond early.

The treatment for relapsed patients usually consists of high-dose chemotherapy followed by autologous stem cell transplant (ASCT). If radiation therapy has not been used in the initial treatment of the disease, it may have a role in the treatment of the relapsed tumor.

2.1.8 Prognosis

The overall survival of children and adolescents with HD is 90% (Schwartz, 2003). Adverse prognostic features include bulky disease, as defined by a mass greater than 10 cm (6 cm in children) in size, and large mediastinal adenopathy. Smith et al. (2003) describe a prognostic factor analysis as reported in two POG studies. They found that stage IV disease and the male gender showed an inferior event-free survival. In Children's Cancer Group (CCG) trials, they found that elevated ESR, liver size, and mediastinal bulk among stage III patients was prognostic for inferior EFS. They also found that advance stage, bulky mediastinal disease, NS histology, and systemic symptoms were prognostic for both inferior disease-free survival and overall survival. Anemia and leukocytosis may also predict an inferior outcome

2.1.9 Follow-up

The follow up for HD must be long term, due to the many late effects that have affected this cohort of patients. Most relapses occur within the first 3 years off therapy; however, relapse has been documented as long as 10 years post-treatment (Hudson and Donaldson, 2002). Disease should be followed with chest x-ray and CT scanning of the primary site. Gallium scans are sometimes used to follow those who are at high risk for recurrence. PET may play a larger role in this regard in the future as more centers gain access to PET scanners. Scans are often carried out every 3 months for the first year off treatment, every 4 months for the second, and then every 6 months up until 5 years, as per POG protocols. Blood work such as CBC and differential, ESR, TSH, T4, LH, FSH, testosterone, and estradiol must all be monitored.

Late effects of therapy must be monitored carefully. Thyroid dysfunction in the form of nodules, hypothyroidism, and hyperthyroidism occur more frequently in patients who have been treated with radiation therapy as compared with the general population. The incidence of hypothyroidism is four to five times higher in patients treated with radiation therapy for HD compared with the general population (Sklar et al. 2000). Thyroid problems usually present within the first 5 years post-therapy but can occur until 20 years post-therapy. TSH and T4 must therefore be monitored. Echocardiogram and pulmonary function tests must be done to monitor for late cardiomyopathies and pulmonary fibrosis, secondary to anthracycline and bleomycin, respectively (with or without radiation). The risks of secondary tumors at various sites can occur in the two to three decades following treatment (Metayer et al., 2000). Patients treated for HD have the highest incidence of second malignancies of all of the pediatric malignancies. Infertility and primary ovarian failure can occur following chemotherapy and pelvic irradiation. Counseling must be done regarding lifestyle behaviors such as smoking.

2.1.10 Future Perspectives

Future trials for HD treatment will continue to focus on tailored disease protocols in an attempt to minimize late effects while continuing to maintain and exceed current excellent survival data. As more advances are made, immunotherapy and vaccine and monoclonal antibody therapy may be of use in he treating HD in the future. Rituximab is being studied now to determine its effectiveness at targeting lymphocyte-predominant HD (Donaldson, 2003).

2.2 Non-Hodgkin's Lymphoma

Non-Hodgkin's lymphomas (NHL) are a group of malignancies that are derived from cells of the immune system and lymphoid tissue. They are an aggressive form of cancer characterized by rapid cell division and an often high tumor burden at diagnosis.

2.2.1 Epidemiology

Lymphomas in general account for about 12 % of all childhood malignancies and are the third most common type of childhood cancer (Sandlund et al., 1996). NHL accounts for 60 % of lymphomas; it occurs at an incidence of approximately 8.4 per million children under the age of 20 per year (Gurney et al. 1995). Males are affected twice as often as females, and whites twice as often compared with blacks in the United States. Burkitt's lymphoma, an NHL subtype, is endemic in equatorial Africa and accounts for approximately 50 % of all childhood cancers. In other areas of the world, Burkitt's lymphoma occurs sporadically and is less common.

2.2.2 Etiology

There are different etiologies of NHL depending on geographical location. It has become apparent that individuals who are immunocompromised are at a higher risk of developing NHL, including those who are HIV infected and those who have undergone bone marrow transplant. EBV has been implicated in most of these lymphomas. Those individuals who

Table 2.2. Summary of major histological categories, immunophenotypes, common cytogenetic abnormalities, and common sites of disease of non-Hodgkin's lymphomas ((Magrath, 2002; Cairo and Perkins, 2000))

Histological category of lymphoma	Immunophenotype	Cytogenetic abnormalities	Common sites of disease
Burkitt's	B-cell (CD 19, CD 20, CD22, CD79, CD77, CD10)	t(8;14), t(8;2) and t(8;22)	Abdomen, head, neck
Large B-cell	B-cell (CD19, CD20, CD22, CD38, CD79, sometimes CD10) TdT neg	Bcl-6 or bcl-2 t(8;14) in 5–10%	Abdomen, mediastinum
Burkitt's-like	B-cell (MIB-1 positivity)	t(8;14)	Abdomen, head, neck
Lymphoblastic	Pre-T (CD77, CD7, CD5, CD2, CD1, CD3, CD4, CD8, TdT pos)	T-cell t(11;14)	Thorax
	CALLA sometimes observed	t(7;14), t(8;14), t(10;14)	Lymph nodes, bone marrow
	Pre-B (CALLA, B4, HLA-DR)	B-cell t(1;19), t(4;11)	
Anaplastic large cell	T-cell or null (CD 30) Ki-1+	t(2;5), and variants	Lymph nodes, skin, soft tissue, CNS, intrathoracic
Peripheral T-cell lymphoma	T-cell	Unknown	Variable

have been previously treated for HD are also at an increased risk for developing NHL due to cumulative effects of treatment; the risk is increased further if the individual has had a splenectomy. In African Burkitt's lymphoma, there is a very high correlation with those who have been previously infected with both EBV and malaria. In the developed world there has been no clear etiology for the development of NHL.

2.2.3 Molecular Genetics

Cytogenetic abnormalities are commonly found in NHL and assist in their diagnosis. A summary of the major histological categories of NHL with their associated cytogenetic abnormalities is shown in Table 2.2.

2.2.4 Symptoms and Clinical Signs

Like many tumors, the presenting signs and symptoms of NHL vary greatly depending on tumor location. NHL usually presents as extranodal disease in children. The primary presentations are as follows:

- Head and neck: 30%
- Abdominal: 30%
- Intrathoracic, mediastinal, or hilar adenopathy: 25% (Cairo and Perkins, 2000)

Localized disease can present as a firm, nontender mass in virtually any location.

Advanced metastatic disease is present in 70% of children who present with NHL (Cairo and Perkins, 2000). Table 2.3 indicates various presentations of NHL.

2.2.5 Diagnostics

A thorough history, physical exam, radiologic imaging, and tumor biopsy are needed to diagnose NHL. NHL is a rapidly growing tumor and often creates major metabolic disturbances that can be life-threatening. Frequent blood work for biochemistry abnormalities is a necessity while monitoring for signs of tumor lysis syndrome.

The sequence of investigations usually depends on the location of the primary tumor. Table 2.4 shows the possible investigations that may be carried out when a diagnosis of NHL is suspected.

Table 2.3. Presentations of non-Hodgkin's lymphoma

Features	Signs and symptoms	Indication
Meningoencephalitis	Headache Cranial nerve palsies Altered level of consciousness	CNS disease found commonly in Burkitt's lymphoma
Waldeyer's ring involvement	Tonsillar hypertrophy	Burkitt's lymphoma
Jaw lesion	Swelling Pain	Endemic Burkitt's
Systemic features	Fever Weight loss Night sweats Anorexia Malaise	Anaplastic large cell lymphoma
Mediastinal mass	Persistent nonproductive cough Dysphagia Dyspnea Chest pain	Intrathoracic disease, common in T-cell lymphoblastic lymphoma
Superior vena cava syndrome	Swelling of the upper extremities Distended neck veins Decreased breath sounds Dyspnea or stridor due to mass pressing on internal structures, pericardial effusion	Intrathoracic lesion Common in T-cell lymphoblastic lymphoma
Acute abdomen	Abdominal distension Pain Rebound tenderness Shifting dullness Nausea Vomiting GI bleeding Change in bowel habits Intussusception	Abdominal lymphoma B-cell (Intussusception is not an uncommon presentation for abdominal Burkitt's lymphoma)
Bone pain	Local pain Swelling	Bony disease, can occur in large cell lymphomas, lymphoblastic lymphomas, and Burkitt's
Skin involvement	Painful lesions	Particularly anaplastic large-cell lymphoma
Testicular involvement	Pain Swelling	Localized anaplastic large-cell lymphoma or lymphoblastic lymphoma.
Pancytopenia	Infection Fatigue Bleeding	Metastatic disease – bone marrow Lymphoblastic lymphoma or Burkitt's lymphoma common

Table 2.4. Possible investigations in the diagnosis of non-Hodgkin's lymphoma

Investigation	Rationale
Chest x-ray	To detect mediastinal mass and pulmonary lesions
CT of the neck, chest, abdomen, pelvis	For staging and evaluating all sites of potential disease (*tracheal compression would also be noted on the CT and is critical to recognize before administering general anesthetics*)
CT of the head	To detect CNS involvement
Ultrasound of the abdomen	To determine if there are abdominal masses and to ensure patency of the urinary tract system before beginning chemotherapy
Bone scan and skeletal survey	To detect bone metastases
Gallium scan	Often lymphomas show avidity for gallium, and scanning after it is administered outlines tumor throughout the body Also used to assess response to treatment
PET scan	As PET scans become more accessible, they will likely be used in the diagnostic workup and monitoring of patients with NHL
Endoscopy	Indicated if gastrointestinal bleeding is a presenting symptom
Complete/full blood count and differential	If cytopenias are present, bone marrow involvement is likely
Renal function tests	Abnormalities may suggest tumor lysis
Liver function studies	Baseline prior to treatment
Lactate dehydrogenase (LDH)	Nonspecific but can be elevated in NHL, possibly indicating a high tumor burden
Blood cultures	If fever present
Coagulation studies such as PTT, INR, fibrinogen, d-dimers	To evaluate possible disseminated intravascular coagulation
Viral studies for EBV, CMV, HSV, hepatitis A, B, and C	To look for evidence of causation (*HIV testing should be considered in a patient with a primary CNS lymphoma because of the high incidence of CNS lymphomas in the HIV population*)
B- and T-cell function tests	If an underlying immunodeficiency is being considered
Bilateral bone marrow aspirates and biopsies	If the bone marrow has greater than 25% blasts, the lymphoma would be treated as a leukemia based on the cellular phenotype of either B or T lineage (Pinkerton et al., 1999)
Lumbar puncture	To examine the cerebrospinal fluid for malignant cells

A biopsy of the node or mass is necessary to make a definitive diagnosis. NHLs are in the class of blue round cell tumors. They are differentiated from other blue round cell tumors based on immunophenotyping, karyotyping, southern blotting, polymerase chain reaction (PCR), and microarray. The presence of leukocyte common antigen CD45 will confirm lymphoid cell proliferation as it is not present in non-hematologic malignancies (Magrath, 2002). See Table 2.2 to view a summary of immunophenotyping and cytogenetic differences in the various subtypes of NHL.

Table 2.5. St Jude staging systems for childhood non-Hodgkin's lymphoma (adapted from Pinkerton et al., 1999)

Stage I	Single tumor (extranodal) or single anatomic area (nodal) with the exclusion of mediastinum or abdomen
Stage II	Single tumor (extranodal) with regional lymph nodes Two or more nodal areas on the same side of diaphragm Two single tumors (extranodal) with or without regional lymph node A resectable primary GI tumor with or without involvement of mesenteric nodes only
Stage III	Two single tumors (extranodal) above and below the diaphragm Two or more nodal areas above and below the diaphragm All primary intrathoracic tumors All extensive primary intra-abdominal disease All paraspinal or epidural tumors
Stage IV	Any of the above with the initial involvement of either the central nervous system and/or the bone marrow (<25%)

Pinkerton et al., 1999

Table 2.6. Non-Hodgkin's lymphoma incidence according to subtype and cell of origin (adapted from Pinkerton et al., 1999)

Cell type	Subgroup	Proportion of NHL (%)
B-Cell	I. Precursor B neoplasm B lymphoblastic	5%
	II. Peripheral B neoplasm	
	Follicular	0.4%
	Diffuse large B cell	3%
	Primary mediastinal	0.4%
	Burkitt's	42%
	High-grade Burkitt's and Burkitt's-like	4%
T-Cell	I. Precursor T neoplasm T lymphoblastic	20%
	II. Peripheral T-cell PTL unspecified	1%
	Anaplastic large cell	15%
	Nonspecific/intermediate	9.2%

Pinkerton et al., 1999

2.2.6 Staging and Classification

The classifications of childhood NHL are divided into three main categories:

- Lymphoblastic (30%)
- Large cell (20%)
- Small noncleaved cell, Burkitt's or Burkitt's like (40%).

Staging normally follows the St Jude Children's Research Hospital schema, which was based on the Ann Arbor Hodgkin's classification (see Table 2.5). This staging and classification system is used for all histologic subtypes of NHL. Incidence can also be defined by the B-cell or T-cell lineage of the tumor (Table 2.6). The National Cancer Institute has provided breakdowns of the incidence in which the various forms of lymphoma can present (Table 2.6).

2.2.7 Treatment

Treatment for NHL depends on the histologic subtype and stage of disease. Most protocols now assign patients to risk groups in order to determine intensity of treatment. Surgery is primarily used for diagnosis and staging of NHL, with the exception of abdominal tumors. Radiation therapy is not generally used in treating these tumors except in emergency situations. NHL is primarily treated with chemotherapy. Emergent complications arise quite often in the treatment of NHL based on the tumor's location and size, and therefore must be anticipated, diagnosed, and treated rapidly.

Debulking surgery has demonstrated no benefit to effective chemotherapy (Patte, 1997). Most abdominal lymphomas are the B-cell immunophenotype, and presentation often mimics an acute abdomen. Bowel obstruction or intussusception can also occur. In these cases, gross total excision of the primary is warranted, followed by adjuvant chemotherapy (Patte,1997).

Radiation therapy is not generally a part of NHL protocols. It is used in the urgent treatment of superior vena cava obstruction and for central nervous system (CNS) involvement causing nerve palsies. Prophylactic radiation has generally been shown to have no advantage in active CNS or limited-stage disease and is not used in multiagent chemotherapy regimens (Cairo and Perkins, 2000).

Chemotherapy regimens are based on the immunophenotype of the lymphoma (B- versus T-cell). In general, T-cell lymphomas receive longer and less intense treatments, and B-cell lymphomas are treated for shorter periods but with higher doses of alkylating agents and antimetabolites. NHLs are sensitive to a variety of chemotherapeutic agents, probably due to the aggressive nature of the disease with its rapid doubling time and high growth fractions.

Lymphoblastic lymphomas are most often treated on protocols similar to leukemia protocols. Treatment involves three phases, induction, consolidation, and maintenance, and generally lasts 2–3 years. Patients are usually not divided into risk groups because most patients have advanced disease. Multiple chemotherapeutic agents are used throughout the treatment course (see Table 2.7).

Small noncleaved cell lymphomas are B-cell lymphomas and have much shorter treatments. Treatment consists of two to six cycles of intense chemotherapy with no maintenance therapy. Large B-cell lymphomas are generally treated as per the small noncleaved cell lymphomas protocols as well. (See Table 2.7.)

Anaplastic large-cell lymphomas have been treated by a variety of approaches. Some of the best results have been from the German BFM group, who have used B-cell lymphoma protocols without local radiation therapy. (See Table 2.7.)

CNS prophylaxis is a necessary part of NHL treatment for most patients. Patients who have completely resected abdominal primaries, or stage I disease that is not in close proximity to the CNS, normally do not require CNS prophylaxis. Generally, all others are treated with varying degrees of CNS prophylaxis that consists of intrathecal methotrexate and/or intrathecal cytarabine (Magrath, 2002).

Autologous stem cell transplant is often used for only partial response to therapy in B-cell lymphomas. Allogeneic transplant is indicated for T-cell relapses after response to salvage therapies has been determined. In anaplastic large-cell lymphoma, relapse therapy using retinoic acid and interferon has been used with some effect at maintaining long remissions (Magrath, 2002).

Treatment and tumor complications can occur emergently and must be anticipated. Tumor lysis syndrome is seen frequently in NHL and specifically in Burkitt's and Burkitt's-like lymphoma because of their rapid doubling times. Other complications include respiratory distress, abdominal emergencies, superior vena cava syndrome, esophageal compression, cardiac tamponade, paraplegia, increased intracranial pressure, obstructive jaundice, pancreatitis, renal failure, and infection. The treatment of these complications is discussed further in other sections.

Table 2.7. Treatment summaries for non-Hodgkin's lymphoma (from Cairo and Perkins, 2000; reprinted with permission)

Stage and histology	Chemotherapy regimen	Cooperative group	Length of therapy	% Survival (3–5 years)
Stages I and II (St Jude) or Group A (FAB)	COPADA	SFOP	6 weeks	95
B large or SNCCL	COMP	CCG	6 months	85
Lymphoblastic	CHOP COMP BFM-NHL	BFM	8 weeks	90
Stages III and IV or Group B and C SNCCL	LMB-89	SFOP	6 months	8090
	Orange	CCG	8 months	7080
	NCI-89-C-41	NCI	6 months	7080
	Total-B	POG	4 months	6070
	BFM-NHL	BFM	4 months	6080
Lymphoblastic	(AD)COMP	CCG	1824 months	70
	LSA-L2	CCG/POG	1824 months	70
	BFM-NHL	BFM	1824 months	90
Large Cell	COMP (D)	CCG	1824 months	6070
B cell	APO(+)	POG	18 months	6070
	LMB-89	SFOP	46 months	90
	ORANGE	CCG	46 months	90
	BFM-NHL	BFM	46 months	7080
	NCI-89-C-41	NCI	46 months	8090
Anaplastic	CHOP/MACOOP-B	ST JUDE'S	6 months	75
	BFM-NHL-B	BFM	6 months	80
	HM 8991	SFOP	68 months	6070

2.2.8 Prognosis

The event-free survival for all stages of NHL ranges widely. The overall survival following the treatment of Burkitt's, Burkitt's-like, and large B-cell lymphoma, including advanced stage disease, is 90% (Magrath, 2002). For lymphoblastic lymphoma and anaplastic large cell lymphoma, the overall survival is 80–90%. Children treated for T-cell acute lymphoblastic leukemia as per the BFM Rez protocol have displayed an event-free survival of 92% (Magrath, 2002).

2.2.9 Follow-up

Follow-up for children treated for NHL needs to consider surveillance for disease recurrence and late effects of treatment. Most relapses of Burkitt's lymphoma occur with 12 months. If children with lymphoblastic lymphoma has not relapsed 30 months from the start of treatment, they have a very high probability of cure (Magrath, 2002).

Surveillance scans of the primary tumor can be done using CT or ultrasound, depending on the tumor's location. These should be carried out every 3 months for the first year off treatment and then with decreasing frequency over several years. Gallium or PET scans are very helpful in the surveillance for NHL recurrence and can be done on a similar schedule to primary tumor imaging. CBCs are necessary, especially in lymphoblastic lymphomas, to look for recurrence of bone marrow disease, which is characterized by blasts in the peripheral smear.

Late effects of chemotherapy for NHL include a variety of potential problems because so many different chemotherapeutic agents are used. Cardiotoxicity from anthracycline therapy is a potential; follow-up echocardiograms should be routinely done at least every 2–4 years in the absence of problems. Appropriate attention needs to be paid to growth and development; for unknown reasons a significant group of children treated for NHL go on to become obese. Children who have been treated with significant amounts of intrathecal chemotherapy may be at more risk for learning problems. Neuropsychological testing may be appropriate so that specific help can be given to these children. Secondary malignancies are always a concern following treatment with VP16 and alkylating agents, so surveillance is paramount. Skeletal sequelae are a potential following the use of high-dose steroids. Osteoporosis is a concern, as is avascular necrosis; no specific follow-up is required for this, but awareness is crucial. Infertility and gonadal dysfunction may be a problem following treatment with alkylating agents.

2.2.10 Future Perspectives

Newer techniques such as microarray analysis might be useful in determining the exact rate of response to therapy. Examining gene expression patterns and proteomic analysis may help to determine therapy response rate so that the appropriate intensity of therapy can be given for each histological subtype of lymphoma. Targeting viral proteins in Burkitt's lymphoma is one area of research; it is hoped that a modified Myc gene may be able to induce tumor lysis of these cells. There are thoughts also that the antisense could cause cell death in DNA sequences involving the (8;14) translocation if targeted appropriately.

2.3 Ewing's Sarcoma Family of Tumors

Ewing's sarcoma family of tumors (ESFT) comprises a group of neoplasms that can arise in bone and soft tissue and that share similar histologic and molecular features. These tumors include Ewing's sarcoma, extraosseous Ewing's sarcoma, peripheral primitive neuroectodermal tumor (PPNET), and Askin tumor (a chest wall tumor). Ewing's sarcoma is the more undifferentiated form of the tumor, whereas PPNET is more differentiated. ESFTs are thought to derive from neural crest cells.

2.3.1 Epidemiology

ESFT is the second most frequently seen primary malignant bone tumor in childhood and represents 3 % of all pediatric malignancies (Venkateswaran et al., 2001). The incidence is approximately 2.8 per million annually in individuals less than 20 years of age. ESFT occurs most often in the second decade of life, with the highest age-specific rates occurring at 13 years of age (Gurney et al., 1995). ESFT is extremely rare in individuals over the age of 30 and in Chinese and black children. There is a slight male dominance in the incidence of this tumor.

2.3.2 Etiology

The cause for ESFT is not known. There does not appear to be strong associations with congenital syndromes or familial cancer syndromes.

2.3.3 Molecular Genetics

ESFTs are in the group of small blue round cell tumors. Molecular genetics is invaluable in helping to distinguish ESFT from other small blue round cell tumors. Fluorescence in situ hybridization (FISH) and reverse transcriptase polymerase chain reaction (RTPCR) are used to detect cytogenetic changes in the tumor for diagnostic purposes. Immunocytochemical staining also helps in this differentiation.

ESFTs display a characteristic t(11;22) (q24;q12) that fuses the EWS and the FLI1 gene; this genetic translocation is found in most tumors (Pinkerton et al. 1999). A second chromosomal translocation consists of a t(21;22)(q22;q12), which fuses the EWS and the ERG gene (Ginsberg et al., 2002). Less frequently observed changes involve trisomy 8 and 2 and deletions of chromosome 22, 16q, and 1p36 (Ginsberg et al., 2002). These aberrations are though to cause dysfunction in tumor suppressor genes, and their presence might be prognostic of poor outcome.

2.3.4 Symptoms and Clinical Signs

ESFT can occur in both long and flat bones. The incidence anatomically is split almost in half, with tumors arising in extremities (53%) and the central axis (47%).

In the central axis

- 45% occur in the pelvis
- 34% occur in the chest wall
- 12% in the spine
- 9% in the head and neck.

In the extremities:

- 52% of tumors are found in distal bones
- 48% in proximal bones

(Ginsberg et al., 2002)

Children typically present with symptoms caused by the primary tumor. Pain and swelling are often present. A palpable mass is frequently seen, and fractures are evident in 5% of cases (Jurgens et al., 1997). It is not uncommon for a child to present after a prolonged history of increasing pain or mass or after a traumatic injury that does not heal. Neurological impairments or weakness may accompany spinal lesions. Urinary and bowel incontinence may accompany large pelvic tumors.

Twenty percent of patients have metastatic disease at diagnosis (Ginsberg et al. 2002). Metastases usually follow a hematogenous route, spreading to lungs, bone, and bone marrow. Fever may indicate systemic or advanced disease. Infections, bleeding, and lethargy may reflect pancytopenia suggesting bone marrow involvement. Respiratory symptoms, such as cough, dyspnea, unequal breath sounds, and rales, may indicate large pulmonary metastases.

2.3.5 Diagnostics

A plain film of the affected area is usually the first diagnostic test ordered. On x-ray, ESFT will show up as a destructive lesion of the diaphysis of the bone that is poorly marginated. It may also have an onion peel characteristic, which is indicative of a periosteal reaction. CT or magnetic resonance imaging (MRI) of the primary should be performed to achieve better delineation of the soft tissue component of the tumor as well as examine its blood supply and tumor extension. Chest x-ray should be done to look for lung metastases; however, a CT of the chest is needed to look for smaller pulmonary nodules. Fig. 2.1 shows the CT of a patient with Askin tumor (chest wall mass). A bone scan is indicated to look for bony metastases. Fig. 2.2 shows a metastatic PNET on bone scan. Bilateral bone marrow aspirates and biopsies are necessary to rule out bone marrow disease.

A biopsy is indicated to determine definitive diagnosis. Tumor histology may be undifferentiated or differentiated showing Homer-Wright rosettes. The tumor specimen should be evaluated with routine staining and immunohistochemistry. Adrenergic, muscle, and lymphoid markers should be negative, and the tumor should stain positive for CD99 and vimentin (Ginsberg et al. 2002). Cytogenetic studies and RTPCR should be ordered to look for the characteristic t(11;22).

There are no definitive blood tumor markers for the ESFT; however, an elevated lactate dehydrogenase (LDH) may indicate a large tumor burden or rapid tumor growth. Elevated LDH has also been associated with a less favorable outcome. An elevated white blood cell count or ESR can also be seen at times with advanced disease.

2.3.6 Staging and Classification

There is not an elaborate staging system for the ESFT. The tumor is described in terms of the presence or absence of metastases.

Figure 2.1

CT of a patient with Askin tumor (chest wall mass)

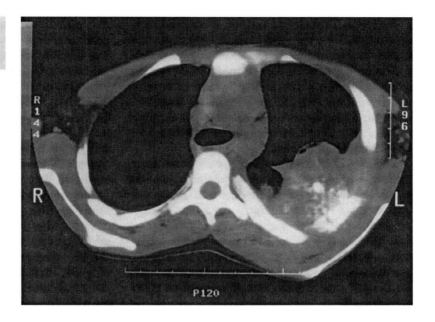

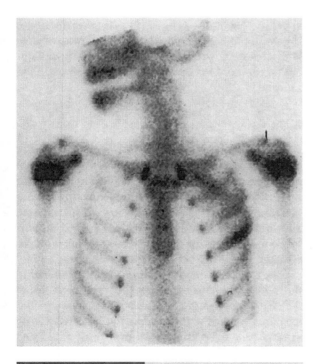

Figure 2.2

Metastatic PNET on bone scan

2.3.7 Treatment

The goals of treatment for the ESFT are threefold:

- Cure the disease
- Preserve useful function in affected area
- Minimize the long-term sequelae

Chemotherapy, radiation therapy, and surgery may all be used in treating this malignancy. Chemotherapy is delivered initially in order to shrink the tumor. Surgery or radiation therapy is then used to establish local control. This is then followed by a maintenance period of chemotherapy. Treatment for ESFT generally lasts up to a year.

Chemotherapy is initially used for cytoreduction in the treatment of the ESFT. After local control has been established, chemotherapy is given to treat micrometastatic disease that may have occurred at the time of surgery or local control. Common chemotherapeutic agents are vincristine, actinomycin, or doxorubicin and cyclophosphamide, alternating with VP16 and ifosfamide. Growth factors such as granulocyte colony-stimulating factor (GCSF) are often used following chemotherapy to hasten white blood cell recovery.

Surgery is the preferred method of establishing local control. It is used most often in local control for tumors of the extremities The entire bony or soft tissue lesion needs to be excised using initial imaging studies ensuring a disease-free margin of approximately 3 cm. Margins of 2 cm are generally acceptable if is near a joint articulation (Ginsberg et al., 2002). Gross or microscopic disease postoperatively is treated with radiation therapy.

Local control following the use of radiation therapy along with systemic chemotherapy delivers a cure rate of 75–90%. Radiation therapy is often the only option that is available for tumors of the central axis, in which radical surgery in not feasible. A total tumor dose of 55–60 Gy is delivered to the whole bony lesion with a 3 cm margin (a smaller margin is used if it avoids radiating an epiphysis); the original imaging studies are used to make this determination (Ginsberg et al., 2002).

Metastases are treated with surgery and/or radiation therapy, depending on the location of the tumors. In the lungs, both surgical resection and radiation therapy can be effectively used, depending on tumor location. Dose intensification regimens for metastatic disease using standard chemotherapy with VACIME (vincristine, adriamycin, cyclophosphamide, ifosfamide, mesna, etoposide) plus peripheral blood stem cell support and GCSF have been attempted with no real increase to disease-free survival (Hawkins et al., 2002). Future Children's Oncology Group (COG) protocols are currently considering the use of antiangiogenic therapies with vinblastine and Celebrex in conjunction with standard chemotherapy therapy for metastatic disease at diagnosis. Angiogenesis is a process by which tumors form new blood vessels; the purpose of antiangiogenic therapies is to target the factors that contribute to the development of new blood vessels, inhibiting or antagonizing them in order to arrest or prevent tumor growth.

2.3.8 Prognosis

Prognosis for the ESFT depends largely on the location of the tumor and the presence of metastases at diagnosis. Cutaneous, subcutaneous, distal bone, and rib tumors tend to have higher cure rates because of the feasibility of surgical resection. Tumors of the pelvis are often associated with poor response. Five-year disease-free survival rates range from 70–75% (Rodriguez-Galindo et al., 2002a). If metastases are present at diagnosis, the 2-year disease-free survival is less than 30% (Hawkins et al., 2002). Prognosis following relapse is poor, with long-term survival less than 25% (Rodriguez-Galindo et al., 2002a). Some children do better with late or local recurrence. Lung metastases tend to respond to treatment more than metastatic disease elsewhere in the body.

The tumor volume, LDH result, and the amount of tumor necrosis at the time of surgery are thought to be of prognostic significance; however, current treatment decisions are not usually based on these criteria. The subtype of fusion gene is also prognostic, with EWS-FLI1 favoring a better outcome than other genetic abnormalities. A retrospective study carried out by Jenkin and colleagues (2002) that looked to determine prognostic factors in localized Ewing's sarcoma and PNET of bone found that age less than or equal to 14, with the primary in a distal extremity or the skull, and tumor volume <200 ml were associated with a favorable prognosis. The amount of neural differentiation did not appear to have a prognostic significance.

2.3.9 Follow-up

Follow-up requires focus on both recurrent disease and late effects of treatment. Recurrent disease is at greatest risk in the first 5 years following treatment for ESFT. Protocols usually request imaging studies including CT or MRI of the primary, CT of the chest, and sometimes bone scan to be done every 3 months following therapy for the first year and then with decreasing frequency over the next several years.

Late effects of therapy must also be considered in the follow-up of these patients. Children are at risk of developing a secondary neoplasm such as a myeloid leukemia (related to the administration of alkylating agents) or a solid tumor in a previously irradiated site. The incidence of secondary malignancies in this group has been reported between 5% and 20% following a period of observation of 20 years (Jurgens et al., 1997). Cardiomyopathy or congestive heart failure can occur following anthracycline therapy; therefore, cardiac function should be monitored with echocardiograms. Toxicities to the liver, kidney, nervous system, and endocrine system must be considered and any symptoms investigated accordingly.

2.3.10 Future Perspectives

Future therapies may involve targeting cytostatic agents or be immunologically targeted therapies. Monoclonal antibody therapies are also currently being researched. The French group is advocating that future studies be tailored to account for prognostic features such as histological response to chemotherapy (percent of tumor necrosis) and tumor volume (Oberlin et al., 2001). Topotecan plus cyclophosphamide shows promise in 35% of recurrent ESFTs and may continue to play a role in the future (Saylors et al., 1999).

2.4 Osteosarcoma

Osteosarcoma is a primary bone tumor that is thought to arise from mesenchymal bone-forming cells. It is characterized by the production of osteoid.

2.4.1 Epidemiology

Osteosarcoma is the third most common solid tumor of children and adolescents and the most frequently occurring primary bone tumor in this population (Wittig et al., 2002). The peak incidence of osteosarcoma is in the second decade of life, a period characterized by rapid bone growth. It occurs at an annual rate of approximately 3 per million children less than 15 years of age (Gurney et al., 1995). The incidence is slightly higher in African-Americans than whites and in males than females.

2.4.2 Etiology

The etiology of osteosarcoma is largely unknown. There appears to be an association between rapid bone growth and the development of osteosarcoma, as evidenced by its high incidence during the growth spurt in adolescence. There are several associations between osteosarcoma and other pathologies. It is known that osteosarcomas can be caused by ionizing radiation, and this is implicated in 3% of osteosarcomas (Link et al., 2002). It has also been found that osteosarcoma can arise in patients with hereditary multiple exostoses, Paget's disease, fibrous dysplasia, chronic osteomyelitis, multiple osteochondroma, and sites of bone infarcts. A genetic predisposition has been found between hereditary retinoblastoma (Rb) and osteosarcoma. The Rb gene is a tumor-suppressor gene and important in apoptosis. It has been estimated that between 8% and 90% of carriers of the Rb1 mutation will acquire a secondary malignancy, including osteosarcoma by the age of 30 (Link et al., 2002). The Rb1 mutation has also been implicated in the pathogenesis of sporadic osteosarcoma. Mutations of p53 have also been found in osteosarcoma, suggesting that inactivation of p53, which is a tumor-suppressor gene, plays a key role in the development of osteosarcoma. There is a higher incidence of osteosarcoma in Li-Fraumeni syndrome.

2.4.3 Molecular Genetics

The diagnosis of osteosarcoma is primarily based on tumor histology. Although there is not a specific cytogenetic or molecular maker for osteosarcoma, there is a great deal of research in the area of genetics that is focusing on better understanding of the disease and determining prognostic criteria.

It is well known that a relationship exists between osteosarcoma and the Rb1 gene mutation as well as p53 mutations. Loss of heterozygosity at the Rb gene occurs in 70% of sporadic osteosarcomas, and loss of heterozygosity at the Rb locus is thought to be a poor prognostic factor (Ragland et al., 2002). Many other genetic abnormalities continue to be examined to determine their role in the disease. C-Myc is expressed more often in those with osteosarcoma who develop metastatic disease. HER2/neu (human epidermal growth factor receptor 2) is expressed in approximately 40% of patients who develop early pulmonary metastases. Important discoveries are starting to be made in identifying the significance of these abnormalities.

2.4.4 Signs and Symptoms

Osteosarcoma commonly affects the metaphyseal growth plates of long bones. Although osteosarcoma can occur in any bone, the anatomic sites most commonly affected are the distal femur, the proximal tibia, and the proximal humerus. Osteosarcoma metastasizes most frequently to the lung, followed by bone. Gross metastatic disease is present at diagnosis in less than 20% of cases (Kager et al., 2003).

Osteosarcoma typically presents with pain and/or soft tissue swelling in the affected area. The mass itself may be warm, and vascularity over the mass may be found. There is often decreased range of motion in the affected limb. The duration of symptoms prior to diagnosis may range up to 6 months. Respiratory symptoms at diagnosis would only be present in very advanced pulmonary disease and are rare. Systemic symptoms of disease, such as fever and night sweats, are uncommon. Lymphadenopathy in proximal lymph nodes is also very rare.

2.4.5 Diagnostics

The workup up of a patient who presents with pain and/or swelling should start with a thorough health history paying special attention to any pain and the duration of the symptoms. Diagnostic imaging, blood tests and tumor biopsy are all needed.

Plain films of the affected area may reveal a lytic lesion with indistinct margins or ossification in soft tissue with a sunburst pattern that is characteristic of osteosarcoma (see Fig. 2.3). Reactive new bone formation can also be seen frequently under the periosteum forming a "Codman's angle" or "Codman's triangle" (Ragland et al., 2002). An MRI of the affected area would further examine the tumor boundaries, the soft tissue component, and the relationship to joints, blood vessels, and neurovascular bundle. A chest x-ray determines the presence of pulmonary metastases, but CT is more sensitive for smaller pulmonary nodules. A bone scan should also be performed to pick up areas of skeletal metastases. Bony metastases occur in 10% of patients with osteosarcoma at diagnosis (Link et al., 2002).

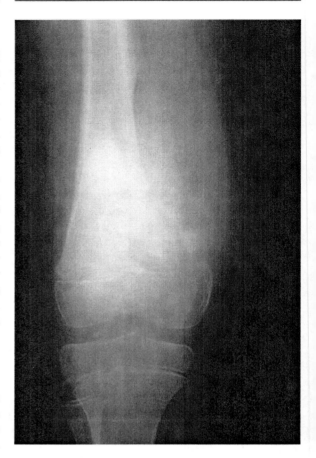

Figure 2.3

Plain fm of patient with osteosarcoma

There are no specific blood tumor markers for osteosarcoma. Elevations of LDH are seen in up to 30% of patients at diagnosis (Link et al., 2002). However, LDH is an acute phase reactant and is not tumor-specific. Elevations of alkaline phosphatase are present in over half of patients, but again do not correlate reliably with disease. Abnormalities cannot necessarily be distinguished between bone and liver etiologies, but experience has shown that they may have a poor prognostic significance.

Table 2.8. Enneking system for staging osteosarcomas

Grade 1	Low-grade osteosarcoma
Grade 2	High-grade osteosarcoma
Grade 3	Osteosarcoma with distant metastases
A	Intracompartmental
B	Extracompartmental

A biopsy is necessary for obtaining definitive diagnosis. Open biopsy is preferred so that contamination of skin and surrounding structures is minimized. Histologically, osteosarcoma is characterized by the presence of spindle cells and the production of tumor osteoid (Jurgens et al., 1997).

2.4.6 Staging and Classification

There are varied histological patterns of osteosarcoma with osteoblastic being the most common, with an incidence of 78%, followed, in descending order of frequency, by chondroblastic, fibroblastic, malignant fibrous histiocytoma-like, giant cell-rich, telangiectatic, low-grade intraosseous, small cell, and juxtacortical (Pinkerton et al., 1999).

Staging in osteosarcoma is generally quite straightforward and considers intra- and extracompartmental factors (whether tumor extends through cortex to bone), as well tumor grade and presence of metastases. Table 2.8 shows the Enneking staging system for osteosarcoma. The tumors are divided into low and high-grade variants depending on the number of mitoses, anaplasia, cellularity, and pleomorphism. Stage IIB is the most common presentation of conventional osteosarcoma.

2.4.7 Treatment

Treatment of osteosarcoma consists of surgical resection of the primary and neo-adjuvant chemotherapy. Historically treatment for osteosarcoma consisted only of amputation of the primary. The outcome was poor with long-term survival at 10% (Ferrari et al., 2003). Currently, with use of adjuvant and neoadjuvant chemotherapy, survival has increased dramatically. Chemotherapy agents that are sensitive to osteosarcoma are doxorubicin, cisplatin, and high-dose methotrexate. Agents such as cyclophosphamide, ifosfamide, and VP16 have also shown to be useful. Typically, chemotherapy is given for 2–3 months prior to local surgical control. Dose intensification regimens have become possible with the use of GCSF post-myelosuppressive chemotherapy cycles.

Local control consists of three options:

1. Amputation: Amputation is usually reserved for tumors that cannot be removed with adequate surgical margins. It is also frequently used in large tumors that do not respond well to chemotherapy and to tumors that have produced skip lesions.

2. Limb salvage: Limb salvage procedures can be done for 90–95% of tumors today (Wittig et al., 2002). They are appropriate when the tumors can be removed effectively with negative margins, meaning that the tumor is removed with a rim of healthy tissue around the tumor. In order to reconstruct the limb and/or joint, an endoprosthesis, allograft, arthrodesis, intercalary allograft, or metallic prosthesis can be used.

3. Rotationplasty: Rotationplasty is another procedure that is used when there is a large tumor around the knee joint. The leg is amputated at the distal femur, and the ankle joint is preserved, rotated 180 degrees, and reattached. This produces an artificial knee joint from which the prosthesis can be effectively secured for a greater range of motion (see chapter 21).

Metastatic disease at diagnosis predicts a poor outcome. Treatment aims should be the same: neoadjuvant chemotherapy and surgical resection of disease. Radiation therapy has been used but is not terribly useful. Bone marrow transplant does not currently have a role in osteosarcoma.

Relapse still occurs in 30–40% of patients despite aggressive chemotherapy and surgical resection in nonmetastatic osteosarcoma of the extremities. The post-relapse survival in this group is poor. The majority of relapses occur in the lung. Accepted strategies for treatment include surgical resection, even when this requires multiple thoracotomies. In a retrospective analysis by Ferrari et al.. (2003), they found that systemic chemotherapy using ifosfamide showed some utility in relapsed osteosarcoma; however, it had little use in pulmonary metastases except in a subset of patients with three or more pulmonary nodules. They also found that relapsed patients with one or two pulmonary nodules did better (5-year event-free survival 24%) than those who had bony metastases or more than two pulmonary nodules. Bony metastases have a poor outcome, but every attempt should be made for complete surgical resection.

2.4.8 Prognosis

The overall survival of patients with nonmetastatic disease at diagnosis, with the tumor located in an extremity, is 60–70%, whereas the survival of patients with metastases at diagnosis remains poor, at 15–20% (Bacci et al. 2002a,b). Prognosis of osteosarcoma depends largely on the extent of disease at diagnosis. Parosteal and intraosseous well-differentiated osteosarcomas tend to have a favorable prognosis. There appears to be no relationship between histological subtypes and overall survival. However, telangiectatic osteosarcomas (which produce lytic lesions) have a poor prognosis (Link et al., 2002). The site of the tumor plays a role in prognosis, with axial tumors faring worse than skeletal, most likely related to the difficulty in surgical resection of axial tumors. The tumor size also has a prognostic significance, with tumors less than 5 cm having better outcomes. Prognosis in children under 10 years old at diagnosis tends to be poorer. Elevations of LDH may have adverse prognosis. Loss of heterozygosity at the Rb gene may indicate that the tumors are more likely to metastasize. HER 2/erbB-2 over expression may be associated with inferior outcome. The response to preoperative chemotherapy is prognostic in that those tumors with greater than 98% necrosis or less than 2% viable tumor at the time of local control have a better outcome. The multidrug-resistance phenotype encodes p-glycoprotein, which if overexpressed may indicate an unfavorable outcome because p-glycoprotein has a propensity to actively pump chemotherapy from tumor cells (Link et al., 2002).

2.4.9 Follow-up

Patients need to be followed for both recurrent and metastatic disease as well as for late effects of the treatment itself. Imaging scans of the primary and the chest are done normally every 3 months for the first year and then at increasing intervals for at least the next several years before finally being done annually.

Late effects of chemotherapy include cardiomyopathies related to anthracycline use and hearing impairments related to cisplatin chemotherapy. Neurological, hormonal, and psychological late effects should also be considered when assessing patients. Infertility and secondary malignancies may result from the use of high-dose alkylating agents.

2.4.10 Future Perspectives

New chemotherapeutic agents have not shown to be effective in phase I and II trials. Dose intensification regimens with current chemotherapeutic agents using cardioprotective agents are being reviewed. There is interest in immunomodulation vaccine therapy and antiangiogenic agents. Antiangiogenic agents are used to target and impede the tumor's ability to form new blood vessels, thereby inhibiting tumor growth. Liposomal muramyl tripeptide-phosphatidylethanolamine (MTPPE) was trialed by the Pediatric Oncology Group (POG) and Children's Cancer Group (CCG) and showed some promise when used with conventional chemotherapy. There are current plans for a Phase II trial using inhaled GMCSF to stimulate macrophage activity for lung metastases. There are also research studies in progress attempting to use monoclonal antibodies to target HER2 receptors (Link et al., 2002). Administration of a bone-seeking radioisotope, samarium, is being tested with autologous stem cell transplant for metastatic bony disease.

2.5 Liver Tumors

Approximately two-thirds of all liver tumors are malignant. The most commonly occurring malignant liver tumor is hepatoblastoma followed by hepatocellular carcinoma.

2.5.1 Epidemiology

Malignant liver tumors occur at an annual incidence of approximately 1.5 cases per million children under the age of 15, and they comprise 1.1% of all childhood cancers (Tomlinson and Finegold, 2002). Hepatoblastoma (HB) is the most common malignant liver tumor affecting children and represents two-thirds of all liver tumors in this population. In infancy, the incidence is 11.2 per million, and this steadily decreases throughout childhood. Ninety percent of HBs occur during the first 5 years of life, 68% present within the first 2 years, and 4% are present at birth (Stocker, 2001). The mean age of diagnosis was found to be 19 months in a POG trial. There is a male predominance ranging from 1.4:1–2.0:1, (Tomlinson and Finegold, 2002), and Caucasians are affected up to five times more often than African-Americans. There is an increased incidence of HB in the Far East.

Hepatocellular carcinoma (HCC) accounts for 23% of all childhood liver tumors. It accounts for less than 0.5% of all pediatric malignancies, with an annual incidence of 0.5–1 case per million children (Czauderna et al., 2002). There is a higher male predominance affected by this tumor, and it most often occurs after the age of 10.

2.5.2 Etiology

Some researchers have suggested in recent years that prematurity is linked to HB development. The cause of this is unknown. In Japan's registry for pediatric malignancy the risk for HB is inversely correlated with birth weight (Tomlinson and Finegold, 2002). There is an association with HB and certain conditions such as Beckwith-Wiedemann syndrome (BWS), familial adenomatous polyposis (FAP), Li-Fraumeni syndrome, trisomy 18, and glycogen storage disease.

Hepatitis B infection has been shown to be pathogenic in HCC. HCC also develops in the presence of cirrhosis and underlying liver disease. There is some suggestion that parenteral nutrition in infancy is associated with HCC in childhood. Maternal exposure to oral contraceptive pills, fetal alcohol syndrome, and gestational exposures to gonadotropins are environmental factors implicated as possibly leading to HCC. The following genetic syndromes that are associated with a higher incidence of HCC include glycogen storage disease, hereditary tyrosinemia, Alagille syndrome, other familial cholestatic syndromes, neurofibromatosis, and ataxia-telangiectasia (Tomlinson and Finegold, 2002).

2.5.3 Molecular Genetics

Several chromosomal abnormalities occur in HB, but very few have been linked to HCC.

In HB the most common chromosomal abnormalities involve trisomy 2 and 20, and a translocation between (1;4)(q12;q34), all of which are of unknown significance (Stocker, 2002). Loss of heterozygosity at 11p15, which is a known tumor suppressor gene, has also been shown in HB and BWS. In a German study, 48% of HBs had a mutation at the B-catenin gene; the significance of this requires further exploration (Tomlinson and Finegold, 2002).

Mutations in the tumor suppressor gene (p53) have been reported in HCC and are associated with a shorter survival (Tomlinson and Finegold, 2002).

2.5.4 Symptoms and Clinical Signs

The presentations of HB and HCC are often quite similar to those of other abdominal tumors. Symptoms depend on the size of the tumor and can arise from the mass effect of space-occupying lesions.

Children most often present with an asymptomatic abdominal mass. On physical examination, a firm, irregular mass may be palpated in the right upper quadrant of the abdomen with extension across the midline or down to the pelvis. Pain, weight loss, anorexia, nausea, and vomiting may occur in advanced disease. Jaundice is quite uncommon, occurring only 5% of the time (Stocker, 2001). Infants can

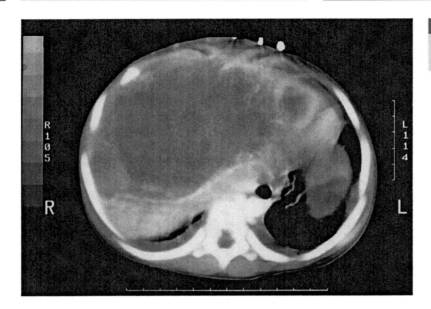

Figure 2.4

CT scan of patient with hepato-blastoma

present with failure to thrive. Severe osteopenia is often seen at diagnosis and is usually picked up incidentally on imaging; however, pathologic fractures occur infrequently. An acute abdomen is present in the case of tumor rupture. Seventy percent of children are anemic at diagnosis, and 35% have thrombocytosis (Stocker, 2001). Precocious puberty may be apparent in children whose tumors secrete beta human chorionic gonadotropin (BHCG). Hypertension can rarely occur in this population due to abnormal rennin secretion. Clinical signs of BWS should be considered, including macroglossia and hemihypertrophy, because of the increased incidence of HB in children with BWS. Patients at risk for developing HB including those with BWS or FAP, are often placed on a surveillance schedule to look for disease.

Metastases tend to spread to lung, bone, and brain.

2.5.5 Diagnostics

The diagnosis of either HB or HCC depends on imaging, blood, physical exam, and ultimately biopsy to determine tumor histology.

x-ray of the abdomen is often one of the first diagnostic tests ordered. A right upper quadrant mass is seen, and sometimes calcification is present. An ultrasound is useful in identifying a mass with increased echogenicity, which is suggestive of malignancy; Doppler will give information about the tumors vascularity. CT or MRI is needed to assess the extent of disease and the presence of local lymph nodes. Fig. 2.4 shows Hb as picked up on CT scan. Tumors often show patchy disease on post-contrast CT, and 50% of tumors show speckled or amorphous calcifications (Tomlinson and Finegold, 2002). CT of the chest is necessary to rule out lung metastases. Bone scan is sometimes ordered to rule out bony metastases, as is MRI of the brain to rule out intracranial spread; however, these are not standard practice.

A biopsy is necessary for definitive diagnosis, and tumor resection at diagnosis is preferred if surgically feasible. HB has two distinct classes based on histology. The first class shows epithelial histology with further variants that include a fetal pattern, a mixed embryonal and fetal pattern, macrotrabecular pattern, and undifferentiated small cell pattern. The second class involves mixed epithelial and mesenchymal histology. Further variants of the mixed histology include variants with teratoid features and those containing mesenchymal elements such as osteoid and cartilage (Stocker, 2001).

Table 2.9. Children's Oncology Group staging of hepatoblastoma (adapted from Tomlinson and Finegold, 2002)

Stage I (favorable histology)	Tumors are those that are completely resected and have a typical histology of a purely fetal histologic pattern with a low mitotic index (<2 per 10 high-power fields
Stage I (other histology)	Tumors that are completely resected with a histological picture other than purely fetal with low mitotic index
Stage II	Tumors are grossly resected with evidence of microscopic residual disease. Such tumors are rare, and patients with this stage have not fared differently from those with stage I tumors. Resected tumors with preoperative or intraoperative spill are classified as stage II
Stage III	(Unresectable) Tumors are those that are considered by the surgeon to be not resectable without undue risk to the patient. This includes partially resected tumors with measurable tumor left behind. Lymph node involvement is considered to constitute stage III disease and may require evaluation with a second laparotomy after the initial four courses of chemotherapy
Stage IV	Tumors that present with measurable metastatic disease to lungs or other organs

HCC has four main histologic types:

- Trabecular pattern is almost always seen in some part of HCC
- Compact and pseudoglandular variants
- Scirrhous is a rare type
- Fibrolamellar carcinoma is another rare variant of HCC that is not associated with cirrhosis; it shows an increased alfa-fetoprotein (AFP) and has a male predilection and a more favorable prognosis (Suriawinata and Thung, 2002)

A CBC should be ordered as well as liver and renal function blood tests. Liver enzymes and bilirubin may be elevated. Coagulation studies should be carried out before any surgical procedure to ensure that liver disease has not interfered with the coagulation pathway. BHCG is sometimes elevated in liver tumors and should be checked; elevations usually correlate with features of precocious puberty. AFP is a protein that is produced by the fetal liver and is elevated in the blood of infants during the first 6–9 months of life (Shafford and Pritchard, 1997). This protein is increased in 90% of HBs and 60% of HCCs (Pinkerton et al., 1999). In infants being worked up for a liver mass, it may be difficult to distinguish between normal AFP and malignant AFP. It is possible to fractionate the malignant and nonmalignant AFP by immunoelectropheresis; however, this lab service in not widely available. The AFP is an important tumor marker in liver tumors and is useful in evaluating response to treatment and recurrent disease. After complete tumor resection, the AFP should return to normal within 6 weeks.

2.5.6 Staging and Classification

Staging of liver tumors has been done by two different methods by two distinct groups. The North American Children's Oncology Group (COG) stages hepatoblastoma by the standard postsurgical tumor status (Table 2.9). The International Society of Pediatric Oncology (SIOP) uses a pretreatment classification schema called PRETEXT, which helps determine feasibility of tumor resection based on the number of liver segments involved using preoperative imaging scans (Tomlinson and Finegold, 2002).

HCC is staged much the same way as HB; however, it is graded differently based on histological differentiation. Stage I HCC resembles normal hepatocytes, stage II and III cells show moderate differentiation, and stage IV tumor cells are very poorly differentiated and often metastatic (Suriawinata and Thung, 2002).

2.5.7 Treatment

For both HB and HCC, surgical resection is crucial for cure and is the single most important factor predicting survival. Chemotherapy often plays a large role postoperatively and sometimes preoperatively if the tumor is unresectable at diagnosis. More recently, liver transplantation is playing a role in unresectable tumors. The use of radiation with these liver tumors is controversial.

Surgery resection is the most important part of curative therapy for children with HB. Forty to 60% of HB tumors are inoperable at diagnosis and 10 to 20% have pulmonary metastases (Stocker, 2001). Surgery is often not possible at diagnosis if both liver lobes are affected, if there is tumor in the porta hepatis, or if bulky lymphadenopathy exists. Presurgical chemotherapy for unresectable lesions renders them resectable 85% of the time (Stocker, 2001). Surgical resection may include a lobectomy or trisegmentectomy based on the extent of disease. Lymph nodes and the porta hepatis should be sampled during surgery; the celiac and paraaortic nodes need

only be biopsied if suspicious for disease. In a COG study, surgery alone is the only treatment for stage I tumors with pure fetal histology, which are completely resected at diagnosis (Rowland et al., 2002). Biopsy of any suspicious pulmonary lesions should occur at diagnosis, and residual lesions should be surgically removed at the completion of therapy.

Chemotherapy agents that have shown utility in the treatment of HB include cisplatin, doxorubicin, ifosfamide, vincristine, and 5 fluorouracil. Irinotecan has showed some activity in phase II trials and recurrent disease. Sequential use of carboplatin, carboplatin-vincristine-5FU, and high-dose cisplatin-etoposide in a POG phase II study showed response in metastatic HB and in patients with unresectable disease at diagnosis, similar to other regimens but perhaps with less toxicity (Katzenstein et al., 2002a,b). Table 2.10 shows the most recent chemotherapy regimens for HB.

HCC has traditionally treated with the same chemotherapy agents used in the treatment of HB but with less success. The results of a Pediatric Oncology Group and Children's Cancer Group intergroup study

Table 2.10. Chemotherapy regimens for hepatoblastoma (adapted from Tomlinson and Finegold, 2002)

Study group	Schema	Overall survival (length of follow-up)	Number of patients	Reference
Children's Cancer Group	Cisplatin Doxorubicin day 1–4 Plan: 4 courses	67[a] (2 years)	26	Ortega et al. (1991)
Pediatric Oncology Group	Cisplatin course 1 and then cisplatin, vincristine, 5 FU courses 2–5	67%[a] (4 years)	60	Douglass et al. (1993)
International Society of Pediatric Oncology	Cisplatin 24-hour infusion and doxorubicin 48-hour infusion Plan: 4 courses-surgery-2 courses	75%[b] (5 years)	154	Pritchard et al. (2000)
German Society of Pediatric Oncology and Hematology	Ifosfamide Cisplatin Doxorubicin Plan: 2 or 4 courses-surgery-2 courses	75%[b] (median 64 months)	72	Von Schweinitz et al. (2000)

[a] Includes only patients with unresectable disease at presentation
[b] Includes patients with all stages at presentation
Refer to references to obtain full schema

using a prospective trial using a uniform treatment approach to HCC were published by Katzenstein and colleagues (2002). The treatment involved cisplatin, vincristine and fluorouracil (5-FU), or cisplatin and continuous infusion doxorubicin as determined by randomization. Neither regimen was effective in controlling residual or metastatic disease in children with HCC. For lack of better treatment, most often patients with HCC are usually treated using the same protocols that are used for HB with poor results. Surgery is vital in these patients, but unfortunately, only 10–20% of these tumors are resectable.

Radiation therapy is sometimes used if there is minimal or gross residual disease, but its utility is controversial and not widely accepted. There are high rates of side effects from tumor irradiation as well.

Liver transplantation is now done in the United States, and malignancies account for 2% of liver transplants in children. Transplant is often considered but not limited to instances where tumors are unresectable and show chemosensitivity. A recent study showed that children who had initially unresectable liver tumors and were treated initially with chemotherapy followed by hepatectomy and liver transplant had post-transplant survival rates at 5 years of 83% for HB and 68% for HCC (Tomlinson and Finegold, 2002).

2.5.8 Prognosis

The most important prognostic factor in HB is complete surgical resection. Pure fetal histology and low mitotic count impart an excellent outcome. Small-cell undifferentiated tumors are associated with poor prognosis independent of any other variable. The cure rate for a patient with HB and lung metastases is 70%.

The overall survival for children with HB is 65–70%. The overall survival rates for the various stages of disease are

Stage I: 100%
Stage II: 75–80%
Stage III: 65–68%
Stage IV: 0–27% (Stocker, 2001)

The survival rates for patients with HCC remain very poor. In all reported HCC series, the therapeutic response to chemotherapy is poor and overall survival is less than 30% (Czauderna et al. 2002).

2.5.9 Follow-up

Follow-up should be similar for both HB and HCC, and must consist of physical examination, abdominal ultrasound for tumor recurrence, and chest x-ray for evidence of pulmonary metastases. CT scan may be a more sensitive way to monitor for recurrence and metastases once off treatment, but this should be decided based on individual patient needs. Surveillance should be done every 3 months for at least the first 2 years and then with decreasing frequency. Monitoring of the AFP is essential and is often the first indication that the tumor has recurred.

Monitoring for late effects of the treatment is also necessary. Audiograms should be done periodically to look for hearing loss resulting from cisplatin therapy. Echocardiograms should be done following anthracycline therapy because the potential for cardiac sequelae from treatment exists. Infertility problems may be an issue once children are older. If the patient has undergone liver transplantation, secondary lymphoproliferative disorders may occur. Psychological, endocrine, and hormonal issues may need to be addressed as well.

2.5.10 Future Perspectives

Clearly there needs to be better treatment available for HCC. Studies have proven that HCC does not respond to chemotherapy as HB does. Novel agents need to be examined for their potential role in treating both these liver tumors.

Effort needs to be placed on developing standardized surveillance programs for those who carry a genetic predisposition to developing a liver tumor, as early intervention would hopefully improve outcomes for this group of patients.

2.6 Neuroblastoma

Neuroblastoma (NBL) is a tumor that arises from neural crest cells that make up the sympathetic or peripheral nervous system and can grow in the sympathetic ganglia, adrenal medulla, and other sites. NBL is an undifferentiated and highly malignant tumor, ganglioneuroblastoma is a more differentiated tumor, and ganglioneuroma is a fully differentiated tumor without malignant potential.

2.6.1 Epidemiology

NBL is the most common pediatric extracranial malignancy and the most frequently occurring cancer in infancy. Although it accounts for approximately 10% of all childhood malignancies, it accounts for 15% of all cancer deaths (Alexander, 2000). The incidence is about 9.7 cases per one million children (Gurney et al. 1995). It affects boys at a slightly higher rate than girls, 1.2:1.0, and is slightly more predominant in white children compared with black. The median age at diagnosis is 17.3 months (Brodeur and Maris, 2002).

2.6.2 Etiology

The cause of NBL is unknown. According to current evidence, environment does not appear to play a role. Correlation with intrauterine exposure to several agents such as alcohol, medications, and maternal use of hair-coloring products has been proposed, but none of these hypotheses have not been confirmed. Although most cases of NBL are sporadic, there seems to be a small group, approximately 1–2%, that are familial (Brodeur and Maris, 2002). NBL has been identified in other disorders of neural crest cells, such as neurofibromatosis, Hirschsprung's disease, Beckwith-Wiedemann syndrome (BWS), and DiGeorge syndrome.

2.6.3 Molecular Genetics

Neuroblastoma is a disease in which enormous advances have been made regarding the molecular and genetic aspects. More recently these results have been used to stratify children into low, intermediate and high-risk treatment protocols. Gene amplification, alterations in gene expression, and tumor suppressor gene inactivation are some of the major factors that influence risk determination.

N-Myc amplification occurs in approximately 25% of all NBLs (Matthay and Yamashiro, 2000). N-Myc is an oncogene found on chromosome 2 band q24, and its amplification is associated with aggressive and advanced disease. It is a powerful predictor of outcome regardless of stage and age. Loss of heterozygosity at chromosome 1p36 has also been shown to have an unfavorable outcome and is a very common chromosomal abnormality. 1p is thought to harbor a yet-to-be-identified tumor suppressor gene, and deletion of this may cause tumors to grow uncontrollably. There appears to be an association between a chromosome 1p deletion and N-Myc amplification (Matthay and Yamashiro, 2000). Chromosomal gains of 17q are also a frequent genetic event and often correlate with 1p deletions, therefore pointing to an unfavorable prognosis (Tomioka et al. 2003). Deletions on chromosome 11 and 14 have also been found in some tumors and again the thought is that they may encode tumor suppressor genes. Ploidy, the number of chromosomes pairs, is another important determination. Infants with NBL who have a DNA index (DI) of >1 (more than 46 chromosome pairs) respond well to standard chemotherapy. A DI equal to 1 would predict a poorer response to standard therapy and often requires more aggressive treatment. Ploidy does not appear to be as significant in children older than 1 year (Brodeur, 2003). Neurotrophin receptor expression is widely correlated with genetic and biologic features. TrkA, TrkB, and TrkC are tyrosine kinases that code for receptors of the nerve growth factor (NGF) family. High TrkA often corresponds with a lack of N-Myc amplification, and therefore a favorable outcome. TrkB, however, is expressed in higher-stage tumors that show N-Myc amplification and have an unfavorable prognosis. The risk classification table takes into account both clinical features such as stage and age as well as biological risk factors to determine an appropriate treatment intensity protocol. See Table 2.11 for proposed NBL risk groups based on clinical and biologic tumor features for Children's Oncology Group protocols.

Table 2.11. Neuroblastoma risk groups based on clinical and biologic tumor features (Children's Oncology Group Protocols [ANBL0032)]; reprinted with permission)

INSS stage	Age	MYCN status	Shimada histology	DNA ploidy	Risk group
1	0–21	Any	Any	Any	Low
2A/2B	<365 d	Any	Any	Any	Low
	>365–21 y	Non-Amp	Any	–	Low
	>365–21 y	Amp	Fav	–	Low
	>365–21 y	Amp	Unfav	–	High-risk
3	<365 d	Any	Any	Any	Intermediate
	<365 d	Any	Any	Any	High-risk
	>365 d-21y	Fav	Fav	–	Intermediate
	>365 d-21y	Unfav	Unfav	–	High-risk
	>354 d-21y	Any	Any	–	High-risk
4	<365 d	Non-Amp	Any	Any	Intermediate
	<365 d	Amp	Any	Any	High-risk
	>365 d-21y	Any	Any	–	High-risk
4S	<365 d	Non-Amp	Fav	>1	Low
	<365 d	Non-Amp	Any	=1	Intermediate
	<365 d	Non-Amp	Unfav	Any	Intermediate
	<365 d	Amp	Any	Any	High-risk

2.6.4 Symptoms and Clinical Signs

Neuroblastoma can occur anywhere along the peripheral nervous system, so the presentations of the disease vary along with the location of the primary tumor or metastases. Neuroblastoma occurs in various anatomic sites as follows:

- 28.4% in the abdomen
- 32% in the adrenals
- 15% in the thorax
- 5.6% in the pelvis
- 2% in the neck
- 16.9% occur elsewhere
  (Ninane and Pearson, 2002)

Infants tend to have more thoracic and cervical spinal tumors than older children. Most children do present before the age of 5 years. Rarely NBL can occur into adulthood.

NBL generally spreads via hematogenous and lymphatic routes and occasionally by regional lymph node invasion. Bone and bone marrow are common areas for metastases, as well as liver and skin in infants. Very rarely, spread to brain and lung occurs.

Extensive involvement of the liver, skin, and/or bone marrow (<10%) in infants reflects stage 4S disease. This clinicopathological staging is reserved for infants who, along with favorable tumor biology, can be considered low risk even with advanced disease.

Clinical signs of NBL vary according to the tumor's location. Various presenting signs of neuroblastoma and the possible causes are listed in Table 2.12.

Skin lesions commonly referred to as "blueberry muffin" can occur in infants.

Paraneoplastic syndromes may sometimes be present at diagnosis. One such syndrome is opsomyoclonus. This involves random eye movements, myoclonic jerking movements, and cerebellar ataxia (Bataller et al., 2003). The phenomenon is though to arise because of the production of antineural antibodies that cross-react with neural cells in cerebellum or elsewhere in the brain (Brodeur and Maris, 2002). Children presenting with opsomyoclonus tend to do quite well from the tumor perspective; however, long-term neurological and developmental deficits can be a large problem. Intractable diarrhea can be a rare presentation caused by tumor secretion

Table 2.12. Various presentation signs of neuroblastoma and their possible causes

Clinical sign or symptom	Possible cause
Abdominal pain, abdominal distension, nausea, vomiting, constipation	Abdominal tumor
Anorexia, weight loss	Mass effect of midline tumors
Horner's syndrome (ipsilateral ptosis, miosis, and anhidrosis)	High thoracic and cervical tumors resulting in compromise of descending sympathetic tracks
Proptosis, periorbital ecchymosis	Periorbital tumor
Anemia, thrombocytopenia, frequent infections	Bone marrow involvement
Hypertension	Renal vascular compression
Limp or leg pain	Metastatic bone disease
Decreased motion in legs, muscle weakness, bowel or bladder disturbances	Spinal or paraspinal disease
Weakness or paraplegia	Compression of spinal cord caused by dumbbell tumors

of vasoactive intestinal polypeptide (VIP); this often has a favorable prognosis.

2.6.5 Diagnostics

Several screening tests are useful in diagnosing NBL. Blood and urine testing are done, in addition to tumor biopsy as part of the workup. Diagnostic imaging is used to evaluate the extent of tumor invasion and any tumor dissemination. The information obtained from imaging and biopsy results is used to determine risk stratification based on both clinical and biological factors.

Initially, imaging studies of the affected area may consist of plain films or ultrasound depending on the presenting symptoms. Fig. 2.5 shows a radiograph of a posterior mediastinal mass found in a patient with NBL. Following this, CT of the chest, abdomen, and pelvis should determine the extent of the disease and the presence of metastases. On imaging the tumors often show calcification. In the case of spinal tumors, an MRI should be ordered. Bone scan should determine the presence of skeletal metastases. Metaiodobenzylguanidine (MIBG) scan, using a dye that is taken up by catecholaminergic cells, is extremely useful in identifying NBL metastases but is not available at all centers.

Neuroblastoma tumors produce several substances that can be measured in the blood. Blood should be sent for LDH and ferritin. Neuron-specific enolase (NSE), GD2 (a cell membrane ganglioside), and chromogranin A are produced by NBL tumors, and although not routinely done at most centers, serum levels of these markers can be measured. Highly elevated ferritin levels may be associated with a worse prognosis. Similarly, elevations of LDH and chromogranin A are associated with unfavorable outcomes. GD2 can be found on the surface of NBL; gangliosides shed from the tumor might be important in accelerating tumor progression (Brodeur, 2003). NSE is a protein associated with neural cells; although nonspecific, overall survival is worse in patients with elevations of NSE and advanced disease (Matthay and Yamashiro, 2000). Other blood tests such as a CBC should also be done; any cytopenias that are present may be the result of bone marrow disease. Renal and liver function tests should also be evaluated to ensure normal functioning and to obtain baseline levels prior to chemotherapy.

Urinary catecholamine metabolites are elevated in NBL in 90–95% of patients (Brodeur and Maris, 2002). Urinary vanillylmandelic acid (VMA), formed from norepinephrine, and homovanillic acid (HVA), formed from dopamine, are considered elevated

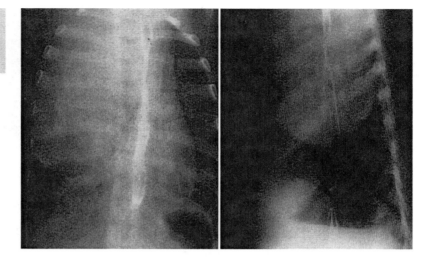

Figure 2.5

Radiograph of a posterior mediastinal mass found in a patient with neuroblastoma

when they are greater than three standard deviations above the upper limit of normal (Brodeur, 2002).

Tumor biopsy and/or tumor resection are done depending on the stage of the tumor. Tissue samples are sent for molecular and histopathological testing. Stage I and II tumors are usually resected at diagnosis, whereas Stage III and IV tumors are only biopsied. Chemoreductive therapy is given in order to facilitate easier removal of higher staged tumors. Bilateral bone marrow aspirates and biopsies are needed to determine the presence of bone marrow disease. It is generally accepted that if tumor is found in the bone marrow studies and the child has an elevated VMA/HVA, it is not necessary to biopsy the primary tumor. However, valuable information gained via biological markers would not be obtained for risk stratification, which may impact patient care.

Histology is an important determinant in risk stratification for these tumors. NBL is a small blue round cell tumor, and Homer-Wright pseudorosettes are often found in the tumor. It can be distinguished from other small blue round cell tumors because of its distinctive monoclonal antibody staining patterns. NBL stains positively for NSE, neurofilament proteins and synaptophysin. Shimada and colleagues (1984) originally developed a pathology staging system; some changes have been made to this earlier system in order to make it internationally useful. The histological determination takes into account the mi-

totic karyorrhectic index (MKI), patient age, the degree of differentiation, and whether the tumor is schwannian stroma poor. Table 2.13 indicates the pathology classification for NBL.

2.6.6 Staging and Classification

Several staging systems exist for NBL. The international NBL staging system (INSS) is based on post-surgical interventions for low-grade tumors according to location and respectability of the tumor; the Pediatric Oncology Group's staging is similar. The Children's Cancer Group's staging is based on tumor location on imaging. Table 2.14 outlines the various staging systems. Most centers, in North America at least, are using the INSS.

2.6.7 Treatment

Surgery, chemotherapy, radiation therapy and autologous stem cell transplant, and more recently immunotherapy and other biological therapies are all used in the treatment of NBL. Treatment intensity depends on risk stratification (Table 2.11). Essentially, the goals of treatment in those children with advanced disease are to

- Chemotherapy to decrease the size of both the primary tumor and metastases
- Surgical resection of the tumor

Table 2.13. Prognostic evaluation of neuroblastic tumors according to the International Neuroblastoma Pathology Classification/Shimada system (taken from Shimada et al., 1999 with permission; *MKI* mitosis-karyorrhexis index)

	International Neuroblastoma Pathology Classification	Original Shimada classification	Prognostic group
Neuroblastoma	(Schwannian stoma-poor)	Stroma-poor	
Favorable		Favorable	Favorable
<1.5 yr	Poorly differentiated or differentiating and low or intermediate MKI tumor		
1.5–5.0 yr	Differentiating and low MKI tumor		
Unfavorable		Unfavorable	Unfavorable
<1.5 yr	Undifferentiated tumor High MKI tumor		
1.5–5.0 yr	Undifferentiated or poorly differentiated tumor Intermediate or high MKI tumor		
5 yr	All tumors		
Ganglioneuroblastoma, intermixed	(Schwannian stroma-rich)	Stroma-rich intermixed (favorable)	Favorable
Ganglioneuroblastoma, nodular ganglioneuroma	(Composite Schwannian stroma-rich/stroma-dominate and stroma-poor)	Stroma-rich nodular (unfavorable)	Unfavorable
Maturing	(Schwannian stroma-dominant)	Well differentiated (favorable)	Favorable
Mature		Ganglioneuroma	

- Myeloablative chemotherapy followed by autologous stem cell transplantation (ASCT)
- Radiation therapy to areas of residual disease

Surgery is a vital aspect of care for children with NBL. For patients with low-risk disease, often stage I and II, surgical resection may be all that is required for treatment. For intermediate and high-risk disease, including stage III and IV tumors, surgery is done after several courses of chemotherapy have decreased the tumor size.

Chemotherapy is used primarily in tumors that are intermediate to high-risk; i.e., in metastatic disease and locally-spread disease. The most common drug combinations known to be effective are some combination of the following: cisplatin, doxorubicin, cyclophosphamide, carboplatin, ifosfamide, and epipodophyllotoxins (Alexander, 2000; Brodeur and Maris, 2002). In metastatic disease and poor-risk stage III disease, myeloablative therapy is used followed by single or double peripheral stem cell rescue. Melphalan is often an integral part of the ASCT conditioning regimen.

NBL is a radiosensitive tumor. In instances where the primary tumor cannot be fully resected, when there are local lymph nodes, and with microscopic residual disease, radiation therapy plays a vital role. Radiation is often also used for palliative pain control and for bony tumors or spinal cord compression that cause distressing symptoms. Accepted treatment doses of ionizing radiation range to 30 Gy, depending on the tumor size, and fractioned doses range between 150 and 400 cGy (Brodeur and Maris, 2002).

Following myeloablative therapy, maintenance therapy often includes treatment with retinoids. Retinoic acid is used to evoke cellular differentiation of NBL in the cases of minimal residual disease; most children receive 6 months of therapy (Matthay and Yamashiro, 2000). Currently, several groups including the North American study group, COG, are trialing targeted therapies using anti-GD2 antibody, Interleukin II (IL2), and granulocyte macrophage colony stimulating factor (GMCSF) after autologous stem cell transplant to target potential minimal residual disease.

Relapsed disease is very difficult to treat following high-risk disease treatment. Chemotherapy agents that have shown response include topotecan, cyclophosphamide, Taxol, and VP16 (Brodeur and Maris, 2002). Targeted therapy using MIBG radioisotope to deliver radiation therapy is being used at some centers and has shown some response to refractory disease.

2.6.8 Prognosis

The prognosis in NBL varies widely depending on the child's age and the tumor's stage, location, and biology.

- Survival rates are as high as 95% in patients with Stage I disease when the tumor has been completely excised (Alexander, 2000)
- Children with stage II disease who are older than 1 year have an 85% disease-free survival with surgery only
- Children older than 1 year of age with stage III disease treated with surgery and chemotherapy have a 50% disease-free survival; however, if radiation is added to treatment the survival may be increased to 70% (Alexander, 2000).
- High-risk patients with metastatic stage IV disease continue to do poorly and the long term survival rate is less than 15% (Brodeur and Maris, 2002)
- Infants, however, with stage IVS disease and good biological features have survival rates approaching 90%

2.6.9 Follow-up

Close observation for recurrent disease is imperative for these children. Most relapse occurs during the first 2 years following the completion of therapy. Diagnostic imaging of the primary using CT or ultrasound depending on location of the tumor is indicated. MIBG scanning is also useful for monitoring for recurrent disease in high-risk patients. Imaging and physical exam should be done every 3 months for the first few years after completing therapy and then with decreasing frequency over several years, or as clinically indicated. Urinary catecholamines should also be measured with the same frequency as radiological imaging. Blood tests such as LDH and ferritin can be monitored easily, and although nonspecific, can be used for screening along with imaging and physical exam. Those children who remain disease-free for 5 years following treatment of NBL are generally considered cured, although with increased intensity of therapy, late recurrences may be possible.

Follow-up must also consider treatment-related toxicity and late effects. Ototoxicity is usually significant following cisplatin therapy, and hearing aids are often necessary. Growth and development may be impacted, especially if radiation therapy has been delivered to the spinal area; this should be monitored carefully. Organ toxicity is a potential following chemotherapy and should be monitored through blood testing where possible. Echocardiograms should be done to screen for cardiomyopathies from anthracycline therapies. If radiation therapy was received, follow-up with a radiation oncologist is imperative. Second malignancies must be considered a risk for long-term survivors of metastatic disease due to the intensive multimodality therapy including radiation these children would have received. Not a lot of data are available on this cohort because they are such a small group.

Table 2.14. Staging systems for neuroblastoma (adapted from Matthay and Yamashiro (2000)

International Neuroblastoma Staging System	Children's Cancer Study Group System	Pediatric Oncology Group System
Stage 1 Localized tumor with complete gross excision and/or microscopic residual disease	**Stage I** Tumor confied to the organ or structure of origin	**Stage A** Complete gross resection of the primary tumor and/or microscopic residual disease
Ipsilateral lymph nodes negative for tumor (nodes attached to the primary tumor may be positive for tumor)		Intracavitary lymph nodes not ad hered to the primary tumor, which are histologically free of tumor (nodes adhered to the surface of the primary tumor may be positive for tumor)
Stage 2A Localized tumor with incomplete gross resection	**Stage II** Tumor extending in continuity beyond the organ or structure of origin but not crossing the midline	**Stage B** Grossly unresected primary tumor
Representative ipsilateral nonadherent lymph nodes negative for tumor microscopically	Possible regional lymph node involvement on the ipsilateral side	Nodes and nodules the same as in Stage A
Stage 2B Localized tumor and/or complete gross excision, with ipsilateral nonadherent lymph nodes positive for tumor		
Enlarged contralateral lymph nodes, which are negative for tumor microscopically		
Stage 3 Unresectable unilateral tumor infitrating across the midline and/or regional lymph node involvement	**Stage III** Tumor extending in continuity beyond the midline	**Stage C** Complete or incomplete resection of primary tumor
Alternately, localized unilateral tumor with contralateral regional lymph node involvement	Possible regional lymph node involvement bilaterally	Intracavitary nodes not adhered to primary tumor, which are positive for tumor histologically Liver as in Stage A
Stage 4 Any primary tumor with dissemination to distant lymph nodes, bone, bone marrow, liver, skin, and/or other organs (except as defied for stage 4S)	**Stage IV** Remote disease involving the skeleton, bone marrow, soft tissue, and distant lymph node groups (see stage IV-S)	**Stage D** Dissemination of disease beyond intracavitary nodes (e.g., extracavitary nodes, liver, skin, bone marrow, bone)
Stage 4S Localized primary tumor (as defied for stages 1, 2A, or 2B) with dissemination limited to skin, liver, and/or bone marrow (<10% involvement)	**Stage IV-S** As defied in stage I or II, except for the presence of metastatic disease confied to the liver, skin, or marrow (<10% involvement) No bone metastases	**Stage DS** Infants <1 year with stage 1 or 2, except for the presence of remote disease confied to the liver, skin, or marrow (<10% involvement) No bone metastases

2.6.10 Future Perspectives

Researchers and clinicians hope to continuously improve risk stratification tools for children with NBL so that treatment intensity may correspond to disease characteristics as more discoveries are made. Gene expression profiling, targeting abnormal transduction pathways, and the use of biologic agents are all areas that are being researched to treat NBL, both in relapsed and primary disease. MIBG therapy is being used at few centers as treatment for refractory disease. Fenretidine, which is thought to induce apoptosis in tumors that may have been resistant to retinoic acid therapy, is being investigated in phase I trials (Brodeur and Maris, 2002). Topotecan has shown activity in relapsed patients and may have a role in first-line therapy. Anti-angiogenic agents, which are used to target and interfere with the tumor's ability to create its own blood supply, are also being researched for a potential role in this disease. Tyrosine kinase inhibitor therapy is being researched to target TRK A, B, and C expression. The intension of current research is to determine agents that are affective against NBL and incorporate these findings into conventional therapy.

2.7 Renal Tumors

The most frequently observed malignant tumor arising from the kidney is Wilms' tumor. Other less frequently occurring renal tumors include renal cell carcinoma, clear cell sarcoma of the kidney, and rhabdoid tumor of the kidney.

2.7.1 Epidemiology

Wilms' tumor is the second most commonly occurring extracranial malignancy in children. It represents about 6% of all childhood cancers (Blakely and Ritchey, 2001). Wilms' tumors can occur bilaterally or unilaterally; bilateral tumors occur either synchronously or at different times. The incidence of Wilms' tumor, or nephroblastoma, in children less than 15 years of age is approximately 7.6 per million. The male to female ratio is 0.92:1 for unilateral tumors and 0.6:1 for bilateral tumors (Grundy et al., 2000). The incidence is slightly higher in African-American children and lower in Asian children compared with Caucasians. Peak age of diagnosis is between 2 and 3 years.

Multiple other tumors arise from the kidney; they are extremely rare and include renal cell carcinoma (RCC), clear cell sarcoma of the kidney (CCSK), and rhabdoid tumor of the kidney (RTK). RCC is a tumor that is distinct from Wilms but also occurs in the kidney at an incidence of 0.1–0.3% of all malignancies, representing 1.8–6.3% of malignant kidney tumors (Indolfe et al.. 2003). CCSK, distinct from Wilms' tumor, was shown to have an incidence of 4% in a National Wilms' Tumor Study (NWTS) (Beckwith, 1998). RTK represents 2% of renal tumors registered with NWTS (Broecker, 2000).

2.7.2 Etiology

Wilms' tumors occur sporadically in 95% of these patients. There is, however, a familial form, comprising 1–2% of all Wilms' tumors, in which tumors tend to occur bilaterally and earlier, suggesting a germ line mutation and a loss of a tumor suppressor gene. The familial form is characterized by an autosomal dominant trait with variable penetrance (Grundy et al. 2002). The disease often occurs in the presence of genetic anomalies or as part of a familial predisposition syndrome. Syndromes often associated with Wilms' are the following:

- Beckwith Wiedemann (BWS) (an overgrowth syndrome)
- Denys-Drash (involving genitourinary abnormalities)
- WAGR (Wilms, aniridia, genitourinary anomalies and mental retardation) (Pritchard-Jones and Mitchell, 1997)

Wilms' tumor has also been described in Bloom syndrome, incontinentia pigmenti, Li-Fraumeni, and genetic instability syndromes, yet no definite link exists (Grundy et al., 2000).

2.7.3 Molecular Genetics

Several genes are described in the development of Wilms' tumor. The first Wilms' tumor suppressor gene, WT1, is located at chromosome (Ch') 11p13. It was cloned in 1990 and is found in patients with WAGR syndrome and involves the PAX 6 gene and WT1 allele (Grundy et al. 2002). Mutations of WT1 have been found also in some sporadic Wilms' cases. WT1 is important in normal kidney development. A second Wilms' tumor putative gene is identified at Ch'11p15, WT2. Children with BWS are predisposed to Wilms' tumor and have mutations at Ch'11p15, the WT2 gene (Neville and Ritchey, 2000). The familial form of the disease has a locus identified at Ch'17q labeled FWT1, and FWT2 is located on chromosome 19q. These genes all appear to have a role in tumor development. Chromosome arms 16q, 1p, 7p, and 17p, the location of p53, have also been associated with Wilms' tumor, but may be linked more to treatment outcome than to tumorigenesis (Grundy et al., 2002). There has been an association also noted between p53 mutations and anaplastic histology in 86% of cases, which may suggest that mutations underlie the anaplastic phenotype (Grundy et al., 2000).

RCC have characteristic translocations involving breakpoint at Xp11.2.

2.7.4 Symptoms and Clinical Signs

Parents are often the first to notice an abdominal mass or abdominal distension in their child. Children are usually asymptomatic. Pain, gross hematuria, fever, and hypertension occur in approximately 25% of children (Grundy et al., 2002). Hypertension is usually attributed to increases in rennin activity. Anemia, fever, and rapid abdominal distension can occur if there has been hemorrhage into the tumor, but this occurs rarely. Syndromes such as BWS and WAGR are linked to Wilms' tumor, so features associated with these syndromes should be noted (e.g., aniridia, GU anomalies, hemihypertrophy). Rarely, extrarenal Wilms' tumors arise; they present as a retroperitoneal mass usually adjacent to the kidney. Symptoms of thrombosis should also be considered and note made of any leg swelling and/or prominent veins over abdomen. Very rarely, a child may present with metastatic disease and may show signs of respiratory difficulty in the presence of advanced pulmonary metastases. Lung, liver, bone, and brain are the major locations of metastases.

2.7.5 Diagnostics

An abdominal ultrasound is usually the first investigation ordered, which will reveal a mass arising from within the kidney. Doppler ultrasound should also be used to assess patency of the renal vein and inferior vena cava, as thrombosis can occur. CT of the abdomen should be ordered to further assess the extent of the mass and assess for smaller lesions in the contralateral kidney. The liver should be thoroughly examined because it is a common site for metastases. A CT of the chest should be ordered to rule out pulmonary metastases. Fig. 2.6 is a chest x-ray demonstrating pulmonary metastases in Wilms' tumor. There is some debate as to whether chest x-ray is sufficient to look for metastases, as smaller nodules are often not picked up.

A CT or MRI of the brain should be done after a diagnosis of CSSK or RTK is made because metastases to the brain can occur. Bone scan and skeletal survey are also indicated in these tumors; bone scan does not always pick up lytic bone lesions, so skeletal survey is also indicated.

Biopsy versus tumor resection at diagnosis remains controversial. There are two major Wilms' tumor study groups: the North American National Wilms Tumor (NWTS) study group and the International Society of Pediatric Oncology (SIOP) in Europe. The NWTS recommends resecting the entire tumor and sampling local lymph nodes at diagnosis. SIOP however, discourages biopsies and recommends chemotherapy with vincristine and actinomycin to shrink the tumor to make surgical resection easier, followed by removal and staging. If pulmonary lesions are noted on CT scan, they should be biopsied at diagnosis prior to treatment.

Histologically, Wilms' tumor can be comprised of blastemal, epithelial, and stromal components, a tumor typically consists of all three components, but one component could predominate. If greater than

Figure 2.6

Chest x-ray demonstrating pulmonary metastases in Wilms' tumor

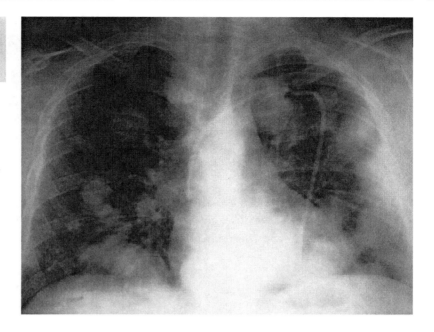

two-thirds of the tumor composition is of one component, the histological type is assigned to the tumor, as they can behave quite differently (Neville and Ritchey, 2000). Monophasic blastemal is a highly invasive type of Wilms' tumor. Cystic or partially differentiated cystic nephroma do extremely well and are often cured with surgery alone. Diffuse or focal anaplasia is associated with unfavorable histology and is seen is approximately 5% of tumors (Neville and Ritchey, 2000). Anaplasia is characterized by large nuclei that are three times the size of nuclei of other cells, hyperchromasia of enlarged cells, and the presence of polyploid mitotic features. Diffuse anaplasia is characterized by more than one area of anaplasia in tumor sample or in regional nodes or metastases (Neville and Ritchey, 2000). Nephrogenic rests are precursor lesions to Wilms' tumor and are comprised of abnormally persistent embryonal nephroblastic tissue with small clusters of blastemal, epithelial, or stromal cells. They are seen in kidneys of 35% of unilateral Wilms' tumors and nearly 100% of bilateral. The term nephroblastomatosis describe a clinical situation in which there are multiple nephrogenic rests. Although they are not malignant, it is important to know this information prior to treating tumors, especially with surgery, because if the contralateral kidney has these nephrogenic rests, a Wilms' tumor may develop in the future.

Histologically, RCC in children tends to have a papillary architecture (Broecker, 2000). CCSK have a distinct histological appearance, but several variant patterns such as epithelioid, myxoid, cystic, and spindling exist. Additionally, CCSK can show anaplastic features. This tumor is often misdiagnosed. RTK is thought to be neurogenic in origin. Cells have a prominent acidophilic cytoplasm, resembling rhabdomyoblasts. They are, however, negative for makers of skeletal muscle (Grundy et al., 2000).

There are no specific tumor markers for Wilms' tumor. For the workup of a patient; however, blood should be sent for CBC, liver function tests, renal function tests, and coagulation screen. It has been noted that acquired Von Willebrand's disease occurs in 8% of Wilms' tumor patients at diagnosis, and treatment with DDAVP may be necessary to correct coagulation prior to surgical intervention (Grundy et al., 2002).

Table 2.15. Staging system for renal tumors developed by the National Wilms' Tumor Study Group

Stage	Description
I	Tumor confined to the kidney and completely resected. No penetration of the renal capsule. No involvement of renal sinus vessels
II	Tumor extends beyond the kidney but is completely resected (negative margins and lymph nodes). At least one of the following has occurred: (i) penetration of the renal capsule (ii) invasion of the renal sinus vessels (iii) biopsy of tumor before removal (iv) spillage of tumor locally during removal

III	Postoperatively, gross or microscopic residual tumor remains, including
	  inoperable tumor
	  positive surgical margins
	  tumor spillage involving peritoneal surfaces
	  regional lymph node metastases, or transacted tumor thrombus

IV	Hematogenous metastases or lymph node metastases outside the abdomen (lung, liver, bone or brain)
V	Bilateral disease at diagnosis (with attempts made to stage each side at diagnosis)

2.7.6 Staging and Classification

The NWTS developed a staging system for Wilms' tumor. It is based on surgical resectability and the presence of bilateral and metastatic disease (see Table 2.15).

2.7.7 Treatment

The treatment for Wilms' tumors always involves surgery and chemotherapy and sometimes radiotherapy. As previously stated, controversy surrounds the treatment of Wilms' tumor. SIOP asserts that if preoperative chemotherapy is given, the tumor is easier to remove and fewer complications arise. Diagnosis is therefore made on clinical and diagnostic imaging only. The wrong diagnosis is made in 5% of cases (Grundy et al., 2002). The approach of the NWTS–V is outlined in Table 2.16. Tumors are completely resected at diagnosis, and nodes are sampled.

A transperitoneal surgical approach is recommended for surgical resection so that the contralateral kidney can be examined intraoperatively and local lymph nodes sampled. Spillage during surgical resection results in a six-fold increase in local abdominal recurrence; these patients are therefore upstaged (Grundy et al. 2002). If a tumor is inoperable at diagnosis due to size or thrombosis, after biopsy the tumor is treated as a Stage III with vincristine, actino-

mycin-D, and doxorubicin, then reevaluated at week 5 and resected as per the NWTS group. Bilateral tumors should be biopsied and staged separately. All efforts should be made to leave any healthy functioning kidney in place by performing a partial nephrectomy and wedge resection; however, this should not be attempted if clear margins are not possible. These patients end up having difficulties with renal dysfunction, and renal failure occurs in 15% of patients 15 years post-treatment, depending on remaining amount of functioning kidney and/or damage related to chemotherapy drugs and radiotherapy (Neville and Ritchey 2000).

Patients with RCC are treated primarily with surgery. There is no standard treatment for advanced stage disease. The tumors are not responsive to radiotherapy, and there is no current chemotherapy that is effective. MacArthur et al. (1994), however, did report complete response to interleukin-2 in one child with metastatic RCC.

2.7.8 Prognosis

The long-term survival is approaching 90% in patients with localized Wilms' tumors and 70% in patients with metastatic disease (Pritchard-Jones, 2002). The results of the NWTS-IV as described by Neville and Ritchey (2000) show 4-year overall survival to be

Table 2.16. Protocol for National Wilms' Tumor Study-V (adapted from Neville and Ritchey, 2000)

Stage of disease	Surgery	Radiotherapy[a]	Chemotherapy
Stage I and II, favorable histology (no anaplasia) Stage I with focal or diffuse anaplasia	Nephrectomy	None vincristine (18 weeks)	Pulse intensive dactinomycin,
Stage III and IV, favorable histology Stage II-IV, focal anaplasia	Nephrectomy	Yes	Pulse intensive dactinomycin, vincristine, doxorubicin (24 weeks)
Stage II-IV, diffuse anaplasia Stage I-IV, CCSK	Nephrectomy	Yes	Dactinomycin, vincristine, doxorubicin, cyclophosphamide, and etoposide (24 weeks)
Stage I-IV, RTK	Nephrectomy	Yes	Carboplatin, etoposide, and cyclophosphamide (24 weeks

[a] Radiotherapy doses are approximately 1,080 cGy for the abdomen and 1,200 cGy for the lung. Only patients with stage IV lung metastases receive whole lung radiotherapy

- 96% in stage I with favorable histology
- 91% for stage II with favorable histology
- 91% for stage III with favorable histology
- 80% for stage IV with favorable histology
- Stages II-IV with diffuse anaplasia was 82%

RTK in the NWTS III series had an overall 4-year survival of 25% and CCSK stages II-IV was 75%. For patients with stage I RCC, the survival is 90%; however, with stage IV disease the survival is about 0% (Broecker, 2000).

2.7.9 Follow-up

Follow-up for Wilms' tumor involves regular physical exams and surveillance scanning, usually with at least abdominal ultrasound and chest x-ray. This is usually done every 3 months for the first 2 years, followed by every 6 months for 2 years and then with decreasing frequency or as clinically appropriate. Renal function does need to be monitored in the remaining kidney quite carefully, especially if bilateral disease existed and radiation therapy was received.

Late effects of radiation therapy and specific chemotherapeutic agents should be assessed. Patients who received anthracycline therapy should be monitored for cardiomyopathy or congestive heart failure; cardiac sequelae might be exacerbated in those patients who also received lung radiation. Patients who have been treated with VP16 need to be screened for second myeloid leukemias, and secondary malignancies are a risk in the radiation field. Ovarian failure is a possible late effect resulting from some of the chemotherapeutic agents.

2.7.10 Future Perspectives

The outcomes for children with Wilms' tumor are relatively favorable. Future efforts will focus on tailoring therapy by decreasing chemotherapy and radiation therapy when possible in order to minimize treatment-related toxicity, based on risk stratification. There is also interest in learning about predisposing factors to Wilms' tumor and whether the use of antiangiogenic agents will have a future role. Topotecan is being currently used in relapsed Wilms' tumors with some effect; it may have a continued role in the future.

New therapies distinct from the protocols for Wilms' tumor need to be developed for RCC and RTK.

2.8 Retinoblastoma

Retinoblastoma (Rb) arises from fetal retinoblasts that normally differentiate into post-mitotic retinal photoreceptor cells and neurons. The tumor tends to outgrow its blood supply, which results in necrosis and calcification.

2.8.1 Epidemiology

Rb is the most frequently diagnosed intraocular malignancy of childhood. It represents 3 % of all pediatric malignancies, with an incidence of approximately 1 in 18,000 live births. Eighty percent of cases are diagnosed before the age of 3 or 4 years. Sixty percent of cases are nonheritable and unilateral. Forty percent of cases are heritable (bilateral or multifocal), of which 5 % are familial and the rest are sporadic. Metastases can occur in up to 10–15 % of patients (Rodriguez and Pappo, 2003).

2.8.2 Etiology

Rb can occur in one or both eyes. Bilateral Rb is generally picked up earlier than unilateral cases. There has been an association between Rb and congenital abnormalities in the 13q- syndrome (Yunis and Ramsay, 1978), and with other abnormalities including cardiovascular defects, cleft palate, infantile cortical hyperostosis, dentinogenesis imperfecta, familial cataracts, Bloch-Sulzberger syndrome, and mental retardation (Hurwitz et al., 2002). The incidence of Rb has been reported to be higher after in vitro fertilization procedures.

The heritable form of Rb is associated with errors in transcription, translocations, or deletions of genetic information on chromosome 13q14. Bilateral Rb can occur at different times, so conservative management should be used in young infants who present with disease in one eye only, as there is potential for tumors to develop in the second eye.

Knudson's two-hit theory of cancer can be used to explain the etiology of Rb. One abnormal chromosome is commonly inherited at conception from an unaffected parent, or rarely inherited from an affect-ed parent, and the second hit occurs after conception. The second hit affects a somatic retinal cell. It can be a mutation in form of a deletion, chromosomal loss by nondysjunction, or somatic recombination (Knudson, 2001). The first hit can either be constitutional (heritable bilateral or multifocal) or somatic (nonheritable unilateral), but the second hit is always somatic. Errors in transcription occur more often in the paternal allele, suggesting that germ line mutations occur more often in spermatogenesis than oogenesis. Predisposition to Rb is imparted by germline mutation in 40 % of cases (Hurwitz et al. 2002). It is transmitted as an autosomal dominant trait; penetrance may be as high as 90 %, but it is not 100 %. There is 50 % chance that a child of an affected parent will inherit the disease. A patient's sibling's can present with the disease even if the parents appear to be unaffected, either because of a low penetrance allele or a germline mosaicism (Hurwitz et al. 2002). The heritable form of the disease, characterized by the errors in the Rb1 gene, predisposes children to a small risk for sporadic secondary malignancies and a much higher risk for radiation-induced secondary malignancies.

2.8.3 Molecular Genetics

Molecular analysis has become increasingly sensitive at picking up chromosomal aberrations, although testing is not routinely done at all centers. The Rb1 gene is located at chromosome 13q14. The Rb1 gene is a tumor suppressor gene and is important in apoptosis. It is a key regulator of the cell cycle and therefore governs the proliferation of tumor cells. In Rb, deregulation of cell proliferation occurs as a result of the inactivated or absent Rb1 protein, and constraint that is normally exerted over the cell cycle is lost (Rodriguez-Galindo and Pappo, 2003).

2.8.4 Signs and Symptoms

The most common signs of retinoblastoma are

- Leukocoria (cat's eye reflex) – caused by the tumor, which is white and occludes the normal red retina

- Strabismus – the tumor's placement over the macula causes loss of central vision and disruption of the fusional reflex, causing the affected eye to drift
- Glaucoma – increased intraocular pressure due to the tumor
- Decreased vision in one eye – caused by the tumor covering the macula or retinal detachment

Some other presenting signs include esotropia, painful eyes, and erythematous conjunctivae. Heterochromia (discoloration of the iris) warrants immediate enucleation because it is a sign of advanced disease. Seventeen percent of patients with Rb and 50 % of children with advanced Rb requiring enucleation, present with rubeosis iridis, which is neovascularization of the surface of the iris (Hurwitz et al., 2002). Hyphema, blood in the anterior chamber of the eye, can occur secondary to rubeosis iridis, so its presence in the absence of trauma warrants an immediate ocular examination. Glaucoma and closed angle glaucoma are also presenting symptoms that usually indicated advanced disease. Endophytic tumors or diffuse infiltrating tumors may produce pseudohypopyon (cells in anterior chamber).

Metastatic spread of Rb occurs through several mechanisms. Tumor can spread posteriorly through the optic nerve to the brain and cerebrospinal fluid. The second method of extraocular spread occurs through lymphatic dissemination; this can occur anteriorly through the iris and ciliary body. Direct extension can occur through sclera into the orbit. Through the choroid, Rb can spread hematogenously to other sites in the body such as bone, bone marrow, lung, and brain.

2.8.5 Diagnostics

The diagnostic workup for Rb begins with a thorough history, paying particular attention to the duration of symptoms and changes in the eye's appearance. Special attention should be given to familial history and incidence of Rb.

Physical examination should assess visual acuity (cranial nerve II), tracking (cranial nerves III, IV, and VI), strabismus, esotropia, and leukocoria. Direct and indirect fundoscopic examination should be done under anesthesia. The pupils should be well dilated to allow for complete visualization of the fundus. CT of the brain and orbits is needed to detect distal spread of tumor and identify areas of calcification. MRI of the brain has been shown to be an excellent method of localizing intraocular extent of disease as well as visualizing tumor extension into the optic nerve and orbital area. A bone marrow aspirate is often done to detect metastatic disease if there is an apparent risk for hematogenous spread (i.e. choroidal involvement). A lumbar puncture may be done to determine if there is metastatic extension to the cerebrospinal fluid; this is especially necessary when there is optic nerve involvement. Ultrasound is a common test that is performed on eyes affected by Rb and shows the tumor in reference to anatomical structures (Servodidio et al., 1991). Fundoscopic pictures are also taken during the exam under anesthesia.

Retinoblastoma can present as trilateral disease. This is rare, with an incidence of 3 %; 6–10 % of those affected have a genetic predisposition to the disease. In addition to bilateral ocular tumors, a tumor is also seen on the pineal gland in trilateral retinoblastoma. It is typically associated with an extremely poor prognosis and usually occurs in children ages 4 and younger (Hurwitz et al., 2002). Trilateral disease can even be seen years after successfully treated ocular disease and is a major cause of mortality for these children in the first 5 years after diagnosis of bilateral Rb.

The diagnosis of Rb is made by ophthalmoscopic, radiologic, and ultrasonographic appearance of the tumor; pathological confirmation is unnecessary. Rb is a small blue round cell tumor consisting of densely packed cells. It is mitotically active, and when the eye is enucleated, there are Flexner-Winterstein rosettes, which are highly characteristic of Rb. See Fig. 2.7 for metastatic Rb in the bone marrow.

2.8.6 Staging and Classification

There are several common growth patterns of Rb tumors. With an endophytic pattern, tumor arises from retina and grows into the vitreal cavity. These tumors usually fill the cavity and float in the vitreous and are known as vitreal seeds. Exophytic tumors grow from

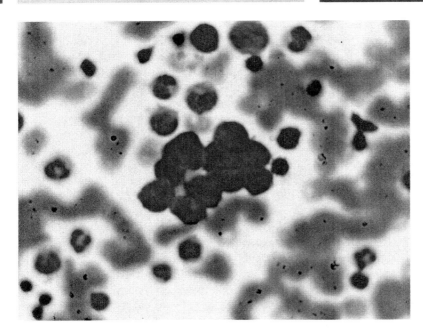

Figure 2.7

Metastatic retinoblastoma in the bone marrow

Table 2.17. The Reese-Ellsworth classification system for retinoblastoma

Group I Very favorable	A: Single tumor, smaller than 4 disk diameters[a] at or behind the equator B: Multiple tumors, none larger than 4 disk diameters, all at or behind the equator
Group II Favorable	A: Solitary tumor, 4–10 disk diameters in size, at or behind the equator B: Multiple tumors, 4–10 disk diameters in size, behind the equator
Group III Doubtful	A: Any lesion anterior to the equator B: Solitary tumors larger than 10 disk diameters behind the equator
Group IV Unfavorable	A: Multiple tumors, some larger than 10 disk diameters B: Any lesion extending anteriorly to the ora serrata
Group V Very unfavorable	A: Tumors involving more than half the retina B: Vitreous

[a] Disc diameter = 1.5–1.75 mm

the retina into the subretinal space and cause serious detachments of the retina. From the retina they can proceed to invade the choroid or the blood supply. A mixed presentation of endophytic and exophytic patterns is the most common occurrence (Hurwitz et al., 2002). Diffuse infiltrating Rb is the least common presentation; it usually occurs in older children and is a diagnostic challenge.

The Reese-Ellsworth classification system is currently the most frequently used tool (Table 2.17). Murphree has developed a simpler staging system, but this has not been adopted widely into practice at this time

2.8.7 Treatment

The goals of treatment for Rb are to preserve useful vision without compromising patient survival. The major treatment modalities for Rb include surgical enucleation, radiation, and chemotherapy, as well as focal cryotherapy and photocoagulation therapy.

Enucleation is used often in the management of Rb. It is used to treat large unilateral tumors with no visual potential. Tumors that invade the optic nerve, choroid, or sclera or those that extend into the orbit need to be removed. Twenty percent of children with bilateral disease lose both eyes eventually (Hurwitz et al., 2002). Enucleation is also used when extensive seeding is evident, as with anterior invasion and secondary glaucoma. When the eye is enucleated, an orbital implant is surgically placed and the rectus muscles are attached to allow for some movement of the eventual prosthesis.

External beam radiation was frequently used in the past treatment of Rb. Its disadvantages include facial hypoplasia, cataract development, retinopathy, and increased risk of secondary tumors in the radiation field. Children who carry the germ line Rb mutation and receive radiation therapy are at a 35% increased risk of developing a secondary malignancy (Gallie et al. 1996). But because Rb cells are very radiosensitive, radiotherapy is sometimes used for the treatment of medium sized tumors. The dose, which ranges 3,500 and 4,500 cGy, is given in 20 fractions (Servodidio et al., 1991). More recently stereotactic radiation has been used to target some intraocular tumors, removing the need to radiate the entire orbit. Incidence of cataracts is lessened with this approach (Hurwitz et al. 2002).

Plaque radiotherapy is another form of radiation therapy. With this form of radiation treatment, cobalt or iodine plaques are surgically implanted at the scleral base of the tumor. The plaque remains in place for 2 to 4 days and then is surgically removed. This treatment is used on medium-sized tumors situated away from the optic nerve and macula (Chan et al. 1996). Plaque radiotherapy is most often used as a secondary treatment after another form has failed.

Focal therapies are used alone or as adjuvant treatment with chemotherapy. Cryotherapy can be effectively used to manage small anterior tumors. Cryotherapy entails freezing the tumor with a probe, allowing the tumor to thaw, and then repeating this process several times. It is usually performed at monthly intervals. Photocoagulation therapy is used for small posterior tumors. Laser burns are made around the tumor, which in effect cut the blood supply to the tumor, ultimately causing cell death.

Until recently, chemotherapy has not played a large role in treating intraocular Rb. A study by Chan et al. (1996) revealed that 30% of already enucleated tumors show resistance to chemotherapy. P-glycoprotein is the multidrug-resistance protein, and was expressed in these chemoresistant tumors (Gallie et al., 1996). P-glycoprotein in vitro has been shown to actively pump chemotherapy out of tumors. Chan et al. (1996) found that high concentrations of cyclosporin reversed this process. A current phase III trial is ongoing to evaluate the efficacy of high-dose cyclosporin in conjunction with the chemotherapy agents vincristine, carboplatin, and etoposide. Preliminary data are showing good results with this approach, which avoids radiation therapy. Adjuvant treatment with photocoagulation and cryotherapy are used in conjunction with the chemotherapy administration. Viable tumor is often left following chemotherapy, so focal therapy is imperative following the cessation of chemotherapy. Other treatment protocols continue to use similar chemotherapy agents in conjunction with focal therapy and without the use of cyclosporin with good success for Reese-Ellsworth eye groups 1, 2, and 3 (Friedman et al., 2000).

Chemotherapy has always played a role in the treatment of metastatic disease. In advanced metastatic disease high-dose chemotherapy followed by stem cell rescue is sometimes being done where available. This is only useful if complete local control of metastatic disease has been obtained. Intrathecal administration of cytarabine and topotecan has also been attempted in efforts to clear metastatic disease in the cerebrospinal fluid.

2.8.8 Prognosis

The overall 5-year survival for Rb is 90 % (Hurwitz et al., 2002). Unfortunately, the survival in patients with metastatic disease remains poor. Optic nerve invasion posterior to the lamina cribrosa at time of enucleation is predictive of poor prognosis.

2.8.9 Follow-up

Ongoing follow-up of children with Rb is needed well after tumor control has been established. Children with hereditary disease are at risk of developing new tumors until retinal differentiation is complete, around the age of 7. Following the treatment of Rb, fundoscopic examinations are imperative to pick up recurrent disease quickly. Eye exams are generally done under anesthesia while the child is receiving active therapy. Once a child is only being monitored and is able to cooperate, eye exams can be moved to the outpatient setting.

A child treated with chemotherapy and/or radiation therapy must be followed up for late effects of their treatment. Carboplatin can cause hearing disturbances, so audiograms must be a regular part of the follow-up regimen. Secondary leukemias are a potential following treatment with VP16. Secondary malignancies can arise in fields of prior irradiation. Children with the Rb1 gene mutation are at an increased risk of developing secondary neoplasms. Families must be taught to be conscientious in reporting any changes in their children's health.

2.8.10 Future Directions

Potential future directions in the treatment of Rb include monoclonal antibody, interferon, and gene therapy. There are also international efforts underway for a clinical trial examining the use of chemotherapy and focal therapy in an effort to avoid radiation therapy. The use of cyclosporine in conjunction with chemotherapy and focal therapy will be trialed on a larger scale to help delineate if cyclosporine reverses multidrug resistance and results in superior outcomes compared with chemotherapy alone in treating intraocular tumors. The development of radiosensitizers may act to diminish the resistance of hypoxic cells to radiation, with the hope of increasing the rate of successful radiation.

2.9 Rhabdomyosarcoma

Rhabdomyosarcoma (RMS) develops from a primitive mesenchymal cell committed to muscle differentiation. They can occur anywhere in the body, even in places where skeletal muscle would not be seen.

2.9.1 Epidemiology

Rhabdomyosarcoma is the most common soft tissue sarcoma that occurs in children. It affects approximately 4.5 per million children less than 15 years of age in age (Gurney et al,. 1995). It is the third most common extracranial solid neoplasm of childhood. Males have a very slightly higher incidence, and whites have a 15 % increased rate of occurrence compared with blacks (Gurney et al., 1995). Two-thirds of children presenting with RMS do so before the age of 6 (Wexler et al., 2002). Younger children tend to present with the embryonal subtype of RMS, whereas the alveolar subtype occurs throughout childhood.

2.9.2 Etiology

The cause of RMS is unknown. There is association with other genetic syndromes including neurofibromatosis, Li-Fraumeni syndrome, and BWS (Wexler et al. 2002). Parental use of marijuana has shown a three-fold increased risk of developing RMS in some studies (Wexler et al., 2002). Other environmental factors that are being considered as adding to the risk are parental use of cocaine, prior exposure to alkylating agents, intrauterine x-ray, and fetal alcohol syndrome. A higher incidence of RMS has also been noted in patients with congenital anomalies of the gastrointestinal, genitourinary, cardiovascular and central nervous systems.

Table 2.18. The prevalence of rhabdomyosarcoma according to primary site and the correlating clinical symptoms (Wexler et al., 2002)

Site of primary tumor	Prevalence	Clinical symptoms
Parameningeal (Ear, nasal cavity, sinuses, infratem poral fossa, pterygopalatine fossa)	16%	Airway obstruction Respiratory symptoms Nasal congestion Pain Cranial nerve palsies
Orbit	9%	Proptosis Periorbital swelling
Other head and neck	10%	Swelling or mass
Extremities	18%	Swelling or mass
Genitourinary	22%	Prostate: bladder and/or bowel difficulties Paratesticular: scrotal swelling, pain, mass above the testes Uterus, bladder, cervix: menorrhagia, or metrorrhagia Vagina: protruding grape-like cluster (typical for botryoid)
Other	25%	

2.9.3 Molecular Genetics

RMS falls into the category of small round blue-cell tumors. They can be differentiated from tumors with similar morphology based on electron microscopy, immunocytochemistry, and cytogenetic analysis. Sixty percent of RMSs are of the embryonal subtype, and 5% of those are considered the botryoid variant, 20% are the alveolar subtype, and the remaining 20% are undifferentiated (Pappo et al., 1997). A solid variant is referred to as a pleomorphic form revealing the presence of anaplastic cells in large sheets.

Alveolar RMS has a characteristic t(2;13) seen in over one-half of patients and a second t(1;13) translocation seen less commonly (Pritchard-Jones and Mitchell, 1997). In the t(2;13) rearrangement, the PAX3 gene is fused with the FKHR gene, whereas the (1;13) rearrangement causes fusion of PAX7-FKHR. It is thought that PAX3 and PAX7 are vital to muscle development during embryogenesis. Patients with metastatic disease and PAX7 fusion gene tend to have a more favorable prognosis than those with the PAX3 (Pappo et al., 1997). N-Myc is amplified in 10% of the alveolar subtype. A tumor should be treated as alveolar even when it displays only scattered alveolar foci because alveolar imparts a worse prognosis and requires treatment intensification.

The embryonal subtypes have not revealed any translocations but characteristically have shown loss of heterozygosity at 11p15.5 (Pappo et al., 1997).

The undifferentiated sarcomas tend to have a t(11;22), which are seen often in the Ewing's sarcoma family of tumors, and tumors are generally treated similarly.

2.9.4 Symptoms and Clinical Signs

RMS can occur anywhere in the body with the exception of bone and is not limited to those places where skeletal muscle exists. The prevalence of the tumors according to primary and the correlating clinical symptoms are listed in Table 2.18.

RMS spreads via hematogenous and lymphatic routes. The most common sites for metastases are lung, lymph nodes, bone, and bone marrow.

Table 2.19. Clinical group staging system for rhabdomyosarcoma

Clinical group		Extent of disease and surgical result
I	A	Localized tumor, confined to site of origin, completely resected
	B	Localized tumor, infiltrating beyond site of origin, completely resected
II	A	Localized tumor, gross total resection but with microscopic residual disease
	B	Locally "extensive" tumor (spread to regional lymph nodes), completely resected
	C	"Extensive" tumor (spread to regional lymph nodes), gross total resection but with microscopic residual disease
III	A	Localized or locally extensive tumor, gross residual disease after biopsy only
	B	Localized or locally extensive tumor, gross residual disease after "major" resection (>50% debulking)
IV		Any size primary tumor, with or without regional lymph node involvement, with distant metastases, irrespective of surgical approach to primary tumor

2.9.5 Diagnostics

Necessary diagnostic tests in the workup of a patient thought to have RMS include

- imaging of the affected area
- imaging of likely areas for metastases
- tumor biopsy
- blood work

Initial workup consists of x-ray or ultrasound of the primary, depending on location. Once a mass is identified, CT or MRI scanning should be ordered to evaluate the extent of the mass and look for evidence of bony erosion. A CT of the chest should be done to look for pulmonary metastases. If the tumor is located in a paraspinal or parameningeal area, an MRI should be ordered to assess the extent of disease. A bone scan is ordered to rule out bony metastases. MRI of the head should be considered if the child is symptomatic at diagnosis or has a paraspinal primary.

A biopsy is done to obtain a tumor specimen; this can be either via core or open biopsy. The specimen should be sent for cytogenetics with FISH (or reverse transcription PCR when FISH is not available). Light microscopy reveals rhabdomyoblasts or cross striations, which are both seen in skeletal muscle. RMS cells stain positive for intermediate filaments, desmin, vimentin, myoglobin, actin, and myoD

(Pappo et al., 1997). A bilateral bone marrow aspirate and biopsy are also done to rule out bone marrow involvement. A lumbar puncture should be done for children with parameningeal primaries to determine whether the cerebrospinal fluid is infiltrated with tumor cells.

Blood work should consist of a CBC, LDH, and liver function tests. Urinalysis is required. There are no specific tumor markers for RMS. In planning for treatment, it is also prudent to do necessary prechemotherapy surveillance studies such as an echocardiogram and audiogram.

2.9.6 Staging and Classification

Staging normally follows two distinct systems. The first involves the TNM (tumor, node, metastases) system, which takes into account not only surgical outcome, which may be dependent on the surgeon's skill, but also site, size, local invasiveness, and presence of nodes and metastases, and then divides patients into distinct prognostic groups (Andrassy, 2002). (See Table 2.19.). The second grouping system, by the Intergroup Rhabdomyosarcoma Study (IRS) group, looks at pretreatment and operative outcome (Table 2.20). Both stage and group are used to determine appropriate therapy. Survival correlates with clinical group, while TNM staging aids in determining risk stratification to allow for risk-based therapy.

Table 2.20. TNM pretreatment staging classification for rhabdomyosarcoma (*T1* confined to anatomic site of origin; *T2* extension; *NO* not clinically involved; *N1* clinically involved; *NX* clinical status unknown; *MO*, no distant metastases; *M1* distant metastasis present)

Stage	Sites	Tumor invasiveness	Tumor size	Regional nodes (N)	Metastases
1	Orbit Head and neck[c] Genitourinary[d]	T1 or T2	a[a] or b[b]	NO, N1, or NX	MO
2	Bladder/prostate Extremity Cranial parameningeal Other[d]	T1 or T2	a[a]	NO or NX	MO
3	Bladder/prostate Extremity Cranial parameningeal Other[e]	T1 or T2	a[a] b[b]	N1 NO, N1, or NX	MO MO
4	All	T1 or T2	a[a] or b[b]	No or N1	M1

[a] a <5 or =5 cm in diameter
[b] >5 cm in diameter
[c] Excluding parameningeal
[d] Nonbladder/nonprostate
[e] Includes trunk, retroperitoneum, and so on
Used in Intergroup Rhabdomyosarcoma Study IV

2.9.7 Treatment

Treatment for RMS includes surgery, radiation therapy (sometimes brachytherapy), and chemotherapy. The full treatment plan for RMS depends largely on the location of the tumor. The IRS group has a stratification schema for tumors according to the primary site, stage, TNM and histology. The timing of each depends on the clinical disease group and study protocols. In general, surgery is often followed by radiation therapy and chemotherapy; in cases of complete surgical resection, chemotherapy alone is used.

Surgery depends largely on the site of disease and the feasibility of complete surgical resection. Surgical resection also helps delineate the clinical grouping to be used. Surgery over the years has become more conservative with each intergroup rhabdomyosarcoma study. Treatments in a recent study have used risk stratification based on the likelihood of disease recurrence, and divided patients into low-, intermediate-, and high-risk groups. Risk is determined by examining the site and size of the tumor, nodal disease, and histology.

Radiation therapy is used for microscopic tumor or residual tumor not removed during surgery. The timing of radiotherapy is variable depending on the protocol used. In the IRS V protocols, radiation therapy begins at week 15 for patients in the high-risk group, week 12 for intermediate risk, week 3 for low risk, and immediately for some high-risk patients with advanced cranial tumors (Wexler et al., 2002).

Chemotherapy is used for cytoreduction prior to a gross total resection and for both gross and micrometastatic disease. Chemotherapeutic agents that are used in treating RMS are vincristine and actinomycin D for low-risk tumors. Vincristine, actinomycin, and cyclophosphamide (VAC) is the gold standard for intermediate-risk RMS, although other agents such as ifosfamide, etoposide, and doxorubicin also show activity. Currently, irinotecan is being used in the IRS V protocol to determine its activity in patients with distant metastases at diagnosis (Wexler et al., 2002). Chemotherapy has traditionally been given longer in RMS than in other solid tumors, sometimes for 12–24 months in IRS studies (McDowell, 2003).

Surgery with adequate margins is the treatment of choice for head and neck tumors where possible, although deforming surgery is not warranted. If complete resection is not possible, then radiation therapy is used. Both of these groups of patients receive chemotherapy. For RMS in the orbit, resection without disfiguration is not possible, so chemotherapy and radiation therapy are the treatment of choice (Andrassy, 2002). For bladder and prostate tumors, surgery, with postoperative radiotherapy for both gross or microscopic residual disease, and chemotherapy are used. Those children with bladder tumors often have dysfunction postoperatively, which is lessened somewhat with more conservative surgical approaches and the use of radiation (Andrassy, 2002). For paratesticular RMS, radical inguinal orchiectomy is recommended along with ipsilateral retroperitoneal lymph node dissection. Adjuvant chemotherapy has favorable cure rates. If nodal resections are positive, retroperitoneal radiation and intensified chemotherapy are warranted. Vaginal, vulval, and uterine RMS used to be treated with radical, mutilating surgery; but the IRS now recommends combination chemotherapy post-biopsy followed by conservative surgery and radiation therapy for incompletely resected disease (Andrassy, 2002). RMS of the extremities is treated when possible with limb-sparing surgical resection. At the time of surgery, aggressive lymph node sampling is warranted or, when available, sentinel node biopsy, and postoperative radiation therapy to these sites is recommended

2.9.8 Prognosis

The overall 5-year survival in RMS is 70% (Pappo et al., 1997). A review article by Andrassy (2002) states that 90% of paratesticular tumors are cured, overall survival for bladder/prostate is 85%, and orbital RMS has survival rates greater than 90%. Patients who have limb primaries have an overall survival of 66%. This is because these tumors are often disseminated and the histology is usually of the alveolar subtype. Patients who are high-risk, who have unresectable tumors in unfavorable sites, have an overall survival of 73% (McDowell, 2003). The improved prognosis and survival in this group of patients is attributed to mul-

timodal risk adapted therapy. Patients with metastatic disease at diagnosis (Group IV disease) continue to have a poor prognosis and a 3-year event-free survival of only 25% (Breneman et al., 2003).

2.9.9 Follow-up

Follow-up protocols for children treated for RMS must look for both local recurrence and late effects of treatment. Most protocols generally require follow-up every 3 months for the first year, with physical exam, as well as chest x-ray or chest CT to look for lung metastases, and CT or MRI of the primary. During the second and third years screening may occur with decreasing frequency as clinically appropriate. Follow-up must consider late effects of all treatments including, site-specific radiation and surgery as well as chemotherapy. These children generally have a high risk for developing secondary tumors later in life if they have been radiated and must continue to be followed (Andrassy, 2002)

2.9.10 Future Perspectives

Patients with metastatic alveolar RMS who are PAX3-FKHR positive continue to do poorly on standard treatment protocols, and new targeted therapy needs to be developed. Molecular gene fusions such as the PAX3-FKHR oncogene may be a therapeutic target in the future (Sorensen et al. 2002). Some clinicians believe that radiation therapy that is hyperfractionated, as well as conventional chemotherapy agents such as VP16 and ifosfamide, may have a role in treating advanced-stage RMS (Kaefer, 2002). Others, however, believe that dose escalation of chemotherapy and radiation therapy is futile because these are not tumor-specific (Pappo et al., 1997).

Studies testing the value of antisense, oligonucleotides, and ribozymes in RMS cell lines currently exist, but their value is yet to be determined (Pappo et al., 1997). Irinotecan and topotecan are being used in some clinical phase II trials in patients with metastatic disease. As with many other solid tumors currently, immunotherapy, antiangiogenic agents, and biological agents are thought to have a future role.

Table 2.21. Prognostic factors in the NRSTS (Miser et al., 2002)

	Factors associated with increased risk of local relapse	Factors associated with increased risk of distant metastases	Factors associated with decreased survival
Microscopically positive margins	X		X
Tumor >5 cm	X	X	X
High histologic grade		X	X
Intraabdominal primary tumor	X		X
No radiotherapy	X		
Invasive tumor		X	

2.10 Non-rhabdomyosarcomatous Soft Tissue Sarcomas

Non-rhabdomyosarcomatous soft tissue sarcomas (NRSTS) are a heterogeneous group of tumors. Collectively they account for approximately 4% of cancers occurring in childhood (Spunt et al., 2002). NRSTS are normally staged according to the Intergroup Rhabdomyosarcoma Study Group surgicopathologic staging system. This staging reflects the postoperative tumor status (Table 2.19). The TNM staging system takes into account the presurgical tumor status, including size, local invasiveness, presence of nodes, and metastases. NRSTS are also graded, 1 through 3, and their grade is of important prognostic significance. Grade is based on histological subtype, amount of necrosis, number of mitoses, the degree of cellularity, and nuclear features. Collectively this information is used to determine appropriate treatment stratification.

The treatment approach for NRSTS is similar regardless of tumor type. Primary treatment consists of wide surgical excision of the tumor. A surgical margin of 1 cm is considered adequate if free of all microscopic disease. Radiotherapy is sometimes used as adjuvant treatment in the presence of microscopic residual disease or in the presence of inadequate surgical margins. The long-term survival of patients with surgically resectable tumors treated with or without radiation therapy exceeds 70% (Spunt et al., 1999).

Although the overall survival of children with completely resected tumors is generally excellent, 20% of these children will relapse and die of their disease (Miser et al. 2002). It is important to recognize those tumors with a high potential for local and distant recurrence so that appropriate adjuvant treatment is utilized in their initial treatment. Prognostic factors in NRSTS are described in Table 2.21.

NRSTS in general are not very chemosensitive tumors; however, in some instances adjuvant chemotherapy is warranted. High-grade tumors that are surgically resected but are large (>5 cm) may benefit from adjuvant chemotherapy regardless of surgical margins. Chemotherapy has also been used as neoadjuvant therapy in unresectable tumors, in those that have been incompletely excised, and in metastatic disease. Vincristine, actinomycin, and cyclophosphamide have been used with good response in inoperable infantile fibrosarcoma (Ninane 1991). Ifosfamide and doxorubicin have been used as adjuvant treatment for some NRSTS (especially with synovial sarcoma), with questionable results. Metastatic NRSTS do poorly and require new therapies.

The most commonly occurring NRSTS in children will be briefly discussed, with typical features unique to each tumor summarized.

Alveolar Soft Part Sarcoma (ASPS) This tumor is found most often in late adolescence, with an incidence higher in females. It represents 0.5–1% of all soft tissue sarcomas in adults and children (Pang et al., 2001). Primary sites of disease are the skeletal muscles of the extremities with the deep soft tissue of the thigh and buttocks being the most common (Coffin et al. 1997). The head and neck regions are more common in children. ASPS metastasizes to lung, bone, and CNS. This disease has an indolent course, and relapses can occur very late. Imaging generally shows a large intramuscular mass with prominent vascularity. Chromosomal abnormalities have been identified at t(x;17)(p11.2q25) (Miser et al., 2002). Prognosis is best for head and neck tumors but poor in general.

Fibrosarcoma This spindle cell tumor has two peaks in incidence. It typically affects young infants and children, with the second childhood peak occurring between the ages of 10 and 15 (Carli et al., 1997). Congenital or infantile sarcomas are generally found in the distal extremities and the head and neck regions; these tumors grow rapidly but rarely metastasize. In the adult form, or in children who are older, presentation typically occurs in the proximal extremities, and the deep thoracic and pelvic regions. Adult-type tumors often have cytogenetic abnormalities such a: t(x;18), t(2;5), and t(7;22) (Miser et al., 2002). These tumors are more aggressive and tend to metastasize more often. The overall 5-year survival with infantile fibrosarcoma is 84–93%, but with older children survival correlates with the adult form of the disease, with the 5-year overall survival being 60% (Coffin et al., 1997; Miser et al., 2002).

Hemangiopericytoma This neoplasm represents approximately 3% of all soft tissue sarcomas in children (Miser et al. 2002). This is a vascular tumor that often display the cytogenetic abnormalities of t(12;19) and t(13;22). It is often found in the oral cavity, chest wall, and head and neck of infants and is termed infantile hemangiopericytoma; it is usually associated with an excellent outcome with complete resection. In older children and adults, the tumor is found more often in the lower extremities and retroperitoneum and is usually more aggressive and associated with metastatic disease and poor outcome (Miser et al., 2002). This tumors can metastasize to lung and bone.

Leiomyosarcoma This malignant smooth muscle tumor accounts for less than 2% of NRSTS in children. Radiation therapy may predispose a child to leiomyosarcoma. Incidences of this neoplasm developing in the radiation field of children previously treated for retinoblastoma have been reported. EBV has been linked to leiomyosarcoma in children with HIV. A t(12;14) translocation has been noted in the tumors of children with leiomyosarcoma (Miser et al., 2002). The most common site of occurrence is the gastrointestinal (GI) tract, specifically the stomach, but it can occur in any vascular structure or soft tissue. Gastric epithelioid leiomyosarcomas can occur as part of Carney's triad. When leiomyosarcoma is diagnosed, regular scanning should be done to rule out the presence or development of paraganglioma and pulmonary chondroma. Patients with tumors arising in the GI tract usually have a poor outcome.

Liposarcoma Liposarcoma most commonly affects adolescents in the second decade of life, with a slight male predominance. The deep soft tissues of the extremities account for about half of pediatric cases, and the second most common site of occurrence is the trunk (retroperitoneum). Metastases are not common but can occur in the lymph nodes, lung, liver, and brain. Liposarcomas can be of myxoid, round cell, well-differentiated, or pleomorphic subtypes (Coffin et al., 1997). In the myxoid variant, which is the most common, a characteristic t(12;16)(q13;p11) is often seen (Swanson and Dehner, 1991). Liposarcomas usually have a low malignant potential, and children generally have a low rate of recurrence (Coffin et al., 1997).

Malignant Fibrous Histiocytoma Malignant fibrous histiocytoma (MFH) comprises 2–6% of all soft tissue sarcomas in children under 20 (Coffin et al., 1997). Males and females are affected equally. It presents most often in the head, neck, and extremities as a painless mass. The lungs are a common site of metastases. Associations have been found between

MFH and children who have received prior radiation therapy, as well as those who have DNA repair defects (Coffin et al., 1997). There are four main subtypes of this neoplasm, with the most common being storiform-pleomorphic; the other subtypes are giant cell, myxoid, and inflammatory. This tumor is characterized by p53 immunoreactivity and the amplification of the MDR2 gene (Coffin et al., 1997). The prognosis for this tumor is poor, with a relapse rate of up to 43 % and tumor death rate of 44 % (Coffin et al., 1997)

Malignant Peripheral Nerve Sheath Tumor (MPNST) MPNSTs arise from the peripheral nerve sheaths, as their name suggests, and they are also referred to as neurofibrosarcomas. They are among the most common of the soft tissue sarcomas occurring during childhood representing 10–20 % of all NRSTS. They most commonly occur in the second decade of life, with males and females being affected equally. There is a well-established association between neurofibromatosis and the development of this tumor. Mutations of p53 on chromosome 17 have been noted. There are, however, no characteristic genetic anomalies in this tumor. The most common anatomic sites of presentation of MPNSTs are the extremities and trunk.

Synovial Sarcoma Synovial sarcoma (SS) is the most commonly occurring NRSTS in older children and young adults (Miser et al. 2002). There is a very slight male predominance in the development of SS. It has three histological subgroups: biphasic, which is the most common and represents 60 % of cases, monophasic-epithelial, and monophasic-fibrous. SS carries a characteristic genetic alteration t(x;18) (p11;q11) (Coffin et al., 1997). SS normally occurs in close proximity to a joint, tendon, or bursa. The most common site of presentation is the leg near the knee or ankle joint, followed by the arm. The lung is a common site for metastases; lymph nodes are less commonly affected. Diagnostic imaging usually shows a mass with calcification. SS is one of the more chemosensitive NRSTSs.

2.11 Germ Cell Tumors

Germ cell tumors (GCTs) are a heterogeneous group of neoplasms that arise from primordial germ cells. They range from benign teratomas to aggressive malignancies. Extragonadal GCTs result from germ cells migrating aberrantly during fetal development. Presumably the differences in stage of germ cell development at the time of tumorigenesis play a role in the malignant potential of this group of tumors.

2.11.1 Epidemiology

GCTs comprise 3 % of all childhood neoplasms and occur at an annual incidence of approximately 2.4 per million children (Gurney et al., 1995). There is a bimodal peak in the ages of occurrence, with the first peak occurring in children less than 5 and the second in adolescents 15–19. Females are affected more often with benign GCTs and males are more often affected by malignant GCTs.

2.11.2 Etiology

Cryptorchidism (undescended testes) and gonadal dysgenesis are known to predispose for GCTs.

2.11.3 Molecular Genetics

Several characteristic genetic abnormalities predominate in GCTs, which can be divided into four groups, each with its distinct molecular characteristics: tumors of the adolescent testes, tumors of infancy, extragonadal tumors of adolescents, and tumors of the adolescent ovary (see Table 2.22).

2.11.4 Symptoms and Clinical Signs

Clinical symptoms of disease depend on the location of the tumor. Tumors arise either in gonadal or extragonadal midline sites. GCTs occur in the ovaries 25 % of the time and in the testes 20 % of the time. They occur in extragonadal locations more than half of the time: 25 % occur in the sacrococcygeal region and 20 % occur in the brain, with other sites includ-

Table 2.22. Common genetic alterations associated with germ cell tumors (Cushing and Marina, 2000)

GCT tumor group	Ploidy	Chromosomal alterations
Tumors of the adolescent testes	Aneuploid	Isochromosome 12p Loss of 13 Gain of 8, 21, 1q
Tumors of infancy		
Teratomas	Diploid	Abnormalities at 1, 3, 6
Yolk sac tumor	Diploid or Tetraploid	Abnormalities at 1, 3, 6
Extragonadal tumors of adolescents		
Brain	Diploid or tetraploid	Loss of 13 and 8
Mediastinum		Some have i(12p)[a]; loss of 13 and 8
Tumors of the adolescent ovary		
Mature teratoma		5% show gain or loss of an entire chromosome
Immature teratoma		No consistent changes
Malignant ovarian GCT	Aneuploid	i(12p)[a]; gains of 21 and 1q

[a] Two copies of 12p exist, both coming from the same parent

ing the retroperitoneal, pelvic, and neck area (Rodriguez-Galindo and Pappo, 2003). GCTs metastasize via both hematogenous and lymphatic spread. Common sites of metastasis are lung and liver.

Testicular tumors usually present as a mass or swelling in the scrotum and are usually not painful. Ovarian tumors usually present with symptoms such as pain, tenderness, and abdominal swelling. Mediastinal disease may cause symptoms of respiratory distress. Sacrococcygeal tumors can present with symptoms of urinary retention and constipation or as a visible gluteal mass. CNS disease may present with headaches, visual disturbances, precocious puberty, hypothyroidism, and diabetes insipidus.

2.11.5 Diagnostics

An ultrasound is usually done initially to investigate abdominal and pelvic tumors and is helpful in differentiating solid from cystic masses. CT of the chest, abdomen and pelvis, is recommended to assess the extent of primary disease and assessing for the presence of metastases. Bone scan may be indicated if bone pain is a presenting feature; however, GCTs rarely metastasize to bone.

There are serum tumor markers for some of the GCTs. Onco-feto-proteins such as alpha feto-protein (AFP) and beta human chorionic gonadotropin (BHCG) are used for screening. Elevations in AFP are seen with endodermal sinus tumor (EST) and embryonal carcinoma; increased BHCG is seen in choriocarcinoma. Serum onco-feto-proteins should decline within a half-life following the removal of a tumor, which for AFP is 7 days,- and for BHCG is 24 hours. Failure of these tumor markers to fall may indicate persistent disease (Pinkerton, 1997a,b). Nonspecific markers such as LDH are often ordered, and elevated levels are thought to correlate with growth of solid tumors (Cushing and Marina, 2000). Placental alkaline phosphatase is the isoenzyme of alkaline phosphatase and is used as a screening test at some centers; increases are seen in seminomas. Pituitary function should be evaluated before and during therapy.

Biopsy and preferably tumor resection (but not mutilating surgery) are necessary for both pathological diagnosis and treatment.

Figure 2.8

Schema for differentiation pathways for germ cell tumors (adapted from Pinkerton, 1997)

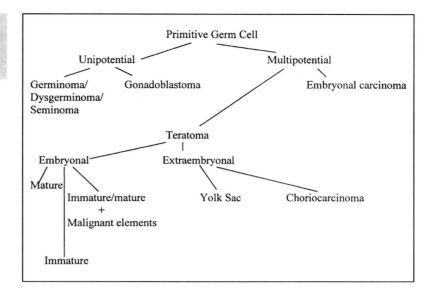

2.11.6 Staging and Classification

Germ cells develop from a primordial germ cell. There are many different morphological subtypes, which reflect the pathway of differentiation to which the cell was dedicated prior to malignant transformation. Fig. 2.8 shows the schema of differentiation pathway for GCTs.

Separate staging systems exist for ovarian and testicular tumors. However, staging of both is similar to that for other solid tumors:

- Stage I indicates localized disease confined to primary site, completely resected
- Stage II implies some degree of microscopic residual disease or nodal involvement (<2 cm)

- Stage III is characterized by gross residual disease or lymph node involvement (>2 cm)
- Stage IV denotes distant metastases (Cushing et al., 2002)

Characteristics that are associated with the different histologic subtypes of GCTs are summarized in Table 2.23.

2.11.7 Treatment

The treatment of both malignant and benign GCTs is surgical resection if feasible. Mutilating surgery should be avoided because GCTs are chemosensitive. Radiation therapy is often used for intracranial GCTs either alone or with chemotherapy. Radiation is also used at times for residual disease post-chemotherapy or in the case of bulky mediastinal disease post-chemotherapy.

For malignant GCTs requiring chemotherapy, platinum-containing regimens (cisplatin or carboplatin) are considered the standard of care. Other chemotherapeutic agents that have been used to treat GCTs include actinomycin, vinblastine, bleomycin, doxorubicin, and etoposide. Low-risk patients, those with stage I gonadal, are treated with surgical resection alone and do not require further treatment upfront but need to be closely followed. Similarly, extragonadal tumors that are completely resected may not require further treatment. Those with an intermediate risk, including stages II–IV gonadal and stage II extragonadal disease are treated with standard chemotherapy such as PEB (cisplatin, etoposide, and bleomycin) or JEB (carboplatin, etoposide, bleomycin) for four courses. High-risk patients, those with stage III and IV extragonadal disease, usually re-

Table 2.23. Germ cell tumors (GCT): subtypes, disease sites, and specific characteristics (Cushing et al., 2002)

Malignant category	Subtype	Sites of disease	Specific characteristics
Benign GCT	Mature teratomas	Ovaries Sacrococcygeal area Mediastinum	Mature elements of all three germ cell layers
Benign GCT	Gonadoblastoma	Dysgenic gonad	Mix of gonadal sex cord cells and immature germ cells
GCT of intermediate behavior	Immature teratoma	Ovaries	Graded based on degree of maturation (0–2 show benign behavior)
Malignant GCT	Germinoma	Ovaries (dysgerminoma) CNS (pineal region) Testes (seminoma)	Chemosensitive Radiosensitive
	Yolk sac tumor (endodermal sinus tumor)	Sacrococcygeal Testes	Elevate serum AFP
	Embryonal carcinoma	Testes Mediastinum Ovaries	Major component of mixed GCT
	Choriocarcinoma	Pineal region Mediastinum Ovary Testes	Elevated serum bHCG

quire 6 months of chemotherapy with cisplatin, etoposide, and bleomycin. Intergroup studies (POG and CCG) in the United States have shown that event-free survival can be improved in the high-risk group of GCTs if high-dose cisplatin therapy instead of the standard dosing is used in conjunction with standard dose etoposide and bleomycin (HDPEB) (Rodriguez-Galindo and Pappo, 2003), but the cisplatin-associated toxicity (ototoxicity predominantly as well as nephrotoxicity) is severe.

2.11.8 Prognosis

The 5-year overall survival of those with mature and immature teratoma is 100% (Cushing et al,. 2002). Results of the COG/POG randomized trials of PEB versus HD PEB have shown that the 3-year event-free survival for those with stage II testicular tumors is 100%, and for stage I and II ovarian tumors it is 96.4% (Rodriguez-Galindo and Pappo, 2003). Those with gonadal stages III and IV and extragonadal

stages I through IV have an event-free survival of 89.6% with HDPEB (Rodriguez-Galindo and Pappo, 2003).

2.11.9 Follow-up

Close surveillance, clinical as well as regular tumor marker assessment, should occur following the surgical resection of teratomas for up to 5 years because disease recurrence is possible. Malignant GCTs should have regular follow-up with either CT or ultrasound of abdominal and pelvic tumors, or MRI of intracranial tumors, every 3 months for the first year, followed by a decreasing frequency of scanning interval over the next several years. CT of the chest is recommended at regular intervals for metastatic surveillance.

Follow-up must also consider late effects of treatment. Cisplatin, especially high-dose cisplatin therapy, is associated with significant hearing loss, and follow-up audiograms are imperative so that hearing aids can be ordered if warranted. Nephrotoxicity can also be a problem during and following cisplatin therapy, and renal function studies should be monitored after the completion of therapy. Pulmonary fibrosis may result from bleomycin therapy, and pulmonary function studies should be done regularly in follow-up. Secondary malignancies including myeloid leukemias have been noted after treatment with chemotherapy, especially etoposide. Those who have undergone cranial radiation should receive regular neuropsychological testing. Screening of thyroid, corticotropin, gonadotropin, and growth hormone should also occur regularly following cranial radiation therapy.

2.11.10 Future Perspectives

The use of high-dose cisplatin has led to increased survival in patients with advanced malignant GCTs. Ototoxicity is a problem for these patients. Preliminary data from the recent POG study are disappointing regarding the effectiveness of amifostine to protect against significant ototoxicity. The formal development of risk groups is needed in order to stratify treatment. The role of carboplatin, ifosfamide, and topotecan may also be used to determine their utility in relapsed GCTs. Effective treatment for high-risk patients remains controversial. Future studies are currently being planned that incorporate new agents such as topotecan and paclitaxel.

2.12 Rare Tumors

There are numerous tumors that occur very infrequently in children and adolescents. Most of the rarely occurring neoplasms are those that are seen most often in the adult population. Several more commonly occurring rare tumors will be summarized here.

2.12.1 Adrenocortical Carcinoma (ACC)

Adrenocortical carcinoma is a very rare and aggressive tumor. It occurs more often in females and peaks in the first and fourth decades of life. The incidence of this tumor is very high in Brazil, 10–15 times that observed in the United States. There is a high incidence of Li-Fraumeni syndrome in the families of the children who acquire ACC. Germline mutations of the p53 gene are found in one-third of patients (Kock et al., 2002). Interestingly, in Brazil, children with ACC typically have p53 mutations but they are not germline. Cushing syndrome, reflecting hormonal excess, is a presenting sign of ACC in 68% of children (Plowman, 1997). Evidence of the development of secondary sex characteristics occurs as a presenting sign in 95% of patients younger than 5 (Kock et al., 2002). Other clinical signs are abdominal pain, fever, anorexia, and weight loss. In children, approximately 40% of patients secrete no active hormones, but their inactive steroid precursors such as pregnenolone, 11-deoxycortisone, and 17-hydroxypregnenolone can be found in blood and urine (Kock et al., 2002). ACC can present as localized disease but presents with regional spread to adjacent lymph nodes or the retroperitoneum 20% of the time. Distant metastases to lung and bone can also occur. Curative treatment depends on early wide total excision of the tumor while it is still encapsulated. Repeated surgeries are warranted if isolated recurrences occur. For patients without surgically curable disease, mitotane therapy is often initiated, which is meant to cause necrosis and disease regression while improving the endocrine system (Plowman, 1997). Chemotherapy agents such as fluorouracil, etoposide, doxorubicin, and cisplatin are also sometimes used. These approaches, although they may increase length of survival, are not usually curative. The prognosis is generally quite poor for ACC.

2.12.2 Melanoma

Melanoma accounts for 1.3% of childhood neoplasms; it represents the second most common carcinoma found in children (Rodriguez-Galindo and Pappo, 2003). There is a much higher incidence in whites compared with blacks and in females. Conditions that are associated with melanoma in children include congenital melanomas, giant congenital melanocytic nevi, xeroderma pigmentosum, immunosuppression, neurocutaneous melanosis, and mole phenotype (atypical moles) (Pratt and Pappo, 2002). Presenting signs may include a mole that has changed in size or color, accompanied by bleeding or itching, with a palpable subcutaneous mass or lymphadenopathy. Common sites are the trunk, head and neck. Metastases generally occur via regional lymph node spread prior to lung, bone, and brain. The American Joint Committee on Cancer staging system of melanoma takes into account tumor thickness, ulceration, nodal disease, and metastases (Balch et al., 2001). Children with thick melanoma >4 mm and those with lymphadenopathy should undergo imaging with CT and MRI to determine the presence of metastatic disease. Wide excision of the lesion is necessary for cure with adequate margins. Interoperative lymphatic mapping with sentinel node biopsy has been shown to be highly sensitive at identifying nodal disease and is usually done for lesions greater than 1 mm in thickness. Alpha interferon therapy has been used in high risk resected melanoma (Pratt and Pappo, 2002). In disseminated disease, agents such as vincristine, dactinomycin, cyclophosphamide, cisplatin, and etoposide, and interleukin 2 have been used with varying rates of success (Pratt and Pappo, 2002). Prognosis depends largely on tumor stage at diagnosis.

2.12.3 Nasopharyngeal Carcinoma

This tumor occurs in the epithelium of the nasopharynx, generally affecting males more often than females. There has been association of EBV infection with this tumor (Plowman, 1997). This tumor has three distinct subtypes, and children are usually affected by the undifferentiated type. It arises in the fossa of Rosenmuller and can spread via direct extension through the oropharynx to the base of the skull and result in cranial nerve palsies (Pratt and Pappo, 2002). The only clinical sign of this disease may be cervical lymphadenopathy, indicating regional metastases. Distant metastases are present in less than 5% of cases, and most common sites include lung and bone (Plowman, 1997). The tumor is staged as per the tumor, node, metastases (TNM) classification system. Surgery is often not possible for nasopharyngeal carcinoma because of its anatomical

location. Radiotherapy is the primary treatment modality. Adjuvant chemotherapy is often used in children, and the tumor shows response to agents such as fluorouracil, cisplatin, carboplatin, methotrexate, and bleomycin. Multiple researchers have noted survival rates to be 75% for T1 and T2 tumors, but only 37% for T3 and T4 tumors (Pratt and Pappo, 2002). Late effects of radiation such as xerostomia, muscle atrophy, fibrosis of the neck, and hypothyroidism may be some of the sequelae that affect this group of children.

2.12.4 Thyroid Carcinoma

Thyroid carcinoma is the most commonly occurring carcinoma in children (Rodriguez-Galindo and Pappo, 2003). It generally occurs more often in females, with a peak in incidence between ages 7 and 12. It is well established that neck irradiation is a causative factor in the development of thyroid carcinoma; however, it does also occur sporadically and is associated with some familial syndromes. Cervical adenopathy and thyroid nodules are often the presenting clinical signs; metastases generally occur in the lung and mediastinum. Twenty percent of patients have metastatic disease at diagnosis (Kock et al., 2002). The tumor is characterized by the secretion of T3 and sometimes T4. There are several different subtypes of thyroid carcinoma: papillary, follicular, and anaplastic (Kock et al. 2002). Imaging is generally done with ultrasound and thyroid scintiscan, and chest x-ray or CT is done to rule out lung metastases. A biopsy is needed to confirm malignancy and histology. Complete surgical resection (thyroidectomy) is the treatment of choice for thyroid carcinoma. Radioiodine therapy is used postoperatively if metastatic disease is present and also to ablate any residual functioning thyroid. Thyroid hormone needs to be supplemented in these patients. The prognosis for thyroid carcinoma is generally quite good, with overall survival in some reports approaching 90%, and metastatic disease does not necessarily impart a poor prognosis with the use of radioiodine therapy (Kock et al., 2002).

References

Alexander F (2000) Neuroblastoma. Urologic Clinics of North America 27 (3): 383–392.

Andrassy, RJ (2002) Advances in the surgical management of sarcomas in children. American Journal of Surgery 184 (6): 484–491.

Bacci G, Ferrari S, Lari S, Mercure M, Donati D, Longhi A, Forni C, Bertoni F, Versari M, Pignotti E (2002a) Osteosarcoma of the limb: Amputation or limb salvage in patients treated by neoadjuvant chemotherapy. Journal of Bone and Joint Surgery 84B (1): 88–92.

Bacci G, Ferrari S, Longhi A, Forni C, Zavatta M, Versari M, Smith K (2002b) High-grade osteosarcoma of the extremity: Differences between localized and metastatic tumors at presentation. Journal of Pediatric Hematology/Oncology 24(1): 27–3

Balch CM, Buzaid AC, Soong SJ, et al. (2001) Final version of the American joint committee on cancer staging system for cutaneous melanoma. Journal of Clinical Oncology 16 (16): 3635–3648.

Bataller L, Rosenfeld MR, Graus F, Vilchez JJ, Nai-Kong V, Cheung NV, Dalmau J (2003) Autoantigen diversity in the opsoclonus-myoclonus syndrome. Annals of Neurology 53: 347–353.

Beckwith JB (1998) Nephrogenic rests and the pathogenesis of Wilms' tumor: Developmental and clinical considerations. American Journal of Medical Genetics 79: 268–273.

Blakely ML, Ritchey ML (2001) controversies in the management of Wilms' tumor. Seminars in Pediatric Surgery 10(3): 127–31.

Breneman JC, Lyden E, Pappo AS, Link MP, Anderson JR, Parham DM, Qualman SJ, Wharam MD, Donaldson SS, Maurer HM, Meyer WH, Baker KS, Paidas CN, Crist WM (2003) Prognostic factors and clinical outcomes in children and adolescents with metastatic rhabdomyosarcoma: A report from the intergroup rhabdomyosarcoma study IV. Journal of Clinical Oncology 21(1): 78–84.

Brodeur GM (2003) Neuroblastoma: Biological Insights into a clinical enigma. Nature Reviews Cancer 3: 203–216.

Brodeur GM, Maris JM (2002) Neuroblastoma. In Pizzo PA and Poplack DG (eds) Principles and Practice of Pediatric Oncology (4th edn.). Philadelphia: Lippincott Williams & Wilkins.

Broecker B (2000) Non-Wilms' renal tumors in children. Urologic Clinics of North America 27 (3): 463–469.

Cairo MS, Perkins S (2000) Non-Hodgkin's lymphoma in children. In Bast RC, Kufe, DW, Pollock RE, Weichselbaum RR, Holland JF, Frei E (eds), Cancer Medicine (5th edn.). Hamilton: B.C. Decker.

Carli M, Guglielmi M, Sotti G, Cecchetto G, Ninfo V (1997) Soft tissue sarcomas. In Pinkerton CR, Plowman PN (eds), Paediatric Oncology Clinical Practice and Controversies (2nd edn.). London: Chapman and Hall.

Chan HSL, DeBoer F, Thiessen JJ, Budnig A, Kingston JE, O'Brien JM, Koren G, Giesbrecht E, Haddad G, Verjee Z, Hungerford JL, Ling V, Gallie BL (1996) combining cyclosporin with chemotherapy controls intraocular retinoblastoma without requiring radiation. Clinical Cancer Research 2: 1499–1508

Chauvenet A, Schwarz CL, Weiner MA (2000) Hodgkin's disease in children and adolescents. In Bast RC, Kufe, DW, Pollock RE, Weichselbaum RR, Holland JF, Frei E (eds), Cancer Medicine (5th edn.). Hamilton: B.C. Decker Inc.

Cheung NK, Kushner BH, Kramer K (2001) Monoclonal antibody-based therapy of neuroblastoma. Hematology Clinics of North America 15 (5): 853–866

Coffin CM, Dehner LP, O'Shea PA (1997) Pediatric Soft Tissue Tumors A Clinical Pathological and Therapeutic Approach Baltimore: Williams & Wilkins

Cushing B, Marina N (2000). Germ cell tumors. In Bast RC, Kufe, DW, Pollock RE, Weichselbaum RR, Holland JF, Frei E (eds), Cancer Medicine (5th edn.). Hamilton: B.C. Decker Inc.

Cushing B, Perlman EJ, Marina NM, Castleberry RP (2002). Germ cell tumors. In Pizzo PA and Poplack DG (eds), Principles and Practice of Pediatric Oncology (4th edn.). Philadelphia: Lippincott Williams & Wilkins.

Czauderna P, Mackinlay G, Perilongo G, Brown J, Shafford E, Aronson D, Pritchard J, Chapchap P, Keeling J, Plaschkes J, Otte JB (2002) Hepatocellular carcinoma in children: Results of the first prospective study of the international society of pediatric oncology group. Journal of Clinical Oncology 20 (12): 2798–2804.

Donaldson SS (2003) A discourse: The 2002 Wataru W. Sutow lecture Hodgkin disease in children – perspectives and progress. Medical Pediatric Oncology 40:73–81.

Donaldson SS, Hudson MM, Lamborn KR, Link MP, Kun L, Billett AL, Marcus KC, Hurwitz CA, Young JA, Tarbell NJ, Weinstein HJ (2002) VAMP and low-dose, involved field radiation for children and adolescents with favorable, early-stage Hodgkin's disease: Results of a prospective clinical trial. Journal of Clinical Oncology 20 (14): 3081–3087.

Douglass EC, Reynolds M, Finegold M, et al. (1993) Cisplatin vincristine and fluorouracil therapy for hepatoblastoma: a Pediatric Oncology Group study. Journal of Clinical Oncology 11:96–99.

Ferrari S, Briccoli A, Mercuri M, Bertoni F, Picci P, Tienghi A, Brach Del Prever A, Fagioli F, Comandone A, Bacci G (2003) Postrelapse survival in osteosarcoma of the extremities: Prognostic factors for long-term survival. Journal of Clinical Oncology 21 (4): 710–715.

Friedman DL, Himelsein V, Shields CL, Shields JA, Needle M, Miller DB, Bunin GR, Meadows A (2000) Chemoreduction and local ophthalmic therapy for intraocular retinoblastoma. Journal of Clinical Oncology 18 (1): 12–17.

Gallie BL, Budnig A, Deboer F, Thiessen JJ, Koren G, Verjee Z, Ling V, Chan HSL (1996) chemotherapy with focal therapy can cure intraocular retinoblastoma without radiotherapy. Archives of Ophthalmology 114: 13211328.

Gallie BL, Dunn JM, Chan HSL, Hamel PA, Phillips RA (1991) The genetics of retinoblastoma. Pediatric Clinics of North America 28 (2): 299–313.

Ginsberg JP, Woo SY, Johnson ME, Hicks MJ, Horowitz ME (2002) Ewing's sarcoma family of tumors: Ewing's sarcoma of bone and soft tissue and the peripheral primitive neuroectodermal tumors. In Pizzo PA and Poplack DG (eds), Principles and Practice of Pediatric Oncology (4th edn.). Philadelphia: Lippincott Williams & Wilkins.

Grundy PE, Green DM, Breslow NE, Ritchey ML, Perlman EJ, Macklis RM (2002) Renal tumors. In Pizzo PA and Poplack DG (eds), Principles and Practice of Pediatric Oncology (4th edn.). Philadelphia: Lippincott Williams & Wilkins.

Grundy PE, Green DM, Breslow NE, Ritchey ML, Thomas PRM (2000) Renal tumors of childhood. In Bast RC, Kufe, DW, Pollock RE, Weichselbaum RR, Holland JF, Frei E (eds), Cancer Medicine (5th edn.). Hamilton: B.C. Decker Inc.

Gurney JG, Severson RK, Davis S, Robinson LL (1995) Incidence of cancer in children in the United States. Cancer 75 (8): 2186–2195.

Gurney JG, Young JL, Roffers SD, et al. (1999) Soft tissue sarcomas. In: Gloeckler Ries LA, Smith MA, Gurney JG, et al., (eds.) SEER Pediatric Monograph: Cancer incidence and survival among children and adolescents, United States SEER program 1975-1995. Bethesda, MD: National Cancer Institute p. 111-124

Hawkins DS, Feigenhauer J, Park J, Kreissman S, Thomson B, Douglas J, Rowley SD, Gooley T, Sanders JE, Pendergrass TW (2002) Peripheral blood stem cell support reduces the toxicity of intensive chemotherapy for children and adolescents with metastatic sarcomas. Cancer 95 (6): 1354–1365.

Hudson MM, Donaldson SS. (2002) Hodgkin's disease. In Pizzo PA and Poplack DG (eds), Principles and Practice of Pediatric Oncology (4th edn.). Philadelphia: Lippincott Williams & Wilkins

Hurwitz Rl, Shields CL, Shields JA, Chevez-Barrios P, Hurwitz MY, Chintagumpala MM (2002) Retinoblastoma. In Pizzo PA and Poplack DG (eds), Principles and Practice of Pediatric Oncology (4th edn.). Philadelphia: Lippincott Williams & Wilkins

Indolfe P, Terenziani M, Casale F, Carli M, Bisogno G, Schiavetti A, Mancini A, Rondelli R, Pession A, Jenkner A, Pierani P, Tamaro P, De Bernardi B, Ferrari A, Santoro N, Giuliano M, Cecchetto G, Piva L, Surico G, Di Tullio, MT (2003) Renal cell carcinoma in children: A clinicopathologic study. Journal of Clinical Oncology 21 (3): 530–535

Jenkin RD, Al-Fawaz I, Al-Shabanah M, Allam A, Ayas A, Khafaga Y, Rifai,S, Schultz H, Memon M, Rifai S, Schultz H, Younge D (2002) Localized Ewing sarcoma/PNET of bone – prognostic factors and international data comparison. Medical and Pediatric Oncology 39 (6): 586–593

Jurgens H, Winkler K, Gobel U (1997). Bone tumours. In Pinkerton CR, Plowman PN (eds), Paediatric Oncology Clinical Practice and Controversies (2nd edn.). London: Chapman and Hall

Kaefer M, Rinck RC (2000) Genitourinary rhabdomyosarcoma: Treatment options. Urology Clinics of North America 27(3): 471–487

Kager L, Zoubek A, Potschger U, Kastner U, Flege S, Kempf-Bielack B, Branscheid D, Kotz R, Salzer-Kuntschik M, Winkelmann W, Jundt G, Kabisch H, Reichardt P, Jurgens H, Gadner H, Bielack SS (2003) Primary metastatic osteosarcoma: Presentation and outcome of patients treated on neoadjuvant cooperative osteosarcoma study group protocols. Journal of Clinical Oncology 21 (10): 2011–2018

Katzenstein HM, Krailo MD, Malogolowkin MH, Ortega JA, Liu-Mares W, Douglass EC, Feusner JH, Reynolds M, Quinn JJ, Newman K, Finegold MJ, Haas JE, Sensel MG, Castleberry RP, Bowman LC (2002a) Hepatocellular carcinoma in children and adolescents: Results from the pediatric oncology group and the children's cancer group intergroup study. Journal of Clinical Oncology 20 (12): 2789–2797

Katzenstein HM, London WB, Douglass EC, Reynolds M, Plaschkes J, Finegold MJ, Bowman LC (2002b) Treatment of unresectable and metastatic hepatoblastoma: A pediatric oncology group phase II study. Journal of Clinical Oncology 20 (16): 3438–3444

Knudson AG (2001) Two genetic hits (more or less) to cancer. Nature Reviews 1: 157–170

Kock CA, Pacak K, Chrousos GP (2002) Endocrine tumors. In Pizzo PA and Poplack DG (eds), Principles and Practice of Pediatric Oncology (4th edn.). Philadelphia: Lippincott Williams & Wilkins

Link MP, Gebhardt MC, Meyers PA (2002) Osteosarcoma. In Pizzo PA and Poplack DG (eds), Principles and Practice of Pediatric Oncology (4th edn.). Philadelphia: Lippincott Williams & Wilkins

MacArthur CA, Issacs H, Miller JH, et al. (1994) Pediatric renal cell carcinoma: A complete response to recombinant interleukin-2 in a child with metastatic disease at diagnosis. Medical and Pediatric Oncology 23: 365–371

Magrath IT (2002). Malignant non-Hodgkin's lymphoma in children. In Pizzo PA and Poplack DG (eds), Principles and Practice of Pediatric Oncology (4th edn.). Philadelphia: Lippincott Williams & Wilkins

Matthay KK, Yamashiro DJ (2000) Neuroblastoma. In Bast RC, Kufe, DW, Pollock RE, Weichselbaum RR, Holland JF, Frei E (eds), Cancer Medicine (5th edn.). Hamilton: B.C. Decker

McDowell HP (2003) Update on childhood rhabdomyosarcoma. Archives of Disease in Children 88 (4): 354–357

Metayer C, Lynch C,F, Clarke EA, Glimelius B, Storm H, Pukkala E, Joensuu T, van Leeuwen FE, van't Veer, MB, Curtis RE, Holowaty EJ, Andersson M, Wiklund T, Gospodarowicz M, Travis, LB (2000) Second cancers among long-term survivors of Hodgkin's diagnoses in childhood and adolescence. Journal of Clinical Oncology 18 (21): 2435-2443

Miser JS, Pappo AS, Triche TJ, Merchant TE, Rao BN (2002) Other Soft Tissue Sarcomas of Childhood. In Pizzo PA and Poplack DG (eds), Principles and Practice of Pediatric Oncology (4th edn.). Philadelphia: Lippincott Williams & Wilkins

Neville HL, Ritchey ML (2000) Wilms' tumor: Overview of national Wilms' tumor study group results Urologic Clinics of North America 27 (3): 435–442

Ninane J (1991) Chemotherapy for infantile fibrosarcoma. Medical Pediatric Oncology 19: 209

Ninane J, Pearson ADJ (1997) Neuroblastomas. In Pinkerton CR, Plowman PN (eds), Paediatric Oncology Clinical Practice and Controversies (2nd edn.). London: Chapman and Hall

Oberlin O, Deley MC, Bui BN, Gentet JC, Philip T, Terrier P, Carrie C, Mechinaud F, Schmitt C, Babin-Boillettot A, Michon J (2001) Prognostic factors in localized Ewing's tumours and peripheral neuroectodermal tumours: the third study of the French Society of Paediatric Oncology (EW88 study). British Journal of Cancer 85 (11): 1646–1654

Ortega JA, Krailo MD, Haas JE, et al. (1991) Effective treatment of unresectable or metastatic hepatoblastoma with cisplatin and continuous infusion doxorubicin chemotherapy: a report from the children's cancer study group. Journal of Clinical Oncology 9:2167–2176

Pang LM, Roebuck DJ, Griffith JF, Kumta SM, Metreweli C (2001) Alveolar soft-part sarcoma: a rare soft tissue malignancy with distinctive clinical and radiological features. Pediatric Radiology 31: 196–199

Pappo AS, Shapiro DN, Crist WM (1997) Rhabdomyosarcoma biology and treatment. Pediatric Clinics of North America 44 (4): 953–972.

Patte C (1997). Non-Hodgkin's lymphoma. In Pinkerton CR, Plowman PN (eds.), Paediatric Oncology Clinical Practice and Controversies (2nd edn.). London: Chapman and Hall Medical

Pinkerton CR (1997a) Malignant germ cell tumours in childhood. European Journal of Cancer 33 (6): 895–902

Pinkerton CR (1997b) Malignant germ cell tumours. In Pinkerton CR, Plowman PN (eds), Paediatric Oncology Clinical Practice and Controversies (2nd edn.). London: Chapman and Hall

Pinkerton CR, Michalski AJ, Veys PA, (eds) (1999) Clinical challenges in Paediatric Oncology. Oxford: ISIS Medical Media

Plowman PN (1997) Rare tumors. In Pinkerton CR, Plowman PN (eds), Paediatric Oncology Clinical Practice and Controversies (2nd edn.). London: Chapman and Hall

Pratt CB, Pappo AS (2002) Management of infrequent cancers of childhood. In Pizzo PA and Poplack DG (eds), Principles and Practice of Pediatric Oncology (4th edn.). Philadelphia: Lippincott Williams & Wilkins

Pritchard J, Brown J, Shafford E, et al. (2000) Cisplatin, doxorubicin, and delayed surgery for childhood hepatoblastoma: a successful approach – results of the first prospective study of the international society of pediatric oncology. Journal of Clinical Oncology 18:3810–3828

Pritchard-Jones K (2002) Controversies and advances in the management of Wilms' tumour. Archives of Disease in Children 87 (3): 241–244

Pritchard-Jones K, Mitchell CD (1997) The genetic basis of children's cancers. In Pinkerton CR, Plowman PN (eds), Paediatric Oncology Clinical Practice and Controversies (2nd edn.). London: Chapman and Hall

Pritchard-Jones K, Mitchell CD (1997) The genetic basis of children's cancers. In Pinkerton CR, Plowman PN (eds), Paediatric Oncology Clinical Practices and Controversies (2nd edn.). London: Chapman and Hall

Ragland BD, Bell WC, Lopez RR, Siegal GP (2002) Cytogenetic and molecular biology of osteosarcoma. Laboratory Investigation 82(4): 365–377

Rodriguez-Galindo C, Pappo AS (2003) Less-frequently encountered tumors of childhood. In Bast RC, Pollock RE, Weichselbaum RR, Gansler TS, Holland JF, Frei E (eds), Cancer Medicine (6th edn.). Hamilton: B.C. Decker

Rodriguez-Galindo C, Billups CA, Kun LE, Rao BN, Pratt CB, Merchant TE, Santana VM, Pappo, AS (2002a) Survival after recurrence of Ewing tumors: The St. Jude Children's research hospital experience, 1979–1999. Cancer 94 (2): 561–569

Rowland JM (2002) Hepatoblastoma: Assessment of criteria for histologic classification. Medical and Pediatric Oncology 39:478–483

Sandlund JT, Downing JR, Crist WM. (1996) Non-Hodgkin's lymphoma in childhood. New England Journal of Medicine 334:1238–1248

Saylors RL, Stine KC, Sullivan J, Bernstein M, Harris MB (1999) Cyclophosphamide plus topotecan in children with recurrent or refractory solid tumors: a Pediatric Oncology Group (POG) Phase II study [abstract]. Journal of Pediatric Hematology and Oncology 21: 332

Schleiermacher G, Peter M, Oberlin O, Philip T, Rubie H, Mechinaud F, Sommelet-Olive S, Landman-Parker J, Bours D, Michon J, Delattre O (2003) Increased risk of systemic relapses associated with bone marrow micrometastasis and circulating tumors cells in localized Ewing tumor. Journal of Clinical Oncology 21 (1): 85–91

Schwartz CL (2003) The management of Hodgkin's disease in the young child. Current Opinions In Pediatrics 15 (1): 10–16

Servodidio CA, Abramson DH, Romanella A (1991) Retinoblastoma. Cancer Nursing 14 (3): 117–123

Shafford EA, Pritchard-Jones, K (1997) Liver tumors. In Pinkerton CR, Plowman PN (eds), Paediatric Oncology Clinical Practice and Controversies (2nd edn.). London: Chapman and Hall

Shimada H, Ambros IM, Dehner LP, Hata J, Joshi VV, Roald B, Stram DO, Gerbing RB, Lukens JN, Matthay KK, Castleberry RP(1999) The International Neuroblastoma Pathology Classification (the Shimada system). Cancer 86(2):364–72

Shimada H, Chatten J, Newton WA Jr, et al. (1984) Histopathologic prognostic factors in neuroblastic tumors: definition of subtypes of ganglioneuroblastoma and an age-linked classification of neuroblastomas. Journal of the National Cancer Institute 73: 405–413

Sklar C, Whitton J, Mertens A, Stovall M, Green D, Marina N, Greffe B, Wolden S, Robinson L (2000) Abnormalities of the thyroid in survivors of Hodgkin's disease: Data from the childhood cancer survivor study. Journal of Clinical Endocrinology and Metabolism 85 (9): 3227–3232

Smith RS, Chen Q, Hudson MM, Link MP, Kun L, Weinstein H, Billett A, Marcus KJ, Tarbell NJ, Donaldson SS (2003) Prognostic factors for children with Hodgkin's disease treated with combined-modality therapy. Journal of Clinical Oncology 21 (10): 2026–2033

Sorensen PHB, Lynch JC, Qualman SJ, Tirabosco R, Lim JF, Maurer HM, Bridge JA, Crist WM, Triche TJ, Barr FG (2002) PAX3-FKHR and PAX7-FKHR gene fusions are prognostic indicators in alveolar rhabdomyosarcoma: A report from the children's oncology group. Journal of Clinical Oncology 20 (11): 2672–2679

Spunt SL, Hill DA, Motosue AM, Billups CA, Cain AM, Rao BN, Pratt CB, Merchant TE, Pappo, AS (2002) Clinical features and outcome of initially unresected nonmetastatic pediatric nonrhabdomyotous soft tissue sarcoma. Journal of Clinical Oncology 20 (15): 3225–3235

Spunt SL, Poquette CA, Hurt YS, Cain AM, Rao BN, Merchant TE, Jenkins JJ, Santana VM, Pratt CB, Pappo AS (1999) Prognostic factors for children and adolescents with surgically resected nonrhabdomyosarcoma soft tissue sarcoma: An analysis of 121 patients treated at St Jude children's research hospital. Journal of Clinical Oncology 17 (12): 3697–3705

Stocker JT (2001) Liver tumors: Hepatic tumors in children. Clinics in Liver Disease 5 (1): 259–281

Suriawinata AA, Thung SN (2002) Malignant liver tumors. Clinics in Liver Disease 6 (2): 527–554

Swanson PE, Dehner LP (1991) Pathology of soft tissue sarcomas in children and adolescents. In Maurer HM, Ruymann FB, Pochedly C (eds), Rhabdomyosarcoma and Related Tumors in Children and Adolescents Florida: CRC Press

Tomioka N, Kobayashi H, Kageyama H, Ohira M, Nakamura Y, Sasaki F, Todo S, Nakagawara A, Kaneko Y (2003) Chromosomes that show partial loss or gain in near-diploid tumors coincide with chromosomes that show whole loss or gain in near-triploid tumors: Evidence suggesting the involvement of the same genes in the tumorigenesis of high- and low-risk neuroblastomas. Genes, Chromosomes and Cancer 36: 139–150

Tomlinson GE, Finegold MJ (2002) Tumors of the liver. In Pizzo PA and Poplack DG (eds), Principles and Practice of Pediatric Oncology (4th edn.). Philadelphia: Lippincott Williams & Wilkins

Venkateswaran L, Rodriguez-Galindo C, Merchant TE, Poquette CA, Bhaskar NR, Rao BN, Pappo AS (2001) Primary Ewing tumor of the vertebrae: clinical characteristics, prognostic factors, and outcome. Medical and Pediatric Oncology 37: 30–35

VonSchweinitz D, Byrd DJ, Hecker H, et al. (1997) Efficiency and toxicity of ifosfamide, cisplatin and doxorubicin in the treatment of childhood hepatoblastoma. European Journal of Cancer 33:1243–1249

Wexler LH, Crist WM, Helman LJ (2002) Rhabdomyosarcoma and the undifferentiated sarcomas In Pizzo PA and Poplack DG (eds), Principles and Practice of Pediatric Oncology (4th edn.). Philadelphia: Lippincott Williams & Wilkins

Wittig JC, Bickels J, Priebat D, Jelinek J, Kellar-Graney K, Shmookler B (2002) Osteosarcoma: A multidisciplinary approach to diagnosis and treatment. American Family Physician 65 (6): 1123–1132, 1135–1136

Yunis JJ, Ramsay N (1978) Retinoblastoma and subband deletion of chromosome 13. American Journal of Diseases of Children 132 (2): 161–163

Bibliography

Abramson DH, Frank CM, Susman M, Whalen MP, Dunkel IJ, Boyd NW (1998) Presenting signs of retinoblastoma. Journal of Pediatrics 132 (3): 505–508.

Abu-Ghosh AM, Krailo MD, Goldman SC, Slack RS, Davenport V, Morris E, Laver JH, Reaman GH, Cairo MS (2002) Ifosfamide, carboplatin and etoposide in children with poor-risk relapsed Wilms' tumor: a children's cancer group report. Annals of Oncology 13 (3): 460–469.

Alexander J, Fizazi K, Mahe C, Culine S, Droz JP, Theodore C, Terrier-Lacombe MJ (2001) Stage I non-seminomatous germ-cell tumours of the testis: identification of a subgroup of patients with a very low risk of relapse. European Journal of Cancer 37: 576–582.

Brichard B, De Bruycker JJ, De Potter P, Neven B, Vermylen C, Cornu G. (2002) Combined chemotherapy and local treatment in the management of intraocular retinoblastoma. Medical and Pediatric Oncology 38: 411–415.

Bussey KJ, Lawce HJ, Olson SB, Arthur DC, Kalousek DK, Krailo M, Giller R, Heifetz S, Womer R, Magenis RE (1999) Chromosome abnormalities of eighty-one pediatric germ cell tumors: Sex-, age-, site-, and histopathologic-related differences – a Children's Cancer Group Study. Genes, Chromosomes and Cancer 25: 134–146.

Carli M, Pinkerton R, Franscella E, et al. (1995) Metastatic soft-tissue sarcomas in children: preliminary results of the second European International group study (EIS). Medical Pediatric Oncology 25 (4): 256.

De Wit R, Roberts JT, Wilkinson PM, de Mulder PHM, Mead GM, Fossa SD, Cook P, de Prijck L, Stenning S, Collette L (2001) Equivalence of three or four cycles of bleomycin, etoposide and cisplatin chemotherapy and of 3- or 5-day schedule in good-prognosis form cell cancer: A randomized study of the European organization for research and treatment of cancer genitourinary tract cancer cooperative group and the medical research council. Journal of Clinical Oncology 19 (6): 1629–1640.

Franzius C, Bielack S, Glege S, Sciuk J, Jurgens H, Schober O (2002) Prognostic significance of 18F-FDG and 99mTc-Methylene diphosphonate uptake in primary osteosarcoma. Journal of Nuclear Medicine43 (8): 1012–1017.

Gobel U, Schneider DT, Calaminus G, Haas RJ, Schmidt P, Harms D (2000) Germ-cell tumors in childhood and adolescence. Annals of Oncology 11:263–271.

Goorin AM, Harris MB, Bernstein M, Ferguson W, Devidas M, Siegal GP, Gebhardt MC, Schwartz, CL, Link M, Grier HE (2002) Phase II/III Trial of etoposide and high-dose ifosfamide in newly diagnosed metastatic osteosarcoma: A pediatric oncology group trial. Journal of Clinical Oncology20 (2): 426–433.

Grier HE, Krailo MD, Tarbell NJ, Link MP, Fryer JH, Pritchard DJ, Gebhardt MC, Dickman PS, Perlman EJ, Meyers PA, Donaldson SS, Moore S, Rausen AR, Vietti TJ, Miser JS (2003) Addition of ifosfamide and etoposide to standard chemotherapy for Ewing sarcoma and primitive neuroectodermal tumor of bone. New England Journal of Medicine 348 (8): 694–701.

Guillermo C, Fandino A, Casak S, Manzitti J, Raslawski E, Schvartzman E (2003) Treatment of overt extraocular retinoblastoma. Medical Pediatric Oncology 40:158–161.

Honavar SG, Singh AD, Shields CL, Meadows AT, Demici H, Cater J, Shields JA (2002) Postenucleation adjuvant therapy in high-risk retinoblastoma. Archives in Ophthalmology 120:923–931

Kullendorff CM, Soller M, Wiebe T, Mertens F (2003) Cytogenetic findings and clinical course in consecutive series of Wilms' tumors. Cancer Genetics and Cytogenetics 140: 82–87

Malogolowkin MH (2000) Hepatic tumors. In Bast RC, Kufe, DW, Pollock RE, Weichselbaum RR, Holland JF, Frei E (eds), Cancer Medicine (5th edn.). Hamilton: B.C. Decker

McLorie G (2001) Wilms' tumor. Current Opinion in Urology 11 (6): 567–570

Pinkerton CR (1999) Hodgkin's disease. In Pinkerton CR, Michalski AJ, Veys PA, Clinical Challenges in Paediatric Oncology. Oxford: ISIS Medical Media.

Pinkerton CR (1999) Osteogenic sarcoma. In Pinkerton CR, Michalski AJ, Veys PA, (eds), Clinical challenges in Paediatric Oncology. Oxford: ISIS Medical Media.

Pinkerton, CR (1999) Hepatoblastoma and hepatocellular carcinoma. In Pinkerton CR, Michalski AJ, Veys PA, (eds), Clinical challenges in Paediatric Oncology. Oxford: ISIS Medical Media.

Pinkerton, CR (1999) Neuroblastoma. In Pinkerton CR, Michalski AJ, Veys PA, (eds), Clinical Challenges in Paediatric Oncology. Oxford: ISIS Medical Media.

Pinkerton, CR (1999) Non Hodgkin's Lymphoma. In Pinkerton CR, Michalski AJ, Veys PA, (eds), Clinical challenges in Paediatric Oncology. Oxford: ISIS Medical Media.

Pinkerton, CR (1999) Retinoblastoma. In Pinkerton CR, Michalski AJ, Veys PA, (eds), Clinical Challenges in Paediatric Oncology. Oxford: ISIS Medical Media.

Pinkerton, CR (1999) Wilms' Tumor. In Pinkerton CR, Michalski AJ, Veys PA, (eds), Clinical challenges in Paediatric Oncology. Oxford: ISIS Medical Media.

Pinkerton, CR (1999). Ewing Sarcoma/primitive neuro-ectodermal tumor. In Pinkerton CR, Michalski AJ, Veys PA, (eds). Clinical challenges in Paediatric Oncology. Oxford: ISIS Medical Media.

Pinkerton, CR (1999). Rhabdomyosarcoma. In Pinkerton CR, Michalski AJ, Veys PA, (eds), Clinical Challenges in Paediatric Oncology. Oxford: ISIS Medical Media.

Reynolds CP, Lemons RS (2001) Retinoid therapy of childhood cancer. Hematology Oncology Clinics of North America 15 (5): 867–910

Rodriguez-Galindo C, Daw NC, Kaste SC, Neyer WH, Dome JS, Pappo, AS, Rao BN, Pratt CB (2002b) Treatment of refractory osteosarcoma with fractionated cyclophosphamide and etoposide. Journal of Pediatric Hematology/Oncology 24 (4): 250–254

Rodriguez-Galindo, C, Wilson MW, Haik BG, Merchant TE, Billups CA, Shah N, Cain A, Langston, Lipson M, Kun LE, Pratt C (2003) Treatment of intraocular retinoblastoma with vincristine and carboplatin. Journal of Clinical Oncology 21 (10): 2019–2025

Rosti F, De Friorgi U, Salvioni R, Papiani F, Sebastiani L, Argnani M, Monti G, Ferrante P, Pizzocaro F, Marangolo M (2002) Salvage high-dose chemotherapy in patients with germ cell tumors. Cancer 95 (2): 309–315

Schleiermacher G, Peter M, Oberlin O, Philip T, Rubie H, Mechinaud F, Sommelet-Olive S, Landman-Parker J, Bours D, Michon J, Delattre O (2003) Increased risk of systemic relapses associated with bone marrow micrometastasis and circulating tumors cells in localized Ewing tumor. Journal of Clinical Oncology 21 (1): 85–91

Shankar AG, Ashley S, Craft AW, Pinkerton CR (2003) Outcome after relapse in an unselected cohort of children and adolescents with Ewing sarcoma. Medical and Pediatric Oncology 40: 141–147

Shields, CL, Honavar SG, Meadows AT, Shields JA, Demirci J, Singh A, Friedman DL, Naduvilath TJ (2002) Chemoreduction plus focal therapy for retinoblastoma: Factors predictive of need for treatment with external beam radiotherapy or enucleation. American Journal of Ophthalmology 133 (5): 657–664

Shields, CL, Honaver SG, Meadows AT, Shields JA, Demirci J, Singh A, Naduvilath TJ (2002) Chemoreduction for unilateral retinoblastoma. Archives of Ophthalmology 120: 1653–1658

Treuner J, Jurgens H, Winkler K (1987) The treatment of 30 children and adolescents of synovial sarcoma in accordance with the protocol of the German Multicenter Study for soft tissue sarcoma. Proceedings of the American Society of Clinical Oncology 6: 215

Uusitalo M, Wheeler S, O'Brien JM (1999) Ocular Oncology: New approaches in the clinical management of retinoblastoma. Ophthalmology Clinics of North America 12 (2) 255–264

Zimmerman A (2002) Pediatric liver tumors and hepatic ontogenesis: Common and distinctive pathways. Medical and Pediatric Oncology 39: 492–503

Common Central Nervous System Tumors

Nicki Fitzmaurice · Sharon Beardsmore

Contents

Primary brain tumors occur in all age groups but are significantly more frequent in children and adolescents under 15 years old (Turini and Redaelli, 2001). In the United States, central nervous system (CNS) tumors are now the most common malignancy of childhood (Copeland et al., 1999); in the United Kingdom (UK), however, leukaemias are still more prevalent, with paediatric brain tumors continuing to be the most common solid tumor and the most common cause of death from childhood cancer (Bouffet, 2000). They account for 25% of all children's cancers, and around 300 children are diagnosed each year in the UK (CancerBACUP, 2002). In comparison with most other childhood cancers, there have been only moderate improvements in survival rates for children with brain tumors in the past 20 years. Mortality in this group of patients is high, with five-year survival estimated at 50% (CancerBACUP, 2002). Treatment options typically involve a surgical approach, radiotherapy, and chemotherapy, applied in isolation or in various combinations or sequences.

Improvements in imaging, neurosurgical techniques, the delivery of radiotherapy, and the inclusion of chemotherapy in treatment regimens have been reflected in improved survival for some specific histological types of tumors, i.e. cerebella medulloblastoma (Radcliffe et al., 1994). However, there remain major challenges unique to the paediatric arena for those involved in planning and delivering treatment strategies. Aggressive, invasive techniques involving an often immature brain are much more likely to result in devastating late effects, with morbidity estimated at 50% (Macedoni-Luksic et al., 2003). In recognition of this, practitioners have now been undertaking more rigorous appraisal of treatment modalities and the potential risks of cognitive, neuroendocrine, and neuropsychological damage (Plowman and Pearson, 1997)

3.1 Causes/Epidemiology

The cause of childhood brain tumors remains largely unknown, although there is correlation with a family history of cancer, and heredity factors have been implicated. Children with neurofibromatosis, for example, have an increased risk of developing optic gliomas.

Environmental factors such as electric and magnetic fields, radio frequency radiation, chemicals, and mobile phones have all been suggested in the development of brain tumors. There remains, however, insufficient evidence to support these claims. Ionising radiation is a known cause of brain tumors, with secondary local malignancies being a small but significant side effect of cranial radiotherapy (Kheifets, 2003).

3.2 Distribution/Classification

Approximately 60% of childhood brain tumors are infratentorial, including medulloblastoma, cerebellar astrocytoma (WHO grades I–IV), brain stem glioma, and ependymoma (Bouffet, 2000). The remaining supratentorial tumors include low-grade astrocytomas, primitive neuroectodermal tumors, germ cell tumors, hypothalamic and optic nerve gliomas, and craniopharyngiomas.

The most common tumors overall are low-grade gliomas, with cerebellar astrocytomas being the largest of this group. Amongst paediatric malignant brain tumors, medulloblastomas occur most frequently. (See Table 3.1.)

Classification of paediatric brain tumors (shown in Table 3.2) can, however, be misleading, as even the most low-grade tumor may have devastating effects because of the nature of its location. It is therefore often unhelpful to use terms such as benign and malignant to describe specific tumors.

Table 3.1. Incidence of most common brain tumors (Bouffet, 2000)

Tumor	Percentage
Low-grade gliomas	25–40%
High-grade gliomas	5–10%
Brain stem gliomas	8–12%
Medulloblastomas	6–20%
Ependymomas	6–11%
Germ cell tumors	3–15%
Craniopharyngiomas	6–15%

Table 3.2. Classification of paediatric brain tumors (Plowman and Pearson, 1997)

Glial tumors

Astrocytoma	Well differentiated cystic cerebellar with mural node Protoplasmic/fibrillary/pilocytic/gemistocytic Intermediate Anaplastic → (glioblastoma multiforme)
Ependymoma	Well-differentiated Intermediate to poorly differentiated
Oligodendroglioma	Well-differentiated Intermediate to poorly differentiated

Mixed gliomas (may include areas with neuroectodermal features)

Neuroectodermal tumors
Medulloblastomas
Other CNS neuroectodermal tumors (PNETs)
Pineoblastoma
Pineocytoma

Germ cell tumors
Other primary CNS germ cell tumors (other sites usually midline third to fourth ventricles)
Craniopharyngioma
Pituitary tumor
Choroid plexus tumors (cyst/papilloma/undifferentiated or carcinoma)
Meningioma
Others

3.3 Staging

Staging remains contentious within neuro-oncology with little consensus regarding universal staging systems. The tumor group however, that does utilise a staging process that has prognostic implication is medulloblastoma. Here the Chang operative system is employed (Laurent et al., 1985). For other tumors, histological grade, age, site of disease, and areas of dissemination are the main prognostic factors.

3.4 Molecular Genetics of Brain Tumors

In contrast to other childhood cancers, the molecular genetics of childhood brain tumors are poorly understood, not only in terms of the pathophysiology but also in terms of the characterisation of tumor-specific molecular abnormalities that predict biologically favourable or unfavourable disease. The latter is particularly important in brain tumors because such knowledge may allow a more judicious use of current therapies such as radiotherapy and may also identify molecular targets against which new therapies can be directed. Mutations of chromosome 17 have been associated with medulloblastoma, and mutations of chromosome 10 associated with astrocytoma. Genetic abnormalities are currently used to predict biological behaviour in neuroblastoma and rhabdomyosarcoma. Similar biologicals of tumor behaviour are now required if we are to improve the movements of childhood brain tumors.

3.5 Diagnosis

Diagnosing the presence of a brain tumor may be difficult. Diagnosis is often complicated by a vague history of symptoms that the parents, general practitioner, or local paediatrician may have attributed to common childhood illnesses. Children who have a long insidious history of symptoms are more likely to have a lower-grade tumor. Those who present with a short history and obvious symptoms are much more likely to have biologically aggressive disease. Clearly

Table 3.3. Sites of tumors in relation to histology (adapted from Plowman and Pearson, 1997)

Tumor site	Most common histological types of tumors
Cerebellum	Astrocytoma Ependymoma Medulloblastoma/PNET
Brain Stem	Astrocytoma
Hypothalmic/pineal4	Astrocytoma PNET NGGCT Teratoma Dysgerminoma
Supratentorial	Astrocytoma PNET Ependymoma

the site (see Table 3.3), severity of disease, and the child's age and development will have an impact on presenting symptoms. For example, those children with posterior fossa disease often have signs of increased intracranial pressure (ICP):

- Headaches
- Early morning vomiting
- Blurred vision
- Ataxia
- Poor concentration
- Changes in vital signs (late sign)

Children with supratentorial tumors, however, are more likely to present with hemiparesis, hemisensory loss, and/or seizures. Table 3.4 outlines the symptoms and treatment of common CNS tumors in relation to the primary site.

Once the child has presented to a specialist paediatrician, the existence of a brain lesion will generally be confirmed via a thorough neurological examination that includes fundoscopy and a visual assessment, followed by magnetic resonance imaging (MRI) of the head and spine. If the presence of an intracranial germ cell tumor is suspected, serum and cerebrospinal (CSF) levels of alpha-fetoprotein (AFP) and human chorionic gonadotropin (HCG) must be

Table 3.4. Symptoms and treatment of CNS tumors in relation to primary site (adapted from Shiminski-Maher and Shields, 1995)

Site	Tumor	Symptoms	Treatment
Supratentorial	Low-grade astrocytoma	Seizures	With gross total resection: surgical removal and observation
		Visual changes	Partial resection: surgical removal and either observation, radiation[a] or chemotherapy
		Endocrinopathies	
		Hemiparesis	
	High-grade glioma/PNET	Seizures	Maximal surgical resection and radiation[a] and/or chemotherapy
		Increased ICP	
		Mental status change	
		Hemiparesis	
Midline	Optic nerve Chiasmal gliomas	Visual disturbances	Observation
		Endocrinopathies	Surgical debulking, radiation, and /or chemotherapy
		Increased ICP	Treatment is age-dependant and related to site of tumor
		Seizures	
	Craniopharyngiomas	Seizures	Gross total resection: observation
		Visual disturbances	Partial resection: observation or radiation[a]
		Increased ICP	
		Endocrinopathies	
Infratentorial/ posterior fossa		Medulloblastoma	Increased ICP Maximal surgical resection and cranial spinal radiation[a] and chemotherapy
		Headache	
		Morning vomiting	
		Cranial nerve deficits	
		Ataxia	
	Ependymoma	Neck pain	Maximal surgical resection and radiation[a] ± chemotherapy
		Increased ICP	
		Cranial nerve deficits	
	Brain stem glioma	Cranial nerve deficits	Malignant tumors diagnosed by MRI requiring radiation ± chemotherapy
		Increased ICP	
		Hemiparesis	
		Usually short history	
		Long history/minimal symptoms/focal lesion on MRI	Low-grade tumor, surgical debulking, and observation or radiation ± chemotherapy

[a] Irradiation should be avoided when possible for children <5 years old

measured. This possibility should be considered in all suprasellar and pineal region tumors. For those tumors with potential to seed along the CSF pathway, CSF cytology should be undertaken at diagnosis or postoperatively.

With some tumors that are impossible to remove, it may be possible to perform stereotactic biopsy to confirm the diagnosis in order to plan treatment.

Figure 3.1

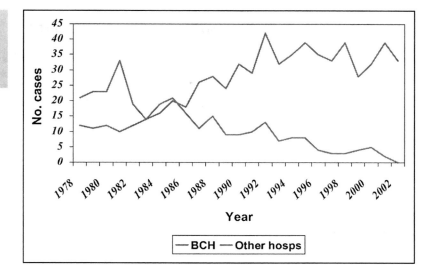

Figure 3.1

West Midlands brain tumor referrals 1978–2002 (permission to reprint given by Birmingham Children's Hospital, UK)

3.6 Specialist Referral

Whilst other childhood tumors have routinely been referred to specialist paediatric oncology centres since the 1970s, many children with brain tumors continued to receive treatment outside of specialist units. This practice resulted in less than 40% being treated within clinical trials until after 1997 (UKCC-SG/SBNS, 1997), when a joint report recommended the centralisation of care for children with brain and spinal disease. Fig. 3.1 demonstrates how the trend has changed in a local region.

3.7 Hydrocephalus

A significant number of children with brain tumors will develop associated hydrocephalus. Noncommunicating hydrocephalus is most commonly seen in paediatric brain tumors and is a result of mass effect. For some children this will present as a surgical emergency around the time of diagnosis, requiring immediate management. The most likely symptoms are headache, early morning vomiting, nausea, and ataxia. The management of hydrocephalus requires the input of a paediatric neurosurgeon with several options available. Debulking or removal of the tumor

may be sufficient to relieve the obstruction and allow normal flow of CSF. Other options are high-dose steroids preoperatively, external ventricular drainage, ventriculoperitoneal (VP) shunting, and ventriculostomy.

For those children with VP shunts, potential complications require consideration. Shunt malformation, infection, and, although rare, tumor dissemination should be taken into account when assessing a child who is unwell. Children may experience problems with their shunts during treatment, during periods of good health, and, should they require it, during palliative care.

3.8 Treatment

It is now widely accepted that the best practice for diagnosing, treating, and managing childhood CNS tumors is through a broad-based multidisciplinary team. Such a team includes the collaboration of paediatric neurosurgeons, oncologists, endocrinologists, psychologists, radiotherapists, social workers, and play, physio-, and occupational therapists. Coordinating these services should be a dedicated neuro-oncology nurse specialist. Nursing children with brain tumors is considered more complex and challenging than generic paediatric oncology, with this patient group often being labelled as the "undesirables" within the discipline (Ryan and Shiminski-Maher, 1995).

Treatment options typically involve surgical removal, radiotherapy, and chemotherapy, applied in isolation or in various combinations or sequences. Tumor type, the extent of disease, the degree of surgical resection, and the individual child will all have an impact on the choice of treatment modality.

3.8.1 Surgery

Primary surgery remains the mainstay of management for paediatric brain tumors. Depending upon the site and extent of the tumor, surgical options range from biopsy alone to complete removal. For most malignant tumors, complete resection is an important surgical goal. There is, however, a balance to be struck between complete excision and the risk of surgical morbidity. For some tumor types, complete surgical excision seems to be of particular prognostic importance (Sutton et al., 1990), i.e. ependymoma medulloblastoma. But in some instances, such as optic nerve gliomas and diffuse brain stem gliomas, surgical excision has little role to play in tumor management.

In other germ cell tumors, chemotherapy now has a primary role, and the indications for surgery are more circumspect (Nicholson et al., 2003).

Increasingly, second-look surgery is an option when it is evident from imaging that excisable tumor remains. Clearly, the surgeon must measure the potential damage to vital structures against the benefits of removing maximum tumor. Debulking alone, however, may relieve local compression and improve the child's symptoms while histology is sought and other treatment modalities are explored.

3.8.2 Radiotherapy

A significant number of children with brain tumors will require radiotherapy, which aims to deliver optimal doses of radiation to tumor cells while sparing surrounding normal tissue.

Conventional Radiotherapy

- 2 cm margin
- Parallel opposed
- Total dose 5055 Gy
- (craniospinal 2535 Gy with boost to tumor bed up to a total of 5055 Gy)

Despite precise planning and delivery of treatment, radiotherapy remains associated with significant long-term sequelae that may lead to significant impairment of quality of life. These sequelae are particularly profound following whole brain treatment and irradiation of pre-school-age children. Internationally, neuro-oncologists recognise the detrimental effects of radiotherapy on the developing brain and have advocated delaying radiation treatment in infants and young children whenever possible (Plowman and Pearson, 1997).

An added complication for young children is their inability to remain still during the delivery of radiotherapy, necessitating the use of daily anaesthetics to ensure dose accuracy. The prolonged use of anaesthetics in an already sick child is not ideal, but it is unavoidable for infants. Every effort should be made via play preparation to obviate the need for anaesthesia

Dose reductions and modified fractionations, to limit the toxicity of craniospinal irradiation, are features of recent investigation

Techniques that have been used to increase the therapeutic index (the tumor to normal tissue dose) include

- Stereotactic radiotherapy
- Brachytherapy
- Radiosurgery

The use of hyperfractionated radiotherapy in medulloblastoma is currently being evaluated in Europe through the SIOP IV trial.

Figure 3.2

BCH brain tumors: cumulative survival 19702002 (permission to reprint given by Birmingham Children's Hospital, UK)

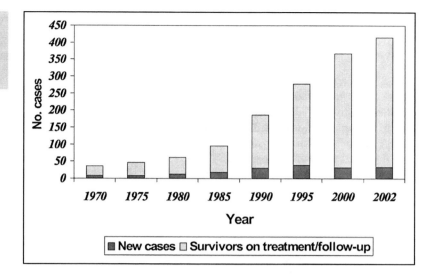

The use of conformal radiotherapy is a subject of on-going debate. Although this type of treatment spares normal brain tissue, an important goal, there is concern that relapse at the margin of the radiotherapy field may increase.

3.8.3 Chemotherapy

The administration of chemotherapy agents to children with brain tumors is a comparatively new treatment development. Until recently, chemotherapy has been considered of little benefit due to the existence of the blood-brain barrier. Recently, however, having established that various degrees of disruption of the blood-brain barrier exist in brain tumors, there has been renewed interest in its role. Significant prejudice did exist regarding the role of chemotherapy and the chemosensitivity of different types of brain tumor, exacerbated by the existence of few randomised and poorly designed trials evaluating the benefits of drug therapy. Chemotherapy is, however, now considered a valuable treatment modality as part of the prospective treatment package facilitating cure. Furthermore, there is now emerging evidence suggesting that chemotherapy is effective in paediatric brain tumor treatment (Taylor, 2002.)

For example, chemotherapy is advantageous in treating those children under 5 years of age who, if diagnosed later in life, would have radiotherapy as a first-line treatment. Multiagent regimens can delay or even obviate the need for radiotherapy and its associated late effects. Likewise, stabilisation of an incompletely resected tumor can be achieved by the use of chemotherapy, allowing second-look surgery.

In addition to management with conventional chemotherapy regimens, children with brain tumors, high-grade gliomas, and medulloblastomas are now being treated with high-dose chemotherapy with stem cell rescue. Intensifying treatment is thought to improve the permeability of the blood-brain barrier, and its role continues to be debated.

3.9 Prognosis

It is prudent to be wary when discussing survival figures. Percentage figures quoted to families can be misleading because they are often based on the evaluation of treatment strategies that lag behind current practice. Fig. 3.2 demonstrates cumulative survival seen at Birmingham Children's Hospital (BCH), UK.

3.10 Specific Tumors

3.10.1 PNETs/Medulloblastomas

Undifferentiated neuroectodermal tumors of the cerebellum have historically been referred to as medulloblastomas, while tumors of identical histology in the pineal region are diagnosed as pineoblastomas, and cerebral tumors are referred to as primitive neuroectodermal tumors (PNETs). Microscopically, both medulloblastomas and PNETs consist of small round cells with disproportionately large hyperchromatic nuclei. These cells are often clustered into rosettes.

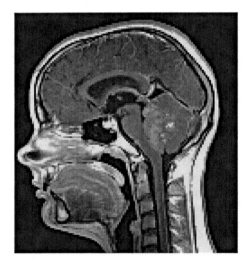

Age at diagnosis   15
Diagnosis   Medulloblastoma
Presenting symptoms   3-4 week of double
                          vision and dizziness
                          Early morning vomiti
                          Reduced conscious level.

Figure 3.3
Craniospinal imaging of medulloblastoma

Medulloblastoma

Epidemiology
- 25 % of paediatric brain tumors
- Most common between 3 and 7 years and in males
- Arises from primitive neuroepithelial cells

Etiology
- Commonly arises in cerebellar vermis
- Invades fourth ventricle with associated hydrocephalus
- Can disseminate via the CSF

Symptoms
- Headache
- Morning vomiting
- Cranial nerve defits
- Ataxia

Diagnostics
- Craniospinal imaging (Fig. 3.3)
- CSF analysis for free-floating tumor cells
- Bone scan and bone marrow aspiration to detect metastatic spread
- Standard risk: >5 years of age
  - Normal risk: >3 years of age
  - Posterior fossa location
  - Total resection or<1.5 cc of residual disease
  - No dissemination
  - Poor risk: <3 years of age
  - Metastatic disease
  - Subtotal resection
    (>1.5 cc of residual disease)
  - Non-posterior fossa location
    (Laurent et al., 1985)

Treatment
- Primary surgery: gross total excision optimal
- Craniospinal radiotherapy + boost to the primary tumor site (optimal dose and mode of administration under investigation) ± chemotherapy
- Children under 5: chemotherapy
- National treatment strategies predominantly seeking to reduce irradiation

Medulloblastoma (continued)

Prognosis
- Nonmetastatic disease: 70 80 % overall survival
- Metastatic disease: trials with craniospinal radiotherapy, high-dose chemotherapy, and stem cell rescue are currently being evaluated

Supratentorial PNETs

These are the supratentorial counterpart of medulloblastoma, having the same histological appearance

- Occur mainly <5 years of age
- The majority arise in the cerebral hemispheres/pineal region
- Treatment considerations are similar to medulloblastoma, with survival being lower

Prognosis
Age-related:

- <3 years: Very poor
- 3 years: Site-dependent

3.10.2 Astrocytomas/Glial Tumors

The majority of these tumors are supratentorial and slow-growing and are referred to as low-grade astrocytomas, pilocytic astrocytomas, oligodendrogliomas, mixed gliomas, or gangliogliomas (Shiminski-Maher and Shields, 1995). Less common are malignant gliomas of the supratentorium, i.e. anaplastic astrocytomas and glioblastoma multiforme.

The Kernohan grading system incorporates grade I to grade IV, with I being favourable histology and grade IV being glioblastoma multiforme that carries a fatal outcome.

Anaplastic astrocytomas are histologically recognisable by more frequent mitosis, cellular pleomorphism, and general cellularity of the tumor. Glioblastoma multiforme is diagnosed when areas of necrosis and peculiar cells forms are present.

Cerebellar Astrocytoma

Epidemiology
- Commonly occurs in the fist decade of life
- More common in boys

Symptoms
- Midline cerebellar signs

Diagnosis
- History
- Neurological examination
- MRI commonly shows cystic tumor with mural node

Treatment
- Complete surgical removal of the tumor is treatment of choice
- Interval MRI scans to monitor for signs of progression
- Radiotherapy

Prognosis
Over 90 % of children with a fully resected pilocytic astrocytoma will survive with only surgical intervention. Those with partially resected diffuse disease who have had radiotherapy have only a 50 60 % chance of survival.
Poor prognostic features include

- Diffuse histology
- Incomplete resection
- Brain stem involvement

Supratentorial Astrocytoma

Epidemiology
- Twice as common in boys

Treatment
- Complete surgical removal is optimal
- Radiotherapy is indicated for all than the lowest-grade, completely resected tumors

Prognosis
- Varies widely

3.10.3 Malignant Gliomas

Account for 5% of new cases of childhood malignancy each year.

Classified primarily by anatomic location and second by histologic phenotype. For those diagnosed within the supratentorium, treatment consists of optimal surgical excision/radiotherapy and chemotherapy. Despite aggressive treatment strategies, survival in this group of patients remains poor.

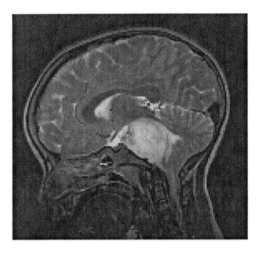

Age	5
Diagnosis	Diffuse pontine glioma
Presenting symptoms	3 week history of gradual onset of left sided weakness
	Headache
	Increasing difficulty swallowing

Figure 3.4

Diffuse pontine glioma

Brain Stem Glioma

Epidemiology
- Gender incidence equal
- Common presenting age: 5–10 years

Etiology
- Arise in the medulla, pons, midbrain, and cerebral peduncles
- Diffuse pontine gliomas are rapidly infiltrative in nature
- Most commonly found in the pons, with equal distribution of histological varieties
- Low-grade tumors constitute <10% of brain stem tumors

Symptoms
- High-grade disease: short history
  - Multiple cranial nerve palsies
  - Ataxia
  - Hemiparesis
- Low-grade disease: long history
  - Minimal or a focal cranial nerve deficit
  - Raised ICP

Diagnostics
Location, radiological appearance, and clinical features are usually diagnostic (Fig. 3.4)

Treatment
- Treat hydrocephalus
- High-grade disease: steroids to alleviate neurological symptoms in short pulses
  - Radiotherapy is palliative, producing a mean survival of 8–10 months. Chemotherapy and hyperfractionated radiotherapy have failed to make an impact on outcome
- Low-grade disease: surgical debulking
  - Observation
  - Radiotherapy and/or chemotherapy may be indicated

Prognosis
- High-grade disease: median survival 8–10 months

3.10.4 Other High-grade Gliomas

The clinical behaviour of supratentorial and cerebellar gliomas is more difficult to predict on the basis of radiological and clinical characteristics, with prognosis being more related to histologic phenotype and grade. After resection, radiotherapy is the treatment of choice. Long-term survival remains poor, with 40% overall survival for grade III and 10% for grade IV (Lashford, 2002).

Intracranial Ependymoma

Epidemiology
- Paraventricular lesions usually occur in the 1st decade of life
- 50% occurring <5 years of age
- Spinal ependymomas present slightly later

Etiology
- Predominantly arise from ependymal tissue within the ventricular system, most commonly the fourth ventricle
- Can disseminate (more frequently with infratentorial and high grade disease)
- Hydrocephalus common at presentation

Are divided into the following categories:

- Subependymoma (WHO grade I)
- Ependymoma (WHO grade II); variants include cellular, papillary, epithelial, clear cell, and mixed
- Malignant/anaplastic ependymoma (WHO grade III)

Symptoms
Depend on site and extent of disease

Typically
- Neck pain
- Increased ICP
- Cranial nerve deficits
- Ataxia

Diagnostics
- MRI (whole brain and spine) to establish extent of disease
- CSF cytology when possible

Treatment
- Surgery
- Treat hydrocephalus
Adjuvant treatment is age-related:
>5 years of age
- No residual disease or disseminated disease: radiotherapy to the tumor bed
- Residual disease, no disseminated disease: re-resection
  - Radiotherapy (no spinal)
  - Trials are ongoing to determine role of chemotherapy
- CNS disseminated disease: radiotherapy to entire CNS
  - Trials underway looking at role of chemotherapy
<5 years of age
- Chemotherapy
- Second-look surgery

Prognosis
- Overall survival: 40–60% at 5 years
- Good prognostic factors: minimal residual disease post surgery
- Poor prognostic factors: young age
  - Subtotal resection

Craniopharyngiomas

Epidemiology
- 8% of all childhood brain tumors
- Most commonly seen <18 years
- Mean age at diagnosis 8 years

Etiology
- Arise from neural ectoderm and epithelial elements in Rathke's pouch
- Can be located anywhere in the primitive craniopharyngeal duct
- 90% suprasellar, 10% intrasellar
- Benign and slow-growing

Symptoms
Presenting symptoms relate to pressure on adjacent structures:
- Visual fields and acuity defects
- Endocrine dysfunction
- Hydrocephalus is possible

Diagnosis
- History
- MRI scan

Treatment
- Presurgical neuroendocrine and ophthalmic work-up are essential
- Treatment of hydrocephalus
- Complete resection optimal

Prognosis
Although classified as benign, they can result in considerable morbidity.

Problems include
- Endocrine dysfunction
- Diabetes insipidus
- Hypothyroidism
- Growth and sex hormone deficits
- Excessive weight gain
- Visual disturbances
- Neuropsychological dysfunction
- Psychosocial problems

Intracranial germ cell tumors

Germ cell tumors arising intracranially are histologically indistinguishable from the gonadal varieties.

Intracranial germ cell tumors can be divided into two main groups:

- Germinomas: 60% of total number of germ cell tumors
- Nongerminomatous germ cell tumors (NGGCTs; also referred to as secreting germ cell tumors)

Both groups have the potential for CSF dissemination.

Epidemiology
- For all intracranial germ cell tumors there is a male prevalence
- Intracranial germinomas primarily present in the 2nd decade of life
- NGGCTs tend to occur earlier

Etiology
- Germinomas occur predominantly in the suprasellar region
- NGGCTs occur mainly as pineal tumors

Symptoms
Pineal tumors
- Raised ICP is commonly seen
- Headache
- Vomiting

Suprasellar tumors
- Visual disturbances (fields/acuity)
- Diabetes insipidus
- Hypopituitarism
- Headache
- Vomiting

Tumors of the basal ganglia-thalamus area

- Hemiparesis
- Precocious puberty
- Failure of puberty
- Short stature

Intracranial germ cell tumors (continued)

Diagnostics
- Germinoma: MRI and biopsy
- NGGCT: MRI (radiological features are characteristic)
- Serum and CSF levels for AFP and HCG

Treatment
Germinomas
- Highly chemo/radiosensitive tumors
- Surgery has a limited role in their management

Current UK treatment is

- Craniospinal irradiation with boost to the primary tumor site
- Chemotherapy followed by local radiotherapy

NGGCTs
- Chemotherapy has improved rates of cure; nevertheless, local radiotherapy is still considered necessary to achieve cure
- Surgery for difficult residual disease

Prognosis
- Germinomas: 90–100%
- NGGCTs: 60–70%

Visual Pathway Gliomas

Epidemiology
- 75% of isolated optic nerve gliomas occur <10 years
- Peak incidence: 2–6 years
- Occurs in 20% of patients with neurofibromatosis (NF1)

Etiology
- Can present anywhere along optic tracts
- May extend to the pituitary fossa, causing hypopituitarism, or to the hypothalamus, resulting in precocious puberty
- Hydrocephalus may be present
- Natural history is unpredictable

Symptoms
Symptoms relate to tumor pressure on the optic nerve and adjacent structures and infiltration:

- Decreased visual acuity or fields
- Squint
- Nystagmus
- Precocious puberty

Diagnostics
- MRI
- Neurological examination
- Frequent neuro-ophthalmological testing (see below)

Treatment
- Treat hydrocephalus
- Observation if disease and symptoms are stable (spontaneous regression has been reported)
- Treatment should be considered to stabilise vision
- Surgery has limited role
- <8 years of age + NF1: chemotherapy
- >8 years of age: radiotherapy
- The lack of randomised trials makes it difficult to know whether chemotherapy and radiotherapy make a difference

Prognosis
- Isolated optic nerve tumors have a better prognosis than those that extend along the visual pathway or involve the chiasm
- Children with neurofibromatosis, particularly those who are asymptomatic at diagnosis, have improved prognosis

Neuro-ophthalmological Testing

Visual assessment is frequently used as the critical tool to determine the need for treatment, with deterioration in visual fields and/or acuity indicating the need for intervention. This can be a particular problem with infants and young children as it can be difficult to get consistently accurate results (particularly regarding visual fields). Experience has shown that even in school-age children, results can fluctuate, and it may be unclear whether this fluctuation relates to disease progression or to variable patient compliance.

Germinoma

Comprise 60% of the total number of germ cell tumors

Epidemiology
- Intracranial germinomas primarily present in the 2nd decade of life

Etiology
- Occur predominantly in the suprasellar region

Symptoms
- Visual disturbances (fields/acuity)
- Diabetes insipidus
- Hypopituitarism
- Headache
- Vomiting

Diagnostics
- MRI
- Biopsy

Treatment
- Highly chemo/radiosensitive tumors
- Surgery has a limited role

Current UK Treatment
- Craniospinal irradiation with boost to the primary tumor site
- Chemotherapy followed by local radiotherapy

Prognosis
- 90–100%

Nonsecreting Germ Cell Tumors (NSGCTs)

Epidemiology
- NGGCTs tend to occur earlier

Etiology
- NGGCTs occur mainly as pineal tumors

Symptoms
- Raised ICP is commonly seen
- Headache
- Vomiting

Diagnostics
- MRI (radiological features are characteristic)
- Serum and CSF levels for AFP and HCG

Treatment
- Sensitive to a range of chemotherapy agents
- Chemotherapy has improved rates of cure
- Local radiotherapy is, however, still necessary to achieve cure
- Surgery for difficult residual disease

Prognosis
- 60–70%

Spinal Tumors

Rare in children. Low-grade astrocytomas are usually intramedullary, requiring extensive surgical removal. Radiotherapy and chemotherapy may be required. High-grade astrocytomas of the spine require radiotherapy and, like similar disease in other sites, surgery has little role. Prognosis for spinal ependymoma (Fig. 3.5) is optimal with total surgical excision. Radiotherapy is routine, with residual disease necessitating chemotherapy.

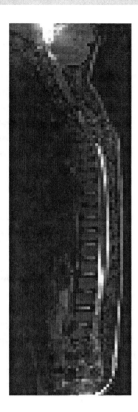

Age	6 years
Diagnosis	Spinal ependymoma
Presenting symptoms	2 month history of intermittent backpain

Figure 3.5
Spinal ependymoma

3.11 Follow-up

Children treated for a brain tumor will require life-long follow-up care in a specialist centre. Interval MRI scanning and neurological examinations will be important indicators of progress in the early months and years following treatment. Late effects of treatment, such as cognitive deficits and endocrine dysfunction, may only become apparent in subsequent years.

3.12 The Late Effects and Rehabilitation of Survivors

It is clear that children who have been treated for brain tumors may have significant long-term problems relating both to the tumor itself and to treatment (Mostow et al., 1991; Plowman and Pearson, 1997). Radiotherapy, prolonged exposure to raised ICP, and often repeated surgical procedures all incur costs. Side effects are both physical and psychological (Glaser et al., 1997) and include growth problems and weight gain relating to endocrine dysfunction, lack of energy, poor body image, low self-esteem, and decreased overall fitness. Adolescent survivors in particular describe feelings of isolation from their peer group and may lack confidence socially. Problems translate into functional difficulties, such as poor attendance at school, attention deficit, and overt eating disorders. Despite the recognition of how devastating brain tumor treatment can be, this cohort of cancer survivors is rarely included in studies of psychological adjustment during and after treatment (Kline, 1996; Radcliffe et al., 1996). If the overall burden of morbidity is to be addressed for this unique patient group, consideration must to be given to strategies that will facilitate development in both physical and psychological well-being (Glaser et al., 1997). Recent work in the UK suggests that adolescent survivors of brain tumor treatment can benefit psychosocially from a rehabilitation programme targeting their unique needs (Fitzmaurice and Beardsmore, 2003).

3.13 Palliative Care

Palliative care is discussed in detail in chapter 30 of this handbook. It is, however, prudent here to refer to the complexities of symptom control for children with brain tumors. Problems such as steroid dependency, spinal involvement, seizure control, reduced mobility, and speech, language, and swallowing difficulties necessitate the input of palliative care nurses who specialise in the care of these children.

3.14 Future Perspectives/New Innovations

New innovations include the following:
- Boron neutron capture therapy, which is an experimental form of radiotherapy that injects a chemical compound containing boron into the bloodstream, which then concentrates in the brain tumor tissue. Radiotherapy with neutrons is then directed at the cancer, and when the neutrons come into contact with the boron, high-energy radiotherapy is released with low penetrance that spares normal tissue.
- Growth factor inhibitors to prevent the effects of the growth factors that allow a cancer to grow.
- Angiogenesis inhibitors to prevent the formation of new blood vessels that nourish the cancers.
- Immunotherapy to stimulate the body's own immune system to fight the cancer.
- Advanced MR techniques such as MR spectroscopy, diffusion MR, and dynamic contrast-enhanced MR to give noninvasive information on tumor function, i.e. metabolism, relation to white matter, and blood flow.
- Conformal radiotherapy that uses three-dimensional planning. The volume of radiation therapy is irregular and "conforms" to the tumor. Shaped fields of treatment are used, which minimise the amount of normal tissue within the radiotherapy field. This in turn results in a decrease in acute and late morbidity.

References

Bouffet E (2000) Common brain tumors in children: diagnosis and treatment. Paediatric Drugs 2(1):57–66

CancerBACUP (2002) www.cancerbacup.uk/childrens-cancer

Copeland D, deMoor C, Moore B (1999) Neurocognitive development of children after a cerebellar tumor in infancy. Journal of Clinical Oncology 17:3476–3486

Fitzmaurice N and Beardsmore S (2003) The rehabilitation of adolescent survivors of brain tumor treatment. Cancer Nursing Practice 2(5):26–30

Glaser AW, Abdul Rashid NF, U CL, Walker DA (1997) School behaviours and health status after central nervous system tumors in childhood. British Journal of Cancer 76(5): 643–650

Kline NE (1996) Neuro-oncology patients and nursing research issues Journal of Pediatric Oncology Nursing 13 (1):40–42

Kheifets LI (2003) EMF and cancer: Epidemiologic evidence to date. World Health Organization. www.who.int.

Lashford LS, Thiesse P, Jouvet A, Jaspan T, Couanet D, Griffiths PD, Doz F, Ironside J, Robson K, Hobson R, Dugan M, Pearson AD, Vassal G, Frappaz D; a United Kingdom Children's Cancer Study Group and French Society for Pediatric Oncology Intergroup Study. (2002) Journal of Clinical Oncology 20(24):4684-4691

Laurent JP, Chang CH, Cohen ME (1985) A classification system for primitive neuroectodermal tumors (medulloblastoma) of the posterior fossa. Cancer 56(7):1807–1809

Macedoni-Luksic M, Jereb B, Todorovski L (2003) Long term sequelae in children treated for brain tumors: impairments, disability and handicap. Pediatric Haematology and Oncology 20(2):89–101

Mostow EN, Byrne J, Connelly RR, Mulvihill JJ (1991) Quality of life in long term survivors of CNS tumors of childhood and adolescents. Journal of Clinical Oncology 9(4):592–599

Nicholson JC, Punt J, Hale J, Saran F, Calaminus G; Germ Cell Tumor Working Groups of the United Kingdom Children's Cancer Study Group (UKCCSG) and International Society of Paediatric Oncology (SIOP) (2003) Neurosurgical management of paediatric germ cell tumors of the central nervous system–a multi-disciplinary team approach for the new millennium. Journal of Clinical Oncology 21(8):1581–1591

Plowman PN, Pearson ADJ (1997) Tumors of the central nervous system. In Pinkerton CR, Plowman PN (eds) Paediatric oncology: Clinical practice and controversies. Chapman and Hall Medical, London

Radcliffe J, Bennett D, Kazak AE, Foley G, Phillips PC (1996) Adjustment in childhood brain tumor survival: Child, mother and teacher report. Journal of Pediatric Psychology 21(4):529–539

Ryan JA, Shiminski-Maher T (1995) Neuro oncology nurses: undaunted, hopeful and enthusiastic. Journal of Pediatric Oncology Nursing 12 (4):179–180

Shiminski-Maher T, Shields M (1995) Pediatric brain tumors: diagnosis and management. Journal of Pediatric Oncology Nursing 12(4):188–198

Sutton LN, Goldwein J, Perilongo G, Schut L, Rorke L, Pa R (1990) Prognostic factors in childhood ependymomas. Pediatric Neurosurgery 16(2):57–65

Taylor RE, Bailey CC, Robinson K, Weston CL, Ellison D, Ironside J, Lucraft H, Gilbertson R, Tait DM, Walker DA, Pizer BL, Imeson J, Lashford LS; International Society of Paediatric Oncology; United Kingdom Children's Cancer Study Group (2002) Results of a randomized study of preradiation chemotherapy versus radiotherapy alone for non-metastatic medulloblastoma: The International Society of Paediatric Oncology/United Kingdom Children's Cancer study group PNET-3 study. British Journal of Neurosurgery 16(2):93–95

Turini M, Redaelli A (2001) Primary brain tumors: a review of research and management. International Journal of Clinical Practice 55(7):471–475

UKCCSG/SBNS United Kingdom Children's Cancer Study Group and Society of British Neurological Surgeons (1997) Guidance for services for children and young people with brain and spinal tumors. Report of working party of UKCCSG and the Society of British Neurological Surgeons

Bibliography

Mulhern RK, Kepner JL, Thomas PR, Armstrong D, Friedman H, Kun LE (1998) Neuropsychological functioning of survivors of childhood medulloblastoma randomized to receive conventional or reduced dose craniospinal irradiation: a pediatric oncology group study. Journal of Clinical Oncology 16:1723–1728

Shiminski-Maher T, Rosenberg M (1990) Late effects associated with treatment of craniopharyngiomas in childhood. Journal of Neuroscience Nursing 22(4):220–225

PART II

Anemias

Rosalind Bryant

Contents

4.1 Anemia

Anemia is defined as a reduction in red cell mass due to decreased production, increased loss/decreased survival, or increased destruction of red blood cells (RBCs). Because most oxygen is transported by the RBCs to the body tissues, a reduction in the red cell mass causes reduced oxygen supply to body cells. Consequently, anemia is a sign of an underlying pathological process, which is usually discovered during a routine health maintenance visit. The investigation of anemia to determine the underlying diagnosis includes a combination of medical history, family history, physical examination, and the initial laboratory assessment, including the evaluation of the full/complete blood count (FBC/CBC), RBC indices/morphology, reticulocyte count, and the peripheral smear (see Table 4.1). More extensive tests may be needed to verify the diagnosis, such as an iron panel, osmotic fragility, hemoglobin (Hgb) electrophoresis, or even a bone marrow examination (see Fig. 4.1).

Table 4.1. Normal red blood cell values in children (adapted from Hastings, 2002a)

Age	Hemoglobin (g/dl)		MCV (fl	
	Mean	2 SD	Mean	2 SD
Birth (cord blood)	16.5	13.5	108	98
1–3 days (capillary)	18.5	14.5	108	95
1 week	17.5	13.5	107	88
2 weeks	16.5	12.5	105	86
1 month	14.0	10.0	104	85
2 months	11.5	9.0	96	77
3–6 months	11.5	9.5	91	74
0.5–2 years	12.0	10.5	78	70
2–6 years	12.5	11.5	81	75
6–12 years	13.5	11.5	86	77
12–18 years, female	14.0	12.0	90	78
12–18 years, male	14.5	13.0	88	78
18–49 years, female	14.0	12.0	90	80
18–49 years, male	15.5	13.5	90	80

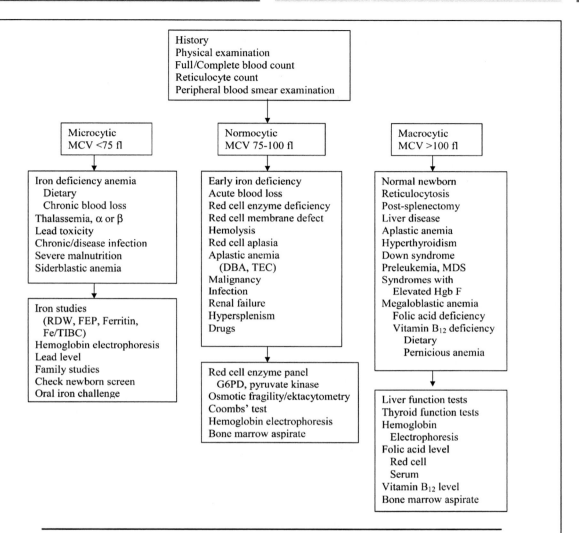

History
Physical examination
Full/Complete blood count
Reticulocyte count
Peripheral blood smear examination

Microcytic
MCV <75 fl

Normocytic
MCV 75-100 fl

Macrocytic
MCV >100 fl

Iron deficiency anemia
  Dietary
  Chronic blood loss
Thalassemia, α or β
Lead toxicity
Chronic/disease infection
Severe malnutrition
Siderblastic anemia

Iron studies
  (RDW, FEP, Ferritin,
  Fe/TIBC)
Hemoglobin electrophoresis
Lead level
Family studies
Check newborn screen
Oral iron challenge

Early iron deficiency
Acute blood loss
Red cell enzyme deficiency
Red cell membrane defect
Hemolysis
Red cell aplasia
Aplastic anemia
  (DBA, TEC)
Malignancy
Infection
Renal failure
Hypersplenism
Drugs

Red cell enzyme panel
  G6PD, pyruvate kinase
Osmotic fragility/ektacytometry
Coombs' test
Hemoglobin electrophoresis
Bone marrow aspirate

Normal newborn
Reticulocytosis
Post-splenectomy
Liver disease
Aplastic anemia
Hyperthyroidism
Down syndrome
Preleukemia, MDS
Syndromes with
  Elevated Hgb F
Megaloblastic anemia
  Folic acid deficiency
  Vitamin B$_{12}$ deficiency
    Dietary
    Pernicious anemia

Liver function tests
Thyroid function tests
Hemoglobin
  Electrophoresis
Folic acid level
  Red cell
  Serum
Vitamin B$_{12}$ level
Bone marrow aspirate

Diagnostic approach to the child with anemia. (Abbreviations: MCV = mean cell volume; DBA = Diamond-Blackfan anemia; TEC = transient erythroblastopenia of childhood; MDS = myelodysplastic syndrome; Hgb F = hemoglobin F; RDW = red cell distribution index; FEP = free erthyrocyte protoporphyrin; Fe/TIBC = iron-/total iron-binding capacity; G6PD = glucose-6-phosphate dehydrogenase.)

Adapted from Hastings C (2002). Anemia. In: The Children's Hospital Oakland Hematology/Oncology Handbook, St. Louis, Mosby Company.

Figure 4.1

Diagnostic approach to the child with anemia. From Wadworth Center, New York State Department of Health. Retrieved 9/13/03 from http://www.wadsworth.org. *From UpToDate webpage. Retrieved 9/17/2003 from www.UpToDate.org

It is important to establish whether the anemia is related to one cell line (i.e., RBCs, white blood cells [WBCs], or platelets) or multiple cell lines (i.e., RBCs, WBCs, and platelets). If multiple cells lines are affected, this may indicate bone marrow production problem (i.e., leukemia, aplastic anemia or metastatic disease). If a single cell line is affected, this usually indicates a peripheral destruction problem such as autoimmune disorders (i.e., immune thrombocytopenic purpura or autoimmune hemolytic anemia).

Anemia is classified into two main categories, which include the morphological and etiological (physiological or functional) basis for the anemia. The mean corpuscular volume (MCV) is the most useful of the RBC indices and is the basis for the morphological category. The morphological category divides the RBC morphology or size into normocytic (normal size RBC), microcytic (smaller than normal RBC), and macrocytic (larger than normal size RBC) anemias (see Fig. 4.1).

These categories are not mutually exclusive for a given anemia because an anemia may present as normocytic and then revert to macrocytic or develop a combination of RBC sizes. The etiological category is divided according to (1) decreased or ineffective production of RBCs, (2) destruction of RBCs, or (3) loss of RBCs. Generally, in the etiological category, there is one basis for the anemia but some anemias may have more than one basis.

Iron deficiency anemia may have more than one basis and more than one morphological presentation (see Fig. 4.1). The usual etiological category for iron deficiency anemia is decreased production of RBCs; however, this anemia may also develop because of an increased loss of RBCs. Iron deficiency is usually morphologically classified as a microcytic anemia, yet early iron deficiency is classified as a normocytic anemia (Fig. 4.1).

Sickle cell hemoglobinopathies represent a group of genetic diseases that are all related to the presence of Hgb S. The most common type of sickle cell disease (SCD) is homozygous Hgb SS, which is morphologically classified as a normocytic anemia when oxygenated but as a macrocytic anemia in the presence of reticulocytosis (an increased number of large immature RBCs). Hgb SS is defined as a protein sub-

stitution on the β globin gene that causes destruction of RBC.

Thalassemia is a type of anemia that lacks alpha or beta production and therefore is etiologically classified as ineffective RBC production. Morphologically the thalassemic RBCs are classified as a microcytic anemia.

Hemolytic anemias are divided into intracorpuscular defects (i.e., glucose-6-phosphate dehydrogenase deficiency hereditary spherocytosis) or extracorpuscular defects (i.e., autoimmune hemolytic anemia) that cause RBC destruction. Hemolytic anemia is morphologically classified as normocytic, but if it has more than 20% reticulocytes, it is then classified as macrocytic.

Lastly, aplastic anemia (AA), which is a bone marrow failure syndrome, is divided into inherited (i.e., Fanconi's anemia, Diamond-Blackfan anemia) or acquired anemia (i.e., moderate or severe) characterized by reduced or absent production of RBCs, WBCs, and platelets. Morphologically it is classified as normocytic but most often as macrocytic anemia. The macrocytosis develops because of stress erythropoiesis, which produces erythrocytes with fetal characteristics that tend to be more pronounced in the inherited types of AA (Shimamura and Guinan, 2003).

4.2 Iron Deficiency Anemia

Iron deficiency anemia is defined as a reduction in red cell mass due to decreased production and/or loss of RBCs (see Fig. 4.1). Infants usually have adequate iron stores at birth unless they were born prematurely or maternal iron stores were inadequate. The iron stores of full-term infants gradually deplete in about four months unless replenished with iron-fortified formula or breast milk supplemented with iron.

4.2.1 Epidemiology

Anemia caused by iron deficiency is a major public health problem, affecting 46% of school children globally (United Nations ACC/SCN, 2000). Iron deficiency is the most common form of nutritional deficiency. Its prevalence is highest among young children between the ages of 12 months and 3 years and women of childbearing age (particularly adolescent girls and pregnant women).

4.2.2 Etiology

Iron is present in all body cells. Iron balance is maintained between dietary intake (approximately 10 % elemental iron is absorbed in the duodenum and jejunum) and iron loss (from sloughing of the skin and mucosal cells). There is no organ that regulates iron excretion (Andrews, 2003). The most common causes of iron deficiency are chronic blood loss and/or inadequate intake of dietary iron during rapid growth periods.

4.2.3 Molecular Genetics

The precise mechanism by which serum iron is loaded onto transferrin (the major protein transporter of iron) as it leaves intestinal epithelial cells or reticuloendothelial cells is unknown. Transferrin binds with the iron (total iron binding capacity = TIBC) and releases the iron into the cell. Once inside the cell, the iron conjugates with free erythrocyte portoporphyrins (FEP or EP) to form heme and binds with the globin protein to form Hgb. The Hgb attracts the oxygen and carries it to body cells for metabolism. The remaining iron is stored as ferritin (soluble protein) or hemosiderin (an insoluble protein complex). Both of these complexes are found in the liver, bone marrow, spleen, and skeletal muscles. Reticuloendothelial cells acquire iron primarily by phagocytosis and breakdown of aging red cells. The iron is then extracted from the heme and returned to the circulation to bind to transferrin and repeat the cycle.

4.2.4 Symptoms/Clinical Signs

Iron deficiency produces a microcytic, hypochromic anemia that impairs tissue oxygen transport to body cells and may cause weakness, fatigue, palpitations, lightheadedness, pallor, lethargy, tachycardia, and tachypnea that may be detected on physical exam and while obtaining a thorough history. Pica, a craving for

unusual substances such as starch, clay, toilet paper, and paint chips, may be detected during the history and is frequently associated with iron-deficiency anemia. Adolescents and children less than 36 months are at the highest risk for developing iron deficiency anemia. Severe iron deficiency anemia is associated with impairment of growth and intellectual development and may cause decreased motor activity and social interaction. The lack of iron causes damaged to epithelial cells, which has been associated with gastrointestinal blood loss and/or increase absorption of heavy metals including lead (Andrews, 2003). Therefore iron deficiency may enhance lead absorption and inadvertently cause lead toxicity. Lead is toxic to the bone marrow and affects erythropoiesis by interfering with the heme synthetic pathway in all cells (Andrews, 2003).

4.2.5 Diagnostic Testing

The smear diagnostic of iron deficiency anemia contains microcytic, hypochromic (decreased iron content) RBCs with poikilocytosis (varying red cell shapes), anisocytosis (different red cell sizes) and target cells (which resemble a bull's eye target; see Fig. 4.1). The lead poisoning smear differs from iron deficiency by consisting of coarse basophilic stippling (coarse granules studding the cytoplasm; see Fig. 4.1) with microcytic hypochromic RBCs. In contrast, a chronic disease anemia smear consists primarily of normocytic and normochromic RBCs (see Fig. 4.1) with approximately 20 % of microcytic cells.

The iron status of the body can be assessed using several laboratory tests. During mild iron deficiency (Hgb >10 gm/dl) when the stores are depleted, the Hgb may not decrease. Consequently, elevated FEP would be a better screening test for early iron deficiency than Hgb concentration (Mei et al., 2003). The FEP is also elevated in lead poisoning but usually to a greater level than in iron deficiency. Moderate iron deficiency occurs with a decreased Hgb of 7–10 g/dl and decreased MCV compared with the age-matched results. Severe iron deficiency is associated with decreased Hgb (<7 g/dl) and decreased MCV compared with age-matched results (see Table 4.1).

The test most commonly used regardless of whether iron deficiency is mild, moderate, or severe is the Hgb/hematocrit (Hct) concentration. Although Hgb concentration and Hct cannot be used to determine the cause of anemia, if Hgb concentration or Hct increases after a course of therapeutic iron supplementation, the diagnosis of iron deficiency anemia can be made even with mild iron deficiency (Segel et al., 2002a). Other laboratory tests (including decreased reticulocytes, increased RBC distribution width [RDW], decreased serum iron, decreased transferrin saturation, elevated total iron binding capacity [TIBC], positive guaiac, and Hgb electrophoresis) can be used to differentiate iron deficiency anemia from anemia of other causes. Serum ferritin concentration is an early indicator of iron store depletion, yet is also an acute-phase reactant to chronic infection, inflammation, or diseases, which may obscure the results. The MCV is the most useful of the RBC indices and is the basis for the classification of the anemias (Fig. 4.1). A decreased MCV and RBC with increased RDW indicates iron deficiency anemia, whereas a decreased MCV and increased or normal RBC with normal RDW indicates thalassemia minor (Demir et al., 2002).

There are nutritional anemias that affect normal red cell production that must be differentiated from iron deficiency (see Fig. 4.1). Megaloblastic anemia (B_{12} and folate deficiency) may be coupled with iron deficiency anemia. Vitamin B_{12} deficiency may develop in the strict vegetarian diet or the totally breastfed infant. It is treated with cobalamin injections 30 µg/day for 5–10 days, then weaned to 100–200 µg monthly; for adolescents, 100 µg daily for 10–15 days then weaned to 60 µg monthly with the addition of B_{12} dietary sources (Lee et al., 2002). The folic acid dose is 50 µg/day in infants and 1 mg/day for children/adolescents coupled with dietary counseling to promote intake of foods containing folic acid.

4.2.6 Treatment

- Treatment requires the identification of the cause of iron deficiency anemia, whether its due to blood loss from intestinal inflammation/malabsorption, surgery, or medications (e.g., chemotherapy, anticonvulsants) and/or lack of adequate iron intake

- The oral iron dose is 2–6 mg/day elemental iron/kg/day divided bid for child/infant and 60–120 mg/day for adolescents. Iron preparations should be given with vitamin C-fortified juice or with water because vitamin C promotes iron absorption from the gastrointestinal tract. Iron should not be taken with milk, milk products, or antacids because they interfere with iron absorption

- Iron fortified cereal (two or more servings) should be added daily to the diet of the exclusive breastfed full-term infant beginning about 4–6 months after birth

- *Preterm or low birth weight* infants who are exclusively breastfed should take iron drops 2–4 mg/kg/day beginning 2–3 months after birth until age 12 months

- The use of low-iron milk (cow, goat, or soy) should be discouraged until after age 12 months

- The intake of solid foods that are rich in iron should be encouraged in children, along with a decrease in milk consumption to <24 ounces daily

- Dietary counseling regarding the intake of iron-rich foods (e.g., meats, bran, lentils, beans, nuts, and some green leafy vegetables) should be reinforced

- Iron treatment should be continued until iron stores are replenished (approximately 4–6 months of oral iron therapy after Hgb normalizes). Side effects of iron therapy should be explained to the child and parents; these include gastrointestinal discomfort, constipation, bloating, stained teeth (to prevent, give liquid iron with a straw) and dark/black stools

Parenteral iron replacement is

- Used when the patient is unable to ingest oral iron or absorb iron from the gastrointestinal tract

- Available in the United States as iron dextran (elemental iron) and administered as intramuscular (IM) using the z-track technique, or intravenously (IV). The preferable route is intravenous (IV) because the intramuscular injection causes pain and skin discoloration

- Composed of iron dextran and contains 50 mg elemental iron per milliliter. The dose of iron (mg) is calculated by wt (kg) × desired increment Hgb (g/dl) × 2.5 (Hastings, 2002a). A peak reticulocytosis will usually occur 10 days after parenteral iron is given with complete correction of anemia in 3–4 weeks
- Given as a test dose of 12.5–25 mg, with observation of the patient for 30–60 minutes after the dose
- Associated with such adverse effects as anaphylaxis, fever, hypotension, rash, myalgias, and arthralgias
- Not recommended in infants less than 4 months old (Lee et al., 2002)

4.2.7 Transfusion

Depending on whether the child is hemodynamically stable, children with severe anemia (Hgb <5 g/dl) may require red cell transfusion. Common practice is to administer the red cells slowly (2–3 ml/kg/hour) in multiple small volumes (aliquots) with careful monitoring of vital signs and fluid balance to prevent pulmonary edema and congestive heart failure (Glader, 2004).

4.2.8 Erythropoietin (Epotin Alfa, Epogen)

Recombinant human erythropoietin may be used as treatment for mild to moderate anemia to stimulate the proliferation and differentiation of erythroid precursors (Andrews, 2003). The usual subcutaneous dose is 150–300 IU/kg one to three times a week. Sufficient erythroid precursors must be in the bone marrow with adequate iron stores and adequate protein intake for erythropoietin to be effective (Carley, 2003). Common practice is to administer 3 mg/kg/day of supplemental iron concurrently. Erythropoietin has shown efficacy in the treatment of anemia of prematurity and in renal failure and is being investigated as a treatment for transient bone marrow suppression induced by chemotherapy.

4.2.9 Prognosis

Once detected, iron deficiency and other nutritional anemias generally respond positively to supplementation. Follow-up Hgb that fails to show improvement within 4–8 weeks after supplementing with oral iron and dietary iron, or an anemia that recurs despite adequate supplementation warrant, further investigation (Segel et al., 2002). Further investigation may include such disorders as malignancy, copper deficiency, inborn errors of iron metabolism, or other rare disorders.

4.3 Sickle Cell Disease

Sickle cell hemoglobinopathies represent a group of genetic diseases that are all related to the presence of Hgb S. Sickle cell trait is a benign condition that involves approximately 35–45% of Hgb S and the remainder Hgb A. Although complications are rare, they have been described and include an increased incidence of hematuria and hyposthenuria. Vaso-occlusive crisis has also been reported, especially under hypoxic conditions such as shock, strenuous physical activity, and flying in an unpressurized aircraft or at high elevations.

4.3.1 Epidemiology

Sickle cell disease (SCD) has been recognized as a worldwide problem. It is a common hereditary disorder, occurring in 1 in 375 births, with 70,000 cases among African-Americans in the United States. SCD affects a variety of nationalities, including Africans, Hispanics, Arabs, Italians, Native Americans, Caribbeans, Iranians, Turks, and, infrequently, American Caucasians (primarily of Mediterranean descent).

4.3.2 Etiology

Sickle cell disease(SCD) is transmitted as an incomplete autosomal-dominant trait (Karayakin, 2000). When both parents carry the sickle cell trait (heterozygous gene or Hgb AS), there is a 25% chance with each pregnancy of producing an infant with

Table 4.2. Diagnostic tests used in sickle cell disease

Test	Interval
Baseline CBC, differential, and reticulocyte count, pulse oximetry	Each visit
Red cell minor antigen phenotype	Visit at 6 months of age
Hgb electrophoresis	Confirmatory 2–6 months, 2 years of age, and if needed, at 5 years age
Renal and hepatitis function tests, amylase, lipase, LDH, liver function tests, urinalysis	Yearly but more often if abnormal.
Human immunodeficiency virus	Yearly post-transfusion
Blood cultures	If febrile ≥38.5 °C
Transcranial cerebral ultrasonography	Yearly (start at age 2 until 16 years in Hgb SS or comparable sickle hemoglobinopathy
Pulmonary function tests	Age 8 and every 2 years unless abnormal
Electrocardiography/echocardiography	Every 2 years unless abnormal
Abdominal ultrasonography	Age 8–10 years or if symptomatic or
Audiogram	Age 8–10 years or if symptomatic
Plain films, MRI of hips/shoulders	Symptomatic
MRI/angiography of brain as needed	Symptomatic
Neuropsychological testing	Age 6 years and repeat as necessary

SCD (homozygous gene – Hgb SS or heterozygous Hgb S variant). The incidence of the sickle cell trait is about 8% in African-Americans in the United States, whereas it has been reported to be as 40% among West Africans.

4.3.3 Molecular Genetics

The molecular defect in Hgb SS occurs due to the substitution of valine for glutamic acid in the sixth position of chromosome 11 of the β-globin chain. The second most common type of SCD is Hgb SC (heterozygous variant) in which the lysine is substituted for the glutamic acid at the sixth position of the β-chain. Other Hgb S variants include a combination of Hgb S trait and β-thalassemia trait, either producing Hgb SB° thalassemia (no normal β-globin production) or Hgb SB+ thalassemia (decreased β-globin production). Another frequently seen variant is the combination of Hgb SS with α-thalassemia trait (usually two or three functional α-globin genes).

4.3.4 Symptoms/Clinical Signs

The basic pathophysiology of sickle cell is directly related to the abnormal Hgb S that polymerizes when deoxygenated. Most of the complications of SCD are the result of entanglement and enmeshing of the sticky, rigid, sickle-shaped cells as they block the microcirculation, causing partial to complete vaso-occlusion of vessels. The resultant decreased blood flow to the tissues causes ischemia and infarction which may result in further complications. A thorough history, physical exam, and periodic diagnostic tests tend to identify existing complications (see Table 4.2).

4.3.5 Diagnostic Testing

The following descriptions of peripheral blood smears are correlated with the type of SCD:

- The typical Hgb SS smear contains mild to moderate normochromic, normocytic to macrocytic

Table 4.3. Neonatal hemoglobin patterns (adapted from Hudspeth and Symons, 2002))

Screening phenotype	Confirmed electrophoresis	Possible genotype
FA	Normal newborn pattern	Hgb AA
FAS	Benign sickle cell trait	Hgb AS
FAC	Benign Hgb C trait	Hgb AC
FAA$_2$	Benign β-thalassemia trait	Hgb AA$_2$
FS	Fetal and sickle Hgb S	Homozygous Hgb SS or Hgb S/β°-thalassemia or Hgb S/B$^+$ thalassemia
FSC	Hgb S and Hgb C	Hgb SC
FSAA$_2$	Heterozygous Hgb S/β$^+$-thalassemia	Hgb S/β$^+$ thalassemia
F	Fetal Hgb F or Hgb F with delayed Hgb A appearance	Homozygous β-thalassemia major or homozygous hereditary persistence of fetal Hgb F
FA Barts	Fetal Hgb, Hgb A, and Barts Hgb (ranges 12% to 30%)	β-thalassemia silent carrier β-thalassemia trait Hgb H disease
AF	May indicate prior blood transfusion	Retest 4 months post-transfusion

Hemoglobin variants are reported in order of decreasing abundance; for example, FA indicates more fetal than adult Hgb. Repeat blood specimen should be done to confm original interpretation

cells with sickled cells and increased anisocytosis and poikilocytosis (see Fig. 4.1, plate 8). The average Hgb range is 5–9 g/dl, with an average reticulocytosis 5–>20%

- The Hgb SC smear contains normochromic, normocytic cells with sickle cells, target cells, and spherocytes (see Fig. 4.1, plate 6). The Hgb SC average Hgb range is 9–12 g/dl, with an average reticulocyte count between normal and 10%

- The Hgb S β°-thalassemia and Hgb SS α-thalassemia smear contains marked microcytosis, and moderate to marked sickle cells with anisocytosis and poikilocytosis. The average Hgb and reticulocytosis are commensurate with Hgb SS

- Hgb S β$^+$-thalassemia smear contains moderate microcytosis, sickle-shaped cells with anisocytosis and poikilocytosis. The average Hgb is 9–12 g/dl with reticulocytosis 5–10%

The differential diagnoses include disorders such as hereditary spherocytosis (HS), glucose-6-phosphate dehydrogenase (G-6PD), pyruvate kinase, thalassemia, leukemia, and juvenile rheumatoid arthritis, which can all be excluded by obtaining the Hgb electrophoresis (see Table 4.3).

About 2,000 infants with SCD born in the United States are identified by neonatal screening (AAP, 2002). Neonatal screening is included in state screening programs that obtain blood via heel prick to identify primarily sickle and thalassemic hemoglobinopathies (see Table 4.3).

4.3.6 Complications of SCD

The chronic destruction of the RBCs in SCD results in acute and chronic complications; however, this chapter will focus on the acute complications of SCD. Complications of SCD may occur suddenly and can rapidly become severe; therefore, the medical provider should consult with a hematologist. The most common complication, which is usually not life-threatening, is vaso-occlusive crisis or episode. Other complications that will be discussed are acute sequestration, aplastic crisis, infection, acute chest syndrome, acute abdominal pain, and acute central nervous system events.

4.3.6.1 Vaso-occlusive Crisis/Episode (VOE)

- Definition: Vaso-occlusive episode (VOE) occurs when deoxygenated sticky, rigid sickled-shaped RBCs block microcirculation completely or partially (infarction) causing tissue ischemia or necrosis.
- Signs and symptoms of VOE: Most children with sickle cell anemia experience some degree of acute pain and may express their pain verbally or by crying, grimacing, or maintaining a stoic expression.

  Most of the children are able to describe their severity of pain by using self-reporting methods such as the faces pain scale or the numeric pain scale (see Fig. 4.2). Other behavior indicators may be helpful in the pain assessment of all children, including infants, such as limited movement of a body part, decreased appetite, or increased irritability. The bones and joints are major pain sites, with tenderness, erythema, warmth and swelling frequently present. The initial site of pain in young children and infants is usually the small bones of the hands and feet, called dactylitis or hand/foot syndrome, and may be accompanied by swelling, erythema, and increased warmth. Severe complications may develop after repeated hip/shoulder infarctions (i.e., avascular necrosis of the fibula, femur, or humerus, known as AVN) or repeated skeletal vertebrae infarctions (i.e., lordosis, scoliosis, or kyphosis).

4.3.6.1.1 Diagnostic Test/Differential
A complete blood count, RBC indices, WBC count and differential, reticulocyte count, renal and liver function tests, and, if needed, bone radiographs are usually obtained during severe VOE. The differential includes VOE versus osteomyelitis, which is difficult to differentiate because both are associated with ery-thema and swelling, low-grade fevers, and joint and bone pain. Osteomyelitis may be excluded by clinical observation, blood cultures, and, occasionally, aspiration of the affected area.

4.3.6.1.2 Treatment
Hydration (oral or intravenous), opioids and NSAIDS (oral or intravenous), incentive spirometry, adjuvant therapy, rest, heat and massage to painful areas, and exercises or diversional activities (school work, friends, meditation, guided imagery) are useful interventions for VOE. Whether VOE is managed by patient-controlled analgesia (PCA) or orally, the pain assessment treatment should be closely monitored to achieve optimal pain management (Jacob et al., 2003).

4.3.6.2 Acute Sequestration Crisis

- Definition: Acute splenic sequestration is a sudden, rapid enlargement of the spleen with trapping of a considerable portion of the red cell mass, leading to acute exacerbation of anemia that drops the Hgb level 2 g/dl or more below baseline
- Signs and symptoms: Sudden weakness, dyspnea, rapidly distending abdomen (spleen or liver enlarging), abdominal pain, lethargy, irritability, pallor, vomiting, headache, tachycardia, and tachypnea are manifestations of acute sequestration. Severe cases of splenic sequestration may lead to circulatory collapse (shock) and death
- Diagnostic tests: Hct may drop to half the patient's usual value. Brisk reticulocytosis with increased nucleated red cells, moderate to severe thrombocytopenia, and leukopenia may be present on the smear
- Treatment: Volume expansion with a fluid bolus and oxygen supplementation are needed immediately. Immediate yet slow transfusion of small aliquots packed RBCs (PRBCs) to restore intravascular volume and oxygen-carrying capacity may be instituted. Prevention of further recurrences is achieved by elective splenectomy after the first major or second minor episode of sequestration, preferably in children >2 years of age

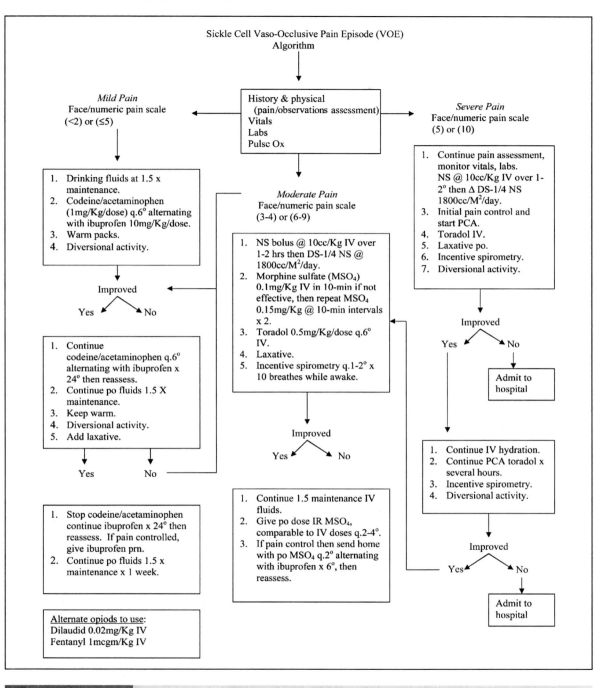

Figure 4.2

Sickle cell vaso-occlusive pain episode (VOE) algorithm

- Education: Parents should be taught splenic palpation and educated about recognizing the signs and symptoms of splenic sequestration to aid in identifying initial episodes of acute sequestration and preventing recurrent life-threatening episodes

4.3.6.3 Aplastic Crisis

- Definition: Temporary cessation of bone marrow activity due to suppression by viral or bacterial infection, which causes a drop in hematocrit without reticulocytosis. Parvovirus B19 is the most common cause of aplastic crisis (Hastings, 2002c).
- Signs/symptoms: Increased pallor, icteric sclera, lethargy, irritability, headache, bone pain, weakness, nausea and vomiting, and dark urine are all manifestations of aplastic crisis.
- Diagnostic tests: The hematocrit decreases as much as 10–15% per day with no compensatory reticulocytosis.
- Treatment: Isolation precautions with oxygen supplementation may be instituted depending on the type of infection. Transfusion of PRBCs may be instituted to prevent congestive heart failure. Folic acid should be given in the recovery phase.

4.3.6.4 Infection

- Definition: The major risk factor for increased susceptibility to infection is splenic dysfunction. The ability of the spleen to clear particles from the intravascular space and provide antibody synthesis is impaired in the patient with SCD. Insidious progressive fibrosis of the spleen (autosplenectomy) occurs in the Hgb SS child, usually by the age of 6 years. Children with splenic dysfunction are 300–600 times more likely to develop overwhelming pneumococcal or *Haemophilus influenzae* sepsis and meningitis than are children without splenic dysfunction. (Karayalcin, 2000).
- Signs/symptoms: Toxic-appearing children with fever ≥38.5 °C, chills, lethargy, irritability, tachypnea, tachycardia, hypoxia, and history of prior sepsis should be treated promptly with parenteral antibiotics after obtaining a blood culture

- Diagnostic tests: A CBC with differential; C-reactive protein (CRP); cultures of blood, throat, and urine; chest x-ray; and oxygen saturation should be obtained. If the chest x-ray shows an infiltrate, a sputum culture should be obtained if possible. After a blood culture is obtained, the child should be started on parenteral antibiotics and admitted to the hospital. If osteomyelitis is suspected, an orthopedics specialist should be consulted regarding needle aspiration and culture of the suspected bone site
- Treatment: A child with SCD and fever ≥38.5 °C must be considered an emergency because of the increased risk for overwhelming sepsis resulting from splenic dysfunction

Children with SCD who have a low risk of sepsis (no high-risk factors, see Table 4.4) and who are older than 2 years of age are treated with outpatient management in several comprehensive sickle cell centers in the United States with close follow-up care (i.e., return clinic visits or telephone contact) (Williams et al., 1996). After blood cultures are obtained, these children are given long-acting parenteral antibiotics such as ceftriaxone (50–75 mg/kg/dose, with maximum dose of 2 g). If the child is allergic to cephalosporin, clindamycin 15 mg/kg is given with a maximum dose of 600 mg. These children are monitored in the clinic or emergency center for several hours prior to being discharged home with close follow-up care (Jakubik and Thompson, 2000).

A SCD child without high-risk factors (see Table 4.4) is discharged on oral antibiotics for 3 days while awaiting blood culture results. The child is prescribed cefprozil 30 mg/kg/day divided twice daily or Pediazole 40 mg/kg/day three times daily if cephalosporin-allergic. Any positive culture obtained from a child being managed on an outpatient basis requires immediate hospitalization and reevaluation of the child. High-risk factors that prevent children from being eligible for outpatient management are listed in Table 4.4.

Table 4.4. Recommended hospital management for the high-risk sickle cell disease patient

Clinically ill-appearing or toxic-looking
Signs of cardiovascular and/or pulmonary compromise
Age less than 12 months
Temperature ≥40 C
White blood count <5,000/mm³ or >30,000/mm³
Platelet count <100,000
Hemoglobin <5 g/dl or reticulocyte count <4%
Dehydration with poor oral flid intake
Pulmonary inftrate and/or previous history of acute chest syndrome
Pulse oximetry <92% or 3% below baseline
Central venous catheter
Prior splenectomy
History of previous sepsis
Evidence of acute SCD complications
Prior noncompliance or evidence of inability to comply with outpatient follow-up

- Prevention
  Morbidity and mortality rates have decreased dramatically since the advent of established newborn screening programs (United States), widespread penicillin prophylaxis, timely administration of immunizations, and parental/caregiver education. Parental/caregiver education is aimed at reducing bacterial septicemia and includes such interventions as immediate medical evaluation of febrile illness (≥38.5 °C), twice-daily administration of prophylactic antibiotic, and compliance with immunization schedules. In addition to standard immunizations, the SCD patient should also receives the 23-valent pneumococcal vaccine, the meningococcal vaccine at 2 years of age with boosters at 5 and 10 years of age, and recommended yearly influenza virus vaccines at 6 months and older. Prophylactic penicillin is started at 2 months of age and continued until 5–6 years of age and indefinitely in the child with a history of pneumococcal sepsis (Jakubik and Thompson, 2000). Currently, the child with SCD should be placed on prophylactic penicillin 125 mg twice daily starting at 2 months of age and increased to 250 mg twice daily at 3 years of age. If the child is allergic to penicillin, then erythromycin is substituted at a dosage of 125 mg twice daily starting at 2 months and increased to 250 mg twice daily at 3 years of age (AAP, 2002). Benzathinepenicillin G 300,000 units intramuscularly may be given monthly to the SCD patient with gastrointestinal dysfunction or who is noncompliant with oral antibiotic prophylaxis.

4.3.6.5 Acute Chest Syndrome

- Definition: Acute chest syndrome (ACS) is a common cause of morbidity and mortality in children with SCD and is characterized by fever, chest pain, and a new infiltrate on chest x-ray
- Signs/symptoms: Clinical manifestations of ACS may include extremity pain, rib or sternal pain, abdominal and chest pain, cough, dyspnea, fever (≥38.5 °C), back pain, tachypnea, wheezing, hypoxia (paO$_2$ <75 mmHg or 3 points of transcutaneous oxygen saturation below baseline) SOB, dyspnea, dullness (palpation), or normal auscultation (Rackoff et al., 1993)
- Diagnostic tests: Chest radiography may be clear initially but should be repeated with increasing respiratory distress or hypoxia. Blood cultures, CBC, differential, reticulocyte count, type and crossmatch, and, if possible, sputum cultures and arterial blood gases should be obtained. It is extremely difficult to differentiate between ACS and pneumonia. The most common organism causing ACS or pneumonia is pneumococcus, followed by *Salmonella, Klebsiella, Haemophilus influenzae,* and *Mycoplasma pneumoniae* and viruses. Martin and Buonomo (1997) reported that pulmonary infiltrates resolve quickly and dramatically in children with ACS not associated with infection, whereas those with infection have a prolonged radiographic course.
- Treatment: Patients may deteriorate rapidly, with progression to pulmonary failure and death; therefore, all patients with ACS should be treated in the hospital. Early recognition of respiratory

Table 4.5. Treatment for acute chest syndrome

Administer oxygen if hypoxic

    Monitor continuous pulse oximetry

    Encourage incentive spirometry

Administer empiric antibiotics

    Cephalosporin (e.g., cefuroxime 150 mg/kg/day divided every 8 h)

    Macrolide (e.g., azithromycin 10 mg/kg/day with 5 mg/kg/day on days 25)

Administer maintenance intravenous fluids (1,500 cc/m²/day)

Administer analgesic for pain (see algorithm)

Administer PRBCs if hemoglobin <10 g/dl

    Simple transfusion (10 cc/kg)

    Exchange transfusion

distress (cough, chest pain, hypoxia with or without fever) and aggressive treatment with oxygen if hypoxic, analgesics (see Fig. 4.2), empiric antibiotics, maintenance intravenous hydration (1,500 cc/m²/day), bronchodilators, respiratory treatments, and simple RBC transfusion (10 cc/kg) or exchange transfusion are instituted immediately (see Table 4.5). Oxygen treatment is monitored closely by pulse oximetry with an ongoing respiratory assessment of the patient. Incentive spirometry is encouraged every hour while awake, with administered analgesics (see Fig. 4.2) to prevent hypoventilation. After a blood culture is obtained, empiric antibiotics are given, which include a cephalosporin such as cefuroxime 150 mg/kg/day divided every 8 hours (maximum dose 2 g) to eradicate possible pathogens such as pneumococcus. A macrolide such as azithromycin 10 mg/kg on day 1 (maximum dose 500 mg) followed by 5 mg/kg/day on days 2–5 (maximum 250 mg) is given to treat possible pathogens such as *Mycoplasma* or *Chlamydia* (see Table 4.5). Hydration at maintenance rate (1,500 cc/m²/day) is administered to avoid overhydration (i.e., pulmonary edema). Bronchodilators such as albuterol aerosols are a common treatment that is given every 4–6 hours to decrease airway hyperreactivity. Transfusion of PRBCs as a simple transfusion of 10 cc/kg may be given. However, if the child's respiratory status continues to deteriorate (worsening hypoxia, anemia, chest pain, and worsening infiltrates on chest radiograph), then an exchange transfusion should be performed (see Table 4.5)

- Preventive: Risk factors related to ACS include young age (2–4 years), lower concentration of Hgb F, higher steady-state Hgb concentration, and higher steady-state WBC count should be assessed to prevent development of ACS (Quinn and Buchanan, 1999). Strategies to prevent ACS also include aggressive pain management and the use of incentive spirometry to prevent hypoventilation. Transfusion is generally recommended to decrease the concentration of Hgb S and can theoretically prevent ACS (Quinn and Buchanan, 1999). Hydroxyurea is an agent that is used to upregulate Hgb F and decrease viscosity and sickling of RBC, which decreases the development of ACS. Stem cell transplant is a therapy only available to limited number of donors but is a known cure of SCD (Quinn and Buchanan, 1999).

4.3.6.6 Acute Abdominal Pain

- Definition: The etiology of acute abdominal pain is unknown, although mesenteric sickling and vertebral disease with nerve root compression have been suggested (Dover and Platt, 2003).
- Signs/symptoms: Guarding, tenderness, rebound, distended abdomen, fever, jaundice, right upper quadrant pain, constipation are all manifestations of acute abdominal pain.
- Diagnostic tests: CBC with differential, reticulocyte count, liver enzymes, pancreatic enzymes, hepatitis panel, urinalysis, chest/abdominal films including upright views for perforated viscus, ultrasonography, or biliary scans may be instituted to determine the etiology of the acute abdominal pain. Differential diagnoses may include ACS, ileus, pneumonia, constipation, surgical abdomen, pancreatitis, urinary tract infection, intrahepatic sickling, and cholecystitis.

Treatment: Maintenance intravenous fluids (1,500 cc/m^2/day), analgesics (see Fig. 4.2), laxatives if constipated, and a surgical consult to rule out surgical abdomen (i.e., appendicitis) are instituted as soon as possible.

4.3.6.7 Acute Central Nervous System Event

- Definition: An acute central nervous system (CNS) event develops from chronically injured cerebral vessels in which the lumen is narrowed or completely obliterated by sickled erythrocytes, causing acute cerebral infarction. Approximately 7–10% of SCD (primarily Hgb SS) patients develop acute cerebral vascular occlusion or stroke, most often between the ages of 2 and 10 years. Cerebral infarction may occur as an isolated event or in combination with such disorders as pneumonia, aplastic crisis, viral illness, painful crisis, priapism, and dehydration
- Signs/symptoms: Sudden and persistent headache, hemiparesis, hemiplegia, seizures, coma, speech defects, gait dysfunction, visual disturbances, and altered mentation are all manifestations of a cerebral infarction
- Diagnostic test: The initial diagnostic test done is a computed tomography scan (CT scan) of the brain without contrast to identify intracerebral hemorrhage, abscess, tumor, or any other pathology that could explain the symptoms. Magnetic resonance imaging (MRI) and angiography aid in assessment of infarcts associated with obstruction of intracranial vessels (i.e., the anterior and/or middle cerebral vessels), and are usually ordered as soon as possible after CT
- Treatment: The standard approach to treating a patient with acute cerebral infarction is exchange transfusion followed by placement on a maintenance monthly transfusion program. The transfusion program is designed to keep Hgb S <30%, which lowers reoccurrence of stroke to 10%. In untreated persons, the mortality rate is approximately 20%, with about 70% of the patients experiencing a recurrence within 3 years of the initial cerebral vascular event (Dover and Platt, 2003). Maintenance monthly transfusion programs are designed to suppress the production of sickle cells, thereby reducing the chance of recurrent strokes. However, the multiple transfusions may cause complications such as hemochromatosis, alloimmunization, and infections such as hepatitis, HIV, and West Nile virus. Hemochromatosis is unavoidable with prolong transfusions and is treated with parenteral desferrioxamine (see section 4.4.6.2)
- Preventive: Transcranial Doppler (TCD) ultrasonography predicts increase risk of stroke in children who have increased flow velocity (>200 cm/sec) in major cerebral arteries that is demonstrated on two consecutive TCDs (Segel et al. 2002; Dover and Platt, 2003). TCDs are done yearly to aid in identifying children who are at high risk for developing stroke or who have asymptomatic brain disease. Neuropsychological testing identifies deficits in intelligence quotient (IQ), which has been instrumental in combination with MRI in discovering SCD children with silent infarcts. Silent infarcts are damage to the brain associated with impaired cognitive abilities secondary to sickling in cerebral vessels without any physical neurological deficits (Dover and Platt, 2003). Recommendations for treatment of silent infarcts may include either hydroxyurea therapy, transfusion program, stem cell transplant or close observation. The best treatment option for silent infarcts is unknown, but the transfusion program is usually recommended as the initial option

4.3.7 Preparation for Surgery

Most children with SCD tolerate chronic anemia well and only require transfusions for severe complications such as splenic sequestration, CNS infarction/ischemia/hemorrhage, aplastic crisis, severe ACS, and preparation for surgery. Because sickling of RBCs is increased during hypoxic periods, it may be necessary to transfuse the patient prior to the surgical procedure that requires anesthesia. If the SCD patient has a history of major complications (i.e., ACS, CNS infarctions, multiple VOE), preoperative transfusion consists of multiple transfusions every 3–4 weeks or exchange transfusion to obtain a goal of <30% Hgb S prior to surgery. Exchange transfusion is used to remove sickled cells and replace them with normal cells without increasing blood viscosity. However, if the SCD patient has not sustained any major complications, the patient is transfused to a Hgb of 10 g/dl irrespective of the percentage of Hgb S. A simple transfusion is usually performed 2–5 days prior to the surgical procedure.

4.3.7.1 Hydroxyurea Therapy

- Hydroxyurea (HU) is an S-phase-specific cytotoxic agent that upregulates Hgb F, which interferes with Hgb S polymerization and increases the lifespan of the sickled RBCs. HU decreases blood viscosity, has an increase affinity for oxygen, and releases a byproduct known as nitrous oxide that acts as a potent vasodilator. Therefore, hydroxyurea will aid in decreasing sickling and promoting unobstructed circulation.
- Children with SCD complications such as repeated ACS, or severe VOE are offered HU therapy
- The initial dose of HU is 15–20 mg/kg/day and is escalated to 35 mg/kg/day while monitoring the platelet, neutrophil, and reticulocyte counts (Powars, 2001; Steinberg et. al., 2003)
- Side effects of HU include neutropenia, leukopenia, reticulocytopenia, elevated liver enzymes, nausea and vomiting, hyperpigmentation, alopecia, and a potential mutagenic and carcinogenic effect. All patients of childbearing age must agree to a contraceptive plan prior to starting HU

4.3.8 Prognosis

SCD patients without a history of major SCD complications will have lifespans 10–15 years shorter than the individual without SCD. In an observational study, Miller and colleagues (2002) found a significant correlation between SCD course and adverse outcomes later in childhood in children who developed dactylitis before age 1 year and had a steady-state of Hgb <7 g/dl and leukocytosis in the absence of infection at an early age of 1 year.

4.3.9 Future Perspectives

- Because HU therapy is a lifetime therapy, more studies are needed to determine its long-term side effects in the SCD patient (Steinberg et. al, 2003). Studies to determine long-term additive effects of HU and erythropoietin on Hgb F production are being researched
- A limited number of umbilical cord blood transplants have been successful; therefore, this area is being researched as a possible cure for SCD
- There are studies focused on gene manipulation to correct the SCD defect and cure the disease

4.4 Thalassemia

Thalassemia is a group of inherited heterogeneous anemias associated with the absence or decreased production of normal Hgb (Table 4.6). Two broad classifications of thalassemia are the alpha (α)- and beta (β)-thalassemias, which contain deficits in α- and β-thal globin production, respectively.

4.4.1 Alpha (α)-Thalassemia

4.4.1.1 Epidemiology

The majority of α-thalassemias are located in Southeast Asia, Malaysia, and Southern China.

4.4.1.2 Etiology

The deficit in α-globin production is due to deletion or mutation of one or more of the four α-globin genes located on chromosome 16.

4.4.1.3 Molecular Genetics

More than 30 different mutations affecting α-globin genes have been described (Nathan and Orkin, 2003).

- Silent carrier has three functional α-globin genes ($-\alpha/\alpha\alpha$)
- α-thalassemia trait has two functional α-globin genes ($-\alpha/\alpha$ or $\alpha\alpha/-$)

Table 4.6. Classification of thalassemias (adapted from Nathan and Orkin, 2003)

Syndrome	Phenotypes	Clinical findings
Silent carrier (α and β-thalassemia)	α: 1–2% Hgb Barts or 1–2% Hgb CS at birth only β: Hgb A$_z$ ≥3.5 80–90% of Hgb F / Hgb A	Normal or slightly microcytic RBCs; no signs or symptoms
Thalassemia trait (α- and β-thalassemia trait)	α: 5–10% Hgb Barts or 1–2% Hgb CS at birth 80–90% Hgb F / Hgb A β: Hgb A$_z$ ≥3.5 80–90% Hgb F / Hgb A	Mild anemia to elevated RBCs; microcytosis/hypochromic
Hgb H or Hgb CS (constant spring)	α: 5–30% Hgb Barts or 1–2% Hgb CS at birth Hgb F 70–90%	Microcytic/hypochromic anemia (7–10 g/dl); pale, icteric, jaundiced; hepatosplenomegaly
Hydrops fetalis	α: combination of Hgb Barts, Hgb H. Hgb Portland usually death in utero	Severe anemia (6.2 g/dl average Hgb); pale, icteric, edematous due to congestive heart failure; hepatosplenomegaly
Thalassemia intermedia	Hgb A$_z$ 2–7% Hgb F 20–100% Hgb A 0–80% (depends on phenotype)	Anemia (6–10 g/dl) microcytosis hypochromic; pale, icteric, and with hepatosplenomegaly; rarely transfused
Thalassemia major	Hgb Az 2–7% Hgb F 20–100% Hgb A 0–80% (depends on phenotype)	Anemia average 6 g/dl with microcytic/hypochromia; pale, failure to thrive, frontal bossing, thalassemic facies, short stature, hepatosplenomegaly; transfusion-dependent

- Hemoglobin H disease has one functional α-globin gene (–/-α) and a Hgb H variant = Hgb constant spring (–/α^{cs}α)
- Hydrops fetalis has no functional α-globin gene (–/–)

4.4.2 Beta (β)-Thalassemia (Cooley Anemia)

4.4.2.1 Epidemiology

β-thalassemia mutations are found worldwide in regions including the Mediterranean, Africa, Southeast Asia, India, Italy, Greece, Spain, and North America, but are uncommon in Northern Europe, Korea, and Japan.

4.4.2.2 Etiology

The deficit in β-globin production is due to mutation of the β-globin genes located on chromosome 11.

4.4.2.3 Molecular Genetics

Within the β-globin gene, 170 mutations affect the transcription, translation of β-globin messenger, and stability of β-globin product (Olivieri, 1999; Nathan and Orkin, 2003). β-thalassemia includes four clinical syndromes (see Table 4.6):

- Silent carrier, which is asymptomatic
- β-thalassemia trait with mild anemia
- Thalassemia intermedia with moderate anemia and usually no transfusion requirement
- Thalassemia major with severe anemia and transfusion-dependent

4.4.3 Diagnostic Testing

Thalassemia testing can be confirmed with Hgb electrophoresis and family studies, or if necessary, DNA analysis can be used to make a definitive diagnosis. In most states of the United States, screening for hemo-globinopathies is performed on newborn infants. Anemias in children who were not screened as newborns but present with hypochromic, microcytic anemias must be differentiated from iron deficiency (see formulas below).

Prenatal diagnosis of α-thalassemia may be done by testing the amniotic fluid or obtaining chorionic villus sampling if there is a suspicion for α-thal trait or a family history of hydrops fetalis. Differentiation between thalassemia trait and iron deficiency can be calculated based on the following formulas:

Formulas for differentiation of thalassemia trait from iron deficiency (adapted from Nathan and Orkin, 2003, p 881)

	Thalassemia trait	Iron deficiency
Mentzer index (655) MCV/RBC	<13	>13
Shine and Lal (665) (MCV)2 × MCH	<1,530	>1,530
England and Fraser (666) (MCV–RBC–[5 × Hb])–8.4	Negative values	Positive values

4.4.4 Treatment

Supportive therapy includes supplementation with folic acid, avoidance of oxidant drugs and iron salts, prompt treatment of infectious episodes, and judicious use of transfusions. β-thalassemia major patients require regular transfusions to sustain life. Thalassemia intermedia patients are able to maintain a Hgb concentration of 6–10 g/dl without transfusions except during periods of infection, surgery, or other stressors. Splenectomy may be considered in Hgb H, thalassemia intermedia, and β-thalassemia major if hypersplenism is present with leukopenia, thrombocytopenia, worsening anemia, or the development of increased requirement for transfusion (>200 ml PRBCs/kg/year). Splenectomy reduces the transfusion requirements by eliminating the organ causing the trapping of the RBCs. At least 2 weeks prior to splenectomy, polyvalent pneumococcal and

meningococcal vaccines should be given. Following splenectomy, prophylactic penicillin 250 mg PO bid is implemented until adulthood. The importance of seeking medical assistance when the splenectomized patient is febrile is emphasized with parents and child to reduce the risk of developing overwhelming infection. Complications of ongoing transfusion therapy regimens are assessed (see section 4.2.7) including hemosiderosis.

4.4.5 Treatment of Hemosiderosis (Iron Overload)

Hemosiderosis is the accumulation of iron in organ tissues such as liver, pancreas, and joints as a result of chronic RBC transfusion therapy received by patients with β-thalassemia, Hgb H, sickle cell (i.e., those with a history of cerebrovascular accident, ACS, retractable vaso-occlusive crisis) or bone marrow failure syndromes (Olivieri, 1999; Beare, 2002). Hemosiderosis may also develop in the frequently transfused patient receiving myelosuppressive chemotherapy and/or radiation treatments. Chronic hemolysis and increased gut absorption of iron can also result in hemosiderosis. Exchange transfusion, phlebotomy, and chelation therapy are the only methods to manage transfusion-related iron overload at present.

4.4.6 Chelation Therapy

The objective of chelation therapy is to remove excess intracellular iron and bind free extracellular iron.

4.4.6.1 Initiation of Chelation Therapy

- Liver biopsy is the most accurate measurement of iron load, so if liver iron is 7 mg/g/dry weight or higher, then chelation should be started
- Ferritin level is helpful but not reliable because it is an acute phase reactant. Ferritin levels >1,000 µg/ml in steady state, then start chelation
- Cumulative transfusions of 120 ml or more PRBCs/kg/year promote hemosiderosis

4.4.6.2 Chelation Regimens

- Desferrioxamine is a complex hydroxylamine with a remarkable affinity to iron
- Desferrioxamine enters cells, chelates iron, returns iron to serum, and excretes the iron via kidney, liver, and skin
- Desferrioxamine 20–50 mg/kg/8–12 hours nightly × 5–6 days weekly
- Desferrioxamine by the IV route accelerates the rate of iron removal
- Supplemental oral ascorbic acid 100 mg daily PO enhances the urinary excretion of iron, particularly in vitamin C-deficient patients

4.4.6.3 Complications of Desferrioxamine

- Local erythema at the infusion site characterized by multiple subcutaneous nodules may be suppressed by including 5–10 mg hydrocortisone in the desferrioxamine solution
- Ototoxicity is a complication of desferrioxamine therefore a hearing test should be done every 6–12 months
- Ocular toxicity is a complication of desferrioxamine; therefore, the eyes should be examined every 6–12 months
- Noncompliance is an ongoing problem particularly with adolescent patients or parents who dread doing the desferrioxamine subcutaneous injections
- Do not administer desferrioxamine during infection or fever because the mobilization of iron aids in bacterial growth, particularly *Yersinia enterocolitica*

4.4.7 Clinical Advances (Hemosiderosis)

MRI of the liver is being studied to determine whether the imaging-measured iron content is comparable to a liver biopsy result, thereby providing a noninvasive means of measuring iron accumulation in the body. Another recent advance is an oral chelator known as deferiprone (L1 or 1,2-dimethyl-3-hydroxy) that has been used in Europe since 1999 in chelating iron in the thalassemia major patient. In July 2003, a new drug application was filed with the U.S. Food and Drug Administration for deferiprone. It is hoped that deferiprone will be available for use by the year 2005.

4.4.8 Prognosis

Bone marrow transplants from HLA-identified donors have been successfully performed worldwide on patients with severe β-thalassemia. A marked increase in survival to the fifth decade of life in the well-managed β-thalassemia patient is seen in developed countries.

4.4.9 Follow-up

All thalassemic β major patients should have 3-month interval appointments with the hematologist medical provider to manage therapies and side effects involving hemochromatosis, vision, hearing, enlarged organs, and dental side effects. Other thalassemic patients (β-intermedia, Hgb H) are usually seen every 6 months provided the patients have not developed any severe complications.

4.4.10 Future Perspectives

Institution of bone marrow transplantation with unrelated phenotypically matched donors and in utero transplantation are being investigated. Development of transduction methods and vectors to transfer genes and correct the genetic defect are being researched.

4.5 Hemolytic Anemia

Hemolytic anemias comprise a group of disorders that cause destruction of RBCs. The reduced RBCs survival may occur as result of intracorpuscular defects due to defective intracellular enzymes (i.e., glucose-6-phosphate dehydrogenase deficiency or pyruvate kinase deficiency) or abnormal membrane structural proteins as in hereditary spherocytosis (HS). The RBC survival is also affected by the extracorpuscular defect of autoimmune hemolytic anemia (AIHA).

4.5.1 Hereditary Spherocytosis (HS)

Hereditary spherocytosis (HS) is the most common congenital RBC membrane disorder. HS is characterized by a deficiency or abnormality of the RBC membrane protein spectrin, one of the major skeletal cell membrane proteins. The HS RBCs are repeatedly trapped by the splenic sinusoids, which causes damage and destruction to the spherocytes.

4.5.1.1 Epidemiology

HS is a common inherited hemolytic anemia, with an estimated incidence in Northern Europe of 1–2 in 5,000 individuals.

4.5.1.2 Etiology

Primary molecular defects in HS reside in membrane skeletal proteins and is a common inherited hemolytic anemia. Approximately 5–10 % of cases of HS are considered new mutations.

4.5.1.3 Molecular Genetics

Microscopically, HS cells show fewer spectrin filaments interconnecting spectrin/actin/protein to junctional complexes, but overall skeletal architecture is preserved except in the most severe forms of HS (Gallagher and Lux, 2003). Typically, HS is associated with approximately 70 % dominant and 20 % recessive inheritance. The membrane protein defects cause instability of the spectrin, which results in membrane instability, loss of surface area, and abnormal permeability, with the average lifespan of the red cell being 90 days.

4.5.1.4 Symptoms/Clinical Signs

A thorough history and physical may elicit a family history of neonatal hyperbilirubinemia, gallstones, splenomegaly or splenectomy, and intermittent jaundice that typically presents in infancy but may present at any age. Anemia is the most frequent presenting complaint, accompanied with reticulocytosis and manifested primarily by pallor, intermittent jaundice, and splenomegaly. Mild to marked jaundice may be present depending on the rate of hemolysis and the ability of the liver to conjugate and excrete indirect hyperbilirubinemia.

4.5.1.5 Diagnostic Testing

Spherocytes are dense, round, and hyperchromic, and lack central pallor on peripheral blood smear (see Fig. 4.1, plate 7). The laboratory findings of HS vary according to the severity and clinical classification. The trait may have a normal Hgb and normal to slightly elevated reticulocyte count (see Fig. 4.1, plate 5). Mild HS Hgb can be 11–15 g/dl, but with an elevated reticulocyte count can be 3–8 %. In moderate to moderately severe HS, the Hgb is 8–12 g/dl to 6–8 g/dl, respectively, with elevated reticulocyte counts above 8 %. Severe HS has a Hgb <6 mg/dl and a reticulocyte count >10. The majority of children with HS are classified as mild to moderate anemia.

Other laboratory findings include anemia (mild to severe) depending upon the HS classification, reticulocyte count, and increased osmotic fragility test (the most sensitive test for diagnosing HS). The spherocytes have a decreased surface area to volume ratio, and when placed in the hypotonic solution, the HS cells lose membrane surface area more readily because their membranes are leaky and unstable, resulting in an increase osmotic fragility test.

The MCV (mean corpuscular volume) is decreased except during reticulocytosis. The red cell distribution width (RDW) is elevated due to the presence of microspheres in proportion to the degree of hemolysis. The Coombs' test is negative, which excludes AIHA. Several other diagnostic tests used to detect HS include the acidified glycerol lysis test, hypertonic cryohemolysis test, and the autohemolysis test. HS must be differentiated from such disorders as AIHA, G-6PD, pyruvate kinase deficiency, elliptocytosis, and pyropoikilocytosis.

4.5.1.6 Treatment

- Because dietary intake of folic acid is inadequate for the increased needs of the erythroid HS bone marrow, the patient routinely receives folic acid 1 mg/day orally to prevent megaloblastic crisis

- The parents and child are instructed regarding signs and symptoms of hemolysis and hypersplenism, such as increased pallor, fatigue, abdominal pain, enlarging spleen, jaundice, and dark urine. The family and child are instructed to avoid trauma to the spleen area and are shown how to monitor spleen size
- If splenectomy becomes necessary, it is delayed until the child is 5 or 6 because the increased risk of postsplenic sepsis is very high in infancy and early childhood. The child should have pneumococcal and meningococcal vaccines at least 2 weeks prior to splenectomy. Prior to splenectomy, an abdominal ultrasonography should be done to determine spleen size and the presence of any accessory spleens and/or cholelithiasis
- After splenectomy, the child should receive prophylactic penicillin therapy 250 mg PO bid until adulthood

4.5.1.7 Prognosis

Splenectomy laparoscopically eliminates hemolysis but exposes the patient to life-long risk for lethal infections. Platelet counts tend to increase to >1,000×10^9/l immediately after splenectomy but will usually decrease over several weeks without any intervention. Penicillin-resistant strains of *S. pneumoniae* have developed, but the use of prophylactic penicillin supersedes this complication because of the increase risk of life-threatening infections.

4.5.1.8 Follow-up

Yearly follow-up is needed for CBC and liver panel and to reinforce penicillin prophylaxis. The splenectomized HS patient should seek medical attention immediately for febrile illness. Healthcare providers should reinforce with the parents and patient that although the hemolysis is eradicated, the HS still exists.

4.5.1.9 Future Perspectives

Management of HS by subtotal splenectomy has shown beneficial results in a small cohort of patients by decreasing hemolysis and maintaining phagocytic function of the spleen (Baden-Meunier et al., 2001).

4.5.2 Autoimmune Hemolytic Anemia (AIHA)

A condition that develops from the interaction between erythrocytes and the immune system is known as autoimmune hemolytic anemia (AIHA). The most common types are AIHA that is composed of warm-reactive autoantibody, usually immunoglobulin (IgG), that binds with the erythrocyte antigen at 37 °C, or cold-reactive autoantibody, usually IgM, that binds to erythrocytes below 37 °C (Ware, 2003). These autoantibodies are recognized by the macrophages, which leads to intravascular destruction of the erythrocyte.

4.5.2.1 Epidemiology

AIHA is estimated to occur at an annual incidence of 1 in 80,000 persons of any age, race, or nationality.

4.5.2.2 Etiology

Children tend to develop AIHA after a recent viral illness or systemic illness because of the development of autoantibodies. The autoantibodies bind to the erythrocyte surface membrane, which results in premature red cell destruction, primarily in the spleen.

4.5.2.3 Molecular Genetics

The antierythrocyte antibodies that develop in most patients with AIHA represent a polyclonal B-lymphocyte response that is poorly understood. Case reports suggest there is an association between AIHA and certain immune response genes.

4.5.2.4 Symptoms/Clinical Signs

Many patients present with signs and symptoms of anemia, such as pallor, weakness, fatigue and light-headedness, with a compensated cardiovascular aspect. Occasionally, the patient develops jaundice, due to accelerated erythrocyte destruction, and dark urine, reflecting intravascular hemolysis. A thorough history must be obtained, including questions regarding medications and the possibility of underlying systemic illness such as any history of newborn jaundice, gallstones, splenomegaly/splenectomy, or episodes of dark urine or yellow sclera. The patient may have a palpable spleen and liver, with tachycardia or a systolic flow murmur manifested on physical exam.

4.5.2.5 Diagnostic Testing

Peripheral blood smear is very useful in establishing the diagnosis of AIHA. It contains numerous small spherocytes, occasional teardrop shapes or schistocytes, polychromasia (common finding), and reticulocytes (see Fig. 4.1, plates 4 and 5). Bone marrow aspiration is not mandatory but may be helpful to exclude a malignant process, myelodysplasia, or bone marrow failure syndrome. The bone marrow reveals erythroid hyperplasia with myeloid/erythroid ratio.

Elevated lactate dehydrogenase and aspirate aminotransferase levels reflect the release of intraerythrocyte enzymes; in contrast, other hepatic enzymes should not be elevated in AIHA. The serum haptoglobin level is typically low because it acts as a scavenger for free plasma Hgb, but haptoglobin is an acute phase reactant and is not synthesized well in infants. The unconjugated bilirubin is elevated and reflects accelerated erythrocyte destruction. The most useful laboratory test is the direct antiglobulin test (DAT or Coombs' test), which identifies antibodies and complement components on the surface of circulating erythrocytes.

The differential diagnosis includes hereditary spherocytosis, which may be excluded by performing the osmotic fragility test. Other rare disorders such as clostridial sepsis, Wilson's disease, hemolytic-uremic syndrome, thrombotic thrombocytopenic purpura, transient erythroblastopenia of childhood, or acquired aplastic anemia are excluded by performing a DAT.

4.5.2.6 Treatment

If the patient has a severe anemia or a decreasing Hgb concentration, then therapy should be instituted. Therapy should begin with close observation, and corticosteroid therapy with the judicial use of erythrocyte transfusions. The corticosteroids are widely accepted first-line therapy. Corticosteroids inhibit the Fc receptor-mediated clearance of sensitized erythrocytes and also inhibit autoantibody synthesis. Corticosteroids, prescribed as 1–2 mg/kg of methylprednisolone IV q.6° × 24–72 hours, and then oral prednisone 2 mg/kg/day divided three times daily, are given until clinically stable. The prednisone is tapered over 1–3 months based on steroid concentration, reticulocyte count, and DAT.

The second line of therapy includes intravenous immunoglobulin therapy, with a systemic benefit at high doses of 5 g/kg/× 5 days, and may be accompanied by plasma exchange transfusion. Exchange transfusion is reasonable with the large IgM antibodies, which are removed by plasmapheresis, whereas the IgG autoantibodies in the extravascular spaces respond better to splenectomy. Transfusion of RBCs is difficult in the AIHA patient due to difficulty in obtaining compatible erythrocytes. The transfusion may result in severe hemolysis, so the transfusion is started at a slow rate, checking both plasma and urine for free Hgb. Other therapeutic modalities include cyclosporin A (suppresses cellular immunity), vinblastine (decrease autoantibody production), danazol (decreased IgG production), azathioprine, and cyclophosphamide (both interfere with autoantibody synthesis).

Splenectomy may be considered late in the disease; it removes the major site of autoantibody production, with a response in about 80% of patients. These children should receive pneumococcal/meningococcal immunizations at least 2 weeks prior to splenectomy. Post-splenectomy patients should seek medical attention immediately if they develop fever >38.5 °C and should take penicillin or erythromycin (if allergic to penicillin) prophylaxis due to the possibility of sepsis.

4.5.2.7 Prognosis

There is a good prognosis for the majority of children who experience the acute self-limiting disease, with a mortality rate less than 10%.

4.5.2.8 Future Perspectives

Rituximab appears to be a promising new treatment for refractory AIHA. Rituximab is a humanized murine monoclonal antibody directed against the human CD20 antigen, which is present only on B lymphocytes (Ware, 2003). A small study treated four chronic AIHA children with Rituximab even though two had prior splenectomies and all were dependent on high-dose steroids and refractory to other immunosuppressive therapy. All four patients became transfusion-independent and were weaned completely off prednisone after being treated with Rituximab, with few reactions.

4.5.3 Glucose-6-phosphate dehydrogenase deficiency (G-6PD)

G-6PD is the most common red cell enzyme deficiency. Because the gene for G-6PD is usually located on the X chromosome, males are either fully deficient or of normal phenotype (Perkins, 2001). However, females can be deficient fully, heterozygous (trait), or of normal phenotype (Lanzkowsky, 2000).

4.5.3.1 Epidemiology

G-6PD deficiency is a worldwide gender-linked red cell enzyme deficiency. The highest incidence is in Africans, African-Americans, Mediterraneans, Native Americans, Southeast Asians, and Sephardic Jews.

4.5.3.2 Etiology

G-6PD variants may be due to deletions or point mutations affecting transcription and processing or the primary structure. Therefore, G-6PD deficiency may not only be caused by mutations in the coding region and a decrease number of normal molecules but also by changes in the primary structure by affecting the catalytic function or by decreasing stability of the protein, or both (Luzzatto H, 2003).

4.5.3.3 Molecular Genetics

Since cloning of the G-6PD gene, nearly all the G-6PD variants possess a single amino acid replacement, which is caused by a single missense point mutation (Luzzatto, 2003). After exposure to an oxidative agent (see Table 4.7), the Hgb and other proteins are oxi-

Table 4.7. Hemolytic oxidants associated with g-6pd deficiency (adapted from Luzzatto, 2003)

Analgesics and antipyretics
Acetanilide
Acetylsalicylic acid (large doses)
Para-aminosalicylic acid
Acetophenetidin (phenacetin)
Nitrofurans
Nitrofurazone
Nitrofurantoin
Furaltadone
Furazolidone
Antimalarials
Pentaquine
Pamaquine
Primaquine
Quinocide
Chloroquine
Pyrimethamine
Plasmoquine
Sulfones
Thiazolsulfone
Diaminodiphenylsulfone
Sulfoxone sodium
Sulfonamides
Sulfanilamide
Sulfamethoxazole
Sulfacetamide
Sulfapyridine
Sulfadiazine
Sulfisoxazole
Sulfathiazole
Sulfacetamide
Miscellaneous
Naphthalene (mothballs)
Methylene blue
Chloramphenicol
Probenecid
Quinidine
Fava beans
Phenylhydrazine
Nalidixic acid
Infections
Diabetic acidosis

dized. The RBC destruction starts hemolyzing the oldest RBCs with the least G-6PD, and then progresses toward younger RBCs and the denatured Hgb precipitates, causing irreversible damage to the membrane, and the red cells lyse.

4.5.3.4 Symptoms/Clinical Signs

A thorough history must be obtained, including the possible precipitant of the acute event. A child with G-6PD deficiency is hematologically normal most of the time until hemolysis occurs secondary to an oxidant (see Table 4.7). Within 24–48 hours after exposure to an oxidant, the child may develop fever (38 °C), nausea, abdominal pain, diarrhea, dark-colored urine, jaundice, pallor, tachycardia, splenomegaly, and possibly hepatomegaly.

4.5.3.5 Diagnostic Testing

The peripheral smear shows moderate to severe normocytic, normochromic anemia, with marked anisocytosis, poikilocytosis, and reticulocytosis with inclusion bodies (Heinz bodies) (see Fig. 4.1, plates 4 and 5). The diagnosis is confirmed by quantitative enzyme assay in reticulocyte-poor red cells or by testing RBCs after reticulocytosis resolves. Other labs that support the G-6PD diagnosis include a reduced haptoglobin, elevated WBCs (predominance of granulocytes), elevated unconjugated bilirubin with normal liver enzymes. Urine is positive for blood (free Hgb).

Studies using polymerase chain reaction (PCR) may identify the abnormal gene as well as the biochemical abnormality (Perkins, 2001). Direct antiglobulin test will be negative in G-6PD and will exclude antibody-mediated red cell destruction. Other disorders to exclude from the differential include blackwater fever (malarial infection), paroxysmal cold hemoglobinuria, paroxysmal nocturnal hemoglobinuria and mismatched blood transfusion (ABO mismatch).

4.5.3.6 Treatment

Treatment depends on the extent of the acute hemolysis. Supportive care during the acute event may require transfusion and must definitely include counseling regarding prevention of future events. Healthcare providers should reinforce to the parents and child the need to avoid the list of oxidants that can possibly trigger a hemolysis (see Table 4.7). For those individuals undergoing chronic hemolysis, dietary supplementation with folic acid (1 mg tab/day) is recommended (Hastings, 2002b).

4.5.3.7 Prognosis

The prognosis is good provided the patient avoids exposure to the oxidants.

4.6 Bone Marrow Failure Syndromes

Bone marrow failure syndromes are a reduction in the effective production of mature erythrocytes, granulocytes, and platelets by the bone marrow, causing pancytopenia. The bone marrow failure syndromes encompass aplastic anemia (AA), Fanconi's anemia, paroxysmal nocturnal hemoglobinuria, Shwachman-Diamond syndrome, dyskeratosis congenita, Diamond-Blackfan syndrome and many other disorders. This section will focus on AA, which is divided into acquired and inherited classifications.

4.6.1 Aplastic Anemia

Aplastic anemia (AA), a bone marrow failure disorder may be acquired or inherited. It is characterized by a reduced or absent production of blood cells in the bone marrow and peripheral blood, causing a decrease of two or more cell lines (i.e., RBCs, WBCs and platelets).

4.6.1.1 Acquired Aplastic Anemia

Aplastic anemia results from an immunologically mediated, tissue-specific, organ-destructive mechanism.

4.6.1.1.1 Epidemiology

An annual incidence of AA was established in European studies as 2 per million per year. The highest mortalities were in Japan, Thailand, and Northern Ireland, with an incidence two or three times higher than in European countries and the United States.

4.6.1.1.2 Etiology

Causative factors of acquired AA include toxins, medications, insecticides, immunologic disorders, irradiation, chemotherapy, and infections (i.e., HIV, CMV, parvovirus, hepatitis); however, most causes are unknown (70% idiopathic). Myelosuppressive drugs such as chemotherapy, antibiotics, insecticides, benzene compounds, and other medications cause dose-related marrow suppression by damaging the DNA and decreasing numbers of progenitors. Radiation injures DNA in the actively replicating progenitor cells, which also causes AA.

4.6.1.1.3 Molecular Genetics

Acquired AA is divided into severe and moderate aplastic anemia. Moderate aplastic anemia has normal to increased cellular marrow with at least two of the following present: granulocyte count >500/µl, platelet count >20 K/µl, and reticulocyte count >1%. Severe aplastic anemia has an aplastic marrow and at least two of the following present: granulocyte count <500/µl, platelet count <20 K/µl, and reticulocyte count <1%.

4.6.1.1.4 Symptoms/Clinical Signs

A detailed history, including medications, infections, radiation exposure, and any family history of aplastic anemia, should be obtained with a thorough physical examination. Thrombocytopenia and hemorrhagic manifestations are usually the first symptoms and are manifested by petechiae, ecchymoses, epistaxis, or oral mucosal bleeding. Neutropenia causes oral ulcerations, bacterial infections, and fever, which are rarely present early in AA. Erythropenia, manifested by pallor, fatigue, headache, and tachycardia, tends to be a late sign since red cells live approximately 120 days compared with platelets that live only 10 days and neutrophils that live 6–12 hours.

4.6.1.1.5 Diagnostic Testing

Blood counts are depressed, and blood smear displays a paucity of platelets, leukocytes, and normal to macrocytic red cells with decreased reticulocytes. Increased fetal Hgb (Hgb F) and red cell I antigen may be present secondary to stress hematopoiesis. Bone marrow examination must be done by obtaining an aspirate and biopsy, which demonstrates the conversion of red bone marrow to yellow fatty marrow. There are decreased numbers of blood and marrow progenitor cells due to a microenvironment that fails to support hematopoiesis.

Laboratory findings include the following:

- Normocytic, normochromic anemia with reticulocytopenia, leukopenia, and thrombocytopenia observed on smear
- Slightly to moderately elevated fetal Hgb noted on Hgb electrophoresis
- Bone marrow denotes marked depression or absence of hematopoietic cells and replacement by fatty tissue containing reticulum cells, lymphocytes, plasma cells, and usually tissue mast cells. Bone marrow biopsy is done to exclude granulomas, myelofibrosis, or leukemia, and a bone marrow chromosomal analysis is done to exclude Fanconi's anemia and myelodysplastic syndromes
- Diepoxybutane test (DEB) is performed on peripheral blood to exclude Fanconi's anemia
- Sugar-water test, Ham test and flow cytometry are done to exclude paroxysmal nocturnal hemoglobinuria (PNH)
- Liver function chemistries are done to exclude hepatitis
- Renal function chemistries are done to exclude renal disease
- Viral serology testing: hepatitis A,B,C antibody panel, Epstein-Barr virus antibody panel, parvovirus B19 IgG and IgM antibodies, varicella antibody titer, and cytomegalovirus antibody titer are done to determine etiology
- Quantitative immunoglobulins, C_3, C_4 and complement and antinuclear antibody (ANA), total hemolytic complement (CH50), and Coombs' test are done to exclude systemic diseases

- HLA typing of the patient and nuclear family is done to determine if bone marrow transplantation match is available
- Blood group typing is performed on the patient for possible transfusion
- Clotting profile including prothrombin time (PT), activated partial thromboplastin time (APTT), and fibrinogen is done to determine any clotting dysfunction

Differential diagnosis for pancytopenia is extensive and includes myelodysplastic syndromes, preleukemias, leukemias, paroxysmal nocturnal hemoglobinuria, myelofibrosis, and some lymphomas. Pancytopenia may occur secondary to systemic diseases such as systemic lupus erythematosus, hypersplenism, vitamin B_{12} or folate deficiencies, alcohol abuse, anorexia nervosa or starvation, and infections such as Sarcoidosis and Legionnaires' disease.

4.6.1.1.6 Treatment
Bone marrow transplant with HLA-matched sibling is the treatment of choice. If no HLA-matched sibling is available and the following indicators are present: bone marrow cellularity <30% with at least two of the following findings: absolute neutrophil count <500/mm^3, platelet count <20 K/mm^3, reticulocyte count <1%, then institute the following immunosuppressive therapy:

- Antilymphocyte globulin (ALG) or antithymocyte globulin (ATG), which are similar products from either horses or rabbits and mixed with human thoracic duct lymphocytes or thymocytes. ALG and ATG preparations contain mixtures of antibodies to lymphocytes and are immunosuppressive and cytotoxic (T-cell depletion). The recommended dose is 40 mg/kg/day × 4 days. The typical adverse reactions to ATG are thrombocytopenia, headache, myalgia, arthralgia, chills, fever, and serum sickness approximately 7–10 days following ATG administration
- Methylprednisolone given as IV boluses on days 1–4 at 10 mg/kg/day, then changed to an oral steroid such as prednisone 1 mg/kg/d until day 30 in order to prevent serum sickness. The toxicities

associated with steroids are hypertension, hyperglycemia, increased susceptibility to fungal infection, potassium wasting, and fluid retention
- Cyclosporine is a specific T-cell inhibitor with a recommended oral dose of 15 mg/kg/day in children to maintain blood trough levels 100–250 µg/ml. Toxic effects from cyclosporine include hypertension, azotemia, hirsutism, gingival hypertrophy, and increased serum creatinine levels
- Hematopoietic growth factors (G-CSF) have shown promise in increasing neutrophil counts. G-CSF are administered subcutaneously at 5–10 µg/kg/day; side effects include fever, chills, headache, and bone pain
- Androgens (i.e., methyltestosterone, oxymetholone) no longer have a primary role in management of aplastic anemia unless the therapies discussed above are unsuccessful. The androgens increase erythropoietin production and stimulate erythroid stem cells. The oral dose is 2–5 mg/kg/day with side effects such as masculinization (hirsutism, deepening voice, genitalia enlargement), acne, nausea, weight gain, and liver dysfunction

4.6.1.1.7 Supportive Treatment
- Blood product support should be used sparingly while the family is HLA-typed
- Thrombocytopenic precautions should be implemented:
  - Promptly report signs and symptoms of bleeding (i.e., excessive bruising/petechiae, oral purpura, melena, prolonged epistaxis or gingival bleeding or hematuria)
  - Avoid contact sports or rough activities (i.e., football, soccer, wrestling, bicycle riding, skating, diving, tree climbing, trampolines)
  - Provide a safe environment to prevent trauma (use side rails, gates, helmets, and knee pads and avoid rectal manipulation, including with thermometers, suppositories, and enemas).
  - Avoid oral mucosa trauma (use soft toothbrushes and avoid dental floss, electric tooth brush and sharp food items)
  - Add stool softeners and increase fiber and fluids in the diet to prevent constipation

4.6.1.1.8 Prognosis

With immunosuppressive therapies or bone marrow transplant, the long-term survival for patients with aplastic anemia has improved to 80%. In the European International Marrow Unrelated Search and Transplant trial, the survival rate from an unrelated donor was about one-half after conventional transplantation, due to a high rate of graft rejection or failure.

4.6.1.2 Inherited Aplastic Anemia

The most common inherited aplastic anemia is Fanconi's anemia (FA) though several others are apart of the category (including Diamond-Blackfan anemia, dyskeratosis congenita, and Shwachman-Diamond syndrome). This section will discuss Fanconi's anemia.

4.6.1.2.1 Epidemiology

All races and ethnic groups have been reported, including American Caucasians, African-Americans, Asians, and Native Americans. The heterozygote frequency may be 1/300 in the United States and in Europe and 1/100 in South African (Alter, 2003).

4.6.1.2.2 Etiology

The incidence is difficult to ascertain. Approximately 25% of childhood aplastic anemia occurs in the presence of known marrow failure genes.

4.6.1.2.3 Molecular Genetics

FA is an autosomal recessive trait with about 10–20% of families having consanguineous marriages (Shende, 2000). There are limited data suggesting a defective gene in FA stem cells.

4.6.1.2.4 Symptoms/Clinical Signs

A detailed history should be obtained that includes toxin and radiation exposure, medications, and any family history of aplastic anemia, and a physical examination done that focuses on identification of any congenital anomalies. Hemorrhagic manifestations such as petechiae ecchymoses, epistaxis, and bleeding of oral mucosa are initially observed. Other signs and symptoms such as pallor, fatigue, headache, tachycardia, or infection are also seen.

Classic anomalies are seen in 75% of FA patients and include short stature, absent thumbs or radii, microcephaly, café au lait spots, skin hyperpigmentation, a broad nasal base, epicanthal folds, micrognathia, hyperreflexia, hypogenitalism, strabismus, ptosis, nystagmus, abnormalities of the ears, deafness, mental retardation, and renal and cardiac anomalies.

4.6.1.2.5 Diagnostic Testing

FBC/CBC with RBC indices, WBC count and differential, platelet count, and reticulocyte count should be obtained. Thrombocytopenia and leukopenia develop before pancytopenia, but severe aplastic anemia develops in most cases. Examination of blood smear shows macrocytic red cells with mild poikilocytosis, anisocytosis, decreased platelets and leukocytes. The bone marrow is a hypocellular fatty bone marrow with decreased myeloid and erythroid precursors and megakaryocytes. Prenatal diagnosis with chorionic villus biopsy and amniotic fluid cell cultures of FA can be made early in the pregnancy. The following labs and tests are usually obtained:

- ANA and DNA binding titer, Coombs' test, rheumatoid factor, liver function tests
- Viral serology: HIV; EBV; parvovirus; hepatitis A, B, C; PCR for virus
- Serum vitamin B_{12} and serum folate levels
- Bone marrow aspirate and biopsy
- Cytogenetic studies on blood lymphocytes (i.e., diepoxybutane (DEB) to diagnose FA)
- Cytogenetic studies on bone marrow to exclude FA
- Acid Ham test and sugar-water test to exclude PNH
- Skeletal x-rays, intravenous pyelogram, chest x-ray to determine congenital anomalies

FA may be differentiated between thrombocytopenia with absent radii (TAR), amegakaryocytic thrombocytopenic purpura, acquired aplastic anemia, and leukemia with a hypoplastic marrow by obtaining the above diagnostic test.

4.6.1.2.6 Treatment

Supportive care includes adherence to thrombocytopenic precautions (see section 4.6.1.1.7). Transfusion of PRBCs and/or platelets, growth factors (G-CSF) for neutropenia, erythropoietin, and e-aminocaproic acid (0.1 mg/kg/dose every 6 hours orally) may be instituted. Antibiotic and antifungal treatment should be used when clinically indicated. A patient without a matched sibling should be treated with androgens, usually oxymetholone 2–5 mg/kg/day. The side effects of androgens are listed in section 4.6.1.1.6. Blood counts, liver function tests, and periodic bone marrow biopsy (to monitor for the development of myelodysplastic syndrome and leukemia) are needed to monitor the patient.

4.6.1.2.7 Prognosis

The prognosis is poor, with projected survival between 20 and 30 years unless the patient receives HLA-matched nonaffected sibling bone marrow, which offers >70% survival. Almost 6% of FA patients develop myelodysplastic syndrome (dysmyelopoiesis and abnormal megakaryocytes), and almost 10% develop acute myeloid leukemia.

References

Alter BP (2003). Inherited bone marrow failure syndromes. In: Nathan DG, Orkin SH, Ginsburg D, Look AT (eds). Nathan and Oski's Hematology of Infancy and Childhood, pp 280–365, Philadelphia, W.B. Saunders

American Academy of Pediatrics [AAP] (2002). Health supervision for children with sickle cell disease. Pediatrics 109(3):526–535

Andrews NC (2003). Disorders of iron metabolism and sideroblastic anemia. In: Nathan DG, Orkin SH, Ginsburg D, Look AT (eds). Nathan and Oski's Hematology of Infancy and Childhood, pp 456–497, Philadelphia, W.B. Saunders

Bader-Meunier B, Gathier F, Archambaud F, et al. (2001). Long-term evaluation of the beneficial effect of subtotal splenectomy for management of hereditary spherocytosis. Blood 97(2):399–403

Beare J (2002). Hemochromatosis. Advance for Nurse Practitioners, pp 63–66

Carley A (2003). Anemia: When is it not iron deficiency? Pediatric Nursing 29:205–211

Demir A, Yarali N, Fisgin T, Duru F, Kara A (2002). Most reliable indices in differentiation between thalassemia trait and iron deficiency anemia. Pediatrics International 44:612–616

Dover GI and Platt OS (2003). Sickle cell anemia. In: Nathan DG, Orkin SH, Ginsburg D, Look AT (eds). Nathan and Oski's Hematology of Infancy and Childhood, pp 762–809, Philadelphia, W.B. Saunders

Gallagher PG, Lux SE (2003). Disorders of the erythrocyte membrane. In: Nathan DG Orkin SH, Ginsburg D, Look AT (eds). Nathan and Oski's Hematology of Infancy and Childhood, pp 560–684, Philadelphia, W.B. Saunders

Glader B (2004). Anemias of inadequate production: Iron-deficiency anemia. In: Behrman RE, Kliegman RM, Jenson HB (eds). Nelson Textbook of Pediatrics, pp 1614–1616, Philadelphia, Saunders

Hastings C (2002a). Anemia. In: The Children's Hospital Oakland Hematology/Oncology Handbook, pp 1–10, St. Louis, Mosby

Hastings C (2002b). Hemolytic anemia. In: The Children's Hospital Oakland Hematology/Oncology Handbook, pp 13–14, St. Louis, Mosby

Hastings C (2002c). Sickle cell disease. In: The Children's Hospital Oakland Hematology/Oncology Handbook, pp 19–38, St. Louis, Mosby

Hudspeth M, Symons H. Hematology (2002). In: Gunn VL and Nechyba C (eds). The Johns Hopkins Hospital: The Harriet Lane Handbook, 16th edn, Philadelphia, Mosby

Jacob E, Miaskowski C, Savedra M, et al. (2003). Management of vaso-occlusive pain in children with sickle cell disease. Journal of Pediatric Hematology/Oncology 25(4):307–311

Jakubik LD and Thompson M (2000). Care of the child with sickle cell disease. Acute complications. Pediatric Nursing 26(4):373–379

Karayalcin G (2000). Hemolytic anemia. In: Lanzkowsky P (Ed). Manual of Pediatric Hematology and Oncology, pp 1157–182, San Diego, Academic Press

Lanzkowsky P (2000). Hemolytic anemia. In: Lanzkowsky P (Ed). Manual of Pediatric Hematology and Oncology, pp 154–157, San Diego, Academic Press

Lee C, Nechyba C, Gunn VL (2002). Drug doses. In: Gunn V and Nechyba C (eds). The John Hopkins Hospital: The Harriet Lane Book, pp 721–742, Philadelphia, Mosby

Luzzatto L (2003). Glucose-6-phosphate dehydrogenase deficiency and hemolytic anemia. In: Nathan DG, Orkin SH, Ginsburg D, Look AT (eds). Nathan and Oski's Hematology of Infancy and Childhood, pp 704–726, Philadelphia, W.B. Saunders

Martin L, and Buonomo C (1997). Acute chest syndrome of sickle cell disease: radiographic and clinical analysis of 70 cases. Pediatric Radiology 27:637–641

Mei Z, Parvanta I, Cogswell ME, Gunter EW, Grummer-Strawn LM (2003). Erythrocyte protoporphyrin or Hgb: which is a better screening test for iron deficiency in children and women? American Journal of Clinical Nutrition 77:1229–1233

Miller ST, Sleeper LA, Pegelow CH, et al. (2000). Prediction of adverse outcomes in children with sickle cell disease. New England Journal of Medicine 342(2):83–89

Nathan DG, Orkin SH (2003). The thalassemias. In: Nathan DG, Orkin SH, Ginsburg D, Look AT (eds). Nathan and Oski's Hematology of Infancy and Childhood, Philadelphia, W.B. Saunders

Olivieri NF (1999). The β-thalassemias. New England Journal of Medicine 341:99–109

Perkins S (2001). Disorders of hematopoiesis. In: Collins RD and Swerdlow SH (eds). Pediatric Hematopathology, pp 105–145, New York:Churchill Livingstone

Perkins S (2001). Disorders of hematopoiesis. In: Collins RD and Swerdlow SH (eds). Pediatric Hematopathology, pp 113–115, Philadelphia, Churchill Livingstone

Powars DR (2001). Hydroxyurea in very young children with sickle cell anemia is not a cure-all. Journal of Pediatrics 139(6):763–764

Quinn CT and Buchanan GR (1999). The acute chest syndrome of sickle cell disease. Journal of Pediatrics 135:416–422

Rackoff WR, Kunkel N, Silber JH, et al. (1993). Pulse oximetry and factors associated with Hgb oxygen desaturation in children with sickle cell disease. Blood 81:3422–3427

Segel GB, Hirsh MG, Feig SA (2002). Managing anemia in pediatric office practice: parts I and II. Pediatrics in Review 23:75–83, 111–121

Shende A (2000). Bone marrow failure. In: Lanzkowsky P (Ed). Manual of Pediatric Hematology and Oncology, pp 93–135, San Diego, Academic Press

Shimamura A, Guinan E (2003). Acquired aplastic anemia. In: Nathan DG, Orkin SH, Ginsburg D, Look AT (eds). Nathan and Oski's Hematology of Infancy and Childhood, pp 256–279 Philadelphia, W.B. Saunders

Steinberg MH, Barton F, Castro O, et al. (2003). Effect of hydroxyurea on mortality and morbidity in adult sickle cell anemia. Journal of American Medical Association, 289: 1645–1651

United Nations Administrative Committee on Coordination Sub-Committee on Nutrition [ACC/SCN] (2000). Fourth report on world nutrition situation. Geneva: ACC/SCN in Collaboration with International Food Policy Research Institute

Wadworth Center, New York State Department of Health. Diagnostic approach to the child with anemia. Retrieved 9/13/03 from http://www.wadsworth.org.

Ware RE (2003). Autoimmune hemolytic anemia. In: Nathan DG, Orkin SH, Ginsburg D, Look AT (eds). Nathan and Oski's Hematology of Infancy and Childhood, pp 521–559, Philadelphia, W.B. Saunders

Williams E, Williams J, Harris S, Day S, Dancy R, Wang W (1996). Outpatient therapy with ceftriaxone and oral cefixime for selected febrile children with sickle cell disease. Journal of Pediatric Hematology/Oncology 18(3):257–261

Neutropenia

Cara Simon

Contents

5.1 Epidemiology

Neutropenia is a condition of inadequate numbers of granulocytes. The absolute neutrophil count (ANC) is calculated by multiplying the white blood cell (WBC) count by the total number of bands plus segmented (mature) neutrophils:

$$ANC = WBC \times \% \text{ neutrophils}$$
$$(\text{bands} + \text{segmented forms})$$

Normal neutrophil counts vary by age and race. Newborn infants usually have an elevated ANC for the first few days of life (range $4.5–13.2 \times 10^3/\text{mm}^3$). Certain populations of blacks and Yemenite Jews will have normally lower WBCs and ANC (men $3.36\pm1.55 \times 10^3/\text{mm}^3$; women $3.13\pm1.47 \times 10^3/\text{mm}^3$) (Baehner and Miller, 1995). Neutropenia is categorized as mild, moderate, or severe, based upon the level of the ANC (Table 5.1). The risk of infection increases as the ANC decreases. Patients with severe neutropenia, especially those with an ANC $<200/\text{mm}^3$, are at significant risk for infection.

Table 5.1. Categories of neutropenia

Category of neutropenia	ANC (mm^3)	Risk of infection
None	>1,500	None
Mild neutropenia	1,000–500	No significant risk of infection
Moderate neutropenia	500–1,000	Some risk of infection
Severe neutropenia	<500	Significant risk of infection

5.2 Etiology

Neutropenia results from four basic mechanisms: decreased production of granulocytes, ineffective granulopoiesis, a shift of circulating granulocytes to the vascular epithelium or tissue pools, or enhanced peripheral destruction. Confirmation of one of these mechanisms is difficult to obtain outside of the research laboratory. Therefore, classification of neutropenia is often based on whether the neutropenia is acquired or congenital.

The most common causes of acquired neutropenia are infection, drugs, and immune disorders. Neutropenia can result from bacterial (typhoid, paratyphoid, tuberculosis, brucellosis), viral (HIV, Epstein-Barr virus [EBV], hepatitis A and B, respiratory syncytial virus [RSV]), measles, rubella, varicella, and rickettsial infections. In most cases, neutropenia that results from infection, especially viral infections, is short-lived and rarely results in serious secondary infections. Congenital neutropenia is rare and may be associated with severe recurrent infections. Congenital neutropenia has been associated with mutations in the neutrophil elastase gene (Table 5.2).

Drug induced neutropenia is the second most common cause of neutropenia. The drugs at the highest risk of producing severe neutropenia are clozapine, the thionamides, and sulfasalazine (Table 5.3).

Table 5.2. Classification of neutropenias

Infection	
Acquired	Collagen vascular diseases
	Complement activation
	Drug-induced neutropenia
	Autoimmune
	Isoimmune neutropenia
	Transfusion reaction
	Chronic benign neutropenia
	Pure white cell aplasia
	Hypersplenism
	Nutritional deficiency
	Bone marrow disorders (neutropenia usually not isolated)
Congenital	Severe infantile agranulocytosis (Kostmann's syndrome)
	Shwachman-Diamond-Oski syndrome
	Myelokathexis/neutropenia with tetraploid leukocytes
	Cyclic neutropenia
	Chediak-Higashi syndrome
	Reticular dysgenesis
	Dyskeratosis congenita

Table 5.3. Common medications that cause neutropenia

Drug Group	Examples
Antibiotics	Chloramphenicol
	Cephalosporins
	Penicillins
	Sulfonamides
	Trimethoprim-sulfamethoxazole
	Macrolides
	Vancomycin
Anticonvulsants	Phenytoin
	Valproic acid
	Carbamazepine
	Ethosuximide
Anti-inflammatory agents	Sulfasalazine
	Nonsteroidal anti-inflammatory drugs
	Gold salts
	Phenylbutazone
Cardiovascular agents	Antiarrhythmic agents
	ACE inhibitors
	Propranolol
	Dipyridamole
	Digoxin
	Ticlopidine
Psychotropic agents	Clozapine
	Phenothiazines
	Tricyclic antidepressants
	Meprobamate
Antithyroid agents (thionamides)	Methimazole
	Carbimazole
	Propylthiouracil

5.3 Symptoms and Clinical Signs

Evaluation of the child with neutropenia should begin with a complete history and physical examination. The history should include the child's family history, drug or toxin exposure, recent illness, age, and ethnicity. Physical examination should pay particular attention to the presence of adenopathy, splenomegaly, evidence of chronic or underlying disease (chronic granulomatous disease [CGD], paroxysmal nocturnal hemoglobinuria, Fanconi's anemia, etc.), and stringent evaluation of the skin and mucous membranes for signs and symptoms of infection.

Recurrent infections are the most significant consequence of neutropenia. The infections can be serious or minor. The organisms responsible for the infection are usually pyogenic or enteric bacteria or certain fungi. The risk of infection is dependent upon the level and duration of neutropenia. Patients who have an ANC <500/mm^3 due to chemotherapy, bone marrow failure, or bone marrow exhaustion are at increased risk for overwhelming bacterial infection. In contrast, patients who have benign chronic neutropenia may have an ANC <200/mm^3 for prolonged periods of time but will not experience serious infections such as bacteremia or pneumonia.

Common sites of infection are the mouth, mucous membranes, skin, and perianal and genital areas. With persistent severe neutropenia, systemic infections can occur in the lungs, blood, and gastrointestinal tract. Common infectious organisms include *Staphylococcus aureus* from the skin and Gram-negative organisms from the gastrointestinal and urinary tracts, such as *Escherichia coli* and *Klebsiella Enterobacter*.

5.4 Diagnostic Testing

Diagnostic testing for neutropenia should start with the evaluation of the full/complete blood count (FBC/CBC) and examination of the peripheral smear. If the WBC differential has been generated by automatic counters, it should be repeated manually. If the child is asymptomatic and the neutropenia is of less than 6 weeks duration, a WBC count with differential should be done twice a week for 2 weeks to assess for cyclic neutropenia. If the neutropenia occurs after a viral illness or if the child is less than 12 months old, viral serologies should be drawn (i.e., cytomegalovirus [CMV], EBV, parvovirus B-19). A neutrophil antigen should be obtained in newborns (present in isoimmune neonatal neutropenia).

If the neutropenia persists longer than 8 weeks and the child remains asymptomatic, additional studies should include HIV antibody, quantitative immunoglobulins, C3, C4, CH50, antineutrophil antibody, ANA, anti-DNA, antiphospholipid panel, and a chest radiograph (to check for thymic shadow). A bone marrow aspiration and biopsy may be necessary to identify granulocyte precursors and defects in myeloid maturation. The bone marrow aspiration and biopsy is also helpful to exclude hematologic malignancies (e.g., leukemia), bone marrow infiltration, and fibrosis.

Suggested testing for the child with chronic neutropenia that lasts longer than 6 months includes quantitative T and B subsets, diepoxybutane (if the patient has dysmorphic features, to rule out Fanconi's anemia), B-12 level, folate level, copper level, radiographs of the long bones, exocrine pancreatic studies (if the patient has a history of diarrhea, short stature, or failure to thrive), CD55/CD59 (for paroxysmal nocturnal hemoglobinuria [PNH]), CBCs of family members, and a leukocyte function test to determine if patient has CGD (if the patient has a history of recurrent infections).

5.5 Treatment

Treatment of neutropenia is dependent upon many factors, including whether the neutropenia is acute or chronic, the severity of the neutropenia, and any underlying immune defects, illnesses, or malignancies. Patients with chronic neutropenia should receive regular dental care at least every 6 months to prevent chronic gingivitis and recurrent stomatitis. In the child with neutropenia, measures to prevent infection, such as good handwashing and protection against food-borne illness (washing and cooking

Table 5.4. Gram-positive and Gram-negative organisms and common antibiotic treatment

Bacteria	Common organisms	Common antibiotics
Gram-positive	Staphylocci (coagulase-negative, coagulase-positive) Streptococci (alpha-hemolytic; group D) *Corynebacterium* *Listeria* *Clostridium difficile*	Cefepime Oxacillin Ticarcillin and clavulanate Clindamycin Vancomycin Cefotaxime
Gram-negative	Enterobacteriaceae (*Escherichia coli, Klebsiella Enterobacter, Citrobacter*) Pseudomonads (multiresistant) Anaerobes (*Bacteroides* sp.)	Cefotaxime Cefepime Ceftriaxone Ticarcillin and clavulanate Amikacin Tobramycin

foods thoroughly) should be observed. The child with severe neutropenia ($<500/mm^3$) should have a monthly physical examination with careful attention to skin and mucous membranes and should observe social isolation (avoiding crowds and persons with infection).

Infections that occur in the child with neutropenia should be treated aggressively. Fever higher than 38 °C may be the only presenting sign of infection, and the child with fever and neutropenia should be treated immediately. The child with fever and an ANC $<500/mm^3$ should be managed as an inpatient. Following culture of blood and urine, the child with severe neutropenia and fever should receive broad-spectrum parenteral antibiotics for coverage of both Gram-positive and Gram-negative organisms (Table 5.4).

A combination of an aminoglycoside and a beta-lactam antibiotic is good for initial coverage. If the child becomes afebrile, the cultures remain negative, and the clinical course improves, antibiotics may be discontinued after 72 hours. Oral antibiotics are unnecessary if there is not a known source of infection, such as otitis media or pneumonia, and if all cultures remain negative after 72 hours. If fever persists, other therapies, especially antifungal therapies (e.g., fluconazole, flucytosine, or amphotericin B) should be initiated. Patients with fever and an ANC $>1,000/mm^3$ can generally be managed on an outpa-

tient basis and treated with a beta-lactam antibiotic such as ceftriaxone and an oral cephalosporin such as Cefzil or Ceftin until all cultures are negative after 72 hours. The child who has fever and an ANC between $500/mm^3$ and $1,000/mm^3$ may be managed on either an inpatient or outpatient basis, depending upon other presenting signs and symptoms such as cough, chills, shortness of breath, or other signs of infection.

Myeloid growth factors, such as granulocyte-colony stimulating factor (G-CSF), can be used to correct neutropenia in patients with severe neutropenia. G-CSF is not indicated for all cases of neutropenia and is most effective when the neutropenia is associated with early myeloid arrest. The child with neutropenia and a serious life-threatening infection or sepsis should be started on G-CSF, 5 mcg/kg/day intravenously (IV) or subcutaneously (SQ), until the ANC is $>5,000/mm^3$ on two occasions. If there is no response after 72 hours, the dose of G-CSF can be increased to 10 mcg/kg/day IV or SQ.

The child with severe neutropenia ($<500/mm^3$) with recurrent symptoms or a past history of life-threatening infection should be started on G-CSF. G-CSF is usually started at a dose of 5 mcg/kg given SQ daily or every other day to maintain an ANC $>1,000/mm^3$. Potential side effects of G-CSF include nausea, bone pain, alopecia, diarrhea, low-grade fever, fatigue, anorexia, rash, and headache. Potential complications of G-CSF therapy include the de-

Table 5.5. Follow-up of acute vs. chronic neutropenia

Type of neutropenia	Interval of follow-up	Studies required
Acute neutropenia	34 weeks	FBC/CBC
Chronic neutropenia	Monthly Yearly	Physical examination, FBC/CBC Bone marrow (if on G-CSF)

velopment of a malignancy such as acute myeloid leukemia (AML) and an increased frequency of osteopenia and osteoporosis. It is unclear whether these are actually complications of G-CSF therapy or are complications of the underlying disease (now evident due to longer life expectancies of children with severe neutropenia). Therefore, the use of G-CSF should be reserved for the child with severe neutropenia who has recurrent symptoms or a past history of life-threatening illness. Patients on long-term therapy with G-CSF should have yearly bone marrow examinations, cytogenetic studies, and measurement of bone density.

Bone marrow transplant has been a successful treatment in some children with severe neutropenia (e.g., severe congenital neutropenia). It should be considered in the child who does not respond to G-CSF, if an appropriate HLA-matched donor is available.

5.6 Prognosis

The prognosis of the child with neutropenia depends on several factors, including the severity of the neutropenia and any underlying immune defects, illnesses, or malignancies. Prognosis also depends on the incidence, quick recognition, and treatment of life-threatening infections and/or sepsis, and is also affected by the potential development of a secondary malignancy due to the use of G-CSF.

5.7 Follow-up

Follow-up of the child with neutropenia is dependent upon many factors, including whether the neutropenia is acute or chronic, the cause of the neutropenia, the severity of the neutropenia, and any underlying immune defects, illnesses, or malignancies (Table 5.5). The child with chronic benign neutropenia of childhood who does not experience severe infections related to his neutropenia will require less follow-up than the child with severe neutropenia who requires G-CSF to prevent serious infections.

Reference

Baehner RL, Miller DR (1995) Disorders of granulopoiesis. In: Blood Diseases of Infancy and Childhood, 7th edn. Mosby-Yearbook, St. Louis, pp. 555–592

Bibliography

Baehner RL (2003) Overview of neutropenia. www.uptodate.com (06/09/2003)
Baehner RL (2003) Cyclic neutropenia. www.uptodate.com (06/09/2003)
Baehner RL (2003) Congenital neutropenia. www.uptodate.com (06/09/2003)
Boxer LA (2003) Neutrophil abnormalities. Pediatrics in Review, 24:52–62
Hastings C (2002) Neutropenia. In: The Children's Hospital Oakland: Hematology/Oncology Handbook. Mosby, St. Louis, pp. 101–106
Lanzowsky P (2000). Disorders of the white blood cells. In: Manual of Pediatric Hematology and Oncology, 3rd edn. Academic Press, San Diego, pp. 207–232

Thrombocytopenia

Cara Simon

Contents

6.1 Epidemiology

A normal platelet count in adults and children ranges from 150,000/mm^3 to 450,000/mm^3. Thrombocytopenia is defined as a platelet count more than two standard deviations below the mean of the general population, or <150,000/mm^3. Thrombocytopenia is not usually detected clinically until the platelet count falls below 100,000/mm^3, and it is rarely associated with bleeding without trauma until the platelet count falls below 30,000/mm^3. A platelet count below 10,000/mm^3 can be associated with severe, often spontaneous, bleeding.

The most common cause of thrombocytopenia in children is immune thrombocytopenia purpura (ITP). The incidence of symptomatic ITP is approximately 3–8 per 100,000 children per year and may be acute or chronic. Acute ITP is defined as ITP that resolves within 6 months of diagnosis. It is more prevalent in children younger than 10 years of age and has a peak incidence at 2–5 years of age. In 80–85% of patients with acute ITP, it will resolve spontaneously in 2–6 months. Acute ITP affects males and females equally. It is more prevalent during the late winter and spring months, and 50–80% of cases are preceded by a viral illness within the previous 3 weeks. ITP has also been associated with live measles vaccination (Lanzowsky, 2000; Steuber, 2003).

Chronic ITP is defined as the persistence of ITP for longer than 6 months. It is more prevalent in adolescents than younger children and affects females more often than males. Up to one-third of patients with chronic ITP will have clinical and laboratory evidence of an underlying autoimmune disorder (Buchanan, 2000). Spontaneous remission of chronic

ITP after 1 year is uncommon but may occur after 4 or 5 years, with or without treatment (Lanzowsky, 2000; Buchanan, 2000).

Immune thrombocytopenia can occur in the newborn period as maternal ITP or as neonatal alloimmune thrombocytopenia (NATP). Both diseases are usually self-limiting and resolve within 6 weeks; however, there are significant differences between the two disorders. In maternal ITP the mother usually has a below-normal platelet count, whereas in NATP the mother usually has a normal platelet count. NATP occurs in approximately 1 in 5,000 newborns. The platelets of the infant contain different antigens than those of the mother; subsequent formation of maternal alloantibodies that cross the placenta result in platelet destruction. Subsequent siblings with NATP are usually more severely affected. NATP is a more serious disorder than maternal ITP and has a higher incidence of intracranial hemorrhage (10–30% versus 1%) (Fernandes, 2003).

6.2 Etiology

The etiology of thrombocytopenia includes disorders of impaired/decreased platelet production, enhanced platelet destruction, and dilutional or distributional thrombocytopenia (Table 6.1). Decreased platelet production occurs when platelet production by the bone marrow is suppressed or damaged, and it can be congenital or acquired. Thrombocytopenia can also occur when the bone marrow produces a normal number of platelets but there is enhanced platelet destruction, which can occur for various reasons. Dilutional or distributional thrombocytopenia occurs when circulating platelets are trapped or sequestered in the spleen.

6.3 Symptoms and Clinical Signs

Patients with thrombocytopenia may be asymptomatic; consequently, the low platelet count is detected on a routine blood test. The most common symptomatic presentation of thrombocytopenia is bleeding, usually mucosal and/or cutaneous (Table 6.2). Mucosal bleeding typically manifests as epistaxis, gingival bleeding, or wet purpura on the buccal mucosa. Cutaneous bleeding manifests as petechiae and ecchymoses. Menorrhagia can occur in adolescent females. Persons with thrombocytopenia may experience profuse bleeding from superficial cuts.

Postsurgical bleeding can be controlled with local measures, but oozing may occur for hours after small injuries such as a minor cut or knee scrape. Bleeding into the central nervous system occurs rarely but is the most common cause of death due to thrombocytopenia. Bleeding in patients with thrombocytopenia can be distinguished from bleeding in patients with coagulation disorders, as patients with coagulation disorders experience more deep bleeding, less bleeding after minor cuts, and tend not to develop petechiae.

A complete history and physical examination should be performed on the child with thrombocytopenia. The health practitioner should obtain a general history (including recent infection, recent immunizations, previously diagnosed hematologic disease, and family history), a bleeding history (both past and present), and a history of drug ingestion. The physical examination should include meticulous examination of the skin and examination for lymphadenopathy and hepatosplenomegaly.

Table 6.1. Differential diagnosis of thrombocytopenia

Etiology	Association	Diagnosis
Destructive thrombocytopenias	Immunologic	ITP Drug-induced Infection-induced Post-transfusion purpura Autoimmune disease Post-transplant Hyperthyroidism Lymphoproliferative disorders
	Nonimmunologic	Microangiopathic disease Hemolytic anemia and thrombocytopenia Hemolytic uremic syndrome Thrombotic thrombocytopenia purpura (TTP)
	Platelet consumption/destruction	Disseminated intravascular coagulation (DIC) Giant hemangiomas Cardiac (prosthetic heart valves, repair of intracardiac defects)
	Neonatal problems	Pulmonary hypertension Polycythemia Respiratory distress syndrome (RDS)/infection (viral, bacterial, protozoal, spirochetal) Sepsis/DIC Prematurity Meconium aspiration Giant hemangioma Neonatal alloimmune Neonatal autoimmune (maternal ITP) Erythroblastosis fetalis (Rh incompatibility)
Impaired production	Congenital and hereditary disorders	Thrombocytopenia-absent radii (TAR) syndrome Fanconi's anemia Bernard-Soulier syndrome Wiskott-Aldrich syndrome Glanzmann's thromboasthenia May-Hegglin anomaly Amegakaryocytosis (congenital) Rubella syndrome
	Associated with chromosomal defect	Trisomy 13 or 18
	Metabolic disorders	Marrow infiltration: malignancies, storage disease, myelofibrosis
	Acquired processes	Aplastic anemia Drug-induced Severe iron deficiency
Dilutional or distributional	Hypersplenism (portal hypertension, neoplastic, infectious, glycogen storage disease, cyanotic heart disease) Hypothermia	

Adapted from The Children's Hospital Oakland: Hematology/Oncology Handbook (2002)

Table 6.2. Clinical manifestations of thrombocytopenia

Mucosal bleeding	Epistaxis
	Gingival bleeding
	Wet purpura
	Menorrhagia
Cutaneous bleeding	Petechiae
	Ecchymoses (bruising)

6.4 Diagnostic Testing

Diagnostic testing for thrombocytopenia should start with the evaluation of the complete blood count (CBC) and examination of the peripheral smear. The peripheral smear is evaluated for estimation of platelet numbers, platelet morphology, and the presence or absence of platelet clumping, and is important to help determine the cause of the thrombocytopenia. Congenital disorders associated with thrombocytopenia can often be diagnosed by platelet morphology on the peripheral smear. Platelets that are of normal size (Fig. 6.1) or small suggest decreased platelet production or bone marrow failure. Large platelets (Fig. 6.2) suggest platelet destruction.

Table 6.3. Additional studies to be considered in thrombocytopenic patients

Viral serologies (EBV, CMV, Parvo)
HIV antibody
Antiplatelet antibody (PAIGG)
Lupus panel
Antiphospholipid antibody
Lupus anticoagulant
C3, C4
Lymphocyte panel
LDH
Direct Coombs
Quantitative immunoglobulins
DEB
PNH
Platelet EMs
X-ray radii
Family members' platelet counts

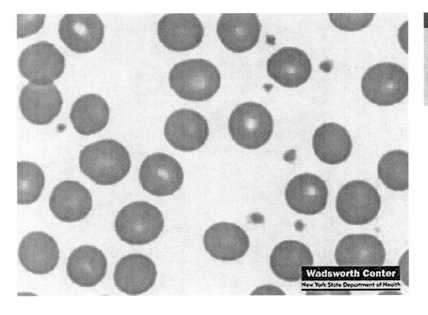

Figure 6.1

Normal platelets. Reprinted with permission from http://www.wadsworth.org/chemheme/heme/microscope/platelets.htm

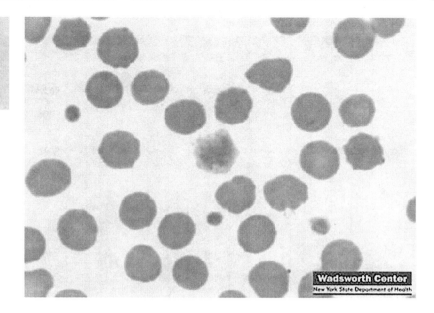

Bone marrow aspiration and biopsy is indicated in patients with unexplained thrombocytopenia. The presence of normal to increased numbers of megakaryocytes in the bone marrow is indicative of increased peripheral destruction of platelets; absent or decreased megakaryocytes in the bone marrow indicate decreased platelet production. In a hypercellular marrow, dysplastic changes are indicative of a myelodysplastic disorder. Bone marrow aspiration may also show the presence of infiltration with malignant cells.

Patients with isolated thrombocytopenia who have a normal physical examination and whose peripheral smear does not suggest other etiologies are diagnosed as having ITP and do not need a bone marrow aspiration and biopsy. However, if ITP persists longer than 6 months, a bone marrow exam may be warranted (Table 6.3).

6.5 Treatment

Treatment depends upon the cause of the thrombocytopenia. Thrombocytopenia that results from decreased platelet production by the bone marrow is treated by platelet transfusion. Platelet transfusion is utilized to correct episodes of bleeding. Bone marrow transplant can be used to treat some disorders of congenital thrombocytopenia, such as Wiskott-Aldrich syndrome and Fanconi's anemia.

Thrombocytopenia that results from increased platelet destruction cannot be treated by platelet transfusion because the immune system will destroy the transfused platelets as well as the patient's own platelets. Treatments for acute ITP include intravenous immune globulin (IVIG), corticosteroids, and anti-Rho(D) immune globulin (Table 6.4). All three of these treatments have advantages and disadvantages. None is curative but will increase the platelet count as the body recovers.

Treatment for ITP does not need to be continued to maintain a normal platelet count, but rather to decrease bleeding complications. Patients with chronic ITP who demonstrate persistent significant episodes of bleeding despite frequent and repeated interventions may require splenectomy. Splenectomy is effective in improving the platelet count in 60–90% of children with chronic ITP. It is recommended that it not be performed until a child is at least 5 years old, and should not be performed in a child less than 2 years of age if possible. Prior to splenectomy, immunizations should be up to date, including Pneu-

Table 6.4. Comparison of ITP treatments

Treatment	Dose	Advantages	Disadvantages	Side effects
IVIG	400 mg/kg IV per day for 5 days, or 1 gm/kg IV per day for 1–2 days	Faster recovery of platelet count	Cost (can be as much as 70 times more expensive than corticosteroids)	Nausea, vomiting, headache, fever, chills Rare: anaphylaxis
Corticosteroids	4 mg/kg/day PO for 4 days (with or without a taper) or 2 mg/kg/day PO for 2–3 weeks, then tapered over 1 week	Easy to administer Relatively inexpensive	Sharp decrease in platelet count after discontinuation	Weight gain, hypertension, Cushing's syndrome, mood changes
Anti-Rho(D) immune globulin	50–75 mcg/kg/day IV; may be divided and given over 2 days	Infusion time less than for IVIG Inexpensive	Must be Rh+ 1–1.5 g/dl or greater fall in hemoglobin as a result of hemolysis (occurs 1–2 weeks after administration)	Fever, chills, headache, anemia Rare: anaphylaxis

movax 23 and Meningovax. The benefit of splenectomy needs to be carefully weighed against the risk of overwhelming post-splenectomy infection that can be life-threatening.

Patients with thrombocytopenia should be instructed on thrombocytopenia precautions. These patients should be discouraged from participating in contact sports, such as football and wrestling, or activities at high altitudes when there is a chance of falling and sustaining a head injury. Children with thrombocytopenia should be instructed to avoid aspirin, ibuprofen, and other aspirin-containing medications that may interfere with platelet function.

The treatment for autoimmune and alloimmune thrombocytopenia in newborns is similar. Both can be treated with IVIG, steroids, platelet transfusions, and exchange transfusions. Platelets should be transfused if the platelet count is <20,000/mm³, but if the infant is premature or ill, they should be given if the platelet count is <50,000/mm³. An adequate platelet count should be maintained for the first 72–96 hours to prevent intracranial hemorrhage. An important distinction is that patients with NATP should be transfused with plasmapheresed or washed platelets from the mother because they lack the alloantigen responsible for the formation of the antiplatelet antibodies. In contrast, infants born to mothers with ITP should not receive platelets from the mother because they contain the antigens responsible for forming platelet autoantibodies.

6.6 Prognosis

The prognosis of the child with thrombocytopenia depends upon several factors, including the severity and underlying cause of the thrombocytopenia, the response to treatment, and the frequency and severity of bleeding complications. Prognosis also depends on the incidence, quick recognition, and treatment of life-threatening bleeding complications such as intracranial hemorrhage.

6.7 Follow-up

Follow-up of the child with thrombocytopenia is determined by the cause and degree of thrombocytopenia, the frequency and severity of bleeding complications, and the response to treatment. The child with chronic ITP with few bleeding complications may be followed in clinic every 3–6 months, whereas the child with congenital thrombocytopenia who requires frequent platelet transfusions to treat bleeding complications may require more frequent follow-up. At each clinic visit or with bleeding episodes, a FBC/CBC should be collected to check the platelet count.

6.8 Future Perspectives

Some medications that are currently being researched for the use of chronic ITP include Rituximab, vinca alkaloids, danazol, cyclophosphamide, and alpha interferon. Cytokines to stimulate platelet production are being studied and include interleukin-3 (IL-3), stem cell factor, IL-6, IL-11, and thrombopoietin.

References

Buchanan GR (2000) ITP: How much treatment is enough? Contemporary Pediatrics 17(4):112–121
Fernandes CJ (2003) Neonatal thrombocytopenia. www.uptodate.com (06/09/2003)
Lanzowsky P (2000) Disorders in platelets. In: Manual of Pediatric Hematology and Oncology, 3rd edn. San Diego: Academic Press, pp. 233–285
Steuber CP (2003) Idiopathic thrombocytopenic purpura in children. www.uptodate.com (06/09/2003)

Bibliography

Chu YW, Korb J, Sakamoto KM (2000) Idiopathic thrombocytopenic purpura. Pediatrics in Review 21(3):95–104
Hastings C (2002) Immune-mediated thrombocytopenia. In: The Children's Hospital Oakland: Hematology/Oncology Handbook. St. Louis: Mosby, pp. 107–116
Hastings C (2002) Non-immune-mediated thrombocytopenia. In: The Children's Hospital Oakland: Hematology/Oncology Handbook. St. Louis: Mosby, pp. 117–118
Landaw SA (2003) Approach to the child with thrombocytopenia. www.uptodate.com (06/09/2003)
Murphy S, Nepo A, Sills R (1999) Thrombocytopenia. Pediatrics in Review 20(2):64–69

Bleeding Disorders

Nicole M. Sevier

Contents

7.1 Hemophilia

7.1.1 Epidemiology

Hemophilia is a condition characterized by a clotting factor deficiency of the intrinsic or plasma pathway of the coagulation cascade. Over 80% of all individuals with hemophilia have a deficiency in factor VIII, also known as hemophilia A, which occurs in one in every 10,000 men. Hemophilia B (previously called Christmas disease), or a deficiency of factor IX, comprises approximately 20% of those with hemophilia and occurs in one in every 34,000 live male births. A deficiency in either of these coagulation factors results in the delayed formation of fibrin and a consequent tendency to hemorrhage. A factor VIII or IX assay of 0–2%, compared with a normal assay of approximately 50–150%, is classified as severe disease, and these patients can have frequent and significant symptoms. Moderate hemophilia is generally noted as a factor level of 2–5%, and these patients have intermittent symptoms. Mild hemophilia indicates a factor assay of greater than 5%; correspondingly, these patients have less frequent bleeding complications. Hemophilia is reported in all races and ethnicities. Other factor deficiencies are possible and infrequent, but some are associated with bleeding symptoms.

7.1.2 Etiology

Factors VIII and IX are integral parts of the intrinsic coagulation pathway that assists in the formation of a fibrin clot. Decreased functional amounts of factor VIII or IX hamper clot formation and hemostasis. Deficiencies of factor VIII or IX are inherited X-linked diseases; the genetic aspects of hemophilia will be reviewed in the upcoming section. It is now recognized that women, who are generally thought of as carriers of hemophilia, can have significantly low factor assays and be symptomatic due to the effects of lyonization.

7.1.3 Genetics

Hemophilia is a sex-linked recessive disease. The genes for both factor VIII and factor IX are located on the long arm of the X chromosome. Heterozygous women are typically asymptomatic, but can transmit the disease to 50 % of their sons and can transmit the carrier state to 50 % of their daughters. Random new mutation is possible, although infrequent, and can result in a carrier state in females or a disease state in males. Affected hemizygous males will transmit the gene to all their daughters, making them carriers. It is possible for a woman to have the disease, or symptoms, by either lyonization of the carrier state, by new mutation, or as a product of the combination of an affected male and a carrier female.

7.1.4 Symptoms and Clinical Signs

There is no distinguishing clinical difference between hemophilia A and B. Presentation of a patient with hemophilia varies, depending on known family history and severity of disease. Obviously, if family history is significant for hemophilia, then the patient's diagnosis is typically made prior to any untoward events. Otherwise, patients with severe hemophilia often present within the first year of life. Approximately 5 % of these patients present with perinatal intracranial or subgaleal bleeding. Use of forceps, suctioning, or traumatic birth may be associated with intracranial hemorrhage. Prolonged bleeding after circumcision is also a common presenting symptom. Otherwise, infants and children with severe hemophilia typically present with significant and excessive ecchymosis with little or no trauma; abnormal bleeding, especially of the mucous membranes; or hemarthrosis (Figs. 7.1, 7.2). There may be no associated injury to produce bleeding in these patients, as hemorrhage can be spontaneous.

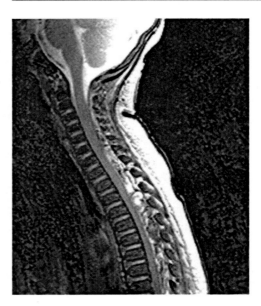

Figure 7.1

CT imaging of a cervical intraspinal epidural hemorrhage in an 8-month-old male with hemophilia A

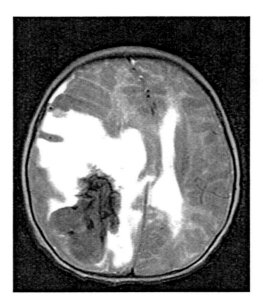

Figure 7.2

CT imaging of a right temporal subdural hemorrhage in a 9-month-old male with hemophilia A

Moderate to mild hemophilia can be associated with bleeding symptoms in later childhood or possibly adulthood. These finding are usually bleeding or bruising thought to be excessive with normal activities or due to some trauma, and hemarthrosis is possible with a significant injuring event. The disease can be so mild that it may not be detected until an adult has an invasive procedure or surgery. It is important to remember that disease genotype does not always accurately correlate with phenotype.

Specific sites of bleeding that are noteworthy include the following:

1. CNS – Intracranial hemorrhage can occur spontaneously in those with severe hemophilia, and is possible with injury or trauma in all classes of hemophilia. Typically, presentation includes symptoms of lethargy, headache, and vomiting. Silent hemorrhage is also possible, however. Head or spinal injury is considered a medical emergency; therefore, factor replacement should occur prior to any diagnostic testing. A CT of the brain is typically performed as it is more immediately available than MRI, but MRI alone may detect some silent intracranial hemorrhages.
2. Head and neck – Epitasis and mouth bleeding after tooth loss, eruption, or trauma is not uncommon in hemophilia. The fibrinolytic activity in mucous membrane areas makes stabilization of clot formation difficult, and prolonged bleeding can occur. Retropharyngeal bleeding, considered a medical emergency because of the possibility of airway obstruction, can be caused by pharyngitis, coughing, vomiting, or trauma to the neck area.
3. Musculoskeletal system – Hematoma development within the muscle causes pain, swelling, and possible decreased muscle function. When bleeding occurs in an extremity, compartment syndrome is possible, and consequent damage to peripheral nerves, vasculature, and tissue can be permanent. Pseudotumor, or encapsulated hematoma, can occur when a muscle hematoma is left untreated, and once developed it is difficult to treat and often recurs. Bleeding into a joint area, or hemarthrosis, is more common in patients with severe disease, but can occur in any patient. Joint swelling, warmth, pain, stiffness, and limp or limited movement are common symptoms of this event. Irritability and refusal to use the affected area may be the only symptoms in infants and small children. Recurrent hemarthrosis to a target joint can culminate in significant chronic arthropathy.
4. Genitourinary system – Hematuria can be spontaneous in severe hemophilia or due to trauma in all types of hemophilia. The patient most often has no symptoms other than the noted hematuria, but pain can indicate clotting in the ureter or renal pelvis. Other diagnoses must be ruled out. Hematoma to the penis can result in urinary obstruction, and testicular hematoma is significant as this may lead to infertility.
5. Post-traumatic bleeding – Most patients, whether with severe or mild disease, will not have significant bleeding after venipuncture. Bleeding post-trauma is related to the trauma itself and the severity of hemophilia. Bleeding can be delayed, occurring hours after the injury or procedure.

Other complications that may occur in a patient with hemophilia include infections due to exposure to blood products or factor replacement and the development of inhibitors.

Unfortunately, prior to 1990 a number of individuals receiving factor products did become infected with hepatitis C and/or HIV. Infections are extremely rare now due to the advent of virucidal treatments such as pasteurization and solvent-detergents and to current screening techniques. Despite treatments and screening, it is still possible for parvovirus B19 to be transmitted, and the newest concern is the possible transmission of Creutzfeldt-Jakob disease (CJD), a transmissible spongiform encephalopathy. There have been no known transmissions of CJD, but there are no current screening tests or treatments for this disease.

The development of inhibitors, or antibodies, to factor VIII or IX is a significant complication that occurs in approximately 25 % of those with severe hemophilia A and up to 5 % of those with severe hemophilia B. Inhibitor development in mild or moderate disease states is possible, but not common. Routine testing for the presence of inhibitors is recommended in all patients with hemophilia who have received factor replacement; testing should be annual or semiannual, or more frequently in high-titer patients. The inhibitor, measured in Bethesda units (BU), removes infused factor replacement at a rate directly proportional to the level of the inhibitor, thus making bleeding episodes difficult to treat. A low-titer inhibitor, or low responder, is usually classified as less than 5 BU, and a high-titer inhibitor, or high responder, as greater than 5 BU. It may be possible to overwhelm a low-titer inhibitor with a high dose of factor replacement, but this is not usually possible with high titers. There is a significant risk, as high as 26 %, that those with hemophilia B who develop inhibitors will have anaphylactic reactions to factor IX replacement.

7.1.5 Diagnostic Testing

Initial evaluation should include a platelet count, prothrombin time (PT), and activated partial prothrombin time (aPTT). The aPTT, as a test of the intrinsic clotting pathway, will be prolonged in most patients with hemophilia (with the exception of some patients with mild factor IX deficiency). The PT and platelet count should be within normal limits. Factor VIII or IX assays will indicate the deficiency state. Several types of factor assays are available. The one-stage clotting assays are commonly used, but two-stage assays are less influenced by variables; the chromogenic assay is very specific but technically complicated. Factor VIII levels can be low in several types of von Willebrand disease, and therefore it is important to distinguish between the two diseases. A von Willebrand panel, to include the ristocetin cofactor assay, von Willebrand factor antigen assay, and multimer analysis, should be done. In addition, type 2N (Normandy) von Willebrand testing, or factor VIII binding assay, should be considered, as in this disease the factor VIII assay is low, but the von Willebrand panel may be normal.

7.1.6 Treatment

There are several options for Factor VIII replacement. The product of choice is typically recombinant factor VIII, a genetically engineered product, as this has the least known risk of viral contamination, but these products are among the most costly treatments available. First-generation recombinant products contain human albumin, which is used to stabilize the factor VIII protein, but the second-generation products have little or no albumin and are stabilized in sucrose. Plasma-derived factor VIII products are less expensive than recombinant products and are most commonly used by those who have previously been exposed to this type of product, or when cost or availability are issues. One unit of factor VIII, either recombinant or plasma-derived, is equal to 2 % of factor activity in vitro. The half-life of plasma-derived or recombinant factor VIII is between 8 and 12 hours. Dosing is reviewed in Table 7.1.

Recombinant factor IX is available for factor IX replacement and is a DNA-synthesized product. This product has no added albumin, is thought to have a very limited risk of viral contamination, and is generally the treatment of choice for this diagnosis. Plasma-derived factor IX is less expensive that recombinant factor IX but carries some risk of viral contamination. Factor IX is dosed in units per kg of body weight; one unit of plasma-derived factor IX is equal to 1 % factor IX activity in vitro, but one unit of recombinant factor IX is equal to about 0.8 % activity in vitro. The half-life of plasma-derived or recombinant factor IX is approximately 16 hours. There is some evidence that if an individual develops an inhibitor, he will likely have an anaphylactic reaction when exposed to factor IX. Because of this risk it is recommended that the first 10–20 infusions of factor IX be done in the clinic or hospital setting (Jadhav and Warrier, 2000).

Table 7.1. Intravenous treatment guidelines for factor VIII and IX deficiency

	Hemophilia A treatment with factor VIII (% activity)	Hemophilia B treatment with factor IX (% activity)	Comments
Hemarthrosis, any joint	4050 units/kg ×1 (80100), followed by 2550 units/kg (50100) q1224h for 25 days	2550 units/kg ×1 (2550), followed by 2550 units/kg (2550) q24h for 13 days	Apply ice/cold pack, immobilize ×48h, then light ambulation; increase dose prn worsening symptoms; consider prednisone 12 mg/kg/day
Hematoma, soft tissue	2535 units/kg ×1 (5070), followed by 25 units/kg (50) qd ×2	2030 units/kg ×1 (2030), followed by 30 units/kg (30) qd ×2	Ice/cold pack
Hematuria	35 units/kg ×1 (70), followed by 25 units/kg (50) q1224h ×27 days	2550 units/kg ×1 (2550), followed by 30 units/kg (30) q24h ×27 days	Hydration is helpful; may use prednisone 12 mg/kg/day ×714 days; consider differential diagnosis; do not use antifibrinolytic (risk of thrombosis)
Gastrointestinal	3550 units/kg ×1 (70100), followed by 35 units/kg (70) q12h ×27 days	50100 units/kg ×1 (50100), followed by 50100 units/kg (50100) qd ×27 days	Determine cause/extent; monitor CBC; potentially life-threatening
Mucosal	3550 units/kg ×1 (70100), followed by 2535 units/kg (5070) q24h ×12 days	2550 units/kg ×1 (2550), followed by 2550 units/kg (2550) q1224h ×12 days	Ice/ cold pack; use antifibrinolytic
Head trauma	50 units/kg ×1 (100), followed by 35 units/kg (70) q12h ×710 days	100 units/kg ×1 (100), followed by 50100 units/kg (50100) q12h ×710 days	First dose to be given immediately, then CT, etc; maintain trough >50% activity
Major surgery	50 units/kg ×1 (100), followed by 35 units/kg (70) q12h ×38 days	50100 units/kg ×1 (50100), followed by 50100 units/kg (50100) q24h ×710 days	Monitor factor activity, trough >50%
Dental extraction	50 units /kg ×1(100), followed by 35 units/kg (70) q12h ×3 days	2550 units/kg ×1 (2550), followed by 2550 units/kg (2550) q24h × 27 days	Use antifibrinolytic
Prophylaxis	2535 units/kg (5070) three times per week	2540 units /kg twice per week	
Immune tolerance	50100 units/kg q2448h	Risk of anaphylaxis	

Table 7.2. Desmopressin challenge

DDAVP IV or SQ	.3 µg/kg in 50 ml of normal saline IV over ~20 min, or same dose for SQ injection
Stimate (150 µg/ml)	<50 kg; one puff intranasally or >50 kg two puffs intranasally, q12‑24h

DDAVP IV may elicit a stronger response than intranasal dosing. An increase in factor VIII levels can be expected in ~30 min
Challenge instructions: Draw factor VIII assay just before dose is given, and repeat 1 hour after dose. A three-fold increase is considered a good response

Table 7.3. Antifibrinolytic medications

Aminocaproic acid (Amicar)	50‑100 mg/kg/dose q6h (maximum 34 doses) IV or PO
Tranexamic acid (Cyklokapron)	25 mg/kg/dose q6‑8h IV or PO

These drugs cannot be used with PCCs or APCC replacement products

In emergency situations when factor replacement is not available, fresh frozen plasma can be used for those with hemophilia A or B. Cryoprecipitate can be used for factor VIII-deficient patients. Both of these products are typically available through local blood banks, and although the risk is small, possible viral contamination is always a concern for patients and families. For dosing recommendations, see Chapter 28.

Prophylaxis is used in hemophilia A and B to decrease the risk of bleeding and involves a strategy of routine administration of factor replacement. Primary prophylaxis refers to the initiation of prophylaxis during the first few years of life, and several studies have shown that this reduces the risk of chronic arthropathy in the future (Panicker et al., 2003; Shapiro, 2003). It is generally recommended that those with severe hemophilia can reap significant benefit from primary prophylaxis. Secondary prophylaxis, which is introduced after the patient has demonstrated frequent bleeding episodes, can minimize joint damage.

Several therapies other than factor replacement can be utilized for adjuvant therapy for bleeding in the patient with hemophilia. Desmopressin, or DDAVP, is a synthetic antidiuretic hormone and can increase available factor VIII levels for 12 and up to 24 hours by stimulating release of factor VIII from storage sites in the endothelial cells. This is typically effective only in those with mild factor VIII deficiency, but it does not work on each individual; therefore, a trial dose (DDAVP challenge) should be given to determine efficacy (Table 7.2). This medication is available in IV form or as a nasal formulation, Stimate (150 µg/ml). Common side effects include flushing, tachycardia, and headache, and uncommonly, hyper- or hypotension. A decreased infusion rate may diminish these effects. Overuse of DDAVP can lead to the antidiuretic effects of this medication, including fluid retention and sodium depletion. Giving more than three doses of DDAVP requires fluid restriction and sodium monitoring. Repeated doses will lead to depletion of stored factor VIII and decreased drug efficacy.

Antifibrinolytic therapies are available for mucous membrane bleeding. Aminocaproic acid (Amicar) and tranexamic acid (Cyklokapron) inhibit the action of fibrinolysis that occurs at mucous membrane sites. Both of these medications stabilize clot formation and are typically used in conjunction with factor replacement, but they may be effective when used alone for minor bleeding in a patient with mild hemophilia. To avoid thrombotic risk, these drugs should not be used concomitantly with prothrombin complex concentrate (Table 7.3). Fibrin glue is being used for wound and tissue sealing with some success in individuals with hemophilia (Kavakli, 1999).

The patient with factor inhibitors presents a significant treatment challenge. The inhibitor may be bypassed by using activated prothrombin complex concentrates (APCCs) for factor VIII inhibitors, and

Table 7.4. Treatment for acute bleeding in patients with factor inhibitors

FEIBA (factor eight inhibitor bypass activity) or Autoplex	Effective for factor VIII inhibitors	75–100 units/kg IV q12–24h	Monitor fibrinogen and D-dimers after 3rd dose due to thrombosis risk; not to be used with antifibrinolytic drugs
Recombinant factor VIIa (NovoSeven)	Effective for factor VIII or factor IX inhibitors	~90 µg/kg IV q2h, weaning to larger intervals as bleeding stabilizes; larger doses may be necessary in some patients	

recombinant factor VIIa for factor VIII or IX inhibitors. Large doses of APCCs are associated with some risk of thrombosis, and there is no in vitro assay to monitor efficacy of APCCs. Porcine factor VIII concentrate can be used to bypass the factor VIII inhibitor and is typically a treatment option for those with high-titer inhibitors. There is the possibility of cross-reactivity between porcine and human factor inhibitor development; therefore, a porcine factor VIII inhibitor assay must be evaluated prior to any treatment with this product. Hypersensitivity is also an issue with porcine factor VIII.

Immune tolerance (IT) strategies or desensitization is used to overwhelm factor inhibitor production in hopes of eliminating the inhibitor. Studies report that this works best if the inhibitor is at low titer levels at the initiation of IT. IT with use of factor IX in the patient with hemophilia B can be complicated by the concomitant development of anaphylactic reaction to factor IX (Jadhav and Warrier, 2000). Additionally, IT is less successful in hemophilia B (~30% success rate) than in hemophilia A (~70% success rate) and is associated with steroid-resistant nephrotic syndrome. Plasmapheresis is used to help rapidly decrease inhibitor levels, such as when the patient requires a surgical procedure, and is usually followed by some combination of IT (Barnes et al., 2000; Jansen et al., 2001). Newer strategies for IT still under investigation include disruption of T-helper cell function, inhibition of antibody receptors, and immunization of anti-idiopathic antibodies.

The therapeutic management of hemophilias A and B are similar and will be reviewed together. Tables 7.1 and 7.4 provide general guidelines for treat-

ment of typical bleeding. Each patient's plan of care must be individualized to reflect any special circumstances or conditions that may require more or less intervention. The patient's dose should be rounded to the nearest vial whenever possible. It is important to note that doses of recombinant factor IX must by adjusted upward by a factor of 1.2 (1 unit = 0.8% activity) to achieve the desired factor IX in vitro percent activity goal.

Supportive treatments are beneficial and include application of an ice or cold pack to the injured area when possible, pressure (local pressure or Ace wrap, if applicable), elevation of the extremity, and rest or immobilization of the affected extremity. Use of nonsteroidal anti-inflammatory drugs should be avoided because they typically diminish platelet function.

7.1.7 Prognosis

Hemophilia is a genetic condition, and as such is a lifelong, chronic condition. Currently there is no cure. In countries where treatment is readily available, individuals with hemophilia typically have normal lifespans, with heart disease as the leading cause of death. Dangers of morbidity and mortality are more significant in those with severe hemophilia.

7.1.8 Follow-Up

The chronicity and multisystem effects of hemophilia lend themselves well to the care provided at a multidisciplinary comprehensive center. Routine surveillance visits to a hemophilia specialist are recommended every 3–6 months for more severe disease and annually for mild hemophilia. Prevention of complications is the key to the care of the individual with hemophilia, and prompt treatment when bleeding or injury occurs is paramount. Management of disease complications and health maintenance are additional aspects of care.

Home care for these patients is an integral aspect of care, as prompt treatment can be given in the home. Additionally, home care can help facilitate the goal of self-infusion, which is especially important in the patient with severe disease. Routine immunizations are necessary; the deep subcutaneous injection route is preferred to intramuscular injections. Hepatitis A and B vaccinations are advised because these viruses are possible contaminates of factor concentrates. Routine surveillance of blood-borne infections should be done in those exposed to factor concentrates. Regular dental care is important, with a focus on preventing caries, infection, and extraction. Dental procedures should be discussed in advance with the treatment team because extraction and, in some cases, cleaning can cause bleeding that would require treatment. Physical therapy evaluation and treatment are required for those with affected joints or musculoskeletal complications. Certainly, education regarding hemophilia, treatment options, and safety precautions must be provided to the patient and family. Exercise is encouraged, but contact sports should be avoided. Genetic counseling should be offered to all parents and patients.

7.1.9 Future Perspectives

The search for a cure for hemophilia continues, and there are several human phase 1 trials ongoing in the United States. The goal of gene therapy is to convert severe factor deficiency to mild, or greater than 5% activity, but one of the difficulties has been how to incorporate the normal gene. Lentiviruses appear promising for future research, as it has been possible to remove the virulent factors and because these viruses infect both nondividing and dividing cells (Lusher, 2002).

7.2 Von Willebrand Disease

7.2.1 Epidemiology

Von Willebrand factor (vWF) is an important component of the clotting system because it acts as a carrier and stabilizer for factor VIII and adhesively binds platelets to subendothelial cells at the site of injury. Von Willebrand disease (vWD) is a group of bleeding diatheses in which there is a quantitative deficiency or qualitative defect in one of the functions of vWF. vWD is thought to be the most common bleeding disorder worldwide, affecting up to 1% of the population. Spread over a continuum of mild to severe disease manifestations, vWD classification includes type 1, type 2 (with several variants), type 3, and pseudo platelet-type. Type 1 vWD is the most common variant; the frequencies of the other types are identified in Table 7.5. This is typically a relatively mild bleeding disorder, and can be so mild as to go undiagnosed until late in life. In a few patients vWD is severe, leading to symptoms comparable to those of severe hemophilia. This is a genetic condition passed on through inheritance, but random mutation is possible. vWD affects males and females equally and is not associated with a specific ethnicity.

7.2.2 Etiology

vWF is a high-molecular-weight adhesive protein (or multimer) that is produced in the endothelial cells of the vasculature and in small amounts in the megakaryocytes. Disease classification is based on the qualitative and/or quantitative defect present in the vWF (Table 7.5).

vWF is an acute phase reactant; therefore, vWF levels rise in individuals during stress, inflammatory processes, pregnancy, exercise, and adrenergic stimulation.

Acquired vWD is possible and is associated with several diseases. Most frequently, acquired vWD occurs in those individuals with clonal lymphoproliferative or autoimmune diseases who have formed an

Table 7.5. Classifications of von Willebrand disease (*hwm* high-weight multimers)

Type	Pathology	Frequency
Type 1	Partial quantitative deficiency of vWF	70–80%
Type 2A	Absence of hwm and associated decrease in platelet binding functions	10–12%
Type 2B	Increased affinity for platelet complex	3– 5%
Type 2M	Decrease in platelet binding functions	<1%
Type 2N	Significantly decreased affinity for factor VIII	<1%
Type 3	Almost complete absence of vWF	<1%
Pseudo platelet-type	Intrinsic abnormality of the platelets, leading to loss of hwm	<1%

Table 7.6. Signs and symptoms of von Willebrand disease

Easy bruising or hematomas	Recurrent epistaxis
Mouth or gum bleeding	Excessive bleeding post-dental extractions
Menorrhagia	Hematuria
Gastrointestinal bleeding (10% of patients)	Bleeding with IM injections
Hemarthrosis	Mild thrombocytopenia
Prolonged oozing from minor wound	Postoperative hemorrhage

antibody to vWF. Other associated causes include absorption of vWF into tumor cells (e.g., Wilms' tumor), destruction by proteolytic enzymes during accelerated fibrinolysis (e.g., pancreatitis), reduced production in hypothyroidism, and associated decreases with certain pharmacological agents (e.g., valproic acid, dextrans, hetastarch).

7.2.3 Genetics

The genetic code for vWF is located on the short arm of chromosome 12 and is a complex single-copy gene. This gene has been sequenced and, more recently, most mutations have been identified. Most types of vWD are autosomal dominant; however, type 2A can be either dominant or recessive, and type 2N and type 3 are autosomal recessive.

7.2.4 Symptoms and Clinical Signs

Logically, symptoms of vWD vary depending on severity of disease. The most common symptoms overall are easy bruising and mucous membrane bleeding. However, the patient with type 1 vWD may have no symptoms at all until an untoward event causes significant injury or until surgery is required. Symptoms of bleeding early in life, hemarthrosis, and significant bruising with normal activities or minor trauma can occur with type 3 vWD. Patients with type 2N vWD can also exhibit more serious bleeding difficulties, such as soft tissue and urinary bleeding, as it is associated with low factor VIII levels and can mimic hemophilia (Schneppenheim et al., 1996) (Table 7.6).

7.2.5 Diagnostic Testing

Diagnostic testing should be done in those who present with clinical symptoms suspicious for a bleeding disorder. The following laboratory tests are common screening tests for vWD: activated partial thromboplastin time (aPTT); a von Willebrand panel, including vWF antigen (vWf:Ag), vWF ristocetin cofactor (vWF activity or functional assay; vWf:RCo), vWF multimers; and factor VIII assay. During screening for bleeding disorders, a prothrombin time (PT) is often done, the results of which should be normal in the patient with vWD. The aPTT, part of the routine screening for bleeding disorders, serves as a measure of the intrinsic pathway. It may be prolonged in an individual with vWD, but if the disease is quite mild, it may be normal. Some centers use a bleeding time (BT) to assist with screening, but this test has fallen out of favor due to variable results and poor correlation with disease. The platelet function analyzer assay, or PFA 100, is a relatively new screening test that identifies patients with poor platelet aggregation, which if noted would place a high index of suspicion on vWD. The PFA 100 appears to be replacing the BT as a screening test. A platelet count is also routinely done and may be abnormally low in those with type 2B, type 2M, type 3, and pseudo platelet-type vWD.

The acute phase reactant qualities of vWF make laboratory evaluation challenging, and repeated testing is commonly necessary, especially in those with mild vWD or type 1. Should repeat von Willebrand panel testing be needed, the tests should be separated by 4 weeks or more. Blood type should be evaluated because those with type O blood have vWF levels approximately 25–30% lower than those with other blood types. Therefore, in those patients with type O blood and no significant personal or family history of bleeding, and with low normal von Willebrand panel assay results, vWD can likely be excluded. Also confounding laboratory evaluation is the issue of vWF (both antigen and ristocetin cofactor) as an acute phase reactant. Consequently, physical stressors such as illness and exercise, and even emotional stressors, can elevate vWF levels; a low normal von Willebrand panel may indeed indicate that disease is present but not demonstrated on that particular day. Estrogen

therapy can increase vWF levels, making it another complicating factor, as women sent for evaluation of a bleeding diathesis often have symptoms of menorrhagia and are being treated with oral contraceptives to control menses (Cordoni, 2000).

Ristocetin platelet aggregation (RIPA) testing is typically used to determine subtypes of vWD after initial von Willebrand panel testing has been abnormal. vWD type 2B and platelet-type vWD both have increased sensitivity to low doses of ristocetin; a low-dose RIPA is performed if either type of vWD is suspected (Table 7.7).

In emergency situations when vWF replacement is not available, cryoprecipitate can be used. Platelet transfusions are the appropriate treatment for pseudo platelet-type vWD. Both of these products are typically available through local blood banks, and although the risk is small, possible viral contamination is always a concern for patients and families. For dosing recommendations, see Chapter 28.

Factors beyond laboratory testing should assist in determining diagnosis. The personal and family history has significant relevance in the patient being evaluated for a bleeding disorder. Patients with vWD may experience easy bruising; bleeding or oozing of blood after dental or surgical procedures, especially tonsillectomy; menorrhagia; or epistaxis. Family history is often remarkable for the same complaints or events. Some female relatives may have undergone hysterectomy for uncontrolled uterine bleeding but were never diagnosed with vWD. Of course, any history of family members as being "free bleeders" or even as having hemophilia should alert the provider to the possibility of vWD. The individual's personal and family history is utilized in conjunction with laboratory reports to determine diagnosis. Should family and personal history be unremarkable, the possibility of acquired vWD should be considered.

7.2.6 Treatment

Treatment of vWD is based on the pathophysiology of the specific variant or type of vWD. Several treatment strategies are available to control bleeding events. Desmopressin, or DDAVP, is a synthetic antidiuretic hormone and can increase available vWF lev-

Table 7.7. Diagnostic testing for von Willebrand disease (*hwm* high-weight multimers, *iwm* intermediate-weight multimers, *lwm* low-weight multimers)

Test	Type 1	Type 2A	Type 2B	Type 2M	Type 2N	Type 3	Platelet-type pseudo
vW ristocetin factor	Normal or decreased	Decreased	Normal or decreased	Normal or decreased	Normal	Decreased or absent	Normal
vWF antigen	Normal or decreased	Decreased	Normal or decreased	Decreased	Normal	Decreased or absent	Normal
Multimer	Normal	Absent hwm and iwm, increased lwm	Absent hwm	Normal	Normal	Absent	Absent hwm
Factor VIII	Normal or decreased	Normal or decreased	Normal or decreased	Normal or decreased	Decreased	Decreased or absent	Normal
Ristocetin-induced platelet aggregation	Poor	Poor	Poor			Poor	Hyper-responsive at low dose
Platelet Count	Normal	Normal	Decreased	Decreased	Normal	Decreased	Decreased

els for 12 and up to 24 hours by stimulating release of vWF from storage sites in the endothelial cells. Desmopressin is usually most effective in those with type 1 vWD and is somewhat effective in types 2A, 2M, and 2N, but it does not work on every individual; therefore, a trial dose should be given to determine efficacy (DDAVP challenge, Table 7.8). DDAVP should not be used in those with type 2B VWD, as the vWF high-molecular-weight multimers have an increased affinity for platelets; thus, increasing the endogenous vWF may cause thrombocytopenia and possibly worsen bleeding.

Once the degree of efficacy is established, DDAVP can be used for minor bleeding events, and for those who respond very well, it may be used for some of the more serious events (epistaxis, menorrhagia, etc). DDAVP should be used in conjunction with vWF replacement therapy for life-threatening injury or when repeated dosing is likely. This medication is available in IV or subcutaneous form or as Stimate, a nasal formulation (150 µg/ml). A lower-concentration nasal spray and pill forms are also available but are not useful for this diagnosis. Common side effects include flushing, tachycardia, and headache, and uncommonly, hyper- or hypotension. A decreased infu-

Table 7.8. Desmopressin dosing guidelines

DDAVP IV or SQ	.3 µg/kg in 50 ml of normal saline IV over ~20 min, or same dose for SQ injection
Stimate (150 µg/ml)	<50 kg; one puff intranasally or >50 kg two puffs intranasally, q12–24h

DDAVP IV may elicit a stronger response than intranasal dosing. Increase in vWF levels can be expected in ~30 min Challenge instructions: Draw factor VIII assay, ristocetin cofactor, and vWF antigen just before dose is given, and repeat 1 hour after dose. A three-fold increase is considered a good response

sion rate may diminish these effects. Overuse of DDAVP can lead to the antidiuretic effects of this medication, including fluid retention and sodium depletion. Giving more than three doses of DDAVP requires fluid restriction and sodium monitoring. Repeated doses of desmopressin will lead to tachyphylaxis (Table 7.8).

Humate-P is considered replacement therapy for vWD, as it contains plasma-derived vWF. This is a pasteurized, solvent-treated product, and the risk of

Table 7.9. Humate-P dosing guidelines

Type	Event	Dosage (IU vWf:RCo/kg)
Type 1	Serious event: Severe epistaxis GI bleeding CNS trauma Traumatic hemorrhage	Loading dose 40–60 units/kg Then 40–50 units/kg q8–12h for 3 days to keep nadir >50% Then 40–50 units/kg QD for ~7 days of treatment
Mild		
Moderate to severe	Minor event: Mucous membrane bleeding Menorrhagia	40–50 units/kg, 1–2 doses
	Serious event: Severe epistaxis GI bleeding CNS trauma Traumatic hemorrhage	Loading dose 50–75 units/kg Then 40–60 units/kg q8–12h for 3 days to keep nadir >50% Then 40–60 units/kg QD for ~7 days of treatment
Type 2 (all variants) and 3	Minor event: Mucous membrane bleeding Menorrhagia	40–50 units/kg, 1–2 doses
	Serious event: Severe epistaxis GI bleeding CNS trauma Traumatic hemorrhage	Loading dose 60–80 units /kg Then 40–60 units/kg q8–12h for 3 days to keep nadir >50% Then 40–60 units/kg qd for ~7 days of treatment

viral transmission is considered low. It is typically dosed in ristocetin cofactor units; dosing recommendations and indications are outlined in Table 7.9 (Aventis Behring, 2000). These recommendations are general guidelines for treatment of typical bleeding. Each patient's plan of care must be individualized to reflect any special circumstances or conditions that may require more or less intervention. The patient's dose should be rounded to the nearest vial whenever possible.

Other similar products are available in the United Kingdom and Europe. Recombinant vWF has been developed and is currently being tested but is not yet available for use in humans.

Antifibrinolytic therapies are available for mucous membrane bleeding. Aminocaproic acid (Amicar) and tranexamic acid (Cyklokapron) inhibit the action of fibrinolysis that occurs at mucous membrane sites. Antifibrinolytics do appear to be effective for menorrhagia and are also used to prepare for dental procedures and oral surgery. Both of these medications stabilize clot formation and are typically used

Table 7.10. Antifibrinolytic medications

Aminocaproic acid (Amicar)	50–100 mg/kg/dose q6h (maximum 3–4 doses) IV or PO
Tranexamic acid (Cyklokapron)	25 mg/kg/dose q6–8h IV or PO

These drugs work best if continued for an additional 3–4 days after bleeding stops

in conjunction with factor replacement, but may also be effective when used alone for minor bleeding in a patient with mild or type 1 vWD (Table 7.10).

Supportive treatments are beneficial and include application of an ice or cold pack to the injured area when possible, pressure (e.g., local pressure or Ace wrap) if needed, elevation of the extremity, and rest or immobilization of the affected extremity. Use of nonsteroidal anti-inflammatory drugs should be avoided because they typically diminish platelet function.

7.2.7 Prognosis

The prognosis for the patient with vWD is excellent. Most patients have very mild symptoms except at times of significant trauma or surgery. Those with type 3 vWD can have more serious symptoms and sequelae, similar to the patient with moderate to severe hemophilia.

7.2.8 Follow-up

Individuals with vWD should be seen at regular intervals by a hematologist who is familiar with vWD management. Routine surveillance visits are recommended every 6–12 months or more frequently for severe disease. Prevention of complications depends on prevention prior to anticipated bleeding events and to prompt treatment when bleeding or injury does occur. Routine immunizations are necessary; in those with more severe types of vWD, the deep subcutaneous injection route is preferred to intramuscular injections. Hepatitis A and B vaccinations are advised because these viruses are possible contaminates of factor concentrates. Routine surveillance of blood-borne infections should be done in those exposed to factor concentrates. Regular dental care is important, with a focus on preventing caries, infection, and extraction. Dental procedures should be discussed in advance with the treatment team because extraction and, in some cases, cleaning can cause bleeding that would require treatment. Home care may be useful for patients with more severe variants, as prompt treatment with Humate-P can be given in the home. Physical therapy evaluation and treatment are required for those with severe disease and those with affected joints or musculoskeletal complications. Certainly, education regarding vWD, treatment options, and safety precautions must be provided to the patient and family. Exercise is encouraged, but contact sports should be avoided. Genetic counseling should be offered to all parents and patients (Cordoni, 2000).

References

Aventis Behring (2000). Dosing schedule for the treatment of bleeding episodes in von Willebrand disease. King of Prussia, PA: Aventis Behring.

Barnes, C, Rudzki, Z. & Ekert, H. (2000). Induction of immune tolerance and suppression of anaphylaxis in a child with hemophilia B by simple plasmapheresis and antigen exposure. Hemophilia, 6, 693–695.

Cordoni, A. (2000). Von Willebrand's disease: Diagnosis and treatment. The American Journal of Nurse Practitioners, 4, 9–16.

Jadhav, M. & Warrier, I. (2002). Anaphylaxis in patients with hemophilia. Seminars in Thrombosis and Hemostasis, 26, 205–208.

Jansen, M., Schmaldienst, S., Banyai, S., Quehenberger, P., Pabinger, I., Derfler, K., Hori, W., and Knobl, P. (2001). Treatment of coagulation inhibitors with extracorporeal immunoabsorption. British Journal of Haematology, 112, 91–97.

Kavakli, K. (1999). Fibrin glue and clinical impact on haemophilia care. Haemophilia, 5, 392–396.

Lusher, J. (2002). Conference report: Highlights from the XXV International Congress of the World Federation of Hemophilia. Medscape General Medicine, 4, 14.

Panicker, J., Warrier, I., Thomas, R. and Lusher, J. (2003). The overall effectiveness of prophylaxis in severe haemophilia. Haemophilia, 9, 272–278.

Shapiro, A. (2003). A global view on prophylaxis: possibilities and consequences. Haemophilia, 9, (suppl. 1), 10–18.

Schneppenheim, R., Budde, U., Krey, S., Drewke, E., Bergman, F., Lechier, E., Oldenbrug, J. and Schwaab, R. (1996). Results of a screening for von Willebrand disease type 2N in patients with suspected haemophilia A or von Willebrand disease type 1. Thrombosis and Haemostasis, 76, 587–602.

PART III

Chemotherapy

Christine Chordas

8.1 Introduction

In the 1940s chemotherapy was introduced as part of standard therapy for childhood cancer. Prior to this time, surgery and radiation therapy were the only treatments available. Following the discovery of nitrogen mustard after World War I, rapid drug development occurred and continues into the 21st century, with novel drug development at the forefront of clinical investigations. Since the introduction of chemotherapy, overall 5-year survival rates for childhood cancers have increased from near 0% to nearly 75%. However, current therapies fail to cure approximately 30% of all children with malignancies (Bernstein et al., 2001), necessitating ongoing investigation of new agents as well as continued improvement of old agents. Today the hallmark approach to treating most childhood cancers is with multimodality treatment that includes some combination of chemotherapy, surgery, and radiation.

8.2 Chemotherapy Principles

The goal of chemotherapy is to eradicate all cancer cells, but chemotherapy is also used for palliation to control disease when cure is not likely and for myeloablation in preparation for stem cell transplant. Chemotherapy agents kill malignant and nonmalignant cells as they move through the five phases of the reproductive cell cycle (Fig. 8.1). Most chemotherapy agents kill cells in the active phases of the cycle (G1, S, G2, M). Malignant and nonmalignant cells in the resting phase (G0) are not dividing and are more resistant to the effects of chemotherapy. Nonmalignant cells that undergo rapid division (e.g., hematopoietic, mucosal, and gastrointestinal cells) are not spared, as demonstrated by some of the side effects exhibited (e.g., bone marrow suppression, mucositis).

Tumors initially grow exponentially, with a high growth fraction and short doubling time (Table 8.1), making them most susceptible to chemotherapy agents. Once in the resting phase, damaged tumor cells may die, become resistant to the particular

Figure 8.1

The reproductive cell cycle

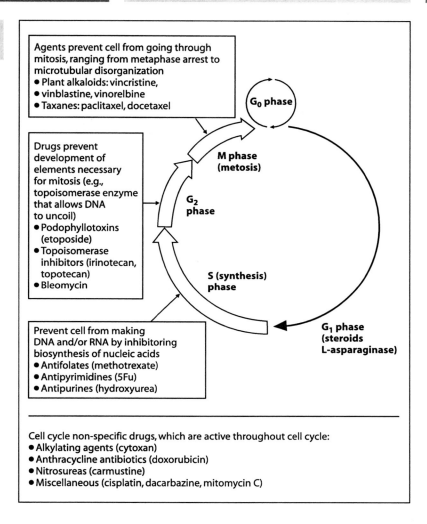

Agents prevent cell from going through mitosis, ranging from metaphase arrest to microtubular disorganization
- Plant alkaloids: vincristine,
- vinblastine, vinorelbine
- Taxanes: paclitaxel, docetaxel

Drugs prevent development of elements necessary for mitosis (e.g., topoisomerase enzyme that allows DNA to uncoil)
- Podophyllotoxins (etoposide)
- Topoisomerase inhibitors (irinotecan, topotecan)
- Bleomycin

Prevent cell from making DNA and/or RNA by inhibitoring biosynthesis of nucleic acids
- Antifolates (methotrexate)
- Antipyrimidines (5Fu)
- Antipurines (hydroxyurea)

G_0 phase

M phase (metosis)

G_2 phase

S (synthesis) phase

G_1 phase (steroids L-asparaginase)

Cell cycle non-specific drugs, which are active throughout cell cycle:
- Alkylating agents (cytoxan)
- Anthracycline antibiotics (doxorubicin)
- Nitrosureas (carmustine)
- Miscellaneous (cisplatin, dacarbazine, mitomycin C)

Table 8.1. Key terms related to the tumor kinetics

Term	Definition
Apoptosis	Programmed cell death
High growth fraction	High percentage of cells in active phases of the cell cycle
Low growth fraction	Few percentage of cells in active phases of the cell cycle
Doubling time	Time for any given number of cells to double

agent, or repair and reenter the proliferation process, whereas nonmalignant cells have a programmed number of cell divisions before apoptosis. To achieve maximum cell kill, a combination of chemotherapy agents with different mechanisms of action to target the various phases of cellular reproduction is given (Table 8.2).

Table 8.2. Classification of agents

Cell cycle phase-specific agents (CCPSA)	Cell cycle phase-non-specific agents (CCPNSA)
Antimetabolites	Alkylating agents
Plant derivatives	Antitumor antibiotics
	Corticosteroids
	Miscellaneous agents

Table 8.3. Key terms related to tumor pharmacokinetics and pharmacodynamics

Term	Definition
Absorption (bioavailability)	Rate and extent of absorption of a drug
Biotransformation	Metabolism of a drug
Clearance	Rate of drug elimination
Half-life	Time to reduce a drug's concentration by 50%
Area under the curve (AUC)	Exposure to drug over time
Excretion	How drug is eliminated from body

8.2.1 Cell Cycle Phase-Specific Agents

- Kill actively dividing cells only during a specific reproductive phase.
- Most effective in tumors with a high growth fraction.
- Typical administration is in small divided doses given at repeated intervals or by continuous infusion to target cells during active phases of reproduction.

8.2.2 Cell Cycle Phase-Nonspecific Agents

- Kill cells actively dividing during any phase of the reproductive cycle.
- Disrupt DNA synthesis, causing cells to die.
- Most effective in tumors with a low growth fraction.
- Typical administration is via single intravenous (IV) bolus dose.

Some malignant cells demonstrate resistance to chemotherapeutic agents. The mechanisms of drug resistance (Ettinger et al., 2002) include the following:

- Decreased drug uptake by the cell.
- Increased efflux of drug out of the cell.
- Detoxification of drugs in the cell secondary to metabolic changes.
- Increased DNA repair.
- Alterations in the structure of drug receptor sites or targets.
- Decreased sensitivity to apoptosis.

- Multidrug resistance gene from genetic mutation following exposure to particular chemotherapeutic agents.

To overcome resistance, most chemotherapeutic agents are administered at the maximum tolerated dose intensity and at consistent intervals. The use of multiple combinations of agents may provide a synergistic effect against the tumor cells. Agents with different toxicity profiles and cell cycle effects are typically part of a treatment regimen to enhance cell kill with minimal side effects.

Other principles used to optimize drug dose and scheduling to achieve maximum cell kill include pharmacokinetics (how the body processes the agent) and pharmacodynamics (how the agent affects the body) (Table 8.3). Physiologic and cellular factors, including concomitant agents, side effects, the child's weight and nutritional status, and organ dysfunction, may alter the agent's pharmacokinetics and pharmacodynamics.

Table 8.4. Types of antimetabolites and indications

Folate analogs	Purine analogs	Purine analogs
Methotrexate (amethopterin, MTX)	Mercaptopurine (Purinethol, 6-MP)	Cytarabine (ARA-C, cytosine arabinoside, cytosar-U)
	Thioguanine (6-thioguanine, 6-TG)	Fluorouracil (5FU, Adrucil)

8.3 Clinical Trials

Regulation of therapeutic products is mandated for all clinical research (Bernstein et. al, 2001). After agents are initially tested in vitro, preclinical studies are then performed in animals to determine toxic effects and safe doses to start clinical trials in human subjects. Before general use, investigational new drugs (INDs) are next given to adult subjects in three phases of clinical trials. Pediatric phase I studies usually follow adult phase I studies, starting at 80% of the adult maximum tolerated dosage (MTD).

8.3.1 Phase I Clinical Trials

- Establish the MTD by administering increasing dosages of the agent until unacceptable side effects are observed. The MTD is the highest dose able to be given without unacceptable side effects.
- Define dose-limiting toxicities as scored by the common toxicity criteria (CTC) scoring system defined by the National Cancer Institute.
- Characterize pharmacokinetics by determining how the agent is metabolized.
- Begin to define antitumor activity.

8.3.2 Phase II Clinical Trials

- Determine efficacy of an agent in a particular type of cancer.
- Further define the safety and toxicity profile of the agent.

8.3.3 Phase III Clinical Trials

- Determine effectiveness of the new treatment compared with existing standard treatment via randomized clinical trials.

8.3.4 Phase IV Clinical Trials

- Evaluate the agent's therapeutic profile following FDA approval for use.

8.4 Types of Chemotherapy Agents

8.4.1 Antimetabolites

8.4.1.1 Mechanism of Action

Antimetabolites are similar in structure (analogs) to normal cellular metabolites. They inhibit essential enzymes from binding in the DNA or RNA pathways, causing nucleic acids to produce the wrong codes (Table 8.4).

Methotrexate is the most widely used antimetabolite for treating childhood cancers. It is used in the treatment of acute lymphocytic leukemia (ALL), non-Hodgkin's lymphoma (NHL), the histiocytoses, and osteosarcoma.

Mercaptopurine is used in the treatment of ALL, chronic myeloid leukemia (CML), and histiocytosis. Thioguanine is used in gliomas. Cytarabine is often used in combination treatment for ALL and lymphoma. Fluorouracil is typically not used for the treatment of common childhood cancers.

Table 8.5. Alkylating agents

Nitrogen mustards	Nitrosoureas	Metal salts	Other
Mechlorethamine (nitrogen mustard)	Lomustine (CeeNU, CCNU)	Cisplatin (Platinol, CDDP)	Dacarbazine (DTIC)
Oxazaphosphorines: Cyclophosphamide (Cytoxan, CTX); ifosfamide (IFOS)	Carmustine (BiCNU, BCNU)	Carboplatin (CBDCA)	Procarbazine (Matulane)
Melphalan (Alkeran)			Busulfan (Myleran)

8.4.1.2 Side Effects

Myelosuppression, mucositis, nausea, and vomiting are the most common side effects following administration of antimetabolites. Other rare effects include dermatitis (characterized by erythema and desquamation), allergic reactions, acute pneumonitis, osteopathy, and neurotoxicity. A syndrome of high fever, malaise, myalgias, joint or bone pain, rash, conjunctivitis, and chest pain has been reported with standard doses of cytarabine.

8.4.2 Alkylating Agents

8.4.2.1 Mechanism of Action

The nitrogen mustards were the first class of alkylating agents used to treat cancer in the 1940s. These antitumor agents act through the bonding of saturated carbon atoms to cellular molecules, causing intracellular alkylation resulting in DNA damage and ultimately cell death (Table 8.5).

Several of the alkylating agents are widely used today as part of multiagent regimens for the treatment of childhood cancer. Cyclophosphamide is used in acute leukemia, a variety of solid tumors, and as part of a preparative regimen before bone marrow or peripheral stem cell transplantation. Phase II trials have demonstrated the activity of ifosfamide alone or in combination with etoposide in sarcomas, lymphoma, germ cell tumors, Wilms' tumor, and neuroblastoma. Melphalan appears to be active against rhabdomyosarcoma. The administration of bone marrow ablative doses of melphalan followed by rescue with autologous bone marrow transplant has resulted in high response rates in children with neuroblastoma, Ewing's sarcoma, and acute leukemia. The nitrosoureas have been used primarily to treat patients with brain tumors or lymphomas, and high-dose carmustine has been incorporated into transplant preparative regimens.

8.4.2.2 Side Effects

Myelosuppression is the primary dose-limiting side effect for most of the alkylating agents. Other common toxicities include nausea, vomiting, alopecia, allergic and cutaneous reactions, and gastrointestinal and neurological toxicity. Hemorrhagic cystitis is a toxicity that is unique to the oxazaphosphorines. It can range from mild dysuria and frequency to severe hemorrhage due to bladder epithelial damage. The reported incidence is 5–10% for cyclophosphamide and 20–40% for ifosfamide. The oxazaphosphorines are also nephrotoxic and can result in water retention, proximal tubular damage resembling Fanconi's syndrome, decreased glomerular filtration rate, and distal tubular damage. Cumulative doses exceeding 70–80 g/m^2 appear to be the primary risk factor. Neurotoxicity related to oxazaphosphorines is greater in children who previously received high cumulative doses of cisplatin. Cardiac toxicity has been reported with high doses of cyclophosphamide (doses >100–200 mg/kg). Ifosfamide has also been implicated as a cause of cardiomyopathy and arrhythmias at doses of 10–18 g/m^2 in patients undergoing transplant. Interstitial pneumonitis is associated with cyclophosphamide and ifosfamide.

Mechlorethamine exerts an anticholinergic effect that can lead to diaphoresis, lacrimation, and diarrhea. It also is a potent vesicant. With cumulative doses of the nitrosoureas of >1,500 mg/m², progressive renal atrophy has been reported. Cumulative doses of carmustine (>=1,500 mg/m²) are associated with progressive, and frequently fatal, pulmonary toxicity. High-dose carmustine (300–750 mg/m² can produce hypotension, tachycardia, flushing, and confusion. High-dose busulfan (600 mg/m²) has a high incidence of severe and persistent ovarian failure.

Busulfan is associated with hepatic venous occlusive disease (VOD) and seizures.

8.4.2.3 Long-Term Effects

Most alkylating agents are carcinogenic, mutagenic, and teratogenic. Gonadal atrophy that permanently affects reproductive function can occur. Nitrogen mustards and nitrosoureas have been linked to pulmonary fibrosis. Nephrotoxicity occurring after treatment with nitrosoureas, cisplatin, and ifosfamide can permanently damage renal function. Secondary leukemia is associated with the administration of melphalan.

8.4.3 Antitumor Antibiotics

8.4.3.1 Mechanism of Action

Antitumor antibiotics interfere with cellular metabolism via various mechanisms to inhibit synthesis of DNA, RNA, or both (Table 8.6). The anthracyclines form free radicals and inhibit topoisomerase II by blocking the rejoining of DNA strands. These agents are used in the treatment of ALL, lymphomas, sarco-

Table 8.6. Types of antitumor antibiotic and indications

Anthracyclines	Chromomycins	Miscellaneous
Daunorubicin	Dactinomycin (actinomycin-D)	Bleomycin
Doxorubicin		Mitomycin
Idarubicin		
Mitoxantrone		

mas of soft tissue and bone, Wilms' tumor, neuroblastoma, and hepatoblastoma. Acute toxicities include myelosuppression, mucositis, nausea, vomiting, and diarrhea. Cardiomyopathy is a late toxicity associated with cumulative drug doses.

Bleomycin chelates metals and binds to DNA to produce DNA breaks. Primary side effects are manifested in pulmonary (e.g., interstitial pneumonitis, pulmonary fibrosis) and skin (e.g., hyperpigmentation) toxicities. Dactinomycin is less widely used today.

8.4.4 Plant Derivatives

8.4.4.1 Mechanism of Action

Plant derivatives are obtained from plant material or manufactured from plant extracts. They interfere with normal microtubule formation and function, causing arrest during mitosis (Table 8.7). Vinca alkaloids extracted from the leaves of vinca plants (e.g., periwinkle) primarily arrest cells during mitosis (M phase) by interfering with microtubule formation and function. Vincristine is used to treat ALL, Hodgkin's and non-Hodgkin's lymphomas, rhab-

Table 8.7. Types of plant derivatives and indications

Vinca Alkaloids	Taxanes	Epipodophyllotoxins	Camptothecins
Vincristine	Paclitaxel	Etoposide	Topotecan
Vinblastine		Tenoposide	Irinotecan
Vinorelbine			
Vindesine			

domyosarcoma, Ewing's sarcoma, Wilms' tumor, brain tumors, and neuroblastoma, and vinblastine is used to treat histiocytosis, testicular cancer, and Hodgkin's disease. Neurotoxicity is the primary dose-limiting toxicity for vincristine. A single dose maximum is 2 mg. The dose-limiting toxicity for vinblastine is myelosuppression.

The epipodophyllotoxins inhibit topoisomerase II, producing DNA breaks during the S and G phases of cellular reproduction. They are used to treat ALL, Hodgkin's and non-Hodgkin's lymphoma, neuroblastoma, rhabdomyosarcoma, Ewing's sarcoma, germ cell tumors, and brain tumors. The primary dose-limiting toxicity is myelosuppression. Secondary leukemia has been reported with use of the epipodophyllotoxins.

The camptothecin analogs are extracts containing camptothecin. This agent was first isolated more than 50 years ago from a native Chinese tree, *Campthotheca acuminate*. Two camptothecin analogs, topotecan and irinotecan, have been approved by the FDA for clinical investigation. These agents target the intranuclear enzyme topoisomerase I and are often referred to as topoisomerase I inhibitors. During cellular reproduction as the DNA helix unwinds, camptothecin analogs cause a single strand of DNA to break. DNA damage occurs during the S-phase of cellular reproduction. Topotecan appears to be active against neuroblastoma and rhabdomyosarcoma. It is currently being investigated in phase III clinical trials. Both agents have demonstrated activity against gliomas and medulloblastomas.

Myelosuppression and diarrhea are the most common toxicities of the camptothecin analogs. Other toxicities include nausea, vomiting, alopecia, mucositis, elevated hepatic transaminases, and rash. Malaise and electrolyte abnormalities have been observed with irinotecan.

Table 8.8. Antiangiogenic agents

| Angiostatin |
| Endostatin |
| Thalidomide (Thalomid) |

8.4.5 Antiangiogenic Agents

8.4.5.1 Mechanism of Action

Antiangiogenic agents are a newer classification of agents that limit tumor growth and development by interfering with proliferating microvessels, a process called angiogenesis. Unlike the classical chemotherapy agents, antiangiogenic agents are not cytotoxic but can be used to limit further tumor growth and metastases (Table 8.8).

The resurgence of thalidomide following its initial use as a sedative in the early 1960s and its quick withdrawal from the market secondary to severe birth defects is due to its therapeutic benefit in the treatment of recurrent myeloma. To avoid birth defects, Celgene Corporation has developed a program called STEPS ("system for thalidomide education and prescribing safety") for controlling and monitoring access to thalidomide (Tariman, 2003). Other side effects include constipation, somnolence, fatigue, skin rash, deep vein thrombosis, peripheral neuropathy, and bradycardia.

8.4.6 Miscellaneous Agents

Miscellaneous agents include those with a wide range of actions that do not fit into a particular class. Miscellaneous agents include corticosteroids, asparaginase, and hydroxyurea.

8.4.7 Corticosteroids

8.4.7.1 Mechanism of Action

Corticosteroids modify the transcription of DNA by interfering with protein synthesis and cellular metabolism. Corticosteroids primarily used in pediatrics include prednisone and dexamethasone. These agents induce cell death by changing the expression of genes by binding to glucocorticoid receptors in the cell, and have a role in treatment regimens for ALL, lymphoma, Hodgkin's disease, histiocytoses, and brain tumors. They may also be used to control side effects (e.g., nausea, vomiting, increased intracranial pressure, anorexia) of other chemotherapeutic agents.

8.4.7.2 Common Side Effects

Common side effects include increased appetite, centripetal obesity, immunosuppression, myopathy, osteoporosis, avascular necrosis, peptic ulceration, pancreatitis, psychiatric disorders, cataracts, hypertension, precipitation of diabetes, growth failure, amenorrhea, impaired wound healing, atrophy of subcutaneous tissue, and osteoporosis.

8.4.8 Asparaginase/Peg-asparaginase

8.4.8.1 Mechanism of Action

A bacterial enzyme derived from *Escherichia coli* or *Erwinia carotovora*, asparaginase depletes asparagine by converting it to the nonessential products aspartic acid and ammonia, inhibiting DNA, RNA, and protein synthesis. Peg-asparaginase is a modified form of L-asparaginase. These agents are used in treatment regimens for ALL, depriving the leukemia cells of amino acids that are essential for survival and replication.

8.4.8.2 Common Side Effects

Allergic reactions occur in 20–30% of patients. Elevated liver enzymes, hepatic toxicity, and coagulopathies can lead to clotting and hemorrhagic complications. General malaise and changes in mental status may occur.

8.4.9 Hydroxyurea

8.4.9.1 Mechanism of Action

Hydroxyurea inhibits DNA synthesis by interfering with the ribonucleotide reductase enzyme system and is administered in the chronic phase of chronic myeloid leukemia (CML). Myelosuppression is a known side effect.

8.5 Administration of Chemotherapy Agents

Chemotherapy can be administered by the oral, intravenous, intramuscular, subcutaneous, and intrathecal routes (Table 8.9). Intraperitoneal and intraarterial routes are rarely used in administering chemotherapy agents to children. Assessment and education of the patient and family are essential before giving any chemotherapeutic agent. Nurses are responsible for giving the patient and family specific information about the treatment's side effects and interventions that can help minimize those effects. Patient education guidelines should consist of four parts: preparation, planning, presentation, and follow-up (Goodman, 2000).

8.5.1 Preparation

- Be available when treatment is explained to better reinforce the information that the physician has given.
- Identify learning needs and give written information regarding medications and prevention of side effects.
- Provide patients and families with self-care guidelines.
- Note the family's primary language and provide for an interpreter if needed.
- Identify any barriers to learning (e.g., anxiety, illiteracy).

Table 8.9. Chemotherapy agents and administration

Bleomycin (Blenoxane)	A test dose of 1–2 units of bleomycin should be given for the first two doses. Monitor vital signs every 15 minutes; wait a minimum of 1 hour before administering remainder of dose Administer IV slowly over at least 10 minutes (no greater than 1 unit/minute) at a concentration not to exceed 3 units/ml Bleomycin for IV continuous infusion can be further diluted in normal saline or dextrose water (D_5W) Administration by continuous infusion may produce less severe pulmonary toxicity Primary route of elimination is via renal excretion
Carboplatin (Paraplatin)	Administer by IV intermittent infusion over 15 minutes to 1 hour or by continuous infusion Compatible with ondansetron Injection site irritation and erythema can occur with infiltration but no ulceration or necrosis Needle or IV administration sets containing aluminum parts should not be used in the administration or preparation of carboplatin. Aluminum can interact with carboplatin, resulting in precipitate formation and loss of potency Maintain adequate hydration to minimize renal toxicity Route of elimination is via renal excretion
Carmustine (BiCNU)	Infusion may burn as it goes in and should be monitored closely Lower the IV rate and apply heat packs to relieve pain along the vein during administration Administer in 100–500 ml D_5W or NS as a 1–2-hour infusion Hypotension can occur if the infusion is given rapidly Avoid contact with skin; a brown stain may result Facial flushing and dizziness occurs infrequently Incompatible with polyvinylchloride infusion bags and sodium bicarbonate Administer by fresh stick if using a peripheral vein. Flush with 5–10 ml NS before and after administration to check vein patency Route of elimination is via renal and biotransformation
Cisplatin (Platinol)	Administer after appropriate hydration with mannitol Do not use sets that contain aluminum parts should not be used for administration of the drug due to loss of drug potency Keep urine output high with adequate hydration and diuresis Monitor hearing loss with audiograms At concentrations greater than 0.5 mg/ml, may act as a vesicant Primary route of elimination is via renal excretion Administer with caution in patients receiving other potentially nephrotoxic drugs
Cyclophosphamide (Cytoxan)	Encourage hydration and frequent voiding or the addition of mesna to help prevent hemorrhagic cystitis Administer IV dose slowly to prevent nasal congestion, headache, and dizziness When taking oral doses, encourage patient to take all pills before 5 pm while oral intake is adequate to minimize bladder contact with toxic metabolites
Cytarabine (Cytosine arabinoside)	Can be administered IM, IVP, IV infusion, or SQ at a concentration not to exceed 100 mg/ml High dose concentrations are usually administered by IV infusion over 1–3 hours or as IV. Continuous infusion For IT use, reconstitute with preservative-free saline or preservative-free lactated Ringer's solution Rotate sites for SQ injections

Table 8.9. (Continued)

Dacarbazine (DTIC)	Irritant; avoid extravasation Could be painful; administer slowly in 50–500 ml of solution over 30–60 minutes. A warm compress applied to the vein may decrease discomfort during infusion Protect drug from the light because it may turn a pinkish color Hypersensitivity reaction can occur with high-dose therapy
Dactinomycin (Actinomycin D)	Vesicant – use extravasation precautions
Daunorubicin (daunomycin)	Vesicant – use extravasation precautions Incompatible with heparin, 5-FU, and dexamethasone Irreversible myocardial toxicity may occur as total dosage approaches 300 mg/m^2 in children older than 2 years or 10 mg/kg in children less than 2 years; 550 mg/m^2 in adults; 400 mg/m^2 if the patient is receiving chest radiation
Dexamethasone	Greater than 80% of oral form is absorbed Hepatic metabolism is primary method of elimination. Small amount via renal clearance Drug interactions include ketoconazole, estrogen-containing oral contraceptives, phenytoin, rifampicin, carbamazepam, barbiturates
Docetaxel (Taxotere)	Monitor liver functions carefully Avoid infiltration – irritant that may cause tissue damage depending upon the concentration
Doxorubicin (Adriamycin)	Vesicant – use extravasation precautions Incompatible with heparin, dexamethasone, furosemide, aminophylline, 5-FU Turns urine reddish-orange for 8–10 hours after administration Local erythematous streaking along the vein and or facial flushing may indicate too rapid a rate of administration Has a similar name and color to daunorubicin. Check to ensure that correct drug given to correct patient
Doxorubicin hydro-chloride liposomal injection (Doxil)	Irritant – use extravasation precautions Total cumulative dose to decrease risk of irreversible cardiac toxicity
5-Fluorouracil (5-FU, Adrucil)	Administer in early morning on an empty stomach Patient should not eat for 2 hours before and after administration Wash hands immediately after topical application
Ifosfamide (Ifex)	Irritant – use extravasation precautions Administer over at least 15–30 minutes with aggressive hydration to reduce the incidence of hemorrhagic cystitis Compatible with mesna and may be infused concurrently when high-dose ifosfamide is given
Irinotecan (CPT-110)	Local irritant Stable for 4 hours at room temperature Refer to hospital protocols for treatment of irinotecan-associated diarrhea Instruct patient and parents to expect diarrhea, nausea, and vomiting Give medications for diarrhea
L-Asparaginase (Elspar)	Observe patient for 1 hour after IM injection for signs and symptoms of hypersensitivity reaction Intramuscular route more commonly used because of its lower risk of severe allergic reactions Consider test dose prior to administration Review standing orders for management of anaphylaxis Teach patient and family symptoms about reactions Route of elimination is via biotransformation Do not infuse through a filter Do not use if solution is cloudy For IV administration, give slow IVP over 30 minutes. Observe for hypersensitivity reaction

Table 8.9. (Continued)

Mechlorethamine hydrochloride (nitrogen mustard)	Avoid extravasation, inhalation of vapors, or contact with skin, mucous membranes, and eyes Potent vesicant, give with extreme caution Must be given within 5 minutes of preparation Administer via IVP via freely running IV line to avoid venous thrombosis and pain
Melphalan (Alkeran)	Administer oral meds on an empty stomach Ensure adequate patient hydration Irritant
Mercaptopurine (6-MP, Purinethol)	Oral administration concurrent with allopurinol results in a five-fold increase in bioavailability, increasing risk for severe hematologic toxicity Do not administer with meals as food decreases bioavailability
Methotrexate (MTX, Mexate)	Lower doses are usually given IVP without leucovorin rescue For high dose methotrexate (>100 mg/m^2) give leucovorin rescue, adequate hydration, and alkalinization. Maintain urine pH >6.5 and <9.0 Timing of leucovorin rescue is critical. Use for all doses >100 mg/m^2 and consider in any case of delayed excretion
Mitomycin (mitomycin C)	Vesicant – use extravasation precautions Skin ulceration may occur at sites distant from the site of drug administration
Mitoxantrone (Novantrone)	Irritant with a low potential for ulceration Extravasation may result in a blue discoloration of the skin Discolors serum and urine green for about 24 hours after administration Dark blue solution in vials. Sclera may turn blue Incompatible with heparin Administer IV over at least 5 minutes
Paclitaxel (Taxol)	Give premedications prior to infusion Irritant with a low potential for ulceration Administer in IV glass bottle or non-PVC IV bag; use non-PVC tubing and filter When administering with doxorubicin, cisplatin, or carboplatin, the doxorubicin, cisplatin, or carboplatin is given first to avoid disruption in elimination of the platinum compound
Teniposide (Vunom, VM-6)	Administer over at least 45 minutes to avoid hypotension Avoid extravasation; local phlebitis may occur Watch for hypersensitivity reactions: hypotension, bronchospasm, tachycardia, urticaria, facial flushing, diaphoresis, periorbital edema, vomiting, fever
Thalidomide (Thalomid)	Oral dosage form Absolute contraindication is pregnancy
Thiotepa (Thioplex)	A 1 mg/ml solution is considered isotonic, not a vesicant May cause local irritation
Topotecan (Hycamptin)	Typically administered daily for 5 days Continuous infusion schedules have been studied Intrathecal investigational use in neoplastic meningitis and recurrent CNS leukemia Synergistic effect if administered simultaneously with cyclophosphamide
Vinblastine (Velban)	Vesicant – use extravasation precautions Maintain adequate hydration Allopurinol may be helpful in preventing uric acid nephropathy Give stool softeners to help prevent constipation
Vincristine (Oncovin)	Vesicant – use extravasation precautions Dose range: 1.0–2.0 mg/m^2 with maximum dose 2 mg Dose by body weight in infants less than 1 year of age: 0.03–0.05 mg/kg Administer over 1 minute at a concentration of 1 mg/ml

Table 8.9. (Continued)

Vinorelbine tartrate (Navelbine)	Venous irritation occurs in about 5 % of patients; symptoms include erythema and pain at the site Administer over 6–10 minutes through a freely-running IV Local tissue damage, necrosis, or phlebitis may occur if the drug infiltrates Pain at tumor site may occur during administration

8.5.2 Planning

- Know the basics about the child's plan of care by reviewing the chart, the protocol, and the information regarding the antineoplastic agents to be given.
- Educate the patient and family about the medications before the treatment is given, and continue to educate with each treatment. Calendars, prescriptions, handouts, and drug information sheets may be useful visual tools to aid with education.

8.5.3 Presentation

- Introduce yourself and explain your role.
- Identify any questions or concerns before proceeding.
- Discuss the treatment process with the parents and give the patient age-appropriate information about the treatment, including the name of the medication, its purpose, the procedure for administering it, the length of the treatment, immediate events, expected follow-up, the medication's side effects, and home care after treatment.
- Describe potential side effects during and after administration, and offer interventions to minimize these effects. Include specific information: what to look for, how to take a temperature, when to call the doctor, how to do mouth care, and other pertinent information related to specific side effects.
- Give written instructions about activity, diet, hygiene, and medications.
- Describe any changes that may occur (e.g., urine color changes, ringing in ears) and identify appropriate interventions.

8.5.4 Follow-up

- Document the encounter and the patient's and family's responses to the teaching.

- Question the patient and parents regarding their understanding.
- Give the patient and family necessary phone numbers for follow-up, including emergency contacts, nurse, physician, home infusion companies, ambulatory clinic, pharmacy, and infusion company.

8.5.5 Nursing Preparation

- Review your institution's policies and procedures for chemotherapy administration.
- Assess response from previous treatments and current lab values.
- Review previous courses for any reactions.
- Assess the patient's prior experience with chemotherapy in order to provide additional medications with this course if needed. Note any monitoring parameters and any premedications that the patient may need.
- Review the treatment plan and orders.
- Compare written orders to formal drug protocol.
- Calculate drug dosages. Review the patient's height and weight and double-check the body surface area (BSA). The BSA is determined by a BSA calculator or nomogram or by calculating the square root of the height (cm) multiplied by weight (kg) divided by 3,600. In obese patients, some institutions use the ideal body weight (IBW) to calculate the BSA. Know your institution's policy regarding the administration of chemotherapy to obese patients. Ascites or edema may affect a patient's weight. Evaluate the prefluid retention weight as a possible basis for dosage calculations. The area under the curve (AUC) is used in patients receiving carboplatin. This dose is calculated based on the glomerular filtration rate (GFR) or the creatinine clearance.

- Review the cytotoxic agents that will be administered and any side effects. Note the emetogenic potential, any premedications needed, or any fluids needed prior to administration.
- Assess the records for any dose modifications. Doses are reduced if there has been severe toxicity with prior treatments. Many protocols or treatment regimens outline how the dose reduction is to be done. Patients may have an increase in the medication if they have tolerated treatment very well. These adjustments will be outlined in the treatment protocols.

8.5.6 Infusion Preparation

- Verify drug order and recheck doses and BSA calculations.
- Obtain agent and double-check for accuracy.
- Obtain supplies and equipment for safe drug administration (e.g., extravasation kit, infusion pump).
- Wash hands and don appropriate protective clothing.
- Assess the child's developmental level and coping mechanisms (Table 8.10).

8.6 Routes of Administration and Practice Considerations

8.6.1 Topical

- Instruct patient and/or parent on the application to the affected area.
- Avoid mucous membranes.
- Use safe chemotherapy handling procedures.
- Observe for adverse reactions (e.g., severe burning or rashes).

8.6.2 Oral

- When preparing oral medications, select the most accurate method to measure medications.
- Give milk or food with oral medications that are irritating to the gastrointestinal mucosa. (e.g., prednisone). Make sure milk products or acidic juices do not interfere with absorption (e.g., 6-MP).

- If the child vomits within 10 minutes of taking the medication, the dose should be repeated (Table 8.11).
- Provide calendars or pill boxes to help patients take the medication on schedule.
- It may be necessary to watch the child take medications.
- During adolescence, teenagers develop more independence and are highly influenced by peers. If the side effects of the medication are unpleasant, the teen may not be compliant.

8.6.3 Intramuscular

- Follow your institutional policy regarding administration of intramuscular (IM) injections.
- Consider appropriate syringe size for small volumes.
- Infants have very few IM injection sites. Usually, 1 ml is the maximum volume that should be injected in a single site for infants and children. The muscles of a small infant may not tolerate more than 0.5 ml.
- The general preferred site for IM injections in an infant is the vastus lateralis.
- The preferred site for IM injections in children of all ages is the ventrogluteal site (Wilson and Perry, 1999).
- The recommendation for using the dorsogluteal site is to wait until after the child has been walking at least 1 year.
- Alternate the injection sites. Repeated use of a single site is associated with fibrosis of the muscle and subsequent muscle contractures. Injections close to large nerves (e.g., the sciatic nerve) may cause permanent disability.
- Use safety precautions in administration, including positive patient identification and confirmation that the medication is not a vesicant.
- Decrease pain by using ethyl chloride or a topical anesthetic (e.g., EMLA) at the injection site. Change the needle if it pierced the rubber stopper on the medication vial, warm medications to room temperature, and use distraction techniques.
- Never give a sleeping child an injection.

Table 8.10. Developmental issues related to the administration of chemotherapy

Ages	Developmental milestones	Nursing interventions
Birth – 1 month	– Reaches toward mouth; strong reflex to grasp objects – Poor head control – Tongue movement may force items out of infant's mouth – Strong suck reflex – Responds to tactile stimuli – Stops sucking when full – Goes from sitting to crawling to walking – Tongue may protrude when swallowing – Responds to tactile stimuli	– Tape lines (central lines, IV lines) out of reach of infants. They like to grasp objects and could pull on lines – Place liquid in an empty nipple, place the nipple in the infant's mouth, and allow the child to suck – Draw medication up into a syringe, place the syringe along the inside of the child's cheek, and administer medication slowly. Infants will suck medicine from a needleless syringe or dropper in small increments (0.5 ml) at a time – Use a nipple or special pacifier with a reservoir for the drug. (e.g., Medibottle) – Raise the child's head slightly during administration to avoid aspiration
1 – 30 months	– Walking to running – Feeds self – Uses cup – Development of 2nd molars – Expresses feelings; may throw temper tantrums – Follows simple directions – Responds to and participates in activities of daily living	– Consider putting medications in a cup rather than a syringe – Secure IV lines – Explain all procedures in age-appropriate language – Use distraction when frustration increases; direct the child to other, less frustrating activities; and reward the child's positive response
30 months – 6 years	– Knows name – Enjoys making decisions – Has fantasies and fears mutilation – More coordinated – Loses teeth	– Explain all procedures in age appropriate language – Allow to have decision-making opportunities – Explain procedures in age-appropriate language – Offer bandages with needle sticks
6 – 12 years	– Strives for independence – Concerned with body image – Tells time – Peer support and interaction are important – Has concern for body mutilation	– Offer praise when they handle a stressful situation – Allow to express feelings – Give the child something to concentrate on during painful procedures – Have the child assist with care
12+ years	– Strives for independence – Understands abstract theory – Reasons are influenced by peers – Questions authority figures – Concerned with sex and sexuality	– Give choices in care – Explain procedures and allow them to ask questions – Provide reasons for medications

Table 8.11. Special tips for giving oral chemotherapy to children (from Meeske and Ruccione, 1987)

Problems administering	Tips and notes
Oral medications to a child who cannot swallow	The ability to swallow pills depends more on the child's past experiences than on age
	Do not use a medication that has an unpleasant taste to teach the child how to swallow a tablet
	Teach child to swallow by starting with small candies (e.g., Tic Tacs or M&Ms)
	When teaching the child to swallow, have him place the tablet on the tongue and concentrate on swallowing the liquid instead of the pill
	Consult child-life or behavioral medicine if available to help the child with swallowing tablets
	Do not crush unpleasant meds and try to administer. Give to patient whole or crush and place in gelatin capsule
Tablets	Tablets may be chewed if palatable
	Do not crush sustained-release tablets
	If a tablet is appropriate for crushing, crush it into a fine powder and mix with a small amount (about 1 teaspoon) of a sweet substance, such as honey (except in infants, due to the risk of botulism), flavored syrups, jam, fruit, pudding, flavored yogurt, sherbet, or ice cream. Make sure food or milk does not interfere with absorption (e.g., 6-Mercaptupurine)
	Avoid using the child's favorite foods to disguise medications
Capsules	Open capsules (e.g., lomustine, procarbazine, hydroxyurea) and sprinkle contents into food
	Not all capsules should be opened; consult with a pharmacist
Medications with an unpleasant taste (e.g. prednisone)	Give a chaser of water, juice, soft drink, or flavored juice after the drug
	Discourage the chewing of tablets
	Mix crushed tablet in juice or food with a strong taste (e.g., peanut butter, maple syrup, fruit-flavored syrup)
	Mix crushed tablet with a small amount of juice or food. Remember that the child must take all to receive the entire dose
	Crush pills and place in a gelatin capsule
	Do not mix tablet powder with essential food items because avoidance may develop through conditioned association
	When the medication has un unpleasant taste, have the child pinch his nose and drink the medicine through a straw (much of what we taste is associated with smell)
Partial doses	Break scored tablets only
	Pharmacy may crush tablets and dispense in unit-dose packages
	If a tablet is appropriate for crushing, crush under BSC hood and put the prescribed in a small amount of juice acceptable to the child
Compliance at home	Negotiation, partnership, empowerment and timing
	Evening administration of 6mp may be easier for families to remember

8.6.4 Subcutaneous Injection

— Some medications (e.g., gCSF, monoclonal antibody) are given daily via subcutaneous (SQ) injection.
— Parents may need to learn injection techniques to administer these medications at home. Begin educating patients and families as early as possible to maximize the amount of practice time.

— Recommendations include offering techniques to decrease the perception of pain, demonstrating the angle for SQ injection, and demonstrating common sites of administration, including the abdomen, the center third of the lateral aspect of the upper arm, and the center third of the anterior thigh.

- It is important to monitor the platelet count. If it is <50,000, additional pressure will need to be maintained at the injection site.

8.6.5 Intravenous

- There are several different ways to administer intravenous chemotherapy: peripheral IVs, PICC lines, and central venous catheters.
- For ease of administration, central lines are commonly used in children receiving chemotherapy.

8.6.6 Peripheral IV Administration

- Prepare the child and parents for the procedure. Medical play is an excellent stress reduction technique and can be used when explaining to a patient what is about to occur. If child life is available at your facility, consult for highly anxious patients and families.
- Arrange for a quiet, private setting for the child during the IV insertion, but avoid safe places such as the child's hospital room, the playroom, or the activity room.
- Provide distraction activities that allow the child to "assist" (e.g., holding the supplies, cleaning the site with alcohol, and assisting with taping).
- Assess whether the child has had an IV inserted before. Some children have never had the experience of an IV catheter, whereas many others will remember the experience quite vividly. If the child has had many IVs, ask the parents or the child which site usually works best.
- Select an appropriate IV site. There are many things to consider regarding peripheral IV insertion sites. Follow institutional guidelines related to starting an IV. Whenever possible, avoid using the child's dominant hand. Foot veins should be avoided in children who are learning to walk or are already walking. Choose a site that restricts movement as little as possible. For veins in the extremities, it is best to start with the most distal site. Avoid using veins in the antecubital fossa for chemotherapy administration. Scalp veins in an infant less than 1 month old can be used as IV sites; however, do not administer a vesicant into a scalp vein.

- A warm pack may be used to distend the veins.
- Maintain the integrity of the vein. In young children the needle or catheter should be firmly secured with tape and protected with a commercial shield. This protects the IV site from any playing and tugging at the IV site that the child may do. This intervention may not be necessary with older children or adolescents. When working with children, padding the undersides of the butterfly wings of the access needle may be necessary if the needle does not lie securely on the skin. Maintain visualization of the site so that infiltration can be identified early.
- Assess for blood return and patency.
- Certain institutional policies state that if a vesicant is to be given, a new IV site must be accessed.
- Pharmacologic interventions: Consider use of an anesthetic for pain during IV insertion. However, it is not advisable to use a topical anesthetic cream (e.g., EMLA) for PIV insertion when a vesicant is to be administered because the cream may leave the patient unable to feel the sensation associated with an extravasation.

8.6.7 Intrathecal/Intraventricular

- For intrathecal or intraventricular administration, the child may require conscious sedation or general anesthesia. Consult your institution's guidelines.
- Have the child lie flat for 30 minutes to an hour after intrathecal administration to facilitate drug distribution throughout the central nervous system and to potentially minimize headache.
- Keep intrathecal medications separate from intravenous medications to reduce the risk of giving the wrong medication intrathecally. Accidental administration of the wrong drug could be fatal.

8.6.8 Post-administration Guidelines

Post-administration documentation should include the following:

- Patient's name, date, and time.
- Site, needle gauge, and length or type of central line.
- Site assessment prior to infusion.

- Presence of blood return before, during, and after the infusion.
- Amount and type of flush used.
- Chemotherapy agent, route, dose, and duration of infusion.
- Patient's response to infusion.
- Patient education.
- Follow-up care required.

8.6.9 Professional Guidelines to Minimize the Risk of Medication Errors

8.6.9.1 Prescribing Errors

- Only a healthcare provider responsible for the care of the patient and most familiar with the chemotherapy regimen should write the orders.
- Use preprinted order sheets, or if these are not available, the generic drug name should be written clearly and in its entirety.
- Avoid using abbreviations.
- The name of the agent, the dose in mg/m², the dose to be given, the total daily dose, and the total number of days that the dose is to be given must be indicated on the order sheet.
- Avoid using ".0" to avoid ten-fold dosing errors.
- The original orders should be sent to the pharmacy. Do not transcribe or rewrite the order before sending it to the pharmacy.

8.6.9.2 Compounding

- Compounding should be performed by a well-trained pharmacist.
- In most settings, computer-generated labels are used. Make sure all information is contained on the label: the child's name, name of medication, amount of drug, and the amount and type of solution the drug is mixed in.
- Label medications with warning labels as needed; for example, "Do not give intrathecally," "Chemotherapy – Handle with care," or "For oral use only."

8.6.9.3 Dispensing

- Dispense medication on trays or in plastic zip-locked bags large enough to hold all the drugs given to one patient.
- Do not combine more than one patient's drugs in the bags or on the tray.

8.6.9.4 Administration

- Administer in a safe, nonhurried environment.
- Chemotherapy should only be administered by a chemocompetent nurse.
- Double-check the treatment plan, medication, and orders prior to administration.

8.7 Safe Practice Considerations

"Safety in the workplace is the prevention of injury by control of the environment and the use of proper work methods" (Harrison, 1996, p. 906). The Occupational Safety and Health Administration (OSHA) requires that healthcare institutions provide safe working conditions for those under their employment. Institutions should develop policies based on OSHA's guidelines for the safe handling of cytotoxic agents. These guidelines are to assist healthcare personnel who may be exposed to cytotoxic drugs through inhalation, skin absorption, or trauma (Table 8.12). The guidelines listed are based upon OSHA recommendations.

8.7.1 Mixing Chemotherapeutic Agents

- In large oncology centers chemotherapy is usually prepared by pharmacy personnel, but in some hospitals and small physicians' offices, chemotherapy may be prepared by physicians and nursing staff. If this is the case, OSHA has guidelines to aid in mixing chemotherapy (OSHA, 2002).
- Chemotherapy should be prepared under a biological safety cabinet (BSC). Even if care is taken, there may be opportunity for absorption through inhalation in areas that are not well ventilated. The blower on the vertical airflow hood should be on at

Table 8.12. Toxic effects of exposure to cytotoxic agents

Dermatologic effects	Nitrogen mustard is a potent irritant. May cause chemical burns. Inhalation of vapors can cause irritation of nasal and bronchial mucous membranes and the eyes BCNU causes inflammation and hyperpigmentation of skin following exposure during administration Doxorubicin causes contact dermatitis 5 FU is a topical irritant
Ocular effects	Doxorubicin may cause intraocular damage after accidental instillation during mixing. Burning and lacrimation, edema of upper lid, conjunctival injection, photophobia, and foreign body sensation may occur 5-FU may cause tear-duct fibrosis ARA-C may cause reversible corneal toxicity Vinblastine causes serious corneal injury
Systemic effects	Symptoms can include lightheadedness, dizziness, nausea, vomiting, flu-like symptoms, headache, cough, wheezing, urticaria rashes. Long-term exposure may cause liver disease

all times. Venting to the outside is preferable if feasible. BSC units should be recertified by a qualified technician every 6 months or any time the cabinet is moved. Technicians servicing these cabinets or changing high-efficiency particulate air (HEPA) filters should be warned of the nature of the cytotoxic agents and should use the same personal protective equipment as an employee dealing with a large spill. The cabinet should be cleaned daily with 70% alcohol and decontaminated weekly, whenever spills occur, or when the cabinet requires service or certification.

- Personal protective equipment should be worn, and hands should be washed prior to donning equipment. Surgical latex gloves should be worn. New research indicates that surgical latex gloves are less permeable to many cytotoxic drugs than the polyvinylchloride gloves previously recommended. A double layer of gloves is substantially less permeable and should be used if double-gloving does not interfere with technique. Gloves should be changed immediately if they are torn or punctured. A protective gown made of lint-free low-permeability fabric with a closed front, long sleeves, and elastic cuffs must be worn. Surgical masks do not protect against the breathing of aerosolized agents. If used in place of a BSC cabinet, a plastic face shield or splash goggles complying with ANSI criteria should also be worn. An eyewash fountain should be made available.

All used gowns, gloves, and disposable materials used in preparation should be disposed of according to the institution's toxic waste procedures.

- Cytotoxic agents should be prepared in one centralized area, and the work areas should be provided with a closable, puncture-resistant, shatterproof container for disposing of contaminated sharps and breakable materials.
- Proper aseptic techniques are essential for worker protection.
- Use the appropriate technique when opening ampules.
- Syringe bottles and IV bottles should be labeled with the patient's name and room number (if applicable), drug name and quantity per total volume, route of administration, date and time prepared, dose, expiration date, and storage requirements (if the drug is not to be transported immediately). All syringes, IV bags, and bottles containing cytotoxic drugs should be labeled with a distinctive warning label such as "Chemotherapy – handle with gloves – dispose of properly."
- Using large-bore needles, #18 or #20, will avoid high-pressure syringing of the solutions.
- Wash hands immediately after handling cytotoxic agents.
- If oral medications are to be crushed, that needs to be done under the BSC cabinet.

- IV tubing should have Luer-Lock connections with the connection sites taped. IV tubing should be primed under a BSC cabinet.
- There should be no eating, drinking, smoking, chewing of gum or tobacco, application of cosmetics, or food storage in areas where antineoplastic agents are used.

8.7.2 Transporting Cytotoxic Agents

- Drugs should be securely capped or sealed and packaged in impervious packing materials for transport.
- Personnel involved in transporting should be cautioned and trained in the necessary procedures should a spill occur.
- All drugs should be labeled with a warning label and clearly identified as a cytotoxic agent.
- Transport methods that produce stress on contents (e.g., pneumatic tubes) should not be used.

8.7.3 Safe Handling After Chemotherapy

- Institute universal precautions when handling the blood, emesis, excreta, or linen soiled with bodily fluids of a patient who has received chemotherapy within 48 hours.
- For children who are incontinent of urine, clean the skin well with each diaper change. Apply a barrier ointment so the patient will not develop chemical burns from contact with contaminated urine. Change diapers frequently.
- Have the patient flush the toilet with the lid down at least twice with each void for 48 hours after receiving chemotherapy.
- Bed linens at home that become contaminated should be washed twice in hot water in a washing machine. No other household garments should be washed with the bed linens.
- Bed linens in the hospital should be placed into a plastic contamination bag. These items need to be prewashed before being washed with other hospital linens.
- Personal protective equipment should be used in handling all linens soiled by someone on chemotherapy.

- If a patient expires within 24 hours of receiving a cytotoxic agent, the mortuary staff needs to be informed of the potential for exposure to chemotherapy (Harrison, 1996).

8.7.4 Disposal of Cytotoxic Materials

- In the hospital, locate and review institutional policies before handling cytotoxic agents.
- Place chemotherapy in a sealable leak-proof plastic bag.
- Use puncture-proof containers for sharps and breakable items.
- Do not break or recap needles.
- Wear gloves when disconnecting the chemotherapy.
- Dispose of the chemotherapy bag and tubing as an intact unit. Capping the end of the infusion tubing after disconnecting it from the patient can decrease the chance of chemotherapy getting onto the skin.
- Only housekeeping personnel who have received instructions regarding the safe handling of hazardous materials should be allowed to handle the containers filled with cytotoxic agents.

8.7.5 Spill Management

- Spill kits should be available in all admixing and administration areas.
- Prior to giving chemotherapy, review the institution's policy regarding spills. Everyone who works with cytotoxic drugs should be trained in spill management (Harrison, 1996); this includes shipment-receiving personnel, physicians, nurses, pharmacists, housekeepers, and employees involved in transporting or storing the drugs. These individuals should receive orientation regarding the known risks of relevant techniques and procedures for spills, for the handling of and proper use of protective equipment, and for medical procedures of cytotoxic drugs.
- In the event of a chemotherapy spill, notify the institutional safety officer and post a sign or have a person available to warn others of the spill. Don protective clothing including heavy-duty gloves, gown, NIOSH respirator, and eye protection.

- In the event of a chemotherapy spill, use the items in the spill kit to prevent the spill from contaminating other areas. Absorb the spill with chemical spill pillows, gauze pads, or absorbent towels. Decontaminate the area if a neutralizing agent is available. Seal and double-bag all contaminated materials for disposal. Broken glass should only be handled with heavy-duty gloves and a disposable scoop. Clean the spill according to the type of spill and the location. A dry powder should be covered with a generous supply of water-dampened absorbent towel or gauze (Harrison, 1996). On hard surfaces, wipe up liquids using absorbent pads. On carpeted surfaces, use absorbent powder to absorb the spill and a vacuum specifically for hazardous clean-up to remove the powder (Oncology Nursing Society, 2001).
- Report and document spill according to institutional policy. Include in documentation the name of the agent and the volume spilled, how the spill occurred and how it was managed, and the names of personnel, patients, and others exposed to the agent.

8.7.6 Procedures Following Accidental Exposure

- If direct skin exposure occurs, rinse immediately with water (Table 8.11). An emergency eyewash or shower should be available.
- For eye exposure, rinse with an eye wash solution for at least 15 minutes (Table 8.11).
- Report all episodes of exposure to employee health.

8.7.7 Storage

- Store chemotherapy drug containers in a location that permits appropriate temperature and safety regulation.
- Label all drug containers to indicate hazardous materials.
- Provide instructions on what to do in case of accidental exposure (e.g., Material Safety Data Sheets).
- Ensure that packaging is intact before removing chemotherapy drug containers.

8.7.8 Medical Management

- Employees who are pregnant or planning to become pregnant, who are breastfeeding, or who have a reason to limit exposure to cytotoxic agents (e.g., hypersensitivity reactions) should be offered work in areas where exposure is not likely.

8.8 Administration of Chemotherapy in the Home

The home care industry is the fastest growing segment of the healthcare industry. Home health agencies provide a wide range of services and can be extremely effective. They can provide intravenous hydration, administer some chemotherapeutic agents, and administer other symptom management drugs. The administration of chemotherapy in the home provides an alternative to hospitalizations and numerous outpatient visits for the pediatric oncology patient.

Studies have shown that home chemotherapy can have a positive impact on patient outcomes, family satisfaction, and the provision of cost-effective care (Close et al., 1995). The frequent hospitalizations and clinic visits required for the treatment of children with cancer disrupt the patterns and flow of family life and the education and socialization of children. Administration of select chemotherapy at home results in lower billed charges, reduced expenses, reduced loss of income for parents, and improved patient and family satisfaction.

The technological advances in equipment and supportive measures (Table 8.13) over the last 20 years have attributed to the increased use of home health agencies.

The National Association of Children's Hospitals and Related Institutions (NACHRI) conducted a patient care oncology focus group. The group developed specific recommendations for home care requirements for children and adolescents with cancer (NACHRI, 2000), and the Association of Pediatric Oncology Nurses reviewed and endorsed these recommendations. A summary of the recommendations follows:

Table 8.13. Functions and equipment provided by home health agencies

Provide central venous access education and care
Administer chemotherapy regimens and antiemetic support
Administer continuous IV infusions, IV hydration, and IV antimicrobial and antifungal treatment
Provide nutritional support
Provide pain management
Provide programmed infusion pumps

- Pediatric health care providers, the payor, and the family must collaborate to select the most appropriate healthcare delivery setting based on assessment of the child and family.
- Families must be given the option to interview and select a home healthcare agency based on the child's specific needs and the agency's expertise (e.g., skilled care requirements, durable medical equipment).
- Home care agencies offering oncology services to children must ensure access to home care nurses and pharmacists with documented competency in pediatrics and oncology.
- Mechanisms must be established to ensure adequate and timely communication between the home care agency, payor, primary care provider, and pediatric oncology specialist about the child's long-term treatment.

8.8.1 Eligibility Guidelines for Home Chemotherapy

The following criteria should be considered before implementing a home treatment plan:
- The medical, nursing, and psychosocial staff should evaluate, with the family, the appropriateness for home chemotherapy
- A comprehensive discharge plan that incorporates all aspects of home health care and supportive services is necessary.
- The child's medical condition should be stable and easily managed in the home by family caregivers partnered with home care professionals.

- Agents that have previously caused an adverse reaction in the patient should not be administered at home.
- Any therapy with a high affinity for anaphylaxis should not be given at home (e.g., L-asparaginase).
- A central venous access device may be required for continuous infusions, vesicants, and parenteral nutrition.
- Prior authorization from the insurance company is necessary for all home administration.
- The best supportive care regimen to prevent and minimize side effects of the therapy in the home should be established.
- The home environment must include general cleanliness, electricity, telephone, refrigeration, plumbing, and heating and cooling systems.
- The caregiver and parent must be physically present in the home during infusions and must demonstrate their ability to operate the infusion pumps and lines.

8.8.2 Home Care Agency Chemotherapy Safety Guidelines

The following are guidelines and criteria to consider for patients and families participating in home chemotherapy:

- The agency should be accredited and licensed by state regulatory agencies.
- There should be a competency program for pharmacists, compounding technicians, and pediatric nurses demonstrating skill with central venous access devices.
- Chemotherapy certification should be required, including safe administration of vesicants and management of side effects.
- Written policies and procedures that address the handling and safe administration of chemotherapy must be in place.
- A system for documentation of double-checking chemotherapy orders must be in place.

8.8.3 Management of Home Chemotherapy Guidelines

- All home care providers must be notified of the planned discharge and start of home therapy. A chemotherapy plan should be sent to the provider.
- The pharmacist must receive the orders the day before discharge in order to process the order safely and communicate questions to the oncology team.
- A visit in the house by the home care nurse should be set up as soon as possible after discharge.
- A chemotherapy spill kit must be available in the home that includes gloves, goggles, a respirator mask, absorbent materials, large plastic disposal bags, and toxic waste labels (Table 8.14).
- Appropriate extravasation interventions and policies must be available.
- Approved laboratory services must be available.
- Family and caregiver education regarding the chemotherapy agent, the treatment schedule, and the method of administration should be ongoing (Table 8.15).
- Patient handbooks, contact numbers, and educational materials should be provided.

Table 8.14. Contents of a home care chemotherapy kit

IV start kit	Normal saline vials
CVL dressing kit	Heparin flush
Implanted catheter access kit	100-cc bag NS
IV tubing	Chemotherapy spill kit
Extension tubing	Oral airway
3-cc syringes	Cold pack and warm pack
5-cc syringes	
10-cc syringes	
Injection cap	
Alcohol preps	Anaphylaxis kit:
Tourniquet	IV diphenhydramine
Latex gloves	IV epinephrine 1:1,000
Mask	IV hydrocortisone
Sharps container	
Gauze	
Bandages	

Table 8.15. Family/caregiver education and information needs for administration of home chemotherapy

Names and indications of all prescribed drugs	Care of the central venous access device
Common side effects of all drugs	Preparation of equipment and working area for giving chemotherapy and medications
Action to take in the event of an allergic reaction	Drug administration procedure
Action to take if child becomes febrile	Technique for taking child's temperature
Safe storage and disposal of drugs and sharps in the home	Monitoring of intake and output
Importance of compliance with prescribed medication	Understanding of how to observe for and report any problems
Details of planned home visit and/or follow-up	Treatment plan, medication record, and allergy sheet in a notebook or folder for ready reference
Knowledge of where to seek advice, with 24-hour contact numbers	Equipment troubleshooting
Handling of antineoplastic agents in the home	Emergency contact numbers (should be displayed near telephones in the home)

Table 8.16. Vesicant (*V*) and irritant (*I*) antineoplastic agents

Alkylating agents	Antitumor antibiotics	Plant alkaloids
Nitrogen mustard (V)	Doxorubicin (V)	Vincristine (V)
Cisplatin (V)	Daunomycin (V)	Vinblastine (V)
Carboplatin (I)	Dactinomycin (V)	Vinorelbine (V)
Ifosfamide (I)	Mitomycin C (V)	Etoposide(I)
		Teniposide (I)

Table 8.17. Key terms related to extravasation

Extravasation	Leakage of a drug into subcutaneous tissue, potentially causing local inflammation, hyperpigmentation, induration, ulceration, pain, sloughing of tissue, damage to nerves and tendons, necrosis
Irritant	Agent that can cause aching, tightness, or phlebitis at the injection site or along the vein (with or without an inflammatory reaction)
Vesicant	Agent that can cause tissue destruction
Delayed extravasation	Extravasation in which symptoms occur 48 hours or more after drug is given
Flare	Local allergic reaction without pain that is usually accompanied by red blotches along the vein. Symptoms subside within 30 minutes with or without treatment

8.8.4 Evaluation of Home Administration of Chemotherapy

Continuous collaboration among the pediatric oncology treatment team, the home care agency, and the family is essential throughout treatment. The treatment team must have a mechanism for evaluating family and treatment center satisfaction with the home care services. Children with cancer should be ensured access to appropriate services for their care.

8.8.5 Immediate Complications of Chemotherapy Administration

Although most immediate complications from chemotherapy are rare, it is important that the pediatric oncology nurse be knowledgeable on how to recognize and manage adverse events. Recognizing side effects that can be potentially damaging or life-threatening is an important skill that at times may be difficult due to the fact that infants and children have difficulty communicating symptoms.

8.9 Extravasation

An extravasation that occurs in a child may lead to an increased risk for injury because of the patient's inability to verbalize pain or changes in sensation during vesicant administration (Tables 8.16, 8.17). Rates of occurrence range from 0.5–6%. Consequences of extravasation can include significant tissue damage, altered limb function, and pain (Table 8.16) and can impact quality of life for long-term survivors (Kassner, 2000).

8.9.1 Pathophysiology of Extravasation

Two major mechanisms are believed to cause tissue damage. Some agents (e.g., anthracyclines) are absorbed by local cells in the tissue and bind to DNA, causing cell death. The vesicant agent is then released into the surrounding tissue, causing further cell death. Healing is inhibited when the process repeats itself and the drug is absorbed by other cells. Doxorubicin at significant levels has been found in surrounding tissues for weeks to months after an extravasation (Albanell and Baselga, 2000).

Other agents (e.g., vinca alkaloids) do not bind to cellular DNA. Local tissue damage is more easily neutralized than damage to surrounding tissues.

8.9.2 Risk Factors of Peripheral Extravasation

Peripheral administration of vesicant agents in children is challenging. Children may be at risk for serious injury due to the difficult access of peripheral veins. Other risk factors include the following:

- Anatomic issues, including site of venous access, venous integrity, vessel size, and blood flow (Kassner, 2000)
- Duration of tissue exposure and the amount of infiltrate (Kassner, 2000)
- Types of intravenous catheters; for instance, steel needles are associated with increased risk of extravasation (Kassner, 2000)
- Smaller-gauge catheters, which allow easier blood flow around the catheter (Beason, 1990)
- Inability of the child to communicate pain or change in sensation during the infusion (Kassner, 2000)

8.9.3 Risk Factors of Extravasation with Central Venous Access Devices

Although the use of central venous access devices (CVADs) in the pediatric oncology population has improved the ease and safety of chemotherapy administration, especially for continuous infusions of vesicants, the risk for extravasation still exists. These factors include the following:

- Needle dislodgement, incorrect needle length, and incomplete or improper needle access technique (Schulmeister and Camp-Sorrell, 2000)
- Increased activity or sleeping on the side of the port-a-catheter (Kassner, 2000)
- Rupture or tear in the catheter or port septum (Kassner, 2000)

- Migration of the catheter tip (Oncology Nursing Society, 2002)
- Fibrin sheath formation at the catheter tip (Oncology Nursing Society, 2002)
- Persistent withdrawal occlusion (e.g., inability to draw blood but able to flush the line without difficulty) or "positional blood draws" (Kassner, 2000)
- Tugging or improper securing of IV tubing

8.9.4 Administration Techniques That May Help Prevent Extravasation

8.9.4.1 Peripheral Administration

- Only nurses who are skilled at venipuncture techniques and know how to assess and intervene in case of extravasation should administer vesicant agents. Competency should be reviewed yearly (Camp-Sorrell, 1998).
- It is recommended that a new peripheral site be used versus an existing IV site, if possible (Camp-Sorrell, 1998).
- Large veins in the nondominant upper extremity should be used whenever possible. The forearm is recommended because this area has more fleshy soft tissue and a decreased risk of physical impairment if extravasation does occur (Kassner, 2000).
- Repeated attempts to place the catheter below the original IV site should be avoided for 24 hours to allow the vein wall to heal (Kassner, 2000).
- Avoid the dorsum of the hand and foot and the antecubital fossa as these areas present an increased risk for serious functional damage because of the proximity of tendons and nerves (Kassner, 2000).
- Select a catheter that is appropriate for the length and rate of the infusion. Small-gauge catheters (0–3 gauge) are recommended by the Intravenous Nursing Society because they cause less trauma to the vein and promote greater blood flow around the needle (Kassner, 2000).
- Short, single-dose infusions can be safely administered through a butterfly catheter, whereas longer infusions should be administered through polyethylene or Teflon catheters (Kassner, 2000).
- Use the two-syringe method, using one syringe to inject the vesicant and the other syringe to check for blood return and patency.

- The vesicant should be given over less than 3 minutes, with blood return being checked after every 1–2 ml of drug administered (San Angel, 1995).
- Avoid using syringe pumps because of the high flow pressure that can increase the risk for extravasation (Kassner, 2000)

8.9.5 Central Venous Access Device Administration

Extravasation into the upper neck or torso can cause serious tissue damage that may require extensive reconstructive surgery. Therefore, administration into a CVAD should be done very carefully.

- CVADs should be used for all continuous infusions of vesicant agents.
- An appropriate size, non-coring needle should be used in patients with a port-a-catheter (Schulmeister and Camp-Sorrell, 2000).
- The nurse's competency to access the port-a-catheter should be reviewed annually.
- A brisk blood return should be noted from the CVAD before starting the administration of a vesicant agent.
- If persistent withdrawal occlusion occurs, alteplase should be administered per institutional policy (Schulmeister and Camp-Sorrell, 2000; Deitcher et al., 2002a).
- For lines that do not clear with alteplase, radiographic studies should be used to determine correct placement of the CVAD before administering a vesicant agent (Schulmeister and Camp-Sorrell, 2000).
- For IV push administration, blood return should be checked every 1–2 ml.
- For continuous infusions into a CVAD, blood return should be assessed every 1 hour (Camp-Sorrell, 1998).
- A clear, occlusive dressing should be placed over the CVAD site, and the tubing should be securely taped (Kassner, 2000).
- Instruct the patient to immediately report any tugging or pulling on the tubing.
- Monitor active children to prevent needle or catheter dislodgement.

- Instruct the child with a port-a-catheter to try to sleep on the opposite side from the needle.

8.9.6 Assessment and Treatment of Extravasation

8.9.6.1 Signs and Symptoms of Extravasation

It is important that anyone who administers vesicant agents be aware of the signs and symptoms of extravasation (Table 8.18) so that quick and appropriate intervention can be done to limit tissue damage. Many of these signs and symptoms are noticeable immediately after the event, but some may occur over several weeks or months. Continued monitoring of the affected site is necessary. Necrosis of tissue may occur up to 6 months after the extravasation and may lead to loss of function in the affected area (Oncology Nursing Society, 2002).

Signs of extravasation include
- Pain at the infusion site
- Any reports of burning or stinging
- Crying or inconsolability in nonverbal children
- Hyperpigmentation
- Induration
- Vesicle formation or ulceration
- Sloughing of skin at injection site

8.9.6.2 Treatment for Extravasation

Knowledge and understanding of the appropriate actions to take in the event of an extravasation may limit its long-term effects (Table 8.19).

8.9.6.3 Peripheral Access

- Stop infusion of vesicant at the first sign of infiltration.
- Notify the physician or nurse practitioner.
- Remove syringe with vesicant agent from tubing, but leave the IV in place.
- Use a 1–3-cc syringe to aspirate any residual drug from the butterfly or catheter.
- Administer the appropriate antidote.
- Instill the appropriate volume into the catheter and discontinue the IV.

Table 8.18. Nursing assessment of extravasation and other reactions

Assessment parameter	Extravasation signs (immediate)	Extravasation signs (delayed)	Vein irritation	Flare reaction
Pain	Severe pain or burning that lasts minutes or hours and eventually subsides; usually occurs while the drug is being given around the needle site	Occurs at least 48 hours post-infusion	Aching and tightness along the vein	No pain
Redness	Blotchy redness around the needle site; not always present at time of extravasation	Occurs 24–48 hours post-infusion	The full length of the vein may be reddened or darkened	Immediate blotches or streaks along the vein, which usually subside within 30 minutes or without treatment
Ulceration	Develops insidiously; usually occurs 48–96 hours later	Occurs late	Not usually	Not usually
Swelling	Usually occurs immediately; is severe		Not usually	Not usually
Blood return	Inability to obtain	Good return during drug administration	Usually present	Usually present
Other		Local tingling and sensory deficits		Urticaria

- Avoid excessive pressure on the site.
- For subcutaneous administration of the antidote, discontinue the IV catheter without putting excess pressure on the site. Use a 25-gauge needle to inject the antidote into the surrounding subcutaneous tissue. Apply heat or cold to the site as appropriate (Oncology Nursing Society, 2001).
- Instruct the patient and family to rest the affected site for 48 hours.
- If blisters appear, instruct the patient and family not to break them.

8.9.6.4 Central Venous Access

- Stop infusion at first report of pain, burning, swelling, color change, change in sensation, or lack of blood return.
- Notify the physician or nurse practitioner.
- If patient has a port, assess for proper needle placement.
- Aspirate residual drug.

- Administer the appropriate antidote and nursing interventions.
- Avoid excess pressure on the site.
- Assess need for radiographic study of the CVAD.

Documentation of extravasation should be very specific and include

- Date and time of occurrence
- Size and type of needle/type of CVAD
- Needle insertion site
- Number of previous venipuncture attempts and sites
- Sequence of chemotherapy agent administration
- Drug administration technique
- Patient complaints/statements/activities
- Appearance of site
- Approximate amount of drug administered
- Physician or nurse practitioner notification
- Nursing interventions at time of the incident
- Follow-up measures
- Patient education provided

Table 8.19. Antidotes for extravasations

Drug	Antidotes	Local care	Comments
Anthracyclines	Dimethylsulfoxide 50% (DMSO); apply topically and allow to air dry every 3 hours. After first 4 hours if extra-vasation area is stable, switch DMSO to every 6 hours	Apply ice for 15 minutes on and 15 minutes off for first 4 hours as tolerated. After 4 hours, ice every 3 hours. Elevate extremity and do not use for several days	Doxorubicin produces severe prolonged tissue necrosis because of the slow release of the tissue-bound drug. Lesions may need surgical consult
Daunorubicin (Daunomycin) without ice	After 48 hours, may use DMSO every 6 hours only		
Doxorubicin (Adriamycin)			
Epirubicin			
Idarubicin (Idamycin)			
Alkylating agents Mechlorethamine (nitrogen mustard)	Sodium thiosulfate Mix 4 ml 10% sodium thiosulfate with 8.4 ml sterile water. Inject 1–4 ml through existing IV line or SQ at extravasation site	Apply cool packs for 3 days	
Cisplatin (Treat cisplatin extravasation only if volume of infiltrate >0 ml and concentration of >0.5 mg/ml)			
Vinca alkaloids Vincristine Vinblastine Vinorelbine	None known	Apply warm compresses for 15–20 minutes four times a day for 1–2 days	Heat increases local blood flow, which enhances absorption and removal of the drug from the site Topical cooling is NOT recommended
Dactinomycin (Actinomycin D) for 48 hours		None known	Elevate and apply ice packs
Mitomycin C (Mutamycin)	Dimethylsulfoxide (DMSO); apply topically and allow to air-dry. Repeat every 4–6 hours for 14 days	Apply ice packs for 24 hours	Protect from sunlight or heat.

8.9.6.5 Follow-Up Guidelines

- Site should be monitored 24 hours after the incident, and then 1 week after the incident, and then 2 weeks after.
- Following up with photographs is recommended.
- Elevate the involved extremity.
- Keep the area clean and dry.
- Do not rupture blisters.
- Consultation with a plastic surgeon may be required depending on the extent of tissue damage or/and functional limitation.

8.9.6.6 Patient Education

- Before administering vesicant agents, educate the patient and family about the possibility of extravasation.
- Instruct the patient to report any symptoms during or after the infusion.
- Provide written instructions on care of the site.

8.10 Acute Hypersensitivity Reactions to Chemotherapy

Although hypersensitivity reactions (HSRs) to chemotherapy are relatively rare, it is important for the pediatric oncology nurse to recognize agents that may have a higher incidence of causing them. Hypersensitivity reactions to chemotherapeutic agents range from a localized immune response that is mild and short, to anaphylaxis, which is a systemic response, severe in nature, and may lead to shock and death. Assessing for the signs and symptoms of an acute HSR and being knowledgeable about the appropriate treatment is imperative.

Hypersensitivity, flare reactions, and anaphylaxis are mediated IgE (Oncology Nursing Society, 2001). These types of reactions can be triggered by four factors (Labovich, 1999): route of entry, amount of antigen received, rate at which the antigen is absorbed, and the individual's degree of hypersensitivity. The clinical manifestations of HSR and anaphylaxis may include

- Urticaria (hives).
- Localized or generalized itching.
- Shortness of breath, with or without wheezing.
- Uneasiness or agitation.
- Periorbital edema or facial edema.
- Lightheadedness or dizziness.
- Tightness in the chest.
- Abdominal cramping or nausea.
- Chills.
- Hypotension.

8.10.1 Risk Factors for Hypersensitivity, Flare Reactions, or Anaphylaxis

- History of allergies, particularly drug allergies.
- Receiving a drug known to cause hypersensitivity reaction (see section 8.9.9).
- Previous exposure to the agent.
- Failure to receive known effective prophylactic premedications.
- Previous exposure to metals (Ciesielski-Carlucci et al., 1997).
- Agent was injected versus being ingested (Labovich, 1999).

8.10.2 Chemotherapy Agents That Can Cause HSRs

8.10.2.1 L-Asparaginase (*E. coli, Erwinia,* Pegaspargase)

- One of the agents *most likely* to cause HSRs (principal side effect that limits treatment).
- Occur in up to 25% of patients (Weiss, 1997).
- Prior exposure to the agent.
- Intravenous route of administration increases.
- Patients that react to *Erwinia* may be switched to PEG-asparaginase without further clinical hypersensitivity (Bryant, 2001).

8.10.2.2 Etoposide/Teniposide

- Approximately 6% of patients will experience a HSR (Carr and Burke, 2001).
- Reactions may occur with any dose (Carr and Burke, 2001).

- Signs and symptoms of an HSR include dyspnea, wheezing, hypotension, hypertension, urticaria, pruritus, angioedema, facial flushing, and rash (Carr and Burke, 2001).

8.10.2.3 Taxanes (Paclitaxel/Docetaxel)

- If given without premedication, paclitaxel administration has been associated with a rate of HSR as high as 16% (Carr and Burke, 2001).
- Mandatory use of premedications has reduced the incidence of HSR to 1–3%, and at the same time has reduced severity of the reaction (Carr and Burke, 2001).
- Suggested premedications before administration of paclitaxel include dexamethasone, diphenhydramine, and an H_2-receptor antagonist such as ranitidine. Oral dexamethasone should be administered at 12 and 6 hours before the first and second infusions (Carr and Burke, 2001).
- HSRs with paclitaxel usually occur within the first 10 minutes of the infusion (Carr and Burke, 2001).
- Reactions to docetaxel may also occur within minutes of starting the first or second infusion (Carr and Burke, 2001).
- Common reactions include generalized pruritus, bronchospasm, generalized urticaria, severe hypotension, angioedema, and fluid retention (Carr and Burke, 2001).
- Premedications are also required before docetaxel infusions. Dexamethasone may be given orally 3 days prior to starting the infusion.

8.10.2.4 Carboplatin

- Allergic reactions may occur in 2–30% of children (Yu et al., 2001).
- Reason for allergic reaction is unclear. May be IgE-mediated (Yu et al., 2001).
- Increased risk for HSR with multiple doses, but risk is not correlated with a single dose (Yu et al., 2001; Schiavetti et al., 1999).
- Weekly dosing schedule is major risk for HSR (Yu et al., 2001; Schiavetti et al., 1999).
- Children with low-grade gliomas treated with carboplatin are at increased risk for HSR (Yu et al., 2001).

- Consider the use of a desensitization protocol in patients with history of HSR to carboplatin.

8.10.3 Recommended Steps to Prevent HSRs

- Obtain baseline vital signs.
- Review patient's allergy and hypersensitivity history.
- Review with parents if any premedications were given prior to arriving for therapy; if so, document when they were given.
- Administer premedications as ordered.
- Be familiar with the location of emergency equipment and medications.
- Obtain orders for anaphylaxis prior to drug administration (Table 8.18).
- Educate the patient and family on signs and symptoms of HSR.
- If patient has high likelihood of hypersensitivity, perform a scratch test or intradermal skin test or administer a test dose before giving the initial dose of the drug. Patient should be observed for any local or systemic reaction for 1 hour or more after the test is performed. If no sign of hypersensitivity, proceed with initial dosing.
- If administering an IV bolus dose of a drug that is associated with hypersensitivity, infuse the drug slowly and observe the patient for signs and symptoms of hypersensitivity.
- Consider medication desensitization. Premedicate with antihistamines and/or corticosteroids. Dilute the drug with additional solution. Increase the infusion time.

Any chemotherapy drugs that are known agents for HSR should only be administered in a controlled setting with appropriate medications and equipment available, not in the home (Bryant, 2001).

8.10.4 Emergency Management of HSR/Anaphylaxis

- HSRs usually occur within the first 15 minutes of the drug's administration.
- Stop the chemotherapy infusion immediately.
- Stay with the patient; call for help.
- Assess airway, breathing, and circulation.

Table 8.20. Emergency drugs for use in case of hypersensitivity or anaphylactic reaction

Drug	Strength	Usage
Epinephrine	0.01 mg/kg IV or SQ or 0.1 mg–0.3 mg q10–15 min for maximum of three doses Epi-pen JR 0.15 mg IM for children </= 15 kg Epi-pen 0.3 mg IM for children >15 kg	Anaphylaxis or allergic reaction
Diphenhydramine hydrochloride	1 mg/kg IV (maximum 50 mg)	Administer IV
Steroids		
Solu-Medrol	0.3–0.5 mg/kg IV	Administer IV
Solu-Cortef (hydrocortisone)	4–8 mg/kg IV (max. 50 mg)	
Dexamethasone	0.1–0. mg/kg IV	
Dopamine	5–0 mcg/kg/min IV	Administer IV; adjust to patient's response

- Maintain an IV line with normal saline or other appropriate solution.
- Place patient in supine position.
- Monitor vital signs every 2 minutes until stable, then every 5 minutes for 30 minutes, then every 15 minutes.
- Administer emergency medications (Table 8.20).
- Provide emotional support for the patient and family.
- Document all treatments and patient's response (Oncology Nursing Society, 2001).

8.10.5 Patient and Family Education

- Explain the importance of being knowledgeable about the patient's history of allergies to medications and remind the family to inform healthcare providers before starting any therapy.
- Explain all side effects of medications and review signs and symptoms of HSRs.
- Instruct family that a delayed reaction to certain medications can occur, and provide them with instructions on how to notify the healthcare team.

References

Albanell, J., Baselga J. (2000). Systemic therapy emergencies. Seminars in Oncology Nursing. 7 (3):347–361

Balinsky, W. (1995). High tech home care. Caring, 14 (5):7–9

Beason, R. (1990). Antineoplastic vesicant extravasation. Journal of Intravenous Nursing, 13 (2):111–114

Bernstein, M.L., Reaman, G.H., Hirschfeld S. (2001). Developmental therapeutics in childhood cancer. Hematology Oncology Clinics of North America,15:631–655

Bryant, R. (2001). Use of a protocol to minimize hypersensitivity reactions with asparaginase administration. Journal of Intravenous Nursing, 4:169–173

Camp-Sorrell, D. (1998). Developing extravasation protocols and monitoring outcomes. Journal of Intravenous Nursing, 1:232–239

Carr, B., Burke, C. (2001). Outpatient chemotherapy hypersensitivity and anaphylaxis. American Journal of Nursing, 27–30

Chapman, D. (1998). Family-focused pediatric home care. Caring 17 (5):12–15

Ciesielski-Carlucci,C., Leong, P., Jacobs, C. (1997). Case report of anaphylaxis from cisplatin/paclitaxel and a review of their hypersensitivity reaction profiles. American Journal of Clinical Oncology, 20:373–375

Close, P., Burkey, E., Kazak, A. Danz, P., Lange, B. (1995). A prospective, controlled evaluation of home chemotherapy for children with cancer. Pediatrics, 95 (6):896–900

Deitcher, S.R., Fesen, M.R., Kiproff, P.M., Hill, P.A., Li, X., McCluskey, E.R., Semba, C.P. (2002a). Safety and efficacy of alteplase for restoring function in occluded central venous catheters: Results of the cardiovascular thrombolytic to open occluded line trial. Journal of Clinical Oncology, 20 (1)

Ettinger, A.G., Bond, D.M., Sievers, T.D. (2002). Chemotherapy. In Baggot C.R., Kelly K.P., Fochtman D., Foley G.V. (eds) Nursing Care of Children and Adolescents with Cancer, pp. 133–176. Philadelphia: WB Saunders

Goodman, M. (2000). Chemotherapy: Principles of administration. In Yarbro C. H, Frogge M. H., Goodman M., Groenwald S. (eds) Cancer Nursing: Principles and Practice, pp. 385–443. Boston: Jones and Bartlett

Harrison, B. R. (1996.) Safe handling of cytotoxic drugs. In Perry M. C. (ed) The Chemotherapy Source Book, 2nd edn. Baltimore: Williams & Wilkins

Kassner, E. (2002). Evaluation and treatment of chemotherapy extravasation injuries. Journal of Pediatric Oncology Nursing, 17 (3):135–148

Labovich, T.M. (1999). Acute hypersensitivity reactions to chemotherapy. Seminars in Oncology Nursing, 15(3):222–231

Meeske, K., Ruccione, K. (1987) Cancer chemotherapy in children: nursing issues and approaches. Seminars in Oncology Nursing, 3:122

National Association of Children's Hospitals and Related Institutions (NACHRI) Patient Care Oncology FOCUS Group (2000). Home care requirements for children and adolescents with cancer. Journal of Pediatric Oncology Nursing, 17:45–49

Occupational Safety and Health Administration: Guidelines for Cytotoxic Drugs (OSHA Directive PUB 8–1.1). Washington, DC, US Department of Labor. Retrieved from the WWW 3/6/2002. http://www.Osha.gov/oshdoc/directive_data/PUB_8–1_1.html

Oncology Nursing Society (2001) ONS Chemotherapy and Biotherapy: Guidelines and Recommendations for Practice. Pittsburg: Oncology Nursing Society Press. (pp. 65–68)

San Angel F (1995) Current controversies in chemotherapy administration. Journal of IV Nursing 18(1):16-23

Schiavetti, A., Varrasso,G., Maurizi, P., Castello, M. (1999). Hypersensitivity to carboplatin in children. Medical and Pediatric Oncology, 3:183–185

Schulmeister, L., Camp-Sorrell, D. (2000). Chemotherapy extravasation from implanted ports. Oncology Nursing Forum, 7:531–538

Tariman, J.D. (2003). Thalidomide: current therapeutic uses and management or its toxicities. Clinical Journal of Oncology Nursing, 7:143–147

Weiss, R. (1997). Hypersensitivity reactions. In Perry M. (ed) The Chemotherapy Source Book, 2nd edn. Williams & Wilkins

Wilson, D., Perry K. A. (1999). Pediatric variations of nursing interventions. In Wong D. L, Hockenberry-Eaton M., Wilson D., M. Winkelstein L., Ahmann E. (eds) Whaley & Wong's Nursing Care of Infants and Children, 6th edn. St. Louis: Mosby

Yu, D., Dahl, G., Shames, R., Fisher, P. (2001). Weekly dosing of carboplatin Increased risk of allergy in children. Journal of Pediatric Hematology Oncology, 3 (6):349–352

Bibliography

Balis, F.M., Holcenberg, J.S., Blaney, S.M. (2002). In Pizzo P., Poplack D. (eds) Principles and Practice of Pediatric Oncology, pp. 237–308. Lippincott William & Wilkins

Bertilli, G., Gozza, A., Forno, G.B., Vidili, M.G., Silvestro, S., Venturini, M., Del Mastro, L., Garrone, O., Rosso, R., Dini, D.(1995). Topical dimethylsulfoxide for the prevention of soft tissue injury after extravasation of vesicant cytotoxic drugs: A prospective clinical study. Journal of Clinical Oncology, 13:2851–2855

Boyle, D.M., Engelking, C. (1995). Vesicant extravasation myths and realities. Oncology Nursing Forum, 22:57–67

Bomgaars, L., Berg, S.L., Blaney, S.M. (2001). The development of camptothecin analogs in childhood cancers. The Oncologist, 6:506–516

Deitcher, S., Fesen, M., Kiproff, P., Hill, P., Li, X., McCluskey, E., Semba, C., Frierdich, S. (2002b). Home Care. In Baggot C.R., Kelly K.P., Fochtman D., Foley G.V. (eds), Nursing Care of Children and Adolescents with Cancer, pp. 391–399. Philadelphia: W.B. Saunders

Durivage, H., Fischer, D., Knobf, M.(1993). The Cancer Chemotherapy Handbook, 4th edn. St. Louis: Mosby

Godson, E. (1997). Behavioral disorders and developmental variations. In Hay, W.W., Groothuis J.R., Hayward, A. R., Levin, M. J. (eds) Current: Pediatric Diagnosis and Treatment, pp. 77–85. Connecticut: Appleton & Lange

Gorski, L.A., Grothman, L. (1995). Home infusion therapy. Seminars in Oncology Nursing, 1 (3), 193–201

Haugen, M., Nuuhhiwa, J. (2002, October). Home alone: safety issues in home chemotherapy administration. Paper presented at the meeting of the Association of Pediatric Oncology Nurses 6th Annual Conference, Denver, CO

Hockenberry, M., Kline, N. (2002). Nursing support of the child with cancer. In Pizzo P., Poplack D. (eds) Principles and Practice of Pediatric Oncology (pp. 134–1343). Lippincott William & Wilkins

Holdsworth, M., Raisch, D., Chavez, C., Duncan, M., Parasuraman, T., Cox, F. (1997). Economic impact with home delivery of chemotherapy to pediatric oncology patients. The Annals of Pharmacotherapy, 31:140–148

Hooke, C., Ellingson, L. (1999). Ifosamide and etoposide: Moving 5-day infusions from inpatient to outpatient. Paper presented at the meeting of the Association of Pediatric Oncology Nurses 2nd Annual Conference

Hooker L., Kohler, J. (1999). Safety, efficacy and acceptability of home intravenous therapy administered by parents of pediatric oncology patients. Medical Pediatric Oncology, 3:421–426

Jacob, E. (2000). Continuing care of the newly diagnosed child with cancer from hospital to home: Part1. Home Health Care Consultant, 7 (6):1A–11A

Joint Commission of Accreditation of Hospital Organizations. (2001). 2001–2002 Comprehensive Accreditation Manual for Home Care. Oakbrook Terrace, Il: Joint Commission Resources

Joint Commission of Accreditation of Hospital Organizations. (2001). The complete guide to the 20021–2002 Home Care Survey Process: Home Health Personal Care, support and Hospice Services. Oakbrook Terrace, IL: Joint Commission Resources

Lawrence, H. J, Walsh, D. (1989). Topical dimethylsulfoxide may prevent tissue damage from anthracycline extravasation. Cancer Chemotherapy Pharmacology, 3 (5):316–318

Lopez, A.M., Wallace, L., Dorr, R.T., Koff, M., Hersh, E.M., Alberts, D.S. (1999). Topical DMSO treatment for pegylated liposomal doxorubicin-induced palmar-plantar erythrodyesthesia. Cancer Chemotherapy Pharmacology, 44:303–306

Martingano, E.C., Ethier, A. (1997). Anaphylaxis to asparaginase preparations: development of a protocol. Leukemia Nursing, 1:6

Moran, P. (2000). Cellular effects of cancer chemotherapy administration. Journal of IV Nursing, 3 (1):44–56

Ogle, S., Rose, M., Wildes, C. (2002). Development and implementation of a carboplatin desensitization protocol for children with neurofibromatosis, type 1 and hypersensitivity reactions in an outpatient oncology clinic. Journal of Pediatric Oncology Nursing, 19:122–126

Rollins, J. A. (1999). Family centered care of the child during illness and hospitalization. In Wong D. L, Hockenberry-Eaton M., Wilson D., M. Winkelstein L., Ahmann E. (eds) Whaley & Wong's Nursing Care of Infants and Children, pp. 1131–1209

Stricklan, L. (ed) (2000). St. Jude Children's Research Hospital Formulary Handbook. Hudson, OH: Lexi-Comp

Taketomo, C.K., Hodding, J.H., Kraus, D.M. (2002). Pediatric Dosage Handbook, 8th edn. Hudson, Ohio: Lexi-Comp

Weaver, J., Simmons, G., Scholfield, R. (1995). The home infusion formula: high tech + high touch = high-quality home care. Caring, 52–56

Wilkes, G.M., Ingwersen, K., Barton-Burke, M. (2000). Oncology Nursing Drug Handbook. Boston: Jones and Bartlett

Wilson, K. (1998). Oncologic emergencies. In Hockenberry-Eaton M. (ed) Essentials of Pediatric Oncology Nursing: A Core Curriculum. Glenview: Association of Pediatric Oncology Nurses

Radiation Therapy

Joan M. O'Brien · Deborah Tomlinson

Contents

Radiotherapy has had a role in malignancies for the last century. X-rays were discovered by Von Roentgen in 1895 and were used diagnostically. The element radium was isolated by Marie and Pierre Curie in 1898. The first therapeutic report of a patient cures by radiation therapy was in 1899.

However it has a diminishing role in childhood malignancies due to more effective chemotherapy regimens and the recognition of late effects of radiation treatment. Children will often be assessed on an individual level regarding the need of radiotherapy. However it is still required for around 20% of children and young people with cancer.

Focus in radiation therapy (XRT) has been on methods of delivery that will minimize injury to normal tissues, to try to avoid long-term negative sequalae.

9.1 Principles of treatment

Radiotherapy causes damage to cells in a localised area. Ionising radiation both causes and treats cancer. Damage is caused by breaking strands of DNA; either double or single strands. This inhibits cell division. It may harm normal cells in the area they pass through or in the area around tumor.

Radiation treatment has three main roles in the treatment of childhood and young person's cancer:

- Radical: Treatment with curative intent
- Adjuvant: "Added on" treatment
- Palliative: Treatment aimed at symptom control.

Radiation is frequently used as part of a bone marrow ablative regimen. At times radiation may be used to ameliorate side effects from tumors that are threaten life or organ function; to quickly reduce the size of a mass that is impinging on the airway, or to relieve pressure on the spinal cord to decrease or prevent paralysis.

Palliative radiotherapy is given to relieve pain in progressive or metastatic disease. It provides shrinkage of tumor to relieve pain and/or obstructions interfering with quality of life. The dose is monitored to ensure minimal toxicities.

9.2 Description of treatment

All radiation emits radiant energy; either in waves and particle form.

- Electrons are electromagnetic and produced from a linear accelerator. They can provide treatment to superficial tumors and have increased absorption to bone. (X-rays are electromagnetic radiation that is produced extranuclearly; electrons are accelerated to high energy and then stopped abruptly at a tungsten target (Farah and Weichselbaum 1994)).
- Gamma rays are electromagnetic radiation produced intranuclearly from a radioactive source. They provide local and wide-field radiation, and are skin sparing. Gamma rays require lead or concrete to absorb them.
- Protons are high energy atoms, emitted from a machine, for the treatment of tumours needing specific dose localization. They are delivered by stereotaxis (a form of radiation that delivers the beam in an extremely precise manner).

9.2.1 Cell radiosensitivity

Factors that contribute to cell radiosensitivity include:

- Phase of cell cycle that cell is in: Studies have shown that cells are most radiosensitive in the M and G2 phases and most resistant in late S phase (Farah and Weichselbaum 1994). Between dose fractions, cells may move through the cell cycle to more sensitive phases. This process is called "reassortment". This allows for a greater cell kill.

- Rate of division: Rapidly dividing cells are more likely to be in the dividing phase of the cell cycle; therefore they are more radiosensitive.
- Oxygenation: Hypoxic cells tend to be radioresistant and only a small quantity of oxygen is required for radiosensitisation. During the course of treatment, oxygenated cells are killed, tumours become smaller, and hypoxic cells move to the well-oxygenated compartments (Farah and Weichselbaum 1994). This is termed reoxygenation. A patient's haemoglobin should be maintained at a minimum of 10 gms/dl.
- Degree of differentiation of cell type: Poorly differentiated cells are more radiosensitive.
- Use of radiosensitizers: Certain chemotherapeutic agents have been known to increase tumor cells' sensitivity to radiation and are often used in combination with radiation to optimize cell kill (Tarbell and Kooy, 2002). These agents include dactinomycin, doxorubicin, etoposide and methotrexate.

9.2.2 Units of radiation

The unit of absorbed radiation dose is a Gray (Gy). A centigray (cGy) is a small fraction (1/100) of a Gy. Prior to the 1990's that unit of energy was referred to as a "rad".

9.3 Methods of delivery

9.3.1 External Beam/Teletherapy (*Tele* comes from the Greek for far)'

- Two-dimensional (2-D) external beam radiation is the most common form. Linear accelerators have mainly replaced cobalt-60 machines in most radiotherapy centers. Linear accelerators generate beams of photons and electrons and can emit megavoltage radiation. Cobalt-60 machines also deliver megavoltage radiation but the machines contain the radioactive material and require to be in thick concreted-walled rooms. Delivery of radiation is faster using a linear accelerator and therefore has obvious advantages in pediatrics.

- Three-dimensional (3-D) conformal and image modulated radiation therapy (IMRT), which allows visualization of radiation in three dimensions. Beams are focused from multiple areas to penetrate the tumor, making the actual radiation field smaller with less "scatter" and damage to normal tissues.
- Stereotactic radiosugery and stereotactic radiation: Stereotactic radiation can be performed as radiosurgery, where multiple beams converge at a point to deliver high dose of radiation to a small area of tumour. This is done as a one time treatment and produces a high degree of tumour necrosis. Tumours must be well circumscribed, < 4 cm in size, and not involve critical structures, such as the brain stem. This type may be carried out using either a linear accelerator or a system frequently referred to as a "Gamma knife" procedure (Swift 2002). For brain tumors, a fixed head frame is secured to the head to ensure precise delivery of the radiation beam. Stereotactic radiotherapy is similar to radiosurgery, but is carried out over multiple fractions and can treat larger tumor volumes. Again, a removable head frame is used to ensure precision of treatment.
- Intraoperative radiation is performed in a fashion similar to radiosurgery, except it is done when the tumour bed is exposed during surgery. It allows a precise treatment field, a higher dose, and potentially less side effects.

9.3.1.1 Fractionation

Fractionation is the process of radiotherapy delivery that divides the total dose into daily doses. The total dose determines the length of treatment. Treatment is normally given Monday to Friday. Fractionation provides better tumor control for a given level or normal tissue toxicity than a single large dose.

Fractionation spares normal tissues because of:

1. the repair of sublethal damage between fractions
2. cellular repopulation.

The normal 2 day rest each week provides time for normal cells to recover.

Tumour damage is increased because of:

1. reoxygenation
2. reassortment of cells within the cell cycle.

However, protracted courses of small doses of radiation may allow for malignant cell re-growth, as they have been given time to repair.

Hyperfractionation is further dividing the daily dose into 2 doses, usually with 6-8 hours between the 2 treatments. Theoretically higher doses may be given with less toxicity and greater tumor cell kill. This technique has been studied for several years and for some tumors, such as brain stem gliomas, no benefit has been found (Mandell et al 1999; Neider et al 1999). Research continues using this technique.

9.3.1.2 Total Body Irradiation (TBI)

The purpose of TBI is to cause bone marrow aplasia, that is to empty out the marrow cavity to allow for new stem cell growth. This is often the preparation for stem cell transplant. It is the aim that TBI will also eradicate malignant cells in sanctuary sites and/or minimal residual disease i.e. it has an antileukemic/antitumor effect.

After TBI, the patient would die of overwhelming infection if stem cells were not given. All organ systems at risk for side effects. TBI is usually given in fractionated doses twice a day for 4 to 5 days.

9.3.2 Interstitial implants/brachytherapy (Sealed source) (brachy comes from the Greek for "short distance")

Interstitial implants are isotopes provided as individually customised "seeds or pellets" that are inserted directly into a body cavity, either close or in contact with the target tissue. They provide a high dose of radiation to a very localised area, while having minimal damage to normal tissue. They may be placed for several days or left permanently in place. Most common uses are for gynecological cancers and supratentorial brain tumors in adults. In children, interstitial implants may be used in retinoblastoma lesions within the eye and removed 72 hours later. Also, in pelvic rhabdomyosarcomas, external beam radiation would have to travel through growing bones and intestines of the child. This could result in major growth retardation. Brachytherapy can minimize the dose delivered to surrounding normal tissue.

9.3.3 Unsealed source of radioisotope

A radioactive isotope is attached to a metabolite or an antigen-specific antibody, for example: iodine-131 – metaiodobenzylguanidine (^{131}I-MIBG). An MIBG scan, using a dye which is taken up by catechoanergic cells, is also useful for diagnostic purposes in children with neuroblastoma in identifying metastases, but this is not available at all centres. I-MIBG is a norepinephrine analog that concentrates in adrenergic tissue and therefore holds promise for cell-specific treatment of neuroblastoma. The MIBG can be labelled with radioactive isotopes of iodine, suitable either for diagnostic imaging or therapy. This is targeted radiotherapy.

9.3.4 Treatment planning

In the delivery of external beam radiotherapy there must be assured accuracy of:

- Dose
- Intensity
- Direction of beam
- Target area.

This will ensure that there is maximum damage to tumour cells with minimal damage to normal, surrounding tissue.

Treatment planning involves:

1. Accurate tumour imaging often using CT scans or MRIs. This outlines a treatment field so that measurements can be collated in order to ascertain the most appropriate form of radiotherapy and the shape and angle of the beams that would be necessary. Margins for treatment are identified that include the tumour and an area of surrounding healthy tissue; this accounts for microscopic tumour extension (Hopkins 1999). Consideration must be given to: limitations of imaging investigations, characteristics of the type of radiation used, and slight changes in body positioning.

2. Determining the dose of radiation energy. This is dependent on protocol, tumour histology and clinical assessment.
3. Identifying the type of radiotherapy. The depth of penetration of the radiation must be considered.

9.3.5 Simulation

Simulation is the process of developing a treatment plan. When planning the shape and angle of the beam it is vital that these factors are simulated with diagnostic radiographic imaging that uses a fluoroscopic unit (Hopkins 1999). This technique uses computer generated fields and simulates the specific number/angle of beams directed at the tumor. Physics calculations enable a computer to simulate the radiation beams that will be delivered.

9.3.6 Protection of health care professionals

Due to the risk of radiation damage to all cells, staff must be protected from any unnecessary exposure. Radiotherapy departments are legally obliged to appoint a radiation protection officer and follow stringent guidelines for radiation monitoring and protection (Byrne 2000). Radiography and radiotherapy staff, and staff caring for patients receiving brachytherapy or unsealed sources of radiation treatments, must wear badges that contain radiographic film that records the cumulative amount of radiation exposure per month.

9.4 Potential side effects

The side effects of radiation therapy are directly related to the amount of radiation received and the location of the field, age of child (younger children more vulnerable to side effects) and adjunctive chemotherapy.

Side effects can be:

- Acute: Acute side effects usually occur within the first few weeks of radiation therapy and are manifested in fast-growing cells located in the radiation field, such as the skin or oral mucosa.

- Delayed (sub)-acute: Delayed acute effects can occur weeks to months after completion of treatment. These are both self-limiting and resolve with time.
- Late: Late effects are the result of irreversible damage. The risk of secondary tumors in the radiation field is also a significant late effect of radiotherapy.

Part 4 of the book will detail the side effects of treatment.

9.5 Special considerations

9.5.1 Ensuring accuracy of treatment: Patient issues

Following planning, the delivery of the angles of the beams must be maintained throughout every treatment. Radiation energy decreases over distance and the energy decreases uniformly along the path. It is therefore possible to calculate the distance the child must be from the radiation source in order that the correct dose is received. Identical body positioning is essential.

9.5.1.1 Marking

External markings using ink or tattoo are applied to the patient's skin to mark the positioning field. These are not easily removed. DO NOT REMOVE markings! If the markings fade the radiographers may need to re-draw the lines. *If the marks fade, while on weekend leave, the family should be asked to redraw over the marks using a different colour of felt tip pen. This will enable the radiographers to distinguish between the two (Hopkins 1999).*

9.5.1.2 Patient immobilisation

Various methods of immobilisation are applied often dependent on the area of the body to be treated. When treating brain tumours or head and neck tumours, a shell is made for individual use to ensure that the head is immobilised. The shell is an exact fit and even small movements will be restricted. These immobilization shells/moulds are also used to reproduce positioning of the child over consecutive treatments. These moulds may sometimes be frightening to the child, depending on his or her developmental level. Developmentally appropriate explanations should be given to the child during radiation planning (McGuire Cullen et al., 2002). To ensure the accuracy and safety of the delivery of radiation treatment, it is also essential during the planning stages to assess the child's ability to cooperate.

Other immobilisation techniques include:

- Head rests, knee rolls
- Vacuum bean bags filled with Styrofoam beads
- Development of immobilizers/blocks
- Plaster of Paris casts.

9.5.1.3 Sedation and general anaesthesia

Because of consecutive days of being unable to eat prior to radiation, the nutritional status of children receiving sedation for radiation should be monitored closely. When possible, it is often best to treat sedation cases early in the morning.

Children may require sedation due to young age, developmental immaturity or extreme distress. Sedation methods range from a mild antianxiolytic to conscious sedation or a short-acting general anesthetic. Short acting drugs such as ketamine may be used. These children will require to be treated early in the day to avoid repeated extended periods of fasting. Hydration and nutrition will need particular attention.

If the child is anaesthetised, an anaesthetist must be present to monitor the child. This will be with the aid of audiovisual monitoring and the electrocardiographic and respiratory monitors for the short period that the child requires to be alone when the radiation treatment is being delivered. Another point to consider is that radiotherapy is usually delivered to children in an adult centre. Adequate, safe recovery must be assured.

If the child requires another procedure such as lumbar puncture, the team will often organise to have these procedures carried out with the same anaesthetic.

9.5.1.4 Preparation of children and young people

Receiving radiation therapy can be a very frightening ordeal. Good preparation will help elicit children's cooperation. Young people may also not be willing to cooperative if they are not adequately informed and prepared for the process involved. Parent's anxiety can also impact the child's anxiety. It may be stressful for everyone that the child is left in the room alone.

9.5.2 Brachytherapy

Although rarely used it may have significant advantages in children and young people due to significant local control and fewer late effects. Initially the mould may need to be inserted or stitched in place using a general anaesthetic.

9.5.3 Unsealed sources of radiation treatment

^{131}I-MIBG is given intravenously under extremely protected conditions. Patent venous access is imperative. The ^{131}I-MIBG contains a specific radioactive isotope of iodine.

Protection of the thyroid gland is imperative. Oral iodine is administered before, during and after the radioactive material is given. This ensures saturation of the thyroid gland with non-radioactive iodine.

All body tissues become radioactive. Therefore all bodily fluids must be handled as radioactive waste (Hopkins 1999). This leads to the need for extreme caution in the care of a child. Unfortunately, the child's contact with family must be kept to a minimum.

9.6 Future Perspectives

There have been several recent advances in the field of radiation oncology. The goal of the research is to deliver the highest tolerated amount of radiation while decreasing exposure to surrounding normal tissue. Several techniques have been developed to reach this goal. Proton radiation therapy is the newest technique that delivers a large dose to the tumor and a smaller dose to normal tissue (Tarbell and Kooy,

2002). The advances in radiation therapy are decreasing side effects, but the cost to update and create new equipment limits the availability of new radiation treatments.

References

Byrne B (2000) Radiotherapy in Alexander MF, Fawcett JN, Runciman PJ (Eds) Nursing Practice: Hospital and Home 2nd Ed, Edinburgh, Churchill.

Farah R & Weichselbaum RR (1994) Principles of radiation biology and radiation therapy, in Pochedly C (Ed) Neoplastic diseases of childhood Switzerland, Harwood Academic Publishers.

Hopkins M (1999) Administration of radiotherapy, in Gibson F & Evans M (Eds) Paediatric Oncology: Acute Nursing Care London, Whurr Publishers.

Mandell LR, Kadota R, Freeman C, Douglass EC, Fontanesi J, Cohen ME, Kovnar E, Burger P, Sanford RA, Kepner J, Friedman H, Kun LE (1999) There is no role for hyperfractionated radiotherapy in the management of children with newly diagnosed diffuse intrinsic brainstem tumors: results of a Pediatric Oncology Group phase III trial comparing conventional vs. hyperfractionated radiotherapy International Journal of Radiation Oncology: Biology and Physics 43(5): 947–94.

McGuire Cullen P, Derrickson JD, Potter JA (2002) Radiation therapy, in Rasco Baggott C, Patterson Kelly K, Fochtman D, Foley GV Nursing care of children and adolescents with cancer Philadelphia, Saunders.

Nieder C, Nestle U, Ketter R, Kolles H, Gentner SJ, Steudel WI, Schnabel K (1999) Hyperfractionated and accelerated-hyperfractionated radiotherapy for glioblastoma multiforma Radiation Oncology Investigations 7(1): 36–41.

Swift P (2002) Novel techniques in the delivery of radiation in pediatric oncology Pediatric Clinics of North America 49(5): 1107–1129.

Hockenberry-Eaton M., Kline N.E. (1998) Radiation therapy. In: Hockenberry-Eaton M.J. (ed) Essentials of pediatric oncology nursing: a core curriculum. Glenview, IL: Association of Pediatric Oncology Nurses, pp 98–100.

McGuire Cullen, P. Derrickson, J.D., Potter, J.A. (2002) Radiation therapy. In: Baggott C. R., Kelly K.P., Fochtman D., Foley G.V. (eds) Nursing care of the children and adolescents with cancer, 3rd edn. Philadelphia: Saunders, pp 116–132

Tarbell N.J., Kooy H.M. (2002) General principles of radiation oncology. In: Pizzo P.A., Poplack D.G. (eds) Principles and practice of pediatric oncology, 4th edn. Philadelphia: Lippincott Williams & Wilkins, pp 369–380.

Hematopoietic Stem Cell Transplantation

Robbie Norville

Contents

10.1 Principles of Treatment

The purpose of hematopoietic stem cell transplantation (HSCT) is to replace diseased, damaged, or absent hematopoietic stem cells with healthy hematopoietic stem cells. In general, allogeneic transplants are used when the hematopoietic stem cells are diseased (e.g., leukemia), damaged (e.g., sickle cell disease), or absent (e.g., severe immunodeficiency disease). Autologous transplants are used to provide stem cell rescue after higher doses of chemotherapy or radiation therapy (e.g., solid tumors).

Higher doses of chemotherapy and radiation therapy can cause dose-limiting myelosuppression. Infusing healthy stem cells allows the bone marrow to recover after intensive therapy. In the allogeneic setting, the new immune system from the donor may be effective in preventing disease recurrence by providing a graft-versus-tumor effect.

HSCT is an important treatment modality for children with aggressive malignancies in first remission or those who have recurrent disease.

Types of HSCT include the following (see Table 1):

- Allogeneic: Stem cells are collected from someone other than the recipient. These donor cells can be obtained from a variety of donor sources. A matched related donor is a family member, usually a sibling, with a 6/6 antigen match. A mismatched related donor is a family member, usually a sibling or parent, with a 3/6, 4/6, or 5/6 antigen match. A matched unrelated donor is one who is not genetically related to the recipient, with a 5/6 or 6/6 antigen match.

Table 10.1. Comparison of advantages and disadvantages of types of HSCT and different donor sources

Type of HSCT	Advantages	Disadvantages
Allogeneic		
Matched related	Healthy source of cells Easy access to donor	Some risk of GvHD 30% likelihood of sibling match
Mismatched related	Healthy source of cells Easy access to donor Availability of donor for most patients	Greater risk of GvHD Risk of graft failure
Matched unrelated	Healthy source of cells	Risk of GvHD 3–6 month waiting period for donor procurement Limited ethnic minority donors Expensive donor charges
Autologous	Easy access to donor No GvHD	No graft versus tumor effect Possible tumor contamination
Syngeneic	Healthy source of cells	Some risk of GvHD
Donor Source	**Advantages**	**Disadvantages**
Bone marrow	Well-tested collection method	General anesthesia risks Pain at harvest site
Peripheral blood	Faster engraftment	Venous access
Cord blood	Easy procurement of cells Decreased chance of viral transmission	Limited number of cells per unit Potential transmission of genetic diseases Costs for cryopreservation and storage

- Autologous: Stem cells are collected (or harvested) from the recipient
- Syngeneic: Stem cells are collected from a donor who is an identical twin of the recipient

If bone marrow is the donor source, the stem cells are collected directly from the bone marrow space, with the posterior iliac crest being the most common harvest site. The collection is done in the operating room, and the donor will usually receive general anesthesia for the procedure. If peripheral blood is used, the stem cells are collected by pheresis, usually in an outpatient setting. Temporary pheresis catheters may be placed prior to the procedure when venous access is difficult. Stem cells may also be collected directly from the umbilical cord at the time of birth. These cells are then cryopreserved (frozen) and stored for use at a later time.

Human leukocyte antigens (HLA) are a complex series of proteins on the surface of human leukocytes used for identifying a donor match (Fig. 10.1). These proteins, called antigens, make up the major histocompatibility complex, which helps the body recognize foreign proteins and cells. One set of antigens is inherited from each parent; therefore, a biological parent will be at least a 3/6 match for a child. The antigens of primary concern for HLA typing are A, B, and DR. The more disparity that exists between the donor and the recipient, the greater the risk of graft versus host disease (GvHD) and graft failure. HSCT is used for a variety of malignant and nonmalignant diseases (Table 10.2).

Figure 10.1

Example of HLA typing

Father	Mother
A1 A2	A2 A1
B8 B44	B7 B57
DR3 DR4	DR2 DR11
Haploidentical Donor	*Haploidentical Donor*

Patient
A1   A2
B8   B7
DR3   DR2

Sibling	**Sibling**	**Sibling**	**Sibling**
A1 A1	A2 A2	A2 A1	A1 A2
B8 B57	B44 B7	B44 B57	B8 B7
DR3 DR11	DR4 DR2	DR4 DR11	DR3 DR2
			Matched Related Donor

Table 10.2. Diseases for which HSCT is a treatment option (from Forte and Norville, 1998)

Disease	Rationale for hematopoietic stem cell transplantation
Leukemias, lymphomas	Chemotherapy, with or without total body irradiation, is used to eradicate tumor cells and to make room for engraftment of healthy cells. Irradiation is often used in mismatched and unrelated transplants.
Solid tumors: neuroblastoma, sarcoma, brain tumor	High doses of chemotherapy or radiation therapy are given to kill tumor cells. An autologous "rescue" is given to prevent prolonged myelosuppression.
Hematologic diseases: thalassemia, sickle-cell disease, severe aplastic anemia, Fanconi's anemia	Chemotherapy is given to eradicate cells in the bone marrow and to make space for engraftment of healthy allogeneic cells. The new donor cells will produce normal white cells, red cells, and platelets.
Immunodeficiency diseases: Wiskott-Aldrich syndrome, severe combined immunodeficiency syndrome (SCIDS), cartilage-hair hypoplasia	Chemotherapy is given to eradicate cells in the bone marrow and to make space for engraftment of healthy allogeneic cells. In the case of SCIDS, chemotherapy may not always be used.
Genetic diseases: adrenoleukodystrophy, metachromatic leukodystrophy, Hurler's syndrome	Chemotherapy is given to eradicate cells in the bone marrow. Donor cells, which will eventually produce the deficient enzyme, are infused.

10.2 Description of Treatment

HSCT can be divided into three phases: pretransplant, transplant, and post-transplant. The pretransplant phase includes donor and recipient evaluation and administration of a conditioning regimen (chemotherapy agents selected for specific activity). Day 0, the day of stem cell infusion, constitutes the transplant phase. Donor stem cells collected on this day are administered as a fresh product infusion. Donor cells collected prior to the initiation of conditioning are cryopreserved for infusion on Day 0. During the post-transplant or engraftment phase, the recipient is monitored for side effects of the conditioning regimen, complications of the transplant, and engraftment, which is the term used to indicate that the donor cells have migrated to and are repopulating the bone marrow space.

Pretransplant evaluation of the donor assures healthy stem cells and a donor who is able to tolerate the collection procedure. The age range of donors varies from infancy (3–4 months) to 65 years. The donor evaluation should include physical examination, complete health history for genetic disorders, and serological testing that includes CBC with differential, confirmatory HLA typing, ABO cross-matching, chemistry profile, coagulation screen, infectious disease testing, and a pregnancy test (if appropriate). Donors may be offered an opportunity to donate, if needed, an autologous unit of blood prior to collection of stem cells for autotransfusion.

The donor should have an opportunity to discuss issues such as testing procedures, health risks, and psychosocial sequelae with appropriate healthcare providers. These issues are especially important in the case of child donors. Consultation with child life specialists, social workers, and clergy may be beneficial and make the procedure less stressful and easier to tolerate.

The purpose of the recipient evaluation is to determine disease status and identify any underlying medical issues such as organ dysfunction or infections that could pose additional risks to the recipient. The recipient will have a more extensive evaluation than the donor. In addition to the studies listed above, the evaluation should include an assessment of the recipient's disease status, which will depend on the type of disease and the areas of previous involvement or treatment. These studies may include diagnostic scans (e.g., CT, MRI) as well as bone marrow aspirate/biopsy and lumbar puncture. Studies useful in evaluating organ dysfunction include chest x-ray, echocardiogram, pulmonary function tests (if age-appropriate), creatinine clearance or glomerular filtration rate, and dental exam. An audiogram may be ordered for patients who have a history of hearing loss or have previously received ototoxic agents. An ophthalmology exam may be done if the recipient is to receive total body irradiation (TBI).

Baseline monitoring for late effects might include baseline neuropsychological testing, endocrine function studies, and bone scans. A central venous access device will be placed, and information regarding sperm banking and egg harvesting should be provided to age-appropriate patients.

Conditioning (preparative) regimens are used to prepare the bone marrow space for the incoming graft, immunosuppress the recipient to prevent GvHD, and eradicate tumor cells when treating a malignant disease. In general, the conditioning regimen is given for 4–10 days prior to the stem cell infusion. The conditioning regimen selection depends on the disease being treated and the type of HSCT.

Conditioning regimens can include chemotherapy, radiation therapy, and immunotherapy. Chemotherapy is the backbone of the conditioning regimen and is used for most HSCT. Commonly used agents include cyclophosphamide, busulfan, cytarabine, melphalan, thiotepa, cisplatin, carboplatin, and etoposide. Radiation therapy in the form of TBI provides immunosuppression as well as treatment for sanctuary sites (central nervous system and testes). TBI is usually delivered in fractionated doses twice a day for 4–5 days. Local control radiation therapy may be given before or after transplant to patients with a history of central nervous system disease. Immunotherapy includes agents such as antithymocyte globulin (ATG) and monoclonal antibodies, such as Campath and CD45 antibody. These agents are usually given once a day for 3–4 days and are used to bind with and destroy recipient circulating T-lymphocytes in an attempt to decrease the risk of nonengraftment and GvHD.

10.2.1 Stem Cell Collection (Harvest)

Hematopoietic stem cells are immature progenitor cells that mature in the bone marrow space. After differentiation and maturation, they are released into the peripheral circulation as mature erythrocytes, lymphocytes, and thrombocytes. Stem cells can be obtained from the bone marrow, peripheral circulation, and cord blood. Stem cells from the bone marrow are most often collected under general anesthesia from the posterior iliac crest. The cells are placed in a sterile collection system, mixed with heparin, and filtered to remove bone spicules, fat globules, and blood clots.

Peripheral stem cells are collected by pheresis. Stem cells are mobilized into the peripheral circulation using granulocyte colony-stimulating factor (G-CSF) or chemotherapy (for autologous HSCT). Using a pheresis machine and large venous catheters, the desired stem cells are selected and removed from the peripheral blood based on weight. The remaining cells (red cells, platelets, and plasma) are then reinfused into the donor. The cells are placed in a sterile collection system, mixed with heparin, filtered, and mixed with a preservative prior to being cryopreserved. Cord blood stem cells are collected from a newborn's cord and placenta immediately after birth and cryopreserved for possible use at a later time.

Stem cell processing can include buffy-coating to deplete volume or erythrocyte contamination and purging to remove any remaining tumor cells. T-cell depletion and CD34$^+$ selection (collection of specific progenitor cells) are techniques used to reduce the number of T-lymphocytes in the final product.

Stem cell infusion is similar to a blood product transfusion, and the patient and family often perceive it as anticlimactic. Stem cells are infused through a central line and should not be filtered or irradiated. Side effects associated with the HCST are listed in Table 10.3. Fresh stem cell products are most often

Table 10.3. Common side effects of hematopoietic stem cell infusions

Type of product	Side effect	Nursing assessment	Nursing interventions
Fresh stem cells	Allergic reaction	Obtain baseline vital signs (VS) and breath sounds. Assess skin for evidence of flushing, itching and urticaria	Premedicate with antihistamine, corticosteroid, and antipyretic. Monitor VS and breath sounds frequently during and immediately after infusion per institutional policy
	Hemolytic transfusion reaction	Assess ABO compatibility of donor and recipient	Administer pre- and post-hydration fluids for ABO incompatibility. Administer diuretic. Maintain brisk urine output (1–2 ml/kg/hr) for 24 hours after infusion. Monitor for fever, chills, chest or back pain, dark urine, dyspnea, tachycardia, hypotension, shock
	Fluid overload	Assess baseline weight and fluid status. Assess baseline breath sounds and pulse oximetry	Monitor fluid status during and immediately after infusion. Monitor for cough, dyspnea, decreased oxygen saturation, hypertension, tachycardia, edema. Administer diuretic. Maintain brisk urine output (1–2 ml/kg/hr) for 24 hours after infusion

Table 10.3. (Continued)

Type of product	Side effect	Nursing assessment	Nursing interventions
	Micropulmonary emboli	Assess preinfusion VS, breath sounds and pulse oximetry	Monitor respiratory rate and pulse oximetry during infusion Monitor for dyspnea, decreased oxygen saturation, sudden severe headache or chest pain
	Infection	Assess baseline VS, including temperature	Monitor temperature frequently during infusion Administer antipyretic for elevated temperature Obtain sample of product and blood sample from patient for cultures
Preserved stem cells	Bad taste in mouth (due to DMSO) Nausea and vomiting		Administer antiemetics prior to infusion Offer hard candy or chewing gum if patient not sedated
	Arrhythmia and hypertension	Assess baseline VS and EKG	Monitor VS and EKG during and immediately after infusion Administer antihypertensive and diuretic
	Hemoglobinuria		Administer pre- and post-hydration fluids Administer diuretic Maintain brisk urine output (1–2 ml/kg/hr) for 24 hours after infusion
	Allergic reaction	Obtain baseline VS and breath sounds Assess skin for evidence of flushing, itching and urticaria	Premedicate with antihistamine, corticosteroid and antipyretic Monitor VS and breath sounds frequently during and immediately after infusion per institutional policy
	Fluid overload	Assess baseline weight and fluid status Assess baseline breath sounds and pulse oximetry	Monitor fluid status during and immediately after infusion Monitor for cough, dyspnea, decreased oxygen saturation, hypertension, tachycardia, edema Administer diuretic Maintain brisk urine output (1–2 ml/kg/hr) for 24 hours after infusion
	Micropulmonary emboli	Assess preinfusion VS, breath sounds and pulse oximetry	Monitor respiratory rate and pulse oximetry during infusion Monitor for dyspnea, decreased oxygen saturation, sudden severe headache, or chest pain
	Infection	Assess baseline VS, including temperature	Monitor temperature frequently during infusion Obtain sample of product and blood sample from patient for cultures Administer antipyretic for elevated temperature

Table 10.4. Timing of potential complications associated with HSCT (adapted from Fort and Norville, 1998)

Early (conditioning to engraftment)	Intermediate (engraftment to first 100 days)	Late (after 100 days)
Bone marrow suppression	Infections	Immunosuppression
Nausea, vomiting, diarrhea, anorexia, mucositis	Acute GvHD	Chronic GvHD
Parotitis	Graft failure	Infections
Infections	Interstitial pneumonitis	Endocrine dysfunction
Skin erythema		Cataracts
Capillary leak syndrome		Disease recurrence
Acute renal insufficiency		Secondary malignancies
Hemorrhagic cystitis		
Veno-occlusive disease		
Seizures		

used for allogeneic transplants, which are generally infused within 48 hours of collection. The stem cell product is infused over 2–4 hours as a slow intravenous (IV) infusion. Red cell or volume depletion prior to infusion is dependent on the donor and recipient's ABO status and the volume of donor cells collected compared to the recipient's body weight.

Stem cells collected from any donor source can be frozen and infused at a later time. In general, frozen stem cells are most often used for autologous transplants. To minimize the destruction of red cells during the freezing and thawing processes, a preservative (dimethyl sulfoxide, DMSO) is added to the stem cell product. DMSO has a garlic-like odor that is excreted from the lungs of the recipient for 24–48 hours after the stem cell infusion. DMSO infusion can cause transient cardiac arrhythmias, most commonly bradycardia, and hypertension. For this reason, many institutions require cardiac monitoring during and immediately after the infusion. Once the product is thawed, a rapid IV infusion is recommended.

10.3 Potential Side Effects

Side effects and complications associated with HSCT can occur at any time during the transplant process (Table 10.4). The side effects commonly associated with the conditioning regimen and time period to engraftment tend to occur early, within the first few weeks of transplant. Side effects that occur from the time of engraftment and during the first 100 days thereafter usually result from the conditioning regimen, prolonged immunosuppression, or early engraftment. Complications occurring 100 days or more after transplant are categorized as late effects.

10.3.1 Early Side Effects

Early side effects of the conditioning regimen can include bone marrow suppression, nausea, vomiting, diarrhea, anorexia, mucositis, parotitis, skin erythema, infections, capillary leak syndrome, acute renal insufficiency, veno-occlusive disease, and seizures. Bone marrow suppression typically occurs 7–10 days after the conditioning regimen begins. Fully ablative conditioning regimens will eradicate all cell lines in the bone marrow, causing anemia, thrombocytopenia, and neutropenia, with an absolute neutrophil count (ANC) of 0. Bone marrow suppression is prolonged and will continue until engraftment occurs. The timing of engraftment is affected by the conditioning regimen administered, the stem cell source, manipulation of the cells, the recipient's past history of prior chemotherapy, and the recipient's clinical condition. An ANC of 500 and a platelet count of

$20,000 \text{ mm}^2$ without transfusions indicate engraftment. The average time to engraftment is, in general, 14–28 days. Typically, platelets are the last cell line to become self-sustaining. As red cells engraft, the recipient's blood type will change to that of the donor when ABO differences are present.

Transfusions of leukocyte-depleted and irradiated red blood cells are often administered when hemoglobin levels fall below 8 g/dl. Leukocyte depletion minimizes the risk of viral contamination, particularly cytomegalovirus (CMV). Irradiation reduces the risk of GvHD from transfused blood products by eliminating the immunocompetent lymphocytes in the product without compromising its functional qualities (Ryan et al., 2002). There is a potential for cardiac and respiratory compromise associated with hemoglobin levels less than 7 g/dl.

Side effects of anemia include fatigue, irritability, pallor, tachycardia, shortness of breath, and dizziness. The administration of blood products or supplemental oxygen may be required. During transfusion, monitor for signs and symptoms of adverse effects.

The risk of bleeding is increased when the platelet count is $<20,000 \text{ mm}^2$. The nurses must assess for signs and symptoms of bleeding or blood loss, including bruising, petechiae, epistaxis, or oozing from the gums or central venous line. If transfusion is required, platelet products should be leukocyte-depleted and irradiated.

When the ANC falls below 500 cells/mm^3, patients are at a significantly increased risk of infection. Physical examination should include detailed inspection of the mouth, rectum, IV sites, and all wounds for evidence of infection. Symptoms including dysuria, sore throat, cough, and rectal pain are particularly worrisome in the neutropenic patient.

Gastrointestinal toxicity in the form of nausea and vomiting can begin within the first 24 hours of starting the conditioning regimen and can continue for several days after the transplant. Antibiotics, infections, and mucositis can exacerbate vomiting. Diarrhea can occur anytime during the conditioning regimen and last as long as 2 weeks after the transplant. Although chemotherapy is the usual cause of diarrhea during this time period, an infectious cause must be excluded. Mucositis usually peaks 7–14 days after the start of the conditioning regimen and resolves as engraftment (return of WBCs) occurs. Anorexia often accompanies the nausea, vomiting, diarrhea, and mucositis and can continue for several months after the transplant, especially in adolescent and young adult patients.

Supportive care for gastrointestinal symptoms includes administering antiemetics on a scheduled basis, as well as nutritional supplements, fluids, and total parenteral nutrition. Meticulous oral hygiene, perirectal hygiene, and skin care to prevent skin breakdown and secondary infections are necessary. Blood and stool cultures may be needed to isolate infectious agents. Pain assessment must be performed each shift and more often if the child is in pain. Oral or IV analgesics, preferably patient-controlled analgesia, may be required for mucositis pain.

Parotitis, inflammation of the parotid gland, usually occurs after the first or second dose of TBI. Common complaints are bilateral swelling and pain in the jaws. This side effect is self-limited, often lasting only a day or two. Applying warm compresses externally to the jaw and administering mild analgesics will usually provide relief.

Skin erythema, darkening, and dryness is not uncommon after TBI. This condition is most often mild and typically responds to moisturizing lotions, creams, and gels. A head-to-toe skin assessment is required daily. To prevent additional skin damage, patients need to be instructed not to use oil-based skin products while receiving TBI.

Infections during the early phase of transplant are a result of neutropenia, immunosuppression, and alterations in mucosal integrity and indwelling central lines. Patients are susceptible to bacterial, viral, and fungal infections. Common bacterial pathogens are *E. coli*, *Klebsiella*, *Pseudomonas*, *Staphylococcus aureus*, and coagulase-negative *Staphylococcus*. Reactivation of herpes simplex virus (HSV) is the predominant viral pathogen complicating mucositis during this time period. *Candida* spp. can infect the gastrointestinal tract, complicate toxicities, and secondarily infect other wounds and IV sites.

Prevention of infections is multifactorial and includes handwashing, limits on the number of visitors, high-energy particulate air (HEPA) filter systems, prophylactic antimicrobials, and administration of CMV-negative blood to CMV-seronegative recipients. A combination of broad-spectrum antibiotics is given from initiation of the conditioning regimen until engraftment as common prophylaxis against bacterial infections. Acyclovir or valacyclovir prophylaxis can reduce the risk of HSV reactivation. Fluconazole, voriconazole, or low-dose amphotericin is effective prophylaxis against fungal infections. Although controversial, intravenous immunoglobulin (IVIG) therapy is administered every 2–4 weeks to provide passive immunity.

Other interventions include monitoring the patient for fever and other signs of infection, obtaining blood and urine cultures at the onset of fever before starting antibiotics, drawing blood cultures daily for subsequent fevers, and obtaining other diagnostic studies (e.g., chest x-ray, CT) as appropriate. Patients who continue to be febrile after 3–5 days should receive treatment doses of amphotericin.

Hemorrhagic cystitis can occur within 24 hours of administration of chemotherapy and as late as several months after HSCT. The primary causes of hemorrhagic cystitis include cyclophosphamide, radiation therapy, and viruses. The active metabolite of cyclophosphamide, when allowed to remain in contact with the bladder mucosa, will cause irritation and bleeding. Viruses that can cause this complication include adenovirus, CMV, and BK virus.

Signs and symptoms of hemorrhagic cystitis include hematuria (microscopic or gross), urinary frequency, dysuria, suprapubic pain, and bladder spasms. A bladder ultrasound and urine cultures for bacteria and viruses are used for diagnosis.

Management includes pre- and post-hydration fluids and mesna for cyclophosphamide administration, placement of a Foley catheter or continuous bladder irrigation, and platelet transfusions.

If a urinary catheter has not been placed, the child must void at least every 1–2 hours during, and for 24 hours after, each dose of cyclophosphamide. Strict measuring of intake and output must be done in addition to platelet counts, coagulation studies, and close monitoring for microscopic hematuria. Administering blood products and providing pain control are other necessary supportive care measures.

Acute renal failure and nephritis are frequent complications after HSCT. Radiation therapy, immunosuppressive agents, and virus and bacterial toxins can cause nephritis. Acute renal failure can result from nephrotoxic drugs, infection, and inadequate renal perfusion.

Common symptoms of renal toxicity include increased weight, edema, decreased urine output, hypertension, elevated creatinine and BUN, and altered sensorium.

Medical management includes administration of diuretics, antihypertensives, vasopressors, and dialysis. Blood chemistries need to be monitored daily, and blood levels of nephrotoxic medications (e.g., cyclosporine, tacrolimus, vancomycin, gentamicin) must be checked until the appropriate dose level is reached and then routinely. Dose and frequency of nephrotoxic medications need to be adjusted as ordered, and renal doses of dopamine are given to promote renal perfusion.

Capillary leak syndrome, a shift of intravascular fluid into the extravascular space, often occurs 7–14 days after HSCT. Tissue damage from the conditioning regimen causes the release of cytokines that cause a capillary permeability. This permeability can lead to weight gain, fluid retention, ascites, cough, shortness of breath, and pulmonary edema. The child must be assessed for signs and symptoms of fluid overload, including weight gain, hypertension, abnormal breath sounds, and intake that is greater than output.

Veno-occlusive disease (VOD) results from the high-dose chemotherapy and radiation therapy administered during the conditioning regimen. The small vessels and central vein of the liver become occluded, causing congestion, venous outflow obstruction, and eventual hepatocyte damage. Onset is usually 7–21 days after transplant. The clinical features of VOD include weight gain, right upper quadrant pain, hepatomegaly, elevated serum bilirubin, ascites, and encephalopathy. Management includes maintaining fluid and electrolyte balance by strictly monitoring intake and output, obtaining accurate daily weights and measuring abdominal girth every shift, minimizing the adverse effects of ascites by restricting oral and IV fluids and administering diuretics and pain medications, adjusting medications to reflect hepatic and renal function, avoiding compounding encephalopathy with medications that alter mental status, and preventing bleeding.

Neurotoxicity can occur anytime during the transplant process. Seizures can result from medication toxicity, infection, hemorrhage, hypertension, and electrolyte abnormalities. In the early phase of transplant, high levels of chemotherapeutic agents (busulfan) and immunosuppressive agents (cyclosporine, tacrolimus) can cause seizures. Cyclosporine and tacrolimus can also cause tremors and peripheral neuropathy. Monitoring blood levels and adjusting doses can prevent and minimize these side effects.

10.3.2 Intermediate Side Effects

Intermediate side effects and complications of HSCT can include infections, graft failure, acute GvHD, and interstitial pneumonitis. Infections during this phase are more common and more severe for allogeneic patients than autologous patients as a result of impaired cell-mediated and humoral immunity, immunosuppressive therapy to prevent GvHD, and the presence of indwelling lines. Common pathogens include gram-negative bacteria (*E. coli, Klebsiella, Pseudomonas, Enterobacter*), gram-positive bacteria (*Staphylococcus aureus,* coagulase-negative *Staphylococcus, Streptococcus pneumoniae*), fungus (*Candida, Aspergillus*), and viruses (adenovirus, CMV).

Predisposing factors associated with infections during this period include neutropenia, central venous lines, immunosuppressive therapy, and GvHD.

Strategies to prevent or minimize the risk of infections include handwashing, HEPA filtration, low-bacterial diets, avoidance of crowded places, and antibacterial, antifungal, and antiviral prophylaxis. Antibacterial and antifungal (fluconazole, low-dose amphotericin B) prophylaxis continues until engraftment (defined as an ANC >500 for 3 consecutive days).

CMV infection is a life-threatening infection that usually occurs within the first 2 months post-transplant. Most centers will provide some form of prophylaxis when the recipient or donor is CMV-seropositive pretransplant, either ganciclovir IV from engraftment through 100 days post-transplant or CMV antigenemia monitoring with ganciclovir treatment when virus is detected. Additional strategies to prevent CMV infection include administration of leukocyte-depleted blood products and CMV-seronegative blood products to seronegative recipients. IVIG may also be given to provide passive immunity during this phase of HSCT.

Treatment is aimed at specific pathogens causing infections. Initial treatment usually includes broad-spectrum antibiotics, followed by specific antimicrobials based on culture and sensitivity results. Treatment of CMV infection can include ganciclovir and IVIG, foscarnet, and cidofovir.

Acute GvHD (AGvHD) is an immune-mediated response in which the immunocompetent donor T-cells recognize the host (recipient) antigens as foreign and mount an attack. It is the consequence of alloreactivity between the donor and recipient. The immunocompetent donor T-cells recognize the alloantigens (major and minor histocompatibility antigens) of the recipient and become activated, which leads to further expansion of alloreactive T-cells. This leads to the release of cytokines, recruitment of other immune system effector cells, and eventual tissue damage.

Incidence and severity depend on the type of transplant and the degree of HLA disparity between the donor and recipient. The recipient's age, the number of T-cells transfused, and the GvHD prophylaxis used are additional risk factors. The onset of AGvHD usually coincides with engraftment and occurs within the first 100 days of transplant.

Clinical presentation typically involves one of three targeted organs: the skin, liver, or gut. Diagnosis can be made clinically based on symptoms and laboratory values. However, tissue biopsy is required for definitive diagnosis. Individual organ involvement is staged for severity, and an overall grade is assigned based on severity and combined organ involvement. Skin AGvHD is the most common initial presenting manifestation. The rash begins as a macular erythematous rash of the palms and soles. It can progress to a maculopapular erythematous rash on the trunk and extremities to bullae and generalized desquamation. Pruritus and pain are common associated symptoms (Table 10.5).

Table 10.5. Acute GvHD stage and grading systems

Staging of individual organ system(s)		
Organ	**Stage**	**Description**
Skin	+1	Maculopapular (M-P) eruption over <25% of body area
	+2	Maculopapular eruption over 25–50% of body area
	+3	Generalized erythroderma
	+4	Generalized erythroderma with bullous formation and often with desquamation
Liver	+1	Bilirubin 2.0–3.0 mg/dl; SGOT 150–750 IU
	+2	Bilirubin 3.1–6.0 mg/dl
	+3	Bilirubin 6.1–15.0 mg/dl
	+4	Bilirubin >15.0 mg/dl
Gut	+1	Diarrhea >30 ml/kg or >500 ml/day
	+2	Diarrhea >60 ml/kg or >1,000 ml/day
	+3	Diarrhea >90 ml/kg or >1,500 ml/day
	+4	Diarrhea >90 ml/kg or >2,000 ml/day; or severe abdominal pain and bleeding with or without ileus

Overall grading of acute GvHD			
Grade	**Skin staging**	**Liver staging**	**Gut staging**
I	+1 to +2	0	0
II	+1 to +3	+1 and/or	+1
III	+2 to +3	+2 to +4 and/or	+2 to +3
IV	+2 to +4	+2 to +4 and/or	+2 to +4

Liver AGvHD causes degeneration of mucosa and small bile ducts and results in hepatitis-like symptoms (fatigue, abnormal liver function tests, right upper quadrant pain, hepatomegaly, jaundice, and pruritus). Increased bilirubin and alkaline phosphatase levels are the earliest and most common abnormalities noted.

Gut AGvHD is characterized by diarrhea and abdominal cramping, which can progress to severe ileus. Degeneration of the mucosal lining of the GI tract results in green, watery, guaiac-positive diarrhea; abdominal discomfort; nausea; vomiting; anorexia; malabsorption; and ascites. Both the upper and lower GI tract can be involved.

Prevention remains the key to effective management of AGvHD. Prevention strategies are aimed at preventing the activation of T-cells and depleting mature alloreactive T-cells from donor grafts. Cyclosporine, used in combination with other immunosuppressive agents, has been standard GvHD prophylaxis, but tacrolimus is being used instead of cyclosporine for unrelated and mismatched transplants because it has proven to be superior to cyclosporine in this group of patients (Ryan et al., 2002). New monoclonal antibodies, Campath and CD45 antibody, are being incorporated into conditioning regimens as GvHD prophylaxis. T-cell depletion, monoclonal antibodies, and CD34+ selection are successful strategies to deplete alloreactive T-cells from donor grafts.

Treatment consists of adding corticosteroids and continuing cyclosporine or tacrolimus (Table 10.6). Antithymocyte globulin and newer monoclonal antibodies are added in cases of steroid-resistant or severe AGvHD.

Table 10.6. Agents used to prevent and treat GvHD (from Forte, 1997)

	Mechanism	Toxicities
Cyclosporine (Sandimmune)	Blocks synthesis of IL-2, suppresses development of cytotoxic T-lymphocytes	Renal toxicity, hypertension, magnesium wasting, hyperkalemia, tremors, seizures, gingival hypertrophy, hirsutism, cortical blindness
FK506 (Prograf)	Is similar to cyclosporine	Are similar to those associated with cyclosporine, hyperglycemia
Methotrexate (Mexate)	Inhibits DNA synthesis by competitively binding with dihydrofolate reductase	Renal toxicity, liver toxicity, mucositis
Glucocorticoids	Prevents production and release of IL-1 from macrophages	Myelosuppression, mood swings, hypertension, hyperglycemia, GI bleeding, osteoporosis, acne, cushingoid syndrome
Antithymocyte globulin (ATG) (an immune globulin)	Acts against human thymocytes	Fever, chills, rash, anaphylaxis, serum sickness
OKT3 (Orthoclone) (a monoclonal antibody)	Is specific for circulating CD3 T-cells dizziness, chest pain, wheezing, tremor	First-dose reaction: fever, chills, diarrhea,
Thalidomide	Decreases the number of helper T-cells and increases the number of suppressor T-cells	Peripheral neuropathies, constipation, sedation
Hydroxychloroquine (Plaquenil)	Reduces secretion of IL-1, IL-6, and tumor necrosis factor	Ocular toxicity, nausea, diarrhea, rash, photosensitivity

Graft failure or rejection occurs when the donor graft is not sustained in the recipient. This complication is relatively uncommon in allogeneic HSCT, with an incidence of approximately 1% with HLA-matched donors and 5–10% with mismatched donors (Guinan et al., 2002). Graft failure can occur when the stem cell dose is too low, the recipient marrow is not completely ablated, or the immunosuppression is inadequate. Infections and tumor recurrence can also cause graft failure. Treatment may include increased immunosuppression or infusion of donor T-lymphocytes.

Interstitial pneumonitis is the leading cause of respiratory failure in HSCT patients. It can result from infection or toxicity of the conditioning regimen. Idiopathic pneumonitis is a noninfectious interstitial pneumonia that often follows engraftment, strongly suggesting an immunologic response involved in the process. Clinical features include dyspnea, nonproductive cough, hypoxia, diffuse alveolar damage, and nonlobar infiltrates on x-ray. The mortality rate for this complication is extremely high despite aggressive treatment with antimicrobials, blood products, steroids, and ventilatory support (Ryan et al., 2002).

10.3.3 Late Side Effects

Late side effects and complications can include immunosuppression and infections, chronic GvHD, endocrine dysfunction, cataracts, disease recurrence, and secondary malignancies. Immunosuppression and infections remain a risk during this time despite neutrophil engraftment. Both cellular and humoral immunity remain depressed until full immune reconstitution occurs. This delayed immune recovery can lead to acute and chronic infections and nutritional deficits (Guinan et al., 2002; Ryan et al., 2002).

Table 10.7. Prophylaxis for PCP

Age	Primary recommendation	Second alternative
Infants (1–12 months)	*TMP-SMZ (150/750 mg/m^2) by mouth twice daily for 3 consecutive days	Dapsone (infants >1 month) 2 mg/kg by mouth daily
Children (>12 months)	TMP-SMZ (150/750 mg/m^2) by mouth twice daily for 3 consecutive days	Dapsone 2 mg/kg by mouth daily, maximum 100 mg by mouth daily
Adolescents	TPM-SMZ (160 mg/800 mg) by mouth three times a week	Dapsone 100 mg by mouth daily

* prophylaxis – sulfomethoxazole/trimethoprim/co-trimoxazole

Several factors contribute to this protracted impaired immunity: patient and donor age, conditioning regimen used, degree of HLA disparity between donor and recipient, presence of GvHD, presence of infection, and type of post-transplant immunosuppression used.

Common post-transplant infections include *Pneumocystis jiroveci* (formerly called *Pneumocystis carinii*), varicella-zoster, CMV, adenovirus, and Epstein-Barr virus lymphoproliferative disease. Management includes *Pneumocystis jiroveci* prophylaxis for 1 year post-transplant (Table 10.7) and frequent monitoring for evidence of infections and immune recovery.

Chronic GvHD (CGvHD) is a chronic autoimmune syndrome that resembles collagen vascular diseases such as scleroderma and systemic lupus erythematosus. The primary effect of CGvHD is the epithelial cell damage to tissue that can lead to fibrosis and atrophy. Chronic GvHD targets the same organs as AGvHD – the skin, liver, and gut – however, it may affect others as well, such as the eyes and lungs. The secondary effect of marked immunosuppression has a significant impact on morbidity and mortality post-transplant.

Risk factors for CGvHD include prior AGvHD, donor and recipient HLA disparity, and increasing patient age. The decreased incidence over the last decade can be attributed to improved HLA matching and effective AGvHD prevention. Chronic GvHD can occur as progression of acute GvHD, follow a period of quiescence after acute GvHD, or occur as de novo disease. Historically, GvHD that occurs 100 days after transplant is considered chronic. The increased use of donor T-lymphocytes in the post-transplant period requires careful assessment and diagnosis of GvHD symptoms.

Clinical presentation is remarkable for sicca syndrome, extreme dryness of mucous membranes and tissues, and infections (Table 10.8). Diagnosis can be made clinically based on symptoms and laboratory values. However, tissue biopsy is required for definitive diagnosis. Chronic GvHD is graded as limited or extensive: Limited is described as localized skin involvement and/or hepatic dysfunction, and extensive is described as generalized skin involvement with multiorgan involvement.

Treatment consists of immunosuppression with many of the same agents used to treat AGvHD (Table 10.6). Initial treatment usually includes cyclosporine or tacrolimus and steroids that are slowly tapered over several months. Several newer agents are now available. For severe CGvHD of the skin, both psoralen and ultraviolet radiation (PUVA) and extracorporeal photopheresis have been beneficial.

Endocrine dysfunction may present as growth failure, thyroid dysfunction, ovarian dysfunction, or testicular dysfunction. Risk factors include TBI and long-term steroid therapy, although fractionated TBI has decreased the incidence of hypothyroidism to 10 % (Guinan et al., 2002). Treatment includes thyroid replacement therapy and growth hormone therapy, respectively, for thyroid dysfunction and growth delays. Females who have chemotherapy after puberty have more permanent infertility and menopausal symptoms than those treated before puberty. Testic-

Table 10.8. Chronic GvHD: clinical effects and nursing interventions

Organ/system involved	Clinical effects	Nursing interventions
Skin	Itching, burning, scleroderma, ulcerations, hyperpigmentation, erythema, dryness Erythema can be activated by sun exposure	Teach patient to use skin moisturizers and nondrying, nonabrasive soaps Teach patient to protect skin from sunlight and avoid prolonged sun exposure; emphasize need to use sunscreens
	Alopecia, nail ridging, joint contractures	Apply topical steroid creams to relieve itching and/or burning Provide range of motion exercises Practice specific exercise regimens recommended by PT/OT to prevent contractures
Liver	Obstructive jaundice	Monitor liver function tests
	Cirrhosis with esophageal varices and hepatic failure	Teach patient low-fat diet, if indicated
GI tract	Xerostomia, stomatitis, ulcerations, lichen planus-like striae and plaques, taste changes, dysphagia, retrosternal pain, diarrhea, malabsorption	Promote oral hygiene and regular dental follow-up Encourage use of artificial saliva or alkaline-saline mouthwash to relieve oral dryness Provide lanolin for lip moisturizing Provide nutritional counseling and dietary referral Monitor weights
Eyes	Decreased tear production Burning, photophobia, itching, sensation of grittiness in eyes	Promote regular ophthalmology exams Provide artificial tears to relieve ocular dryness Suggest use of sunglasses to decrease discomfort of photophobia
Lungs	Obstructive and restrictive lung changes Cough, dyspnea, pneumothorax	Provide chest PT and incentive spirometer, if indicated Monitor pulmonary function tests on a regular basis
Immunosuppression	Increased risk of infection Slowed immune recovery	Maintain measures to prevent infections Promote good general hygiene Administer immunosuppressive therapy and monitor for side effects Monitor compliance with infection prophylaxis medications

ular dysfunction includes sterility, azoospermia, and premature ejaculation in males treated with TBI. Regardless of age, TBI may result in primary gonadal failure in both genders. Treatment may include hormone replacement therapy.

Cataracts, usually posterior and bilateral, can occur several years post-transplant in patients who receive TBI. Fractionated TBI has significantly reduced

the incidence. Treatment is surgical removal of the cataracts.

Disease recurrence remains the primary cause of treatment failure after autologous and allogeneic HSCT. Patients at increased risk for relapse include those with high-risk diseases, poor response to initial therapy, unfavorable cytogenetic abnormalities, and significant disease/tumor burden at time of transplant. Treatment can include donor lymphocyte infusions, second transplants, and discontinuing immunosuppressive therapy.

Secondary malignancies are potential problems for both autologous and allogeneic transplant recipients. High-dose chemotherapy, TBI, and immunosuppression are the primary etiologies. Myelodysplastic syndrome and leukemia occur at an incidence of 4–20% at 5–6 years after autologous transplant. Patients receiving an allogeneic transplant are at risk of developing post-transplant lymphoproliferative disease, which can occur within 6 months after transplant, and a variety of solid tumors at an incidence rate eight times higher than the normal (Guinan et al., 2002).

10.4 Special Considerations

Discharge planning and teaching become focused once engraftment begins. Discharge can be anticipated once engraftment has occurred. Engraftment is generally defined as an ANC >500 for 3 consecutive days. In general, patients are required to remain in close proximity to the transplant center for the first 100 days after allogeneic transplant. Autologous transplant patients may be referred to their primary physician once engraftment has occurred and HSCT complications have resolved.

General discharge criteria include the following:

- ANC >500
- Afebrile for 24 hours
- Able to take oral medications
- Oral intake of calories and fluids is 50% of nutritional needs
- Patient is on total parenteral nutrition or nasogastric feedings
- Any transplant complications are resolved or controlled
- Primary caregiver is able to care for central venous line and provide any nutritional support that is needed.

Instructions to patient and caregiver should include the following topics:

- Infection control practices: handwashing, social isolation, face masks, temperature monitoring, and avoidance of new pets and plants
- Activities of daily living: diet, personal hygiene, mouth care, sun exposure, exercise, and school reentry
- Central line care and parenteral medication administration
- Importance of oral medication compliance
- Reportable signs and symptoms: fever, cough, rash, vomiting, diarrhea, bleeding, pain, and inability to take oral medications.

Outpatient follow-up will be tailored to the patient's needs. The frequency of clinic appointments is based on type of transplant, engraftment status, and unresolved complications. Regular monitoring will include physical assessment, routine blood counts, serum chemistries and medication levels (cyclosporine and tacrolimus), symptom and toxicity management, medication compliance, and nutritional assessment.

Annual evaluations of recipients of allogeneic transplants are required for monitoring engraftment status and assessing for late effects. Typical tests performed on an annual basis include

- Complete blood count with differential
- Serum chemistries
- Immunoglobulin levels
- Immune function tests
- Endocrine function tests
- Pulmonary function tests
- Cardiac function tests
- Ophthalmologic examination
- Renal function tests
- Neuropsychological evaluation.

Psychosocial issues faced by patients and their families are numerous, with different issues presenting during each stage of transplant. Some of these include prolonged hospitalization, emotional isolation from family and friends, role changes within the family dynamics, invasive medical procedures, treatment-related side effects and complications, fear of relapse, and financial concerns. All of these can have a significant impact on the quality of life experienced by the patient and the entire family. Consequently, a diverse multidisciplinary team of healthcare providers is required to assist the patient and family in successfully dealing with these issues.

10.5 Future Perspectives

Future direction in HSCT will consist of optimizing graft versus leukemia (GvL) effects, minimizing toxicity, engineering more precise grafts, moving to outpatient procedures, and combining stem cell transplantation with gene therapy.

GvL is an immune response to donor cells against recipient leukemia. There is evidence for GvL effect with the infusion of unmanipulated donor lymphocytes to relapsed patients after allogeneic HSCT. The future holds identification of minor antigens and their roles in GvL and GvHD.

Minimizing regimen-related toxicity would broaden the use of HSCT to nontraditional disorders such as autoimmune and degenerative diseases and improve long-term survival of transplant recipients. Monoclonal antibodies, such as Campath, CD45, and Rituxan, are being incorporated into conditioning regimens to substitute in part or in whole for the traditional cytotoxic and immunosuppressive drugs currently used. Many centers are developing submyeloablative conditioning regimens with less toxic chemotherapy. The use of adoptive immunotherapy in the form of cytotoxic T-lymphocytes has been demonstrated to prevent and treat transplant infections and post-transplant lymphoproliferative disorders.

T-cell depletion and CD34$^+$ selection are examples of more precise graft engineering to reduce complications such as graft failure and GvHD. Further identification of minor antigens could lead to more selective T-cell depletion techniques that might allow GvHD prevention without significant loss of GVL effect.

Several centers are exploring the possibility of providing stem cell transplants in the outpatient arena. This could have a significant impact on length of hospitalization and financial costs of HSCT in the future. As technology and basic science advance, HSCT will be combined with gene therapy as a vehicle for gene insertion, which will enhance applicability of stem cell transplantation, provide less toxic therapy, and improve survival.

References

Forte K (1997) Alternative donor sources in pediatric bone marrow transplant. Journal of Pediatric Oncology Nursing 14:221.

Forte K, Norville R (1998) Hematopoietic stem cell transplantation. In Hockenberry MJ (ed) Essentials of Pediatric Oncology Nursing: A Core Curriculum, 2nd edn. Glenview, IL: Association of Pediatric Oncology Nurses, p.103

Guinan, E. C., Krance, R. A., Lehmann, L. E. (2002) Stem cell transplantation in pediatric oncology. In Pizzo P. A., Poplack D. G. (eds) Principles and Practice of Pediatric Oncology. Philadelphia: Lippincott Williams & Wilkins, pp. 429–451

Ryan, L. G., Kristovich, K. M, Haugen, M. S., Hubbell, M. M. (2002) Hematopoietic stem cell transplantation. In Baggott C. R., Kelly K. P., D. Fochtman, Foley G. V. (eds) Nursing Care of Children and Adolescents with Cancer. Philadelphia: WB Saunders, pp. 212–255

Bibliography

Centers for Disease Control and Prevention (2000) Guidelines for preventing opportunistic infections among hematopoietic stem cell transplant recipients. Retrieved April 22, 2003, from http://www.phppo.cdc.gov/cdcrecommends/

Foss, F. M., Gorgun, G., Miller, K. B. (2002) Extracorporeal photopheresis in chronic graft-versus-host disease. Bone Marrow Transplantation 20:719–725

Gonzalez-Ryan, L., Van Syckle, K., Coyne, K. D., Glover, N. (2000) Umbilical core blood banking: Procedural and ethical concerns for this new birth option. Pediatric Nursing 26(1):105–110

Gross, T. G., Egeler, R. M. Smith, F. O. (2001) Pediatric hematopoietic stem cell transplantation. Hematology/Oncology Clinics of North America 15(5):795–808

Jacobsohn, D. A., Vogelsang, G. B. (2002) Novel pharmacotherapeutic approaches to prevention and treatment of GvHD. Drugs 2002 62(6):879–889

Kapustay, P. M. Buchsel, P. C. (2000) Process, complications, and management of peripheral stem cell transplantation. In Buchsel P. C., Kapustay P. M. (eds) Stem Cell Transplantation: A Clinical Textbook. Pittsburgh: Oncology Nursing Press, pp. 5.3–5.28

Kemp, J., Dickerson, J. (2002) Interdisciplinary modular teaching for patients undergoing progenitor cell transplantation. Clinical Journal of Oncology Nursing 6(3):157–160

McCarthy, P. L., Williams, L. A., Holmes, M. (2000) Stem cell transplantation: Past, present, and future. In Buchsel P. C., Kapustay P. M. (eds) Stem Cell Transplantation: A Clinical Textbook. Pittsburgh, PA: Oncology Nursing Press, pp. 1.3–1.18

Mills, S. B., Appel, B. (2000) Umbilical cord blood transplantation. In Buchsel P. C., Kapustay P. M. (eds) Stem cell transplantation: A Clinical Textbook. Pittsburgh: Oncology Nursing Press, pp. 10.3–10.12

Norville, R., Bryant, R. (2002) Blood component deficiencies. In Baggott C. R., Kelly K. P., Fochtman D., Foley G. V. (eds) Nursing Care of Children and Adolescents with Cancer. Philadelphia: WB Saunders, pp. 347–364

Norville, R., Monroe, R., Forte, K. (in press) Hematopoietic stem cell transplantation. In Kline N. J. (ed) Essentials of Pediatric Oncology Nursing: A Core Curriculum. Glenview, IL: Association of Pediatric Oncology Nurses

Secola, R. (2001) Hematopoietic stem cell transplantation: A glimpse of the past and a view of the future. Journal of Pediatric Oncology Nursing 18(4):171–177

Taketomo, C. K., Jodding, J. H., Kraus, D. M. (2002–2003) Pediatric Dosage Handbook, 9th edn. Hudson, OH: Lexi-Comp

Zaia, J. A. (2002) Prevention and management of CMV-related problems after hematopoietic stem cell transplantation. Bone Marrow Transplantation 29:633–638

Surgical Approaches to Childhood Cancer

Jill Brace ONeill

Contents

11.1 Principles of Treatment

A multimodal treatment approach has improved survival rates of children with cancer. This multifaceted approach may include surgery, chemotherapy, radiation, or a combination of these. Many advances in the treatment of childhood cancers have been through development of intensive chemotherapy and radiotherapy regimens. Due to this multimodal approach to pediatric malignancies, there has been a decreased need for radical surgical procedures. However, the surgical team is still required to be an integral part of many aspects of pediatric oncology care, particularly supportive care and related complications. Common surgical techniques in the management of childhood malignancies include, but are not limited to, those listed in Table 11.1.

11.2 Description of Treatment

A local and regional determination of the extent of disease, or staging, is performed at diagnosis and relapse (Leonard, 2002). A system of staging exists for many pediatric tumors and helps to determine both prognosis and treatment, relating the extent of disease at diagnosis to the subsequent clinical course. It is based on the premise that cancer of similar histologic features and sites of origin grows and metastasizes in a similar manner. All treatment protocols are based on stage of the tumor, which determines such factors as use of radiotherapy and intensity of chemotherapy. Correct staging allows the medical team to minimize therapy and yet maximize cure. This further provides the opportunity to limit thera-

Table 11.1. Common surgical techniques for management of childhood malignancies

Procedure	Description
Biopsies, including fine needle aspiration, core biopsy, and incisional/open or excisional biopsy	Biopsies include taking a sample of the desired tissue by means of a Biopsies include taking a sample of the desired tissue by means of a needle aspiration, a core biopsy for larger specimens, and open procedures to remove entire sections of tumor and/or lymph nodes.
Staging and second-look surgery	Staging is used when treatment depends on the location of the cancer and the extent of disease involvement. "Second-look" procedures are used to assess response to nonsurgical treatment.
Debulking	Debulking involves removing a portion of the tumor mass when it is not possible to remove the entire mass. This may be done as first-line therapy or after receiving chemotherapy or radiation.
Management of metastasis	Provides pathologic confirmation of metastasis via biopsy and can include staging and/or debulking efforts.
Supportive care surgery	Surgeries necessary for placement of central venous access devices/catheters or feeding tubes vital to supportive care measures.
Palliative surgery	Palliative surgery is done to relieve the symptoms caused by tumors that have been unresponsive to medical therapy. It may also be done to relieve pain and bleeding.

py to minimize the long-term sequelae of different treatments.

Similar to staging of the disease, use of the correct biopsy technique is critical to the childhood cancer patient. The diagnosis of childhood cancer requires a multimodal tumor analysis carefully planned before the biopsy by the pediatric oncologist, pathologist, and surgeon. Biopsy is best performed in a pediatric cancer center because optimal use of the surgical specimen can be performed only in specialized childhood cancer centers. Considerations when selecting the method and type of incision include the creation of an incision that may be incorporated in the future incision used for resection, the need to avoid contaminating an uninvolved body cavity, the need to avoid contaminating otherwise uninvolved lymphatic drainage, and adequate staging at the time of biopsy if the child is to receive preoperative chemotherapy.

Because pediatric cancers include a diverse group of malignancies, there is no single surgical procedure that can be used in all cases. Regardless, the goal of treatment is cure that will best be achieved with multimodal treatment (i.e., chemotherapy, radiation therapy, surgery, or a combination of these).

11.3 Method of Delivery

11.3.1 Preoperative Evaluation

The pediatric oncology patient undergoing surgery warrants detailed consideration with regard to perioperative and anesthetic management. Clinically, this includes coagulation and transfusion evaluation and support, evaluation of tumors that result in an anterior mass, and immunization of those patients undergoing splenectomy. For patients already treated with chemotherapy, assessment of cardiac, pulmonary, renal, and electrolyte status is also critical (Shamberger et al., 2002). Close coordination between services will avoid duplication of studies and decrease the need for repeated sedation for procedures or diagnostic tests.

A complete blood count, including hemoglobin, white blood cell count, platelet count, and coagulation studies, is necessary prior to surgery. Low blood counts can be corrected using granulocyte colony stimulating factor and red blood cell and/or platelet transfusions when indicated. It is difficult to discern, however, particularly in the leukemic patient, whether neutropenia may be functional or a result of

Table 11.2. Ideal blood counts prior to surgical procedure

Platelets >50,000/mm³
Hemoglobin >6–8 g/dl
Absolute neutrophils >1,000/mm³
Normal coagulation studies (including thrombin time, fibrin degradation products, fibrin monomers, and D-dimer levels)

a bone marrow "packed" with leukemic cells. The clinical situation will mandate the need for transfusion support of the oncologic surgical patient. Immunodeficient patients should receive irradiated and leukocyte-reduced blood products. Patients who are serologically cytomegalovirus (CMV)-negative should receive CMV-negative blood products as well.

Most often, elevations in prothrombin time (PT) and partial thromboplastin time (PTT) are acquired defects. For the patient with a normal platelet count and fibrinogen, an injection of vitamin K – or for immediate correction, fresh frozen plasma – can correct these abnormalities. For the patient with other associated abnormal laboratory values (e.g., fibrinogen), disseminated intravascular coagulation (DIC) or liver disease should be considered (Table 11.2).

A child with a mediastinal mass is at risk for respiratory collapse due to airway compression during induction of general anesthesia. Anterior mediastinal masses may also compress the superior vena cava, causing some or all manifestations of superior vena cava syndrome. These symptoms include orthopnea, headache, dizziness, fainting, plethoric facial swelling, jugular venous distension, papilledema, and pulsus paradoxus. Computed tomography (CT) is helpful in diagnosing the mediastinal mass and the degree of tracheobronchial compression (Shamberger, 1999). Pulmonary function testing can also be important in evaluating this type of patient. Those patients with a mediastinal mass that will not shrink with chemotherapy, emergency radiation therapy, or steroids may have conscious sedation considered for obtaining diagnostic biopsy material.

A child needs to be immunized at least two weeks before undergoing a splenectomy. The spleen contains macrophages, which provide defense against infections. Necessary vaccines include *Haemophilus influenzae* type B (Hib), pneumococcal vaccine, and meningococcal vaccine.

Patients who have a history of receiving bleomycin, anthracycline agents, or radiation therapy will be assessed differently prior to surgery than those children who have not been exposed to these treatments. Pulmonary fibrosis with a loss of lung volume, compliance, and diffusing capacity can occur as a result of bleomycin, BCNU, or radiation therapy to the lung; therefore, these patients need to be identified to the anesthesiologist as high-risk. All patients who have a history of receiving anthracycline agents (cardiotoxic) or mediastinal radiation will also need further preoperative evaluation, which can include an echocardiogram (ECHO) and/or multigated angiography (MUGA).

Preparation of the patient and his or her family cannot be overemphasized as a vital part of preoperative nursing management. Besides ensuring adequate nutrition, confirming no evidence of infection, and checking that laboratory criteria are met or within normal limits, the child and family will need education to support them. Play therapy is often used to help prepare children for surgery. This may include allowing the child to handle medical equipment, providing developmentally appropriate explanations, and giving a tour of the operating room if time permits; these measures can positively influence the operative experience. Assessing the patient and family's learning needs is an important part of this preparation phase before surgery.

11.3.2 Postoperative Nursing Care

The child with cancer is often a high-risk surgical patient. Postoperative care of these patients must include attention to the following areas: prevention of infection, airway maintenance and oxygenation, fluid and electrolyte balance, pain control, nutritional support, and wound care.

11.4 Potential Side Effects

Immunosuppression related to cancer therapy presents the increased potential for complications due to infectious causes. A secondary problem related to this is that signs and symptoms of infection are often delayed in these patients because of their immune suppression. Therefore, surgical oncology patients require close monitoring postoperatively.

11.4.1 Complications of Medical Therapy Requiring Surgical Evaluation

Bowel obstruction can be partial or complete and may be caused by tumors, adhesions, constipation, ileus as a result of vincristine, or graft-vs.-host disease in hematopoietic stem cell transplant patients. Perforation and necrosis are rare but can occur. Treatment usually includes hydration, antibiotics, and laxatives for first-line therapy. A nasogastric tube is inserted to relieve pressure, and subsequent surgery is used if the obstruction persists despite the previous interventions.

Pancreatitis is an inflammation of the pancreas. Symptoms are nausea, vomiting, and right-sided tenderness, and the diagnosis is confirmed by physical examination and elevated lipase and amylase. CT or ultrasound shows an enlarged and inflamed pancreas. The cause is tumor lysis and/or chemotherapy (asparaginase or, less frequently, steroids). Treatment includes stopping the causative agent and restricting the diet. Necrotizing pancreatitis may require surgical debridement in extreme cases. Maintenance of nothing-by-mouth status with total parenteral nutrition until symptoms resolve is the usual first-line therapy, with a subsequent low-fat diet prescribed.

In neutropenic children, inflammation of the cecum (typhlitis) can occur postoperatively and can progress rapidly to gangrene or perforation of the bowel. Symptoms include abdominal pain in the right lower quadrant, fever, distention, diarrhea, and vomiting (see chapter 15). An x-ray film can demonstrate bowel wall thickening, and a CT scan confirms inflammation and its extent. Treatment includes antibiotics and bowel rest. Laparotomy is a surgical intervention to remove the diseased bowel if there is clinical deterioration, persistent gastrointestinal bleeding, uncontrolled sepsis, or evidence of perforation.

Different types of infections can occur and are not uncommon in the immunosuppressed pediatric oncology patient. Surgical site infections are the leading type of infection among hospitalized patients. Infections of the surgical wound/site or the central line site often can be treated with antibiotics without having to remove the newly-planted central venous access device. Symptoms of wound infection are tenderness, erythema, fever, and wound drainage. Wound infections usually occur after 5–7 days postoperatively. Other than antibiotics, wound infection treatment may also include excision and drainage, particularly when symptoms of cellulitis are present. The surgeon may debride a wound when infection interferes with healing. Temporary drains are used to remove fluid accumulation.

Currently clinical practice standards for the prevention of surgical site infections have been derived from guidelines prepared by the American College of Surgeons and the Centers for Disease Control (CDC) (Nichols, 2000). These guidelines include educational preparation of the patient/family; antisepsis of the surgical team; management of infected surgical personnel; antimicrobial prophylaxis; intraoperative ventilation; intraoperative cleaning and disinfection; microbiologic sampling; sterilization of surgical instruments, surgical attire, and drapes; and asepsis and sterile technique, incision care, and surveillance.

Incision care is defined per the aforementioned guidelines as following recommendations during the postoperative phase to prevent surgical site infections. Specifically, these recommendations include the following:

- Protect incision with sterile dressing 24–48 hours postoperatively
- Wash hands before and after any contact with the surgical site
- Use sterile technique when changing dressing
- Educate patient and family regarding proper incision care, symptoms of an infection, and the need to report these symptoms.

Pneumothorax is the collapse of a lung and can be spontaneous, a presenting symptom of metastatic lung disease, or a direct result of an invasive procedure (e.g., thoracotomy). The most common symptoms of pneumothorax are shortness of breath and chest pain. A chest x-ray revealing lung collapse will confirm the diagnosis. Symptoms can develop within 24 hours postoperatively. The treatment includes lung expansion via insertion of a chest tube. The tube is left in place until the x-rays and the clinical condition of the patient show that the lung has re-expanded.

11.4.2 Complications Arising from Surgical Management of Solid Tumors

Operations for solid tumors can present risks unique to the type of tumor being approached. Specific tumor considerations include, but are not limited to, neuroblastoma and Wilms' tumor. Surgery is a cornerstone of treatment in neuroblastoma. Neoadjuvant chemotherapy has made surgical resection of locally advanced tumors more feasible and has improved local control and survival (Rubie et al., 2001). With advanced tumors, injury to major vessels occurs and the need for extended resections becomes necessary. The most common intraoperative complication is the need for nephrectomy. In addition, extensive dissection of renal vessels can lead to ultimate damage that may not become apparent until the postoperative period. Renal impairment is evidenced by anuria/oliguria.

In children with Wilms' tumor, surgical complications are potential causes of significant morbidity. However, with the introduction of preoperative chemotherapy and standardization of surgical techniques, the rate of surgical complications has been markedly reduced. Risk factors for the development of surgical complications in patients with Wilms' tumor include advanced local tumor at time of diagnosis, intravascular tumor extension, and resection of other organs at the time of nephrectomy. The most common complication is intestinal obstruction, followed by hemorrhage, wound infection, and vascular injury. Furthermore, two risk factors related to local recurrence of Wilms' tumor are directly related to the type of surgical resection performed: The presence of microscopic tumor at the margin of the surgical resection and intraoperative tumor spill are both factors that can predict disease recurrence. Other childhood cancers that are benefiting from advances in surgical techniques and coordination with multimodality treatment regimens include rhabdomyosarcoma, Ewing's sarcoma, germ cell tumors, and hepatoblastoma.

11.5 Special Considerations

11.5.1 Vascular Access Devices

Vascular access devices (VADs) are vital in managing and treating childhood cancer. Central venous catheters provide for the long-term delivery of prolonged courses of chemotherapy as well as parenteral nutrition, blood products, intravenous fluids, antibiotics, pain medications, and other agents. Furthermore, they are useful devices for repeated blood sampling. There are three types of devices most commonly used in the pediatric cancer population: peripherally inserted central venous catheters (PICCs), tunneled external central venous catheters (CVCs), and the implanted vascular access device or port-a-catheter. The CVC uses a flexible silicone tube placed in a central vein that exits thorough a subcutaneous tunnel. The CVC has historically been placed surgically, but more recently is also being inserted by the interventional radiology service with the use of ultrasound image guidance. Totally implanted devices or ports consist of a reservoir implanted in a subcutaneous pocket connected to a silicone catheter placed in a central vein.

Despite the fact that the central VAD has greatly improved the quality of care received by pediatric oncology patients, these devices are not without the potential for complications, including pneumothorax, hemothorax, arterial perforation, air embolism, nerve injury, catheter malposition, infection, and occlusion or thrombosis.

The most common complications of these devices are infection and occlusion. The incidence of intravascular catheter infection varies considerably by type of catheter, frequency of catheter manipulation, and patient-related factors (e.g., underlying disease and acuity of illness). The majority of serious catheter-related infections are associated with central venous catheters (O'Grady et al., 2002). Migration of skin organisms at the insertion site into the cutaneous catheter tract with colonization of the catheter tip is the most common route of infection for peripherally inserted catheters. The majority of catheter-related bloodstream infections in children are caused by coagulase-negative staphylococci. Exposure to lipids has also been identified as an independent risk factor in certain pediatric populations. Because of the limited vascular sites in children, attention should be given to the frequency with which catheters are replaced in these patients. One study found no relationship between duration of catheterization and the daily probability of infection, suggesting that routine replacement of VADs does not reduce the incidence of catheter-related infection (O'Grady et al., 2002). Indicators that reduce the incidence of catheter-related bloodstream infections are

1. Implementation of educational programs that include didactic and interactive components for those who insert and maintain catheters
2. Use of maximal sterile barrier precautions during catheter placement
3. Use of chlorhexidine for skin antisepsis
4. Removal of the catheter when it is no longer required for treatment (O'Grady et al., 2002).

Catheter occlusions can be intermittent, sluggish, partial, or complete/total and can result from several different mechanisms. Patency may be affected by anatomical obstruction due to compression of the catheter between the first rib and clavicle or by improper catheter tip placement. Occlusion may also result from precipitation caused by the administration of incompatible drugs or infusates; however, this is a less common cause.

The most common cause of catheter occlusion is thrombus formation within the lumen of the catheter, in the portal reservoir, or at the catheter tip. Venous stasis, hypercoagulability, and local trauma of the intima of the vein wall are contributing factors to the development of catheter thrombosis. The majority of thrombi causing central catheter occlusion de-

velop without symptoms. Warning signs of catheter malfunction are most often recognized by an experienced clinician. One study found that persistent asymptomatic vascular occlusion was a late complication of CVC placement for treatment of childhood malignancies, although the frequency was low among patients treated primarily for solid tumors (Wilimas et al., 1998).

Catheter occlusions due to the formation of a thrombus are treated by instilling a thrombolytic agent. Currently, recombinant tissue plasminogen activator (rt-PA) or alteplase is used to restore patency to occluded catheters. Rt-PA is a fibrin-specific thrombolytic agent produced through recombinant DNA technology. The optimal rt-PA dose, solution volume, and dwell time for the clearance of thrombosed CVCs is 2 mg (1 mg/ml), with a 30-minute to 2-hour dwell time. For the persistent occlusion, this dose may be repeated once. Clinical experience has demonstrated that increasing the dwell time (e.g., allowing the rt-PA to remain in the catheter overnight) has also had success for persistent occlusions.

Two common complications associated with the use of VADs, infection and occlusion, can be diminished by adhering to institutional protocols for catheter insertion, catheter site dressings, and drug and fluid administration. However, compliance with catheter care regimens also needs to occur in the home care setting. Standardization of line care between the treating institution and the home care agency is key to reducing confusion and anxiety in the child and family. Teaching is based on the educational level of the child and parents as well as on their preferred methods of learning.

11.6 Future Perspectives

11.6.1 New Surgical Techniques and Directions for Future Research

The past decade has brought significant changes to the surgical management of the child with cancer. Currently, pediatric surgical oncology has become extremely complex, requiring advanced technical skills using newly developed equipment. Minimally invasive surgery (MIS) is an example of one of the most recent additions to the surgical armamentarium. MIS is used for a variety of abdominal and thoracic procedures and describes a surgical procedure accomplished with instruments directed through cannulas. The advantages of MIS for certain types of operations include smaller wound size, less tissue exposure, and minimal tissue and organ manipulation. Because the body's response to MIS is different from its response to open surgical procedures, there is less stress imposed on the body, postoperative pain is decreased, and respiratory management and activity restrictions are also decreased. Examples of MIS include, but are not limited to, fundoplication, colon pull-through for Hirschsprung's disease, splenectomy, and thoracoscopic procedures.

The surgical oncology team now includes not only physicians and nurses but also scientists, computer specialists, and bioengineers. This is critical as new surgical procedures and devices are directed by computer technology, including robotics, telepresence, and virtual reality. Several types of surgical robotic systems have been developed that allow the performance of surgery with a higher degree of accuracy than that capable by human hands (Bagnall et al., 2002). Telepresence is the ability to perform a task or procedure using a remote manipulator and video image. This remote-controlled system was developed to solve deficiencies of MIS such as the absence of three-dimensional imaging, poor dexterity, and loss of sensory feedback. Lastly, virtual reality permits surgical intervention on imaginary patients. For pediatric surgical oncology, the implications of this new technology are immense. Tumors that were once deemed inoperable can now be excised with the use of robotics. Similarly, surgeons who are specialists in a particular tumor type will be able to perform surgical procedures from afar.

Today the surgeon administers vital services in the care of children and adolescents with malignant disease. Managing vascular access and its complications, as well as providing supportive care and appropriate intervention for medical complications of chemotherapy, have become the standards for the modern pediatric surgical oncologist.

References

Bagnall-Reeb H., Perry, S. (2002) Surgery. In Rasco Baggott, C., Patterson Kelly, K., Fochtman, D., Foley, G.V. (eds) In Nursing Care of Children and Adolescents with Cancer (3rd edn, pp. 91–115). Philadelphia: Saunders

Leonard, M. (2002) Diagnostic evaluations and staging procedures. In Rasco Baggott, C., Patterson Kelly, K., Fochtman, D., Foley, G.V. (eds) In Nursing Care of Children and Adolescents with Cancer (3rd edn, pp. 66–89) Philadelphia: Saunders

Nichols, R. (2000) Guidelines for prevention of surgical site infection. Bulletin of American College of Surgeons 85:23–29

O'Grady, N.P., Alexander, M., Patchen Dellinger, E., Gerberding, J.L., Heard, S.O., Maki, D.G., Masur, H., McCormick, R.D., Mermel, L.A., Pearson, M.L., Raad, I.I., Randolph, A., Weinstein, R.A. (2002) Guidelines for the prevention of intravascular catheter-related infections. Pediatrics 110:1–24

Rubie, H., Plantaz, D., Coze, C., et al. (2001) Localized and unresectable neuroblastoma in infants: Excellent outcome with primary chemotherapy. Medical Pediatric Oncology 36:247–250

Shamberger, R.C., Jaksic, T., Ziegler, M.M. (2002). General Principles of Surgery. In Pizzo P.A., Poplack D.G. (eds) In Principles and Practice of Pediatric Oncology (4th edn., pp. 351–367). Philadelphia: Lippincott Williams & Wilkins

Shamberger, R.C. (1999) Preanesthetic evaluation of children with anterior mediastinal mass. Seminars in Pediatric Surgery 8:61–68.

Wilimas, J.A., Hudson, M., Rao, B., Luo, X., Lott, L. Kaste, S.C. (1998) Late vascular occlusion of central lines in pediatric malignancies. Pediatrics 101:E7

Bibliography

Andrassy, R.J. (2002) Advances in the surgical management of sarcomas in children. The American Journal of Surgery 184:484–491

Miller, S.D., Andrassy, R.J. (2003) Complications in pediatric surgical oncology. Journal of the American College of Surgeons 19:832–837

Gene Therapy

Kathleen E. Houlahan · Mark W. Kieran

Contents

12.1 Introduction

Gene therapy, also known as gene transfer, is a novel approach of altering the genetic basis of normal or cancerous cells in order to modify their function. The manipulation of genes may help fight cancer and prevent genetic diseases as well as increase the body's ability to receive intense treatment that would be impossible otherwise. The first gene therapy clinical trial was conducted in 1990 on two children with adenosine deaminase (ADA) deficiency and today is being evaluated with the hopes of curing diseases such as cancer, cystic fibrosis, and hemophilia.

One of the major goals of gene therapy is to supply cells with healthy copies of missing or altered genes. Gene therapy remains in its infancy, with limited success up to this point, and is viewed by many in the same way that chemotherapy was viewed in the 1950s. To date, more than 200 cancer patients have received genetically modified cells (Brenner, 2002). Many of these trials involved removing the patients' tumors, infecting them with the new genes, and then irradiating the cells to kill the gene therapy vector so that it could no longer spread or cause illness. Other experiments have involved genetically modifying the hematopoietic stem cells so that the blood-forming cells could withstand a much greater intensity of chemotherapy.

Finally, many patients have had their tumors directly injected with gene therapy vectors containing suicide genes that, when picked up by the dividing tumor cells, would allow them to be selectively killed. Throughout these experiments, minimal procedure-related toxicity has been seen in most patients, although severe reactions to this approach, including death, have been observed in rare cases.

12.2 Principles of Treatment

To date, four major strategies have been adopted for incorporating gene transfer into cancer therapy:

1. The tumor cell itself is modified, either by repairing one or more of the genetic defects associated with the malignant process, by introducing a gene that triggers an antitumor response, or by delivering a pro-drug metabolizing enzyme that renders the tumor sensitive to the corresponding agent (Brenner, 2002). An example of this approach is adding back key regulatory genes that have become dysfunctional in the tumor, such as p53, whose normal function is to prevent abnormal (cancer) cells from dividing. Oncogenes are genes that typically stimulate tumor formation when abnormal, and inserting new genes that turn off or counteract these oncogenes might therefore also stop tumor growth. There are, of course, some inherent limitations with this approach. Tumor cells that don't pick up the vector will not be killed or affected. Others will react to the therapy by altering (mutating) genes not treated by the inserted gene that allowed them to escape.

   Over the last 50 years, it has been discovered that tumors have an almost unlimited ability to rapidly and effectively develop resistance to whatever modality we treat them with. A form of gene therapy known as suicide gene therapy uses the delivery of the herpes simplex virus thymidine kinase (TK) gene by a replication-defective adenoviral vector injected directly into the tumor. Ganciclovir, a nucleoside analog, is then administered intravenously to the patient. The expressed TK phosphorylates the ganciclovir within the tumor cells. The resulting nucleotide analog is a potent inhibitor of deoxyribonucleic acid (DNA) synthesis and causes the death of the dividing tumor cells (Hurwitz et al, 2002). Normal cells throughout the rest of the body that did not pick up the vector will be exposed to ganciclovir, but because this pro-drug cannot be activated unless TK is expressed, they will not be affected. Furthermore, by virtue of a phenomenon called the "bystander effect," if the gene is picked up by a few cells and causes their death, some of the adjacent cells will die as a result of the localized destruction.

2. The immune response to the tumor is modified by altering the specificity or effector function of immune system cells (Brenner, 2002). Tumors are able to grow in part because the immune system fails to recognize them as abnormal. Two strategies that have been implemented are to insert genes into the tumor cells, acting like large neon signs that help the immune system "see" the tumor, and to introduce genes into the immune cells so that they are better able to detect the tumor. For example, expression of major histocompatibility antigens (MHC) on a cell is an excellent way to help the immune system reexamine not just the MHC protein but also other proteins on the cell surface. Once aware of these new "tumor antigens," the immune system can then aggressively go after all of the tumor cells, including those that failed to pick up the vector. On the other side, transferring the immune cells themselves with genes that wake up the immune system (cytokines such as IL-2 and GM-CSF, for example) are other ways of getting a previously subdued immune response up and running.

3. The drug sensitivity of normal host tissue is decreased by delivering cytotoxic drug-resistant genes to marrow precursor cells, thereby increasing the therapeutic index of chemotherapy (Brenner, 2002). Certain alkylating drugs such as CCNU and BCNU damage the DNA of both tumor and normal cells by adding methyl groups onto the DNA, preventing the cells from properly duplicating it at the time of cell division. An enzyme called MGMT reverses this damage. As a result, one approach has been to infect normal blood-forming stem cells with the MGMT gene. When a patient receives a standard dose of chemotherapy, the observed myelosuppression may be significantly reduced if the blood-forming genes express the MGMT protein, making the therapy better tolerated and allowing for more frequent or higher doses

of therapy to be administered against the tumor. A potential concern with this approach relates to the consequences if a tumor cell inadvertently picks up the "resistant" gene vector because it, and all of its progeny, would be highly resistant to this kind of therapy.

4. Normal or malignant cells are marked (tagged) so that the efficacy of conventional therapies can be monitored more closely (Brenner, 2002). Humans have between 50,000 and 100,000 genes (National Cancer Institute, 2004). A gene, which is a stretch of sequence of the DNA molecule, is the basic unit of heredity. Genes determine traits such as height, hair, and eye color, and carry the instructions that allow the cells to produce specific proteins and enzymes. Each protein has a certain function in the body. The pattern of active and inactive genes in a cell and the resulting protein composition determine the type of cell and its capabilities. Genes that protect against cancer are referred to as tumor suppressor genes. Mutated genes that are capable of causing cancer when expressed at the wrong place or time are known as oncogenes. Although the last 50 years of cancer-directed therapy (i.e., radiation and chemotherapy) have targeted cells that divide, researchers are now realizing that cancer therapy may be more effective if therapy is directed at the abnormal genes and their signaling pathways.

Gene therapy, or gene transfer, is defined as the transfer of genetic material, including complementary DNA, full-length genes, RNA, or oligonucleotides, into somatic or germline cells (Albelda et al., 2002). Gene therapy changes the cell function dependent on the selection of the gene. A simple explanation of gene therapy is to take a virus that has evolved to effectively penetrate cells and remove the parts of the virus that code for propagating the infection and the genes that cause illness. The virus acts as a Trojan horse, easily able to penetrate dividing cells. Once the bad part of the gene is removed, the gene of interest is inserted, the cell is infected, and the cell begins to translate it into a protein. While viruses are a common "vehicle," a large number of different structures are now being evaluated, although the principle for all of them is the same. As previously mentioned, more than 200 patients have received genetically modified cells. Although most of these patients received irradiated gene-modified tumor cells that would be expected to have little safety risk, more than 60 children have received genetically modified hematopoietic progenitor cells with no adverse events attributable to the gene transfer process. There are more than 100 clinical protocols approved thus far, most open only to patients with advanced malignancy in whom highly experimental therapies such as this can be justified (Brenner, 2002).

12.3 Method of Delivery

Gene therapy has two methods of delivery that are essential in the process of successful gene transfer. The first essential mode of delivery is transferring the gene in the cell. The second essential mode of delivery is transferring the cell into the patient. In most gene therapy clinical trials, cells from the patient's blood or bone marrow are removed and grown in the laboratory. The cells are exposed to the virus that is carrying the desired gene. The virus enters the cells, and the desired gene becomes part of the cells' DNA. The cells grown in the laboratory are extensively washed to remove any unincorporated virus and are then returned to the patient by injection into a vein. This type of gene therapy is called ex vivo (outside the body) gene transfer because the gene is transferred into the patient's cells while the cells are outside of the body.

In the last few years researchers have developed several methods of delivering the gene into the cell, including transfer via viruses, plasmids, tumor cells, and immune system cells. The most successful mode of delivery is the use of virus as a vector to deliver the gene into the cell. This likely results from the millions of years that viruses have used to evolve specifically to infect human cells and insert their DNA into ours so that they can make new virus and continue to survive. However, other viral and nonviral vectors that can achieve similar functions are also being tested. Retroviral, adenoviral, and vaccinia are examples of viral vectors. An example of a nonviral vector is plasmid DNA (naked chunks of DNA). Examples of the viral vectors are the adenovirus (AV), the adeno-associated virus (AAV), the herpes virus (HV), and the AIDS virus. The use of these natural vectors, all of which demonstrate significant ability to infect human cells, requires specialized knowledge in terms of how to inactivate them from causing human disease before reinjecting them into patients.

The most widely used vector system in cancer gene therapy has been the replication-incompetent recombinant adenovirus. Adenoviruses are respiratory tropic viruses with a double-strand DNA genome and a naked protein capsid coat. Recombinant vectors have been created by genomic deletion of viral gene functions involved in replication and provision of these functions in trans by a packaging cell line (Zhang, 1999). The deleted gene regions then can be replaced with expression cassettes containing the desired gene under the control of general or tumor-specific promoters. This vector system offers a number of advantages, including high-efficiency transduction in a wide range of target cells (including nondividing cells) and high expression levels of the delivered transgene (Yeh and Perricaudet, 1997). Other vectors are plasmids, which are small particles of raw DNA. The advantage of using plasmids is that there is less chance of the patient becoming infected by a virus particle that regenerates the ability to become infectious. The disadvantage of using plasmids is that they are often limited to skin cancer, where they can be delivered directly and easily to the patient's cancer cells. The most common viruses used as vectors in pediatric oncology gene therapy are AAV and HV.

12.4 Potential Side Effects

It would be unrealistic not to expect genetic therapies to produce side effects. Gene therapy continues to require informed use in controlled clinical studies, with a clear consideration of the risks and potential benefits. Current vector systems may need to be modified, and additional efforts are required to better understand the biology of the diseases that are candidates for therapeutic genetic intervention. Together this in-

formation will enable risk classifications for specific vectors and transgenes, as well as assessment of the risk factors that are unique to each clinical trial. With this approach, the therapeutic potential of somatic gene transfer may be realized through the application of appropriate prevention strategies (Williams and Baum, 2003).

Some of the potential side effects of gene therapy include viruses infecting more than one type of cell, being inserted in the wrong location in the DNA (for example, in the middle of a critical gene), and possibly causing cancer or other cellular damage. Other concerns include the possibility that the transferred genes could be "overexpressed," producing so much of the missing protein as to be harmful, resulting in inflammation or immune reaction (National Cancer Institute, 2004).

12.5 Special Considerations

Given the considerable risk and unproven nature of this approach, most institutions have a number of local and national regulatory bodies that oversee the design and conduct of gene therapy trials. In the USA, gene therapy protocols must also be approved by the U.S. Food and Drug Administration (FDA), which regulates all gene therapy products. In addition, trials that are funded by the National Institute of Health (NIH) must be registered with the NIH Recombinant DNA Advisory Committee (RAC) (National Cancer Institute, 2004).

There have recently been two documented cases of children diagnosed with severe combined immunodeficiency disease (SCIDS) who developed leukemia after participating in a gene therapy trial. In both cases the retrovirus was the vector, and the gene wrongfully inserted itself into a piece of DNA that can cause leukemia. As a result of those cases, gene therapy and clinical trials face intense scrutiny, with the recommendation from the NIH that gene therapy should be used only as a last resort.

12.6 Future Perspectives

Gene therapy is a new approach to treating children with cancer, and despite some recent setbacks, it holds significant promise for the future. Scientists have made great progress in the last decade in understanding the molecular architecture of viruses used for gene therapy, and based on these advances, more sophisticated vectors have been designed. The progress in hand is hopeful; however, there remains a need for continued advancement in this field.

In addition to identifying disease-specific risk factors, there are three ways to limit the possible deleterious side effects of genetic interventions. The first is to develop vectors with improved safety profiles, including a reduced propensity for insertional "genotoxicity." The second is to define "safe integration sites" in the genome and to design integration vectors that are targeted to these sites. The third is to reduce the number of vector-exposed cells (and thus vector integrations) that are infused into the patient; for example, by correcting a very small number of stem cells ex vivo and genetically characterizing them before they are infused back into the patient (Williams and Baum, 2003)

One exciting possibility for the future is to harness homologous recombination that will either target viral vectors or directly correct genetic defects. Homologous recombination enables the introduction of foreign genetic material at specific locations on the chromosome. For instance, it would enable the replacement of a defective gene by inserting a normal copy of the gene into the locus (Pellman, 2004). However, it is important to remember that most advances in medicine proceed incrementally, and gene transfer is already being used successfully to complement conventional therapies for malignant hematologic disorders. The benefits of this new technology can only increase as current limitations are progressively, albeit slowly, surmounted (Brenner, 2002).

Gene therapy is still in the early phases despite the fact that it has been an area of research and clinical trials since 1990. It is hoped that although barriers and challenges remain, gene therapy will someday be FDA-approved and offer successful cancer treatment as well as reduce the impact that the disease has on pediatric patients.

References

Albelda S, Wiewrodt R, Sternman D (2002) Gene therapy for lung neoplasms. Lung Cancer 23:265

Brenner M (2002) The applications of gene transfer to pediatric malignant disease. In Pizzo P, Poplack Principles and Practice of Pediatric Oncology, 4th edn (pp 453–461) Philadelphia: Lippincott Williams & Wilkins

Hurwitz R, Shields C, Shields J, Chevez-Barrios P, Hurwitz M, Chintagumpala M (2002) Retinoblastoma. In Pizzo P, Poplack Principles and Practice of Pediatric Oncology, 4th edn (p 841) Philadelphia: Lippincott Williams & Wilkins

National Cancer Institute. Questions and answers about gene therapy. http://cis.nci.nih.gov (accessed January 1, 2004)

Pellman D. Dana-Farber Cancer Institute, Boston. Personal communication. January 8, 2004

Williams D, Baum C (2003) Gene therapy: new challenges ahead. Science 302:400–401

Yeh P, Perricaudet M (1997) Advances in adenoviral vectors: from genetic engineering to their biology. The FASEB Journal 11:615–623

Zhang WW (1999) Development and application of adenoviral vectors for gene therapy of cancer. Cancer Gene Therapy 6:113–138

Complementary and Alternative Therapy

Nancy E. Kline

13.1 Principles of Treatment

Complementary and alternative medicine (CAM) therapy includes diverse medical and holistic practices and products that are not presently considered to be part of conventional medicine. Although some scientific evidence exists regarding some CAM therapies, for most there are scientific questions that have not been answered, such as whether they are safe and whether they work for the diseases or medical conditions for which they are used.

The list of what is considered to be CAM changes continually as those therapies that are proven to be safe and effective become adopted into conventional health care and as new approaches to health care emerge. These therapies may be used in conjunction with conventional, or modern, medicine (complementary) or in place of modern medicine (alternative):

- Complementary medicine is used together with conventional medicine. An example of a complementary therapy is using massage to help lessen nausea and vomiting while receiving chemotherapy.
- Alternative medicine is used in place of conventional medicine. An example of an alternative therapy is using a special diet to treat cancer instead of undergoing surgery, radiation, or chemotherapy that has been recommended by a conventional doctor.

Table 13.1. Types of complementary and alternative therapies

Type of therapy	Examples
Alternative medical systems	Homeopathic and naturopathic medicine
Mind-body interventions	Medication, prayer, art, music
Biologically-based treatments	Herbs, dietary supplements
Body manipulation	Chiropractic or osteopathic manipulation
Energy therapies	Therapeutic touch, electromagnetic fields

Factors that prompt parents to choose complementary or alternative therapy for their children include the following:

— Desire to avoid toxicities of conventional therapy
— Ability to provide treatment at home
— Preference for natural over synthetic medicine
— Failure of conventional therapy to provide a cure
— Serious or chronic illness that carries a poor prognosis

13.2 Description of Treatment

Complementary and alternative therapy can be separated into five categories: (a) alternative medical systems, (b) mind-body interventions, (c) biologically-based treatments, (d) manipulation and body-based methods, and (e) energy therapies (Table 13.1) (National Center for Complementary and Alternative Medicine, 2003).

13.3 Method of Delivery

13.3.1 Alternative Medical Systems

In homeopathic medicine, small, highly diluted quantities of medicinal substances are given to cure symptoms. However, when the same substances are given at higher or more concentrated doses, they cause those symptoms. Naturopathic medicine is based on the theory that natural healing forces exist within the body. These forces help the body heal from disease and attain better health. Practices may include dietary modifications, exercise, and acupuncture, which is a method of treating pain injuries and diseases by inserting solid, extremely thin needles into precise points on the body. This insertion may be accompanied by manual, electrical, or heat stimulation of the needles.

13.3.2 MindBody Interventions

Mind-body interventions use a variety of techniques designed to enhance the mind's capacity to affect bodily function and symptoms. Several that were previously considered alternative therapy have become mainstream (e.g., patient support groups and cognitive-behavioral therapy). Other mind-body techniques still considered complementary or alternative therapy include meditation, prayer, mental healing, and therapies that use creative outlets such as art, music, or dance.

Meditation, relaxation, and guided imagery facilitate the mind's capacity to affect bodily function and symptoms. Meditation is practiced throughout the world but has its origins in India, China, and Japan. It is often part of a religious practice (Chiaramonte, 1997). Meditation is self-directed and is aimed at relaxing the body and mind. The person focuses on a particular object, sound, or image for a period of time, thereby cleansing the mind of stressors. Several studies have shown that meditation yields positive results for stress reduction and effective coping mechanisms (Greene et al., 1999).

Relaxation is the absence of anxiety and skeletal muscle tension. Relaxation techniques include deep breathing exercises, autogenic relaxation, music, and progressive muscle relaxation. The techniques are easy to learn and perform and can be done alone or in a group. Relaxation is often used in combination with guided imagery, which deliberately introduces healthful images to encourage relaxation or to alleviate a symptom. Relaxation and guided imagery can be used to decrease acute symptoms, stress, fatigue, pain, blood pressure, pulse, and respiration; to induce sleep; to increase endorphins; and to stimulate the immune system (Chiaramonte, 1997).

13.3.3 Biologically Based Treatments

Biologically-based therapies in CAM use substances found in nature, such as herbs, foods, vitamins, dietary supplements, and other so-called "natural" but as yet scientifically unproven therapies (e.g., shark cartilage). Dietary supplements are widely available through many commercial sources, including health food stores, grocery stores, pharmacies, and by mail. Dietary supplements are provided in many forms, including tablets, capsules, powders, geltabs, extracts, and liquids. A wide array of supplement products are available worldwide and include vitamins, minerals, other nutrients, and botanical supplements as well as ingredients and extracts of animal and plant origin.

13.3.4 Body Manipulation

Body-based methods are based on manipulation and/or movement of one or more parts of the body. Therapeutic massage may bring relief to patients who are suffering from pain, have pathological tightening of skeletal muscle, or have not responded to more traditional physical therapies. Examples include massage and chiropractic or osteopathic manipulation.

13.3.5 Energy Therapies

Healing touch is one of a long line of healing traditions based on the belief in a universal healing energy. Therapeutic touch is derived from an ancient technique called laying-on of hands. It is based on the premise that it is the therapist's healing force that affects the patient's recovery, that healing is promoted when the body's energies are in balance, and that, by passing their hands over the patient, healers can identify energy imbalances. Therapeutic or healing touch uses light, gentle touch to affect the energy system physically, mentally, emotionally, and spiritually. Therapeutic touch has been used to increase the body's own healing potential; accelerate healing; decrease pain, swelling and spasms; and induce relaxation, peace, and well-being (Lorenzi, 1999).

Magnetic therapy was used thousands of years ago by the Egyptians and Greeks. There are several theories regarding the mechanism of how magnetic therapy works. It is believed that magnets enhance blood flow to the affected area, thereby decreasing inflammation and pain and speeding healing. Magnets are also thought to activate electrical activity in the body and cause the release of certain neurotransmitters to decrease pain. Lastly, magnets are believed to realign and balance the body's own electromagnetic field to facilitate self-healing by improving circulation, cellular oxygenation, and metabolism (Lorenzi, 1999).

Electromagnetic fields (EMFs, also called electric and magnetic fields) are invisible lines of force that surround all electrical devices. The earth also produces EMFs; electric fields are produced when there is thunderstorm activity, and magnetic fields are believed to be produced by electric currents flowing at the earth's core.

13.4 Potential Side Effects

Herbs and spices have been used for common and chronic ailments for centuries. Many of the conventional medicines used today are made from elements found in nature. Substantial research exists to support the use of some herbal and spice remedies for common illnesses, such as chamomile for colic, goldenseal for diarrhea, and tea tree oil and aloe vera for skin infections. Others require judicious use because of the risk of serious toxicity with overdose. The ingredients used in emetics may damage the mouth, tongue, esophagus, stomach, and duodenum. Perianal excoriation, hemorrhagic ulcerative proctocolitis, and electrolyte imbalance have been reported following colonic enema therapy.

Table 13.2. Common dietary and herbal supplements

Supplement	Common uses	How taken	Side effects
Chamomile (flowers)	Anxiety, sedation Antispasmodic Colic Anti-inflammatory	Tea or tincture taken internally	Allergic reaction Botulism
Aloe vera (pure gel from leaves)	Burns Constipation Skin ulcers Oral ulcers Immune stimulant	Gel applied topically or taken internally	Diarrhea Gastric cramping Contact dermatitis
Black tea Green tea	Antioxidant	Brewed, taken internally	Nausea Diarrhea
Goldenseal (roots)	Diarrhea Antiseptic Acne Immune stimulant	Tincture taken internally or applied topically DO NOT USE IN INFANTS <1 MONTH OF AGE	Hypotension Hypertension Local irritation Nausea, vomiting
Echinacea (leaves, roots, flowers)	Immune stimulant Colds Ear infection	Tinctures, capsules, or tablets taken internally	None reported
Cayenne	Improves circulation Improves appetite Heals ulcers	Used in cooking Added to fruit juice for an energizing drink	None reported
Cinnamon	Diarrhea Nausea Improves digestion Oral ulcers	Used in soups, stews, fruit juice, tea	None reported
Cloves	Stimulates appetite Diarrhea Nausea Vomiting	Used in soups, stews, fruit juice, tea	None reported
Coriander	Indigestion Stimulates appetite	Flavoring used in salads, stews, soups	None reported
Fennel	Abdominal cramps Flatulence Stimulates appetite	Used in stews, tea	None reported
Ginger	Improves digestion Nausea Diarrhea Abdominal cramps Stimulates appetite Colds	Used in stir-fried foods, stews, soups, tea	None reported

Table 13.2. (Continued)

Supplement	Common uses	How taken	Side effects
Turmeric	Improves digestion Antiseptic Antioxidant	Used in stir-fried foods	None reported
Shark cartilage	Angiogenesis inhibitor Anti-inflammatory Immune stimulant	Liquid Powder Injectable form Topical preparation	Nausea Vomiting Abdominal cramping Constipation Hypotension Hyperglycemia Hypercalcemia

Alternative remedies appear to be relatively safe. A review of 19 clinical trial reports, 19 case (or case series) reports, and 15 homeopathic pathogenetic trials were reviewed. The mean incidence of adverse effects was higher with homeopathy than with placebo, but all were mild and transient. Perhaps more striking is the fact that 36 reports did not report on collection or incidence of adverse effects at all. However, adverse event data are poorly and inconsistently collected and reported, so this conclusion should be interpreted with caution (Dantas and Rampes, 2000).

Examining acupuncture for life-threatening adverse reactions revealed a number of potential problems, not all of which are recognized commonly. Fifty-six articles were reviewed (including overviews, epidemiological surveys, and case reports) examining two main areas: rate of infection and traumatic injury (Ernst and White, 1997). Infections linked to acupuncture and the improper handling of needles or their reuse without adequate sterilization included hepatitis B and C, HIV, bacterial endocarditis, and staphylococcal septicemia. Other traumatic events included cardiac tamponade and punctured heart, including at least one actual death.

Table 13.2 provides a brief list of some dietary and herbal therapies used for symptom management, the conditions they are used to treat, and the side effects they may produce.

13.5 Special Considerations

Complementary and alternative therapies may be usefully incorporated into the patient's treatment regimen for pediatric cancer. Various dietary supplements, herbs, and magnetic therapy are often used in hopes of boosting immune function and providing a cure. However, as a single therapy for malignancy, these treatments may jeopardize recovery and would be regarded as dangerous if other treatments of established effectiveness were delayed or rejected.

Many patients use complementary or alternative treatments but may be reluctant to share the information. One study showed that 40% of patients who utilized CAM therapies did not disclose the information with their health care providers (Eliopoulos, 1999). It is very important for parents to know whether a certain alternative therapy they are considering may cause a serious reaction when taken in conjunction with conventional treatments. The following questions may be useful to ascertain whether a parent has opted to use therapies in addition to the prescribed regimen:

- What unacceptable side effects has your child had from the medicines that we have prescribed?
- Dietary supplements or other nonprescription therapies are very commonly used by people who have cancer. Do you have any questions regarding these treatments?

13.6 Future Perspectives

Clinical trials of complementary and alternative therapy are taking place throughout the world. Although many of these treatments have already been in use for years, there is not appropriate scientific knowledge available about them similar to that gained from studies of conventional medicine. However, many patients are already using CAM, and without this scientific knowledge, they may be at risk for serious effects from taking the wrong dose, using the treatment in the wrong way, or using it with another treatment with which it adversely interacts.

A few therapies for which studies are underway include acupuncture; herbs such as Ginkgo biloba; dietary supplements such as green tea glucosamine, chondroitin, saw palmetto, and soy; and massage. Examples of diseases and conditions for which these CAM therapies are being studied include arthritis, neurological disorders, cardiovascular disease, and cancer.

References

Chiaramonte D.R. (1997) Mind-body therapies for primary care physicians. Primary Care 24:787–807

Dantas F., Rampes H. (2000) Do homeopathic medicines provoke adverse effects? A systematic review. British Homeopathic Journal 89(1):S35–38

Eliopoulos C. (1999) Using complementary and alternative therapies wisely. Geriatric Nursing 20:139–143

Ernst E., White A. (1997) Life-threatening adverse reactions after acupuncture? A systematic review. Pain 71:123–126

Greene K.B., Berger J, Reeves C, Moffat A, Standish L.J., Calabrese C. (1999) Most frequently used alternative and complementary therapies and activities by participants in the AMCOA study. Journal of the Association of Nurses in AIDS Care 10:60–73

Lorenzi E.A. (1999) Complementary/alternative therapies: So many choices. Geriatric Nursing 20:124–133

National Center for Complementary and Alternative Medicine (2003) Understanding complementary and alternative medicine. http://nccam.nih.gov/health

PART IV

Metabolic System

Deborah Tomlinson

Contents

14.1 Cancer Cachexia

14.1.1 Incidence

Cancer cachexia can be described as a syndrome characterised by weight loss, anorexia, muscle loss and atrophy, asthenia (general weakness including physical and mental fatigue), and anaemia that occurs in cancer patients. Weight loss or the failure to gain weight are common adverse effects of cancer in children. Picton et al. (1995) studied the nutritional status of 25 children with leukaemia and 42 children with leukaemia. Nutritional status can be assessed using weight-for-height index, triceps skinfold thickness, and mid-upper arm circumference. Table 14.1 shows the rates of cachexia seen in children in this study. Undernutrition has also been found to be significant (around 7%) in newly diagnosed children with acute lymphoblastic leukaemia (ALL) (Reilly et al., 1999). In adults a cachectic state at diagnosis is associated with a poor prognosis, but in children this association seems to be cause for debate and may be of more importance in developing countries when associated with socioeconomic status and in social groups with relevant nutritional deficits (Weir et al., 1998; Viana et al., 1994; Reilly et al., 1994).

Table 14.1. Rates of cachexia seen in children with cancer (Picton, 1995)

	Cachexia at presentation	Cachexia during treatment
Solid tumours (*n*=42)	33%	57%
Leukaemias (*n*=25)	12%	28%

Halton and colleagues (1993) studied intestinal malabsorption in children treated for ALL. No generalised malabsorption was reported; however, intestinal lactose intolerance was seen in four of 12 patients.

14.1.2 Etiology

Fundamentally, weight loss or growth failure is caused by a negative energy balance as a result of caloric/food intake that is inappropriate to meet energy expenditure. In growing children, energy balance should be positive to ensure adequate growth. Reduced intake commonly results from treatment-associated nausea and vomiting, gastrointestinal dysfunction, and/or taste disturbances. Anorexia of cancer may also be due to the disruption of the central nervous system appetite centre by cancer metabolites. Other factors that contribute to cachexia in cancer patients include competition for nutrients between the tumour and the host and altered metabolism of nutrients.

Normally, a negative energy balance means that the body adapts to low nitrogen intake by reducing protein synthesis and breakdown, causing an overall reduced protein turnover. In children with cancer, the body does not adapt sufficiently, so protein turnover increases and muscle breakdown occurs. The increase in protein turnover in these children may be related to tumour, chemotherapy, or related conditions such as febrile neutropenia. Lipid metabolism is altered, with depletion of lipid stores, increased lipid in circulation, and increased free fatty acid turnover. Changes in carbohydrate metabolism include an increased whole body glucose turnover. Tumours appear to consume glucose, producing lactic acid that the liver must then metabolise and convert back to glucose. Energy is lost in this cycle. Carbohydrate metabolism may also be affected by chemotherapy. Endogenous mediators of cancer cachexia are undetermined but are thought to include tumour necrosis factor (TNF-α), also called cachectin, interleukin 1 (IL-1α), and interleukin 6 (IL-6). These cytokines are regarded as anorexigenic cytokines and have been reported to act on cells in the central nervous system and peripheral tissues in various conditions

Severe and prolonged undernutrition may result in atrophy of intestinal villi and can create lactose intolerance.

14.1.3 Treatment

Nutritional assessment is essential to identify nutritional status and anticipated problems. Picton (1998) reported that some patients at high risk of developing cachexia could be identified at presentation by raised energy expenditure. Aggressive nutritional intervention for these patients may help to prevent subsequent weight loss. This intervention may also be important for children on intensive chemotherapy regimes.

Symptom management of anorexia and cachexia should focus on

- Improving caloric intake
- Decreasing energy expenditure and minimising factors that create a negative energy balance

The oral intake of energy, protein, and carbohydrates for hospitalised children with cancer has been found to be below a recommended level (Skolin et al., 2001). When enteral, parenteral, and treatment-related glucose were taken into account, the level came close to that recommended for healthy children. However, children with malignant disease are likely to have increased energy and nutrient requirements.

Chapter 26 will detail nutritional requirements of the child and adolescent with cancer.

14.1.4 Prognosis

Weight loss is a serious complication of childhood cancer. Fortunately, developing strategies for providing enteral and parenteral nutrition can prevent major morbidity and mortality from this complication. Occasionally, nutritional strategies are insufficient to reverse a cachectic state. Metabolic changes can result in growth failure in paediatric cancer patients. Body tissue is then catabolised to meet the nutritional demands of the tumour, and nutritional death could be a possibility. Future treatment approaches may be able to combine different pharmacological approaches that target the cytokine factors involved.

The resulting effects would be to reverse the metabolic derangements associated with the tumour and to ameliorate anorexia.

14.2 Obesity

14.2.1 Incidence

Children and adolescents treated for leukaemia, particularly ALL, have a tendency to gain excessive weight during and following treatment, and a high proportion of young adult survivors is obese (Reilly et al., 2001a). This finding is more pronounced in girls than in boys, with cranial irradiation being an important factor (Odame et al., 1994; Mayer et al., 2000; Sklar et al. 2000). Obesity in children treated for other malignancies has not been reported in the literature.

14.2.2 Etiology

The most significant abnormality in energy balance identified in the current literature regarding ALL is reduced total energy expenditure as a result of reduced physical activity during and following therapy (Reilly et al., 2001a).

The effect of glucocorticoid therapy on energy balance and body weight control is accepted; however, there is little evidence of this effect, particularly in children with ALL. A study by Reilly and colleagues (2001a) was the first to show that energy intakes increased significantly when children were treated with glucocorticoids during the long-term maintenance phase of therapy. No significant difference was found between patients treated with prednisone and those treated with dexamethasone. This study concluded that glucocorticoid therapy substantially increases energy intake in patients with ALL and that this contributes to the development of obesity characteristic of these patients.

Another study carried out by Reilly et al. (2001b) found that adiposity rebound (AR) occurred much earlier in patients with ALL than in healthy children. AR occurs when body mass index begins to increase after its nadir in childhood (usually between 5 and 7 years of age). This period is important for the regulation of energy balance and adult obesity risk, and early AR is associated with an increased risk of adult obesity.

Other effects on energy balance may include growth hormone status derangements (Van Dongen-Melman, 1995) and resting energy expenditure, although differences between patients treated for ALL and healthy controls have not been observed (Reilly et al., 1998). In patients who receive cranial irradiation as part of ALL therapy, the parameters of resting metabolic rate, physical activity, and growth hormone levels tend to be lower than normal, which would indicate causes for obesity in this group of patients. However, nonirradiated patients also have a tendency to obesity, which confounds the conclusions surrounding the etiology of obesity in this patient group (Mayer et al., 2000).

14.2.3 Treatment

Body mass index (weight/height^2), resting metabolic rate (measured by indirect calorimetry), caloric intake (24-hour recall), and physical activity (questionnaire) are suggested parameters that can be used to identify and manage overweight and obesity (Mayer et al., 2000).

The main focus of treatment (and prevention) should concentrate on

- Achievable increases in habitual physical activity, working towards a more active lifestyle
- Modest restriction of dietary intake
- Monitoring of excess weight gain

Nutritional screening would identify patients who may require intervention and referral to specialist services.

14.2.4 Prognosis

Obesity can be an adverse effect for ALL survivors that may have considerable consequence because of their already higher risk for various health outcomes, including cardiovascular factors as well as general health, social, and emotional well-being.

With the current emphasis on the quality of survival, it is vital that these patients and their families

Table 14.2. Risk factors associated with tumour lysis syndrome in children

Disease-related	Patient-related	Treatment-related
Bulky tumours (0.8–10 cm)	Increased uric acid level prior to treatment	Chemotherapy (main association)
High proliferative rate	Renal insufficiency leading to oliguria	Ionising radiation therapy
Hematopoietic malignancies	Dehydration	Corticosteroids
Chemosensitive tumours	Male gender	Hormonal therapy
ALL (T-cell most commonly)	Immature tubular function (age <1 year) results in inefficient sodium and water regulation	Immunotherapy
Burkitt's lymphoma (and other non-Hodgkin's lymphomas)	Children may have a decreased glomerular filtration rate	
AML with high WBC	Greater fluid needs per kilogram of body weight	
Neuroblastoma (on occasion)	Increased pretreatment lactic dehydrogenase	

be educated about preventing later obesity. These efforts may take the form of encouraging a more active lifestyle.

14.3 Tumour Lysis Syndrome

Tumour lysis syndrome (TLS) is a potential life-threatening emergency that results from rapid spontaneous or treatment-related tumour cell death. The cell lysis releases large amounts of uric acid, potassium, phosphate, and other purine metabolites into the blood circulation. When these quantities of intracellular electrolytes exceed the excretory capacity of the renal system, TLS can occur.

14.3.1 Incidence

The incidence of TLS appears to be undefined, emphasising identification of individual risk factors and preventative measures. Factors that influence the risk of TLS are shown in Table 14.2. Risk for renal failure may also be increased if there is kidney tumour infiltration or tumour compression on the ureters or renal veins. Farley-Hills et al. (2001) reported a rare case of a 2-year-old girl with suspected lymphoproliferative disorder who developed TLS during anaes-

thesia. This case highlights a need for suspicion if a patient known to be at risk of TLS deteriorates suddenly during anaesthesia.

TLS typically occurs within 24–48 hours after cytotoxic therapy begins, with rising serum potassium levels seen. It can then persist over 4–7 days as phosphate and urate levels rise. TLS normally occurs after commencement of the first treatment only.

14.3.2 Etiology

TLS is characterised by four metabolic abnormalities (Fig. 14.1):

- Hyperuricaemia
- Hyperphosphataemia
- Hypocalcaemia
- Hyperkalaemia

These abnormalities may ultimately lead to seizures, acute renal failure, cardiac arrhythmias, and, in some cases, multiorgan failure and death.

Acute renal failure associated with TLS may be attributable to several factors. Uric acid, phosphorus, and potassium are primarily excreted by the kidneys. The release of intracellular purines from the nuclei of tumour cells increases the levels of uric acid in the blood. Uric acid crystals are formed when uric acid

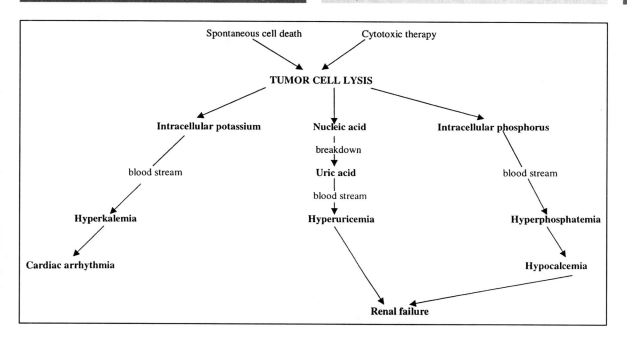

Figure 14.1

Metabolic consequences of tumour cell lysis

enters the acidic urine environment of the collecting ducts and ureters, causing precipitation of xanthine. (Xanthine is a by-product of nucleic acid destruction.) This can lead to a renal obstruction. Serum uric acid levels of 10–15 mg/dl can cause symptoms of lethargy, nausea, or vomiting, with renal failure usually seen as the level increases to 20 mg/dl (Allegreta et al., 1985). The drugs used to prevent TLS in these circumstances may also present a predisposition to renal failure. Allopurinol lowers the production of uric acid by inhibiting xanthine oxidase. Xanthine oxidase acts as a catalyst in the conversion of hypoxanthine to xanthine and xanthine to uric acid (see Fig. 14.2). Therefore, increased levels of xanthine and hypoxanthine are excreted in the urine. These products may then precipitate, especially in alkaline urine, and pose another contributing factor in acute renal failure.

Lymphoblasts are very rich in phosphorus compared with normal lymphocytes. Lysis causes increased serum phosphorus, which can lead to hypocalcaemia or to calcium phosphate precipitation. Calcium phosphate precipitation may lead to tissue damage. Table 14.3 lists the clinical features associated with the metabolic abnormalities that occur in TLS.

Hyperkalaemia is the most rapidly occurring, dangerous consequence of TLS. Potassium levels can rise because of its release during cell lysis and quickly reach life-threatening levels if there is associated acute renal failure. Serum potassium levels of 7.0 mEq/l (mmol/l) can show changes in electrocardiograph (ECG) readings with QRS widening and peaked T-waves. Ventricular arrhythmias and death can occur if there is no intervention to lower the serum potassium levels. However, the incidence of serum potassium reaching this level is particularly uncommon due to conventional hydration and acid-base management.

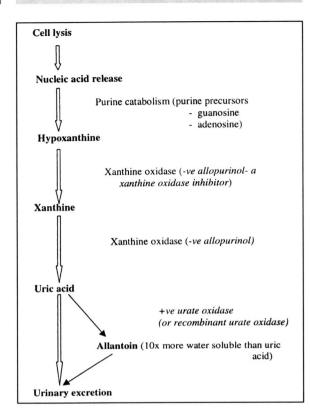

Cell lysis

⇩

Nucleic acid release

Purine catabolism (purine precursors
- guanosine
- adenosine)

⇩

Hypoxanthine

Xanthine oxidase (-*ve allopurinol- a
xanthine oxidase inhibitor*)

⇩

Xanthine

Xanthine oxidase (-*ve allopurinol*)

⇩

Uric acid

+*ve urate oxidase
(or recombinant urate oxidase)*

Allantoin (10x more water soluble than uric
acid)

⇩

Urinary excretion

◄ **Figure 14.2**

Uric acid metabolism (adapted from Nicolin, 2002)

14.3.3 Treatment

The main treatment strategy for TLS concerns prevention. Nurses have a key role in the management of paediatric patients at risk of developing TLS. The main areas of focus are

- Patient assessment prior to treatment administration
- Preventative measures
- Management of metabolic abnormalities

14.3.3.1 Patient Assessment

Identifying patients at risk should allow for prompt administration of prophylactic measures to avoid the complications associated with TLS. Patient assessment should include a patient history with respect to clinical features as described in Table 14.3. Physical examination should assess blood pressure, heart rate and rhythm, neurological status, and respiratory sta-

Table 14.3. Clinical features of tumour lysis syndrome

Hyperuricaemia	Hypocalcaemia	Hyperphosphataemia	Hyperkalaemia	Acute renal failure

Gastrointestinal
– Nausea
– Vomiting
– Diarrhoea
	Neurological
	– Tetany, demonstrated
	  by Trousseau or
	  Chvostek's signs
	– Irritability
	– Tingling of extremities
		Renal
		– Oliguria or anuria
		– Elevated blood urea
		  and creatinine
			**Gastrointestinal
			symptoms**
			
			Neuromuscular
			– Weakness
				Oliguria or anuria
				
				Oedema
				Hypertension

Renal
– Anuria or oliguria
– Oedema
– Haematuria
– Lethargy
	– Carpopedal spasm
	– Confusion
	– Laryngospasm
	– Convulsions
	– Alterations in consciousness
			– Paraesthesias
			– Paralysis
			
			Cardiovascular
			– Widening QRS and
			  peaked T-waves
			– Blood pressure
			  changes
			– Ventricular
			  arrhythmias	

	Cardiovascular – Prolonged QT interval in the ECG – Hypotension			

tus. Children should also be examined for lymphadenopathy, abdominal mass, ascites, oedema, and weight changes. Radiological examinations including chest x-ray, renal ultrasound, or computerised tomography may be indicated. A renal scan is indicated to anticipate renal infiltration that could add to the risk of TLS.

Baseline laboratory assessment should include a full/complete blood count, blood urea nitrogen, and electrolytes, including lactate dehydrogenase. If the serum potassium level is higher than 6.0 mEq/l, an ECG should be performed to rule out any cardiac abnormality. Blood urea nitrogen and electrolytes may need to be obtained every 6–8 hours in the first few days of cytotoxic treatment.

14.3.3.2 Preventative Measures

Metabolic stability should ideally be achieved prior to administration of cytotoxic treatment as long as there is not too long a delay. The preventative measures are

1. Hydration
2. Alkalisation
3. Uric acid reduction

Table 14.4 indicates the interventions that may be employed to achieve these three goals. Laboratory values should be monitored on a regular basis as the patient's condition requires and should include the following:

Table 14.4. Preventative measures in the management of tumour lysis syndrome (Truini-Pittman and Rossetto, 2002; Nicolin, 2002; Kelly and Lange, 1997)

Preventative measure	Method
Hydration	IV fluids of 0.45% (or 0.225%) saline with 5% dextrose. NO POTASSIUM ADDED Generally two to four times the usual maintenance requirements[a] with approximately 3 l/m^2/day Maintain urine specific gravity at <1.010 and urinary output ≥3 ml/kg/hr To avoid fluid overload, diuretics may be necessary: Furosemide/frusemide 1 mg/kg slow IV bolus q6h; mannitol 0.5 g/kg IV over 30 minutes q6h may also be required. Avoid diuretics if hypovolaemia present
Alkalisation	Maintain urine pH at 7.0–7.5 Sodium bicarbonate 50–100 mEq/l (mmol/l) added to IV maintenance fluids if advocated. *NOTE: Excess alkalisation may be life-threatening as it may encourage precipitation of calcium phosphate and xanthine (phosphate precipitates at pH >7.5). Symptoms of hypocalcaemia may also be aggravated by shifting ionised calcium to its nonionised form.* Reduce sodium bicarbonate if serum bicarbonate >30 mEq/l (mmol/l) or urine pH>7.5
Uric acid reduction	Allopurinol 100 mg/m^2 orally q8h (maximum 800 mg/day) or IV 200 mg/m^2/day in one to three divided doses (maximum 600 mg/day). IV allopurinol is compatible with dextrose and saline but not sodium bicarbonate. See Fig. 4.2. Uric acid production is blocked. Reduce dose of allopurinol in established renal failure. *Allopurinol has a drug-drug interaction with 6-mercaptopurine and cyclophosphamide.* Alternatively, urate oxidase 50–100 units/kg IV infusion over 30 minutes daily or recombinant urate oxidase (rasburicase) 0.15–0.2 mg/kg IV over 30 minutes four times daily for 5 days. This will convert uric acid to allantoin, which is 10 times more soluble than uric acid and promotes excretion by the kidneys. Use of urate oxidase targets a different step in uric acid metabolism that avoids build-up of xanthine and hypoxanthine. See Fig. 4.2. Do not administer urate oxidase as a bolus or through a filter. Infuse through a dedicated line. Patients receiving either of these drugs should be monitored for hypersensitive-related adverse reactions (Brant, 2002).

[a] Paediatric daily maintenance fluids are determined as follows: 100 ml/kg for the first 10 kg of body weight, 50 ml/kg for the second 10 kg of body weight, 25 ml/kg for any remaining kg of body weight over 20 kg, Divide the sum of these three numbers by 24 to establish the hourly rate for maintenance fluids

Table 14.5. Approaches in the management of electrolyte imbalances associated with tumour lysis syndrome (Truini-Pittman and Rossetto, 2002; Nicolin, 2002; Kelly and Lange, 1997)

Electrolyte imbalance	Treatment
Moderate hyperkalaemia Serum potassium > 5.0–6.0 mEq/ml (mmol/ml)	Stop the intake of potassium-containing food and fluids, e.g. bananas, chocolate Ensure that potassium is removed from IV fluids including parenteral nutrition Potassium-binding resin: polystyrene sulphonate resin 1 g/kg orally mixed with 50% sorbitol (0.25 g/kg q6h)
Severe hyperkalaemia Serum potassium >6.0 mEq/ml (mmol/ml) or ECG shows arrhythmia or significant widening of QRS complex	Calcium gluconate 10% 0.3–0.5 ml/kg or 100–200 mg/kg/dose slow IV bolus (monitor for bradycardia); this augments myocardial conduction and shifts potassium intracellularly Consider IV furosemide/frusemide 1 mg/kg (loop diuretic) if appropriate Rapid reduction of potassium levels may be achieved by IV 25% glucose 2 ml/kg with IV insulin 0.1 units/kg; this promotes intracellular flow of potassium Salbutamol 2.5–5 ml nebulised or 4 mcg/kg as slow IV bolus (5 minutes) to promote intracellular potassium flow Sodium bicarbonate 1–2 mEq/l (mmol/l) IV (diluted); this induces hydrogen efflux, leading to potassium influx Consider dialysis
Hyperphosphataemia Serum phosphate ≥6.5 mg/dl	Low-phosphate diet Aluminium hydroxide 50 mg/kg q8h Maintain urine output ≥3 ml/kg/hour
Symptomatic hypocalcaemia Calcium ≤8.0 mEq/l (mmol/l) or Ionised calcium ≤1.5 mEq/l (mmol/l)	Hyperphosphataemia treated first Maintain serum bicarbonate ≤30 mEq/l (mmol/l) IV calcium gluconate 10% 0.3–0.5 ml/kg slow bolus-5–10 minutes. Monitor for bradycardia. *Only used for symptomatic patients due to risk of calcium phosphate precipitation.* Consider dialysis

- Complete/full blood count
- Blood urea nitrogen
- Electrolytes
- Creatinine

Nurses are in a position to perform the necessary assessments and interventions. Nursing intervention should also include communication regarding physical findings and overall patient status while ensuring support and education for the patients and their families.

14.3.3.3 Management of Metabolic Abnormalities

The early identification of electrolyte imbalance along with prompt and aggressive treatment are essential and will minimise the need for hemodialysis.

Table 14.5 outlines approaches in managing electrolyte imbalances.

When these methods are ineffective in correcting imbalances and improving urinary flow, some patients may require dialysis. Indications for dialysis include

- Volume overload
- Anuria
- Symptomatic hypocalcaemia with hyperphosphataemia
- Hyperkalaemia (>6.0 mEq/l or mmol/l) with cardiac changes
- Hyperuricaemia
- Elevated serum creatinine with low urinary output

Haemodialysis, peritoneal dialysis, and continuous haemofiltration with or without dialysis have all been used to treat acute renal failure associated with TLS.

Conventional haemodialysis is most efficient at correcting imbalances, but the continuous haemofiltration may benefit patients who cannot tolerate the osmotic shift of haemodialysis (Bishof et al., 1990). Peritoneal dialysis is much less efficient at clearing uric acid and is ineffective for removing phosphates. Peritoneal dialysis is also contraindicated in patients with abdominal tumours (Stapleton et al., 1988). Dialysis should continue until metabolic stability is achieved.

Note that other concomitant therapies may contribute to metabolic abnormalities in patients with TLS:

- Oral and intravenous (IV) electrolyte and/or dietary supplements
- Thiazide and potassium-sparing diuretics
- Aspirin
- Probenecid
- Angiotensin-converting enzyme (ACE) inhibitors (associated with increased potassium), e.g. captopril
- Nephrotoxic agents, e.g. aminoglycosides
- Radiographic contrast media (Morris and Holland, 2000)

14.3.4 Prognosis

Life-threatening metabolic abnormalities may be observed at presentation in children with leukaemia and lymphoma. TLS has a high morbidity, and rare cases may lead to multiorgan failure and death. However, if children at risk are identified, properly assessed, and treated with correct prophylactic measures, TLS can be prevented and/or treated before it reaches the stage of life-threatening complications.

14.4 Hypercalcaemia

14.4.1 Incidence

Hypercalcaemia can be defined as a serum calcium concentration >3.24 mEq/l (mmol/l) or 13 mg/dl. The incidence of hypercalcaemia of malignancy is cited as approximately 0.4–0.7% (McKay and Furman, 1993). It is observed most frequently in children with ALL or alveolar rhabdomyosarcoma but has been associated with other types of malignancy in children. The incidence of hypercalcaemia varies for each type of malignancy and has been noted to be as high as 18% in children with renal rhabdoid tumours (Vujanic et al., 1996).

Table 14.6. Symptoms of hypercalcaemia

Mild hypercalcaemia	Severe hypercalcaemia
Generalised weakness	Profound muscle weakness
Poor appetite	Severe nausea and vomiting
Nausea	Decreased levels of consciousness
Vomiting	Bradyarrhythmias
Constipation	
Abdominal or back pain	
Polyuria	
Drowsiness	

14.4.2 Etiology

The cause of hypercalcaemia may be multifactorial:

- Release of calcium from sites of skeletal metastases
- Production of humoral factors from tumour, including ectopic production of parathyroid hormone-related peptide, prostaglandin E_2, tumour necrosis factor, osteoclast-activating factor, interleukin 1, and growth factor alpha.
- Hypercalcaemia interferes with the mechanisms of urinary concentration, with subsequent dehydration and a reduction in glomerular filtration rate. This causes reduction in renal calcium excretion and further hypercalcaemia (Kelly and Lange, 1997; Ralston, 1987)

Symptoms of hypercalcaemia are listed in Table 14.6. These symptoms are not always recognised in children because they may be attributed to other problems.

Table 14.7. Management of hypercalcaemia (Nicolin 2002; Kelly and Lange 1997)

Treatment aim	Management	Comments
Increase renal calcium clearance	Increase IV fluid intake (3–6 l/m²/day)	Associated vomiting and polyuria will have caused hypovolaemia
	Increase output with IV furosemide/frusemide (1–3 mg/kg q6h)	Promotes excretion of calcium and blocks its renal reabsorption in the loop of Henle
	Monitor fluid balance and electrolytes	*Treatment will cause fluid shifts and loss of sodium, potassium, and magnesium*
Inhibit osteoclastic bone resorption	Administer bisphosphonates (pamidronate) 1 mg/kg as an IV infusion with a rate not exceeding 1 mg/minute	Bind to hydroxyapatite crystals, induce osteoclastic activity, and induce deposition of calcium into bone
		Use may be limited by severe diarrhoea
	Correct hypophosphataemia with oral phosphate 10 mg/kg/dose two or three times a day	*IV phosphate is not recommended due to risk of calcium phosphate deposition*
Reduce or eliminate the tumour burden	Glucocorticoids (prednisolone) 1.5–2.0 mg/kg/day	Interfere with tumour-induced osteoclast-stimulating factors (osteoclast-activating factor and prostaglandins) Reduction in serum calcium may not be seen for 2–10 days
	May be used in conjunction with calcitonin (4 units/kg subcutaneously q12h)	Acts within hours by blocking bone resorption and promoting calcium excretion; *resistance develops within days*
	Alternatively: mithramycin, an antitumour antibiotic, given IV 25 mg/kg in 5% dextrose 50 ml over 3 hours	Inhibits osteoclastic activity. *Significant toxicity, including thrombocytopenia, azotaemia, proteinuria*

14.4.3 Treatment

Treatment for hypercalcaemia focuses on the following:

1. Increasing renal calcium clearance
2. Inhibiting osteoclastic bone resorption
3. Reducing or eliminating the tumour burden

Table 14.7 outlines the approaches that may be taken in the management of hypercalcaemia. Should approaches fail to reduce serum calcium levels, dialysis may be necessary.

14.4.4 Prognosis

Hypercalcaemia is rare; however, it is difficult to correct. Immediate attention and appropriate treatment are essential to prevent a life-threatening situation.

14.5 Impaired Glucose Tolerance Following Bone Marrow Transplant

14.5.1 Incidence

Although there are few documented studies regarding insulin-related metabolism glucose intolerance post-bone marrow transplant (BMT), the reported incidence in surviving patients is significant (Taskinen et al., 2000). Diabetes mellitus has also been reported following abdominal irradiation for Wilms' tumour (Teinturier et al., 1995). Growth hormone therapy has been reported as a potential risk factor for type-2 diabetes (Cutfield et al., 2000).

Transfer of diabetes mellitus type-1 by bone marrow transplant (from donor to recipient) has also been observed (Beard et al., 2002; Lampeter et al., 1998).

14.5.2 Etiology

Type-2 diabetes mellitus (DM) is caused by a combination of genetic causes and acquired factors. This type of DM is more common in adults, many of whom are overweight. Observations by Traggiai and colleagues (2003) suggest that radiation may compromise pancreatic α-cell function without the presence of autoantibodies.

In insulin resistance, a normal amount of insulin produces a subnormal biological response in peripheral target tissues. The impaired biological response to insulin means that the serum insulin level rises to sustain normal blood glucose concentrations (Taskinien et al., 2000). Eventually, abnormal responses lead to the exhaustion of the pancreatic islet cells and to type-2 diabetes.

Type-1 DM is thought to be transferable because the immune system of the recipient destroys the B-cells of the recipient due to the myeloablative therapy received prior to the BMT. However, the risk of contracting type-1 DM from BMT is small, and type-1 DM in an otherwise eligible donor is not thought to be reason for exclusion (Lampeter et al., 1998).

14.5.3 Treatment

Given that diabetes can be symptom-free, follow-up for BMT patients should include monitoring for glucose intolerance. Laboratory investigations should include

- Serum lipids
- Fasting blood glucose
- Serum insulin

A diagnosis of DM requires urgent referral to a paediatric endocrinologist, and treatment will include dietary advice and possibly insulin therapy.

14.5.4 Prognosis

A diagnosis of DM presents challenges along with the other potential late effects of cytotoxic therapy. Early recognition may lead to early therapy and prevention of death from resulting coronary heart disease.

References

Allegretta GJ, Weisman SJ, Altman AJ (1985) Oncologic emergencies 1: Metabolic and space occupying consequences of cancer and cancer treatment. Pediatric Clinics of North America 32(3): 601–611

Beard ME, Willis JA, Scott RS, Nesbit JW (2002) Is type 1 diabetes transmissible by bone marrow allograft? Diabetes Care 25 (4): 799–800

Bishof NA, Welch TR, Strife CF, Ryckman FC (1990) Continuous hemofiltration in children. Pediatrics 85(5): 819–823

Brant JM (2002) Rasburicase: an innovative new treatment for hyperuricemia associated with tumor lysis syndrome. Clinical Journal of Oncology Nursing 6(1): 12–16

Cutfield WS, Wilton P, Bennmarker H, Albertsson-Wikland K, Chatelain P, Ranke MB, Price DA (2000) Incidence of diabetes mellitus and impaired glucose tolerance in children and adolescents receiving growth-hormone treatment. Lancet 355: 610–613

Farley-Hills E, Byrne AJ, Brennan L, Sartori P (2001) Tumour lysis syndrome during anaesthesia. Paediatric Anaesthesia 11: 233–236

Halton J, Atkinson SA, Bradley C, Dawson S, Barr RD (1993) Acute lymphoid leukemia. No evidence of consistent chemotherapy-induced intestinal malabsorption. American Journal of Pediatric Hematology and Oncology 15(3): 271–276

Kelly KM, Lange B (1997) Pediatric oncology: oncologic emergencies. Pediatric Clinics of North America 44(4): 809–830

Lampeter EF, McCann SR, Kolb H (1998) Transfer of insulin-dependent diabetes by bone marrow transplantation. Lancet 351: 568–569

McKay C, Furman WL (1993) Hypercalcemia complicating childhood malignancy. Cancer 72: 256–260

Mayer EI, Reuter M, Dopfer RE, Ranke MB (2000) Energy expenditure, energy intake and prevalence of obesity after therapy for acute lymphoblastic leukemia during childhood. Hormone Research 53(4): 193–199

Morris JC, Holland JF (2000) Oncologic emergencies. In Bast RC Jr, Hellman S, Rosenberg SA (Eds) Holland Frei Cancer Medicine, 5th edn. Hamilton, Ontario: BC Decker

Nicolin G (2002) Emergencies and their management. European Journal of Cancer 38(10): 1365–1377

Odame I, Reilly JJ, Gibson BE, Donaldson MD (1994) Patterns of obesity in boys and girls after treatment for acute lymphoblastic leukemia. Archives of Disease in Childhood 71(2): 147–149

Picton SV (1998) Aspects of altered metabolism in children with cancer. International Journal of Cancer Supplement 11: 62–64

Picton SV, Eden OB, Rothwell NJ (1995) Metabolic rate, interleukin 6 and cachexia in children with malignancy. Medical Pediatric Oncology 5(249): (abstract o-63)

Ralston S (1987) Pathogenesis of humoral hypercalcemia of malignancy. Lancet ii: 1443–1445

Reilly JJ, Odame I, McColl JH, McAllister PJ, Gibson BE, Wharton BA (1994) Does weight for height have prognostic significance in children with acute lymphoblastic leukemia? American Journal of Pediatric Hematology and Oncology 16(3): 225–230

Reilly JJ, Ventham JC, Ralston JM, Donaldson M, Gibson B (1998) Reduced energy expenditure in preobese children treated for acute lymphoblastic leukemia. Pediatric Research 44(4): 557–562

Reilly JJ, Weir J, McColl JH, Gibson BE (1999) Prevalence of protein-energy malnutrition at diagnosis in children with acute lymphoblastic leukemia. Journal Pediatric Gastroenterology Nutrition 29(2): 194–197

Reilly JJ, Brougham M, Montgomery C, Richardson F, Kelly A, Gibson BES (2001a) Effect of glucocorticoid therapy on energy intake in children treated for acute lymphoblastic leukemia. The Journal of Clinical Endocrinology and Metabolism 86(8): 3742–3745

Reilly JJ, Kelly A, Ness P, Dorosty AR, Wallace WHB, Gibson BES, Emmett PM, Alspac Study Team (2001b) Premature adiposity rebound in children treated for acute lymphoblastic leukemia. The Journal of Clinical Endocrinology and Metabolism 86(6): 2775–2778

Sklar CA, Mertens AC, Walter A, Mitchell D, Nesbit ME, O'Leary M, Hutchinson R, Meadows AT, Robison LL (2000) Changes in body mass index and prevalence of overweight in survivors of childhood acute lymphoblastic leukemia: role of cranial irradiation. Medical and Pediatric Oncology 35(2): 91–95

Skolin I, Hernell O, Whalin Y B (2001) Energy and nutrient intake and nutritional status of children with malignant disease during chemotherapy after the introduction of new mealtime routines. Scandinavian Journal of Caring Sciences 15 (1): 82–91

Stapleton FB, Strother DR, Roy S 3rd, Wyatt RJ, McKay CP, Murphy SB (1988) Acute renal failure at onset of therapy for advanced stage Burkitt lymphoma and B cell acute lymphoblastic lymphoma. Pediatrics 82(6): 863–869.

Taskinen M, Saarinen-Pihkala UM, Hovi L, Lipsanen-Nyman M (2000) Impaired glucose tolerance and dyslipidaemia as late effects after bone-marrow transplantation in childhood. Lancet 356:993–997

Teinturier C, Tournade MF, Caillat-Zucman S, Boitard C, Amoura Z, Bougneres PF, Timsit J (1995) Diabetes mellitus after abdominal radiation therapy. Lancet 346: 633–634

Traggiai C, Stanhope R, Nussey S, Leiper AD (2003) Diabetes mellitus after bone marrow transplantation during childhood. Medical Pediatric Oncology 40(2): 128–129

Truini-Pittman L, Rosseto C(2002) Pediatric considerations in tumor lysis syndrome. Seminars in Oncology Nursing 18(3): 17–22

Van Dongen-Melman JEWM, Hoekken-Koelaga ACS, Hakler K, de Groot A, Tromp CG, Egeler RM (1995) Obesity after successful treatment of acute lymphoblastic leukemia in childhood. Pediatric Research 38 (1): 86–90

Viana MB, Murao, Ramos G Oliveira HM, de Carvalho RI, de Bastos, Colosimo EA, Silvestrini WS (1994) Malnutrition as a prognostic factor in lymphoblastic leukaemia: a multivariate analysis. Archives of Disease in Childhood 71 (4): 304–310

Vujanic GM, Sandstedt B, Harms D, Boccon-Gibod L, Delemarre JF (1996) Rhabdoid tumour of the kidney: a clinicopathological study of 22 patients from the International Society of Paediatric Oncology (SIOP) nephroblastoma file. Histopathology 28: 333–340

Weir J, Reilly JJ, McColl JH, Gibson BE (1998) No evidence for an effect of nutritional status at diagnosis on prognosis in children with acute lymphoblastic leukemia. Journal of Pediatric Hematology/Oncology 20(6): 534–8

Gastrointestinal Tract

Anne-Marie Maloney

Contents

To some degree, gastrointestinal (GI) complications are experienced universally by paediatric oncology patients. The rapidly dividing cells of the GI tract predispose patients to toxic sequelae of chemotherapy and radiation therapy; destruction of the protective mucosal barrier may lead to opportunistic infections; and the primary malignancy may invade or impinge on the function of the organs of the GI tract.

15.1 Mucositis

15.1.1 Incidence

The mucosal lining of the GI tract, including the oral mucosa, is a prime target for treatment-related toxicity by virtue of its rapid cell turnover rate. Mucositis is an inflammation of the oral mucosa. Breakdown of the mucosal barrier can predispose patients to potentially fatal systemic infection. Estimated rates of the incidence of oral mucositis from standard cancer chemotherapy range from 31% to 40% and rise to 76% in haematopoietic stem cell transplant patients (Panzarella et al., 2002). Chemotherapeutic agents differ in their potential for causing mucositis. Mucositis can also vary in intensity of pain and discomfort. Several grading systems have been developed to rate this common toxicity to cancer therapy. A common toxicity grading criteria for mucositis is detailed in Table 15.1.

15.1.2 Etiology

15.1.2.1 Iatrogenic

The many oral complications associated with the chemotherapy are the result of

- the direct stomatotoxicity of the antineoplastic agents on the oral mucosa in the form of mucositis
- the indirect effects of myelosuppression, consisting of haemorrhage and infection

The onset of oral mucositis secondary to chemotherapy is usually within 3–7 days of therapy with complete resolution at 14 days post-onset of this condition, coinciding with blood count recovery. Mucositis

Table 15.1. Common toxicity criteria grading for mucositis (Berger and Kilroy, 2001)

Grade	Criteria
0	Mouth pink No bleeding Mucosa moist No oedema or infection No limit to eating or drinking
1	Slight increase in redness of mouth One to four oral lesions Thinning of mucosa No bleeding or infection Mucosa moist Mild discomfort or burning sensation Possible avoidance of hot, harsh, or spicy foods
2	Moderate increase in mouth redness More than four oral lesions, not coalescing Mucosa bleeds with manipulation Mucosa slightly drier Salvia slightly thicker Moderate oedema White or yellow patches, infection present Eating only bland soft foods Avoidance of hot, spicy, or acid liquids Moderate continual pain, necessitating intermittent, usually topical analgesics
3	Severe redness throughout oral cavity Multiple confluent ulcers Possible total denudation of oral cavity Marked xerostomia Severe oedema White, yellow, or purulent patches Inability to eat or drink Inability to swallow salvia Severe, constant pain, necessitating system analgesia

Table 15.2. Chemotherapeutic agents commonly associated with mucositis

Alkylating agents	Antitumour antibiotics
Busulfan	Actinomycin D
Cyclophosphamide	Amsacrine
Mechlorethamine	Bleomycin
Procarbazine	Mithramycin
Thiotepa	Mitomycin

Anthracyclines	Taxanes
Daunorubicin	Docetaxel
Doxorubicin	Paclitaxel
Epirubicin	

Antimetabolites	Vinca alkaloids
5-Fluorouracil	Vinblastine
Hydroxyurea	Vincristine
Methotrexate	Vinorelbine
Cytosine arabinoside	
6-Mercaptopurine	
6-Thioguanine	Vinorelbine

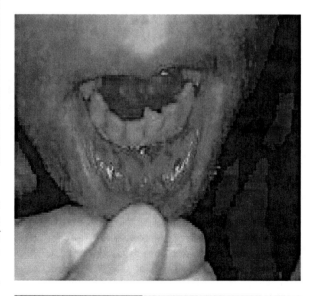

Figure 15.1

A case of ulcerative oral mucositis lesions of the labial mucosa and floor of the mouth (Woo and Treister, 2001)

secondary to head and neck radiation therapy is the most common oral complication of this treatment modality (Steinle and Dock, 1994). Combination of certain chemotherapeutic regimens along with radiation therapy can magnify the resulting mucositis.

Chemotherapeutic agents that are commonly associated with mucositis are listed in Table 15.2.

Fig. 15.1 shows a case of ulcerative oral mucositis lesions of the labial mucosa and floor of mouth (Woo and Treister, 2001).

15.1.2.2 Bacterial

Oral bacterial infections occur in 10–20% of patients being treated with antineoplastic agents. The majority of these infections are caused by opportunistic aerobic Gram-negative bacilli, which are seldom pathogenic in an immunocompetent host. Other bacterial aetiologies of mucositis include *Klebsiella, Enterobacter, Serratia, Proteus* and *Escherichia coli.* These lesions typically are creamy to yellow-white in colour. They appear as moist, glistening, nonpurulent, smooth-edged surfaces seated on painful red superficial mucosal ulcers (Steinle and Dock, 1994).

15.1.2.3 Viral

The oral cavity is affected primarily by four different viral strains: herpes simplex (HSV), which is the most common; cytomegalovirus (CMV); varicella zoster; and Epstein-Barr virus (EBV). The incidence of HSV infection varies in studies from 3% to 85%. These lesions may present as painful scabbed blisters typically on the lips but may be found on any surface in the oral cavity. Scraping of the lesion for viral cultures will confirm the etiology of the infection

15.1.2.4 Fungal

Fungal superinfection of mucositis is mostly caused by *Candida albicans,* although other *Candida* species may be the causative agent. Oral candidiasis presents as small, white, pearly patches firmly adhered to the oral mucosa.

15.1.3 Prevention

Protocols and algorithms for preventing and treating mucositis vary among institutions, and many preparations have been investigated in the prevention of chemotherapy-induced mucositis. In a Cochrane Database review, Clarkson et al. (2000) concluded that the only preventive measure for chemotherapy-induced mucositis that is supported in the literature is sucking on ice chips during chemotherapy administration. Certainly, this approach is not a viable option in very young patients.

15.1.4 Treatment

It is generally agreed that good oral care is an important adjunct to the management of oral mucositis. A limited study by Cheng et al. (2003) supported a standardised oral care protocol to reduce the incidence and severity of oral mucositis, but this study did not include a randomised comparison of agents. Given that the literature does not support the superiority of any particular agent in oral care, a simplified approach may be the best course of action.

Saline or sodium bicarbonate mouthwashes are nonirritating solutions that provide mechanical rinsing (Rogers, 2001). These solutions have the benefit of being very cost-effective. Parents should be instructed to have their child rinse his mouth a minimum of four times a day. Young children may have their mouths cleaned with a saline-soaked sponge Toothette or gauze. Good oral hygiene should be emphasised throughout the child's treatment. Tooth brushing should continue with a soft-bristle toothbrush for as long as the patient's oral condition allows. A recent case study reported that toothbrushes may become colonised with pathogenic organisms, so frequent replacement is recommended (Kennedy et al., 2003). Lips may be lubricated with petroleum jelly or lip balm to help prevent cracking.

If feasible, a dental consultation should be obtained before the start of intensive chemotherapy, head and neck radiation therapy, and stem cell transplant (Shaw et al., 2000). Orthodontic appliances should be removed because they can harbour bacteria. If dental work is required during chemotherapy, it should be scheduled for a period when the patient is not expected to be pancytopenic.

Frequent assessment of the oral cavity is essential. Chemotherapy-induced mucositis can become further infected with *Candida* or HSV. Oral thrush caused by *C. albicans* appears as whitish plaques with slightly raised indurated boards. Herpetic lesions usually appear as clear vesicular eruptions, frequently in clusters or "crops" on an erythematous base, either periorally or intraorally (Alexander et al., 2002). Scrapings of suspicious lesions should be sent for culture. Culture-proven infections are treated with appropriate antimicrobials.

Pain is managed with topical anaesthetics initially; opioid analgesics may be required. The patient's nutritional status must be carefully assessed because the inability to maintain adequate oral intake can quickly evolve into dehydration and nutritional deficits. A soft diet with cool and bland foods may be best tolerated. Ice chips and Popsicles can be soothing and help in hydration. In severe cases intravenous hydration or parenteral nutrition may be required.

15.1.5 Prognosis

Mucositis typically resolves with the resolution of neutropenia. In severe causes of mucositis, future chemotherapy cycles may need to be dose-reduced.

15.2 Dental Caries

15.2.1 Incidence

Dental side effects of cancer therapy can be of concern in the acute treatment period and in long-term follow-up. Although chemotherapy has little permanent effect on oral health, there is evidence that chemotherapy alone may result in an increased incidence of dental developmental disturbances (Chin, 1998). In a recent study, Minicucci et al. (2002) described dental abnormalities, most frequently dental hypoplasia, in childhood leukaemia survivors treated with chemotherapy alone. Radiation to the head and neck predisposes patients to dental decay (Steinle and Dock, 1994).

15.2.2 Etiology

15.2.2.1 Iatrogenic

The late effects of radiation therapy to the oral cavity are well established. The nature and severity of the potential side effects of radiation on the developing tooth vary with

- the child's age at diagnosis
- the stage of tooth development
- the doses and schedules of treatment
- the anatomic region treated

The principal dental abnormalities caused by radiation include destruction of the tooth germ with failure, stunted growth of the whole tooth or root, and incomplete calcification (Minicucci et al., 2002). Radiation caries is a rapidly progressive and destructive disease that develops between 2 and 10 months posttreatment when radiation has been delivered to the head and neck. When the major salivary glands are irradiated, all teeth within the field of radiation, as well as those outside the field, have an increased risk of developing rampant caries. Depending on the reversibility of the salivary gland dysfunction, the patient can develop a lifelong susceptibility to severe dental caries. A decrease in salivary flow will decrease the buffering and diluting function of saliva on acids produced by bacteria in the mouth. A lowered saliva pH initiates the demineralisation process that leads to tooth decay (Steinle and Dock, 1994).

15.2.3 Prevention and Treatment

Nurses can play a vital role in establishing good oral hygiene practices in paediatric cancer patients. In the acute treatment period, the development of mucositis can often preclude the practice of effective oral hygiene practices. Poor baseline oral hygiene can be a predisposing factor for the development of infections. Gingivitis should be considered as a likely site for systemic entry of oral bacteria (Kennedy et al., 2003). This would suggest that dental cleanings should optimally be scheduled prior to chemotherapy or during periods of anticipated satisfactory blood counts. Ideally, all potential foci of dental infection and bleeding should be removed before the start of cancer therapy. Grossly carious teeth should be removed before the start of therapy, and other carious teeth should be restored (Chin, 1998)

Xerostomia can lead to an increased susceptibility to dental caries and erosion of tooth structure (Shaw et al., 2000). Interventions directed at increasing oral moisture and avoidance of refined sugar can help to prevent tooth decay. Patients and families should be instructed regarding the increased risk of dental caries secondary to xerostomia. Strategies to achieve satisfactory oral hygiene during periods of painful mucositis should be addressed with the patient and family. Adequate pain control will help facilitate tooth brushing or at least oral cleansing with Toothettes. Children should continue to have regularly scheduled dental examinations and cleanings during non-neutropenic periods in their therapy if possible.

15.2.4 Prognosis

For the child receiving chemotherapy, the oral side effects tend to be temporary. There is evidence, however, that chemotherapy alone may result in increased dental development disturbances (Chin, 1998). Given that increased susceptibility to dental caries can be a lifelong problem following radiation therapy to the oral field, nurses involved in late-effects clinics should counsel patients regarding these dental late effects. Preventive dental hygiene must be reinforced, and referral to a dentist familiar with the dental late effects of cancer therapy is indicated.

15.3 Nausea and Vomiting

15.3.1 Incidence

Nausea and vomiting are symptoms experienced by nearly all childhood cancer patients and are most commonly associated with chemotherapy and radiation therapy. However, the disease process, constipation, abdominal obstruction, infections, opioids for pain control, and other pharmacologic interventions can also contribute to nausea and vomiting in the paediatric oncology patient. Recent advances in the understanding of the mechanisms involved in nausea and vomiting and the development of 5-hydroxytryptamine ($5-HT_3$) receptor antagonist have greatly improved antiemetic management of patients.

15.3.2 Etiology

The neurophysiological mechanisms that control nausea and vomiting are mediated by the central nervous system (CNS) by different mechanisms. Nausea is mediated through the autonomic nervous system. The vomiting centre, located in the medullary lateral reticular formation, mediates vomiting. This centre receives afferent input from five main sources:

Figure 15.2 ▶

The emesis pathway
(adapted from Panzarella et al., 2002)

1. Chemoreceptor trigger zone (CTZ)
2. Vagal and sympathetic afferents from the viscera
3. Midbrain receptors that detect changes in intracranial pressure
4. Labyrinthine apparatus which detects motions and position
5. Higher CNS structures (e.g. the limbic system)

The vomiting centre in turn activates a series of efferent pathways, which include phrenic nerves to the diaphragm, spinal nerves to abdominal musculature, and visceral nerves to the centrally mediated stimulation in the vomiting centre which act to induce actual vomiting (Berde et al. 2002). (See Fig. 15.2.)

The vomiting centre contains neurotransmitter receptors of the serotonergic (especially $5-HT_3$), dopaminergic (especially D2), histaminergic (especially H1), muscarinic cholinergic, endorphin cannabinoid, neurokinin (NK_1), and benzodiazepine types. The exact site and type of neurotransmitter involved in the pathogenesis of vomiting caused by each emetic stimulus is not known. The present understanding of pharmacologic control of emesis suggest that by blocking the effects of specific neurotransmitters for each stimulus, vomiting can be prevented or decreased. Blocking more than one type of receptor has the potential to further enhance vomiting control (Kris and Pizzo, 1997). Currently, evidence indicates that acute emesis following chemotherapy is initiated by the release of neurotransmitters from cells that are susceptible to the presence of toxic substances in the blood or cerebrospinal fluid (CSF). Area postrema cells in the CTZ and enterochromaffin cells within the intestinal mucosa are implicated in the initiating and propagating of afferent stimuli that ultimately converge on the vomiting centre.

Nausea and vomiting secondary to treatment experienced by paediatric oncology patients can be divided into three major categories:

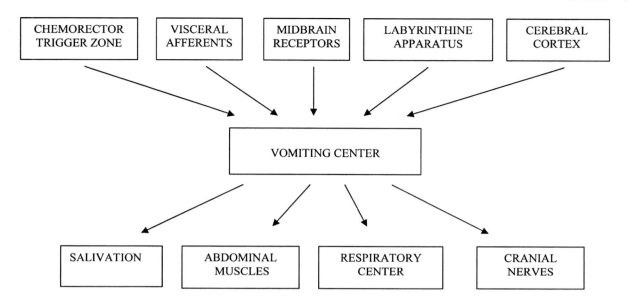

Table 15.3. Acute emetogenic potential of chemotherapeutic agents (Roy and Griffiths, 2003)

Very high Rank 4	High Rank 3	Moderate Rank 2	Mild Rank 1	None Rank 0
Carmustine 250 mg/m²	Carboplatin	Amsacrine	Etoposide <60 mg/m²	Bleomycin
Cisplatin 50 mg/m²	Carmustine 250 mg/m²	Cyclophosphamide <750 mg/m²	Methotrexate 51–249 mg/m²	Busulfan
Cyclophosphamide >1,500 mg/m²	Cisplatin <50 mg/m²	Daunomycin 60 mg/m²		Chlorambucil <1000 mg/m²
Dacarbazine	Cyclophosphamide >750–1,500 mg/mg²	Doxorubicin 60 mg/m²		Cytarabine <1000 mg/m²
Mechlorethamine	Cytarabine >1,000 mg/m² Dactinomycin Daunomycin >60 mg/m² Doxorubicin >60 mg/m² Methotrexate >1,000 mg/m² Procarbazine	Epirubicin Etoposide 60 mg/m² Fludarabine Idarubicin Ifosfamide Methotrexate 250 mg–1,000 mg/m² Mitoxantrone		Hydroxyurea Lomustine Mercaptopurine Methotrexate 50 mg/m² Teniposide 6-Thioguanine Vinblastine Vincristine

- Acute: nausea and vomiting experienced in the first 24 hours following therapy
- Delayed: nausea and vomiting that occurs 24 hours following therapy
- Anticipatory: nausea and vomiting that occurs before the start of subsequent cycles of chemotherapy

Table 15.3 indicates the emetogenic ranking of common chemotherapeutic agents.

Table 15.4. Frontline antiemetics commonly used in paediatric oncology

Classification/drug	Dosing	Therapeutic considerations
5-HT₃ antagonist: Ondansetron	5 mg/m² PO/IV q8–12h Maximum dose 8 mg PO/IV	May cause headache, constipation with prolonged use Expensive; oral form more cost-efficient
Granisetron	10–20 mcg/kg IV q12h	Adult oral dose 2 mg PO daily. Currently no paediatric oral dosing available. Some literature to support up to 40 mcg/kg/dose IV in paediatric patients; more research needed
Steroids: Dexamethasone	8 mg/m² PO/IV Maximum dose 20 mg/dose	May be contraindicated in patients with brain tumours and patients on concurrent steroid therapy Risk of avascular necrosis

15.3.3 Prevention

Preventing nausea and vomiting is a cornerstone of good patient care. Good antiemetic control is best achieved by medicating with appropriate antiemetics before therapy begins; it is very difficult to break the cycle of nausea and vomiting once it starts. Patient response to the previous course of chemotherapy should be assessed with each subsequent course, and alterations to the antiemetic regimen should be implemented if a history of antiemetic failure is detected. Effective management of acute nausea and vomiting from the first exposure to treatment is important in preventing anticipatory nausea and vomiting.

15.3.4 Treatment

Successful management of chemotherapy-associated nausea and vomiting requires an accurate assessment of the emetic potential of the chemotherapy regimen. The initial combination of antiemetics for a given chemotherapeutic regimen must be tailored to the emetogenic potential of that drug combination. Appropriate antiemetics must be given before chemotherapy begins and given around the clock, not on a prn schedule. Prevention is essential in the treatment of nausea and vomiting, as it is very difficult to treat nausea once it starts.

In paediatrics, commonly used antiemetic drugs include

- 5-HT₃ antagonists
- steroids (see Table 15.4)

The use of steroids may be contraindicated based on the patient's disease, past medical history, or treatment protocol.

One method to determine the appropriate initial antiemetic combination is to assign ranks to the emetogenicity of the individual chemotherapeutic agents, starting with the highest emetogenic agent and then adding one rank order for each additional emetogenic agent, to a maximum of five. Table 15.5 indicates the antiemetic selection based on emetogenicity of the cytotoxic drugs prescribed. An agent with an emetogenic rank of 0 will not add a rank. For example, cisplatin 50 mg/m² (rank 4) plus daunomycin 50 mg/m² (rank 2) would equal an emetogenic rank of 5 (very high). Thus, this patient would receive an initial combination of a serotonin 5-HT₃ blocker plus twice-daily dexamethasone. Limited evidence suggests that if a patient fails one 5-HT₃ antagonist, switching to another drug in this class for subsequent chemotherapy cycles may be of benefit (de Wit et al., 2001). Thus, if the patient were initially treated with ondansetron on his first cycle of chemotherapy and suffered an antiemetic failure, he would be switched

Table 15.5. Initial antiemetic selection based on emetogenicity of chemotherapeutic regimen (Roy and Griffiths, 2003)

Emetogenicity rank of single agent or combination	Recommended antiemetic regimen
Very high (rank 4)	Serotonin (5-HT$_3$) antagonists IV or PO pre-chemo and around the clock for 24 hours after last dose of chemo PLUS dexamethasone 8 mg/m^2 (max dose 20 mg) PO/IV 12 hours
High (rank 3)	Serotonin (5-HT$_3$) antagonists IV or PO pre-chemo and around the clock for 24 hours after last dose of chemo PLUS dexamethasone 8 mg/m^2 (max dose 20 mg) PO/IV daily
Moderate (rank 2)	Serotonin (5-HT$_3$) antagonists IV or PO pre chemo and around the clock for 24 hours after last dose of chemo
Mild (rank 1)	Serotonin (5-HT$_3$) antagonists IV or PO pre-chemo
None (rank 0)	None

Table 15.6. Other antiemetics used in paediatric oncology

Classification/antiemetic	Indications
Benzodiazepine Lorazepam	Useful in treating anticipatory and breakthrough nausea and vomiting. Route IV/PO/SL, dosing 0.025 –0.05 mg/kg; give 1 hour pre-chemo and q6h prn max dose 4 mg. Start with lower dosing and increase as necessary. Monitor for excessive sedation
Oral cannabinoids Nabilone Marinol	Useful in treating anticipatory nausea and breakthrough nausea and vomiting. Some patients may not tolerate the euphoria associated with cannabinoids. Optimal dosing starts the night before chemotherapy
Phenothiazines Chlorpromazine Prochlorperazine Thiethylperazine Perphenazine	Major side effects are extrapyramidal reactions and agitation, especially in younger children. Slow administration over 30–60 minutes and concurrent administration with antihistamines for 24 hours after last phenothiazine dose will minimise these effects. Phenothiazines may be added to frontline antiemetic regimens with 5- HT$_3$ antagonist when these regimens fail
Procainamide derivative Metoclopramide	Major side effects extrapyramidal reactions, which are minimised with slow administration and concurrent antihistamine administration. Metoclopramide has both antiemetic and gastric-emptying effect 1 mg/kg q2–4h
Antihistamines Diphenhydramine Dimenhydrinate	Mild antiemetic properties. May be used in combination with other antiemetics. Sedating properties of antihistamines may be desirable for some patients

to granisetron for his next cycle of therapy. The management of acute nausea requires preventive around-the-clock dosing of antiemetics for 24 hours following the last dose of chemotherapy when the emetogenic potential is moderate or greater. Ideally, breakthrough antiemetics are ordered in case of antiemetic failure. Other antiemetics that may be used in paediatric oncology are listed in Table 15.6.

15.3.4.1 Delayed Nausea and Vomiting

Delayed nausea and vomiting (DNV) occurs 24 hours after the last dose of chemotherapy and may last up to 5 days following a cycle of chemotherapy. It is most often associated with cisplatin, carboplatin, and high-dose cyclophosphamide. Serotonin 5HT$_3$ antagonists have not been found effective in treating DNV;

dexamethasone alone or in combination with meto-clopramide has some support in the literature (Dupuis and Greenberg, 2001).

15.3.4.2 Anticipatory Nausea and Vomiting

Anticipatory nausea and vomiting (ANV) can occur at any time following the first cycle of chemotherapy. ANV can best be treated by preventing nausea and vomiting with the first administration of chemotherapy. Sights, sounds, or people that the patient associates with chemotherapy can precipitate ANV. Treatment of ANV can be pharmacologically managed with lorazepam or cannabinoids given the evening before chemotherapy. Assessment of the factors that trigger ANV can be helpful in developing nonpharmacological approaches to treatment. Guided imagery, relaxation therapy, music therapy, and art therapy may be beneficial in treating ANV.

15.3.4.3 Radiation-Induced Nausea and Vomiting

Total body, abdominal, craniospinal, mantle, and hemibody irradiation have been associated with significant radiation-induced emesis. 5-HT$_3$ antagonists have been found to be effective when given prior to each fraction and for 24 hours following the treatment (Gralla et al., 1999).

15.3.4.4 Other Causes of Nausea and Vomiting

In paediatric oncology, nausea and vomiting can be attributed to factors other than treatment. Metabolites of many tumours (especially in advanced disease), increased intracranial pressure (secondary to brain tumours), constipation, bowel obstruction, and opioid administration for pain control are some of the potential causes in these patients. Treatment is ideally achieved by controlling the underlining cause of the nausea and vomiting. If this is not feasible, symptom control may be achieved with standard antiemetic therapies. 5 HT-$_3$ antagonists may be of benefit in opioid-induced nausea.

15.3.4.5 Nonpharmacological Management

Nonpharmacological approaches to the management of nausea and vomiting include controlling the patient environment and reducing strong odours, bright lights, and noise. Patient education regarding strategies to mange nausea and vomiting and the potential for delayed nausea are essential. Parents must be instructed to closely monitor their child for signs of dehydration. Small frequent bland meals are best tolerated. Families should be counselled that children may develop food aversions to favourite foods after therapy; taste alterations are common in this population. Relaxation therapy, guided imagery, and other psychological supports may all be beneficial in emesis management.

15.3.5 Prognosis

Nausea and vomiting are self-limiting sequelae to cancer therapy. They also can be the most dreaded and debilitating consequences of therapy. Effective antiemetic control is an essential component for a high quality of life for a paediatric oncology patient.

15.4 Constipation

15.4.1 Incidence

Constipation is a common sequela of childhood cancer and its therapy. It is defined as a decrease in an individual's normal pattern of defaecation. Constipated stool is often hard, difficult to pass, and accompanied by straining, abdominal pain or cramping, and rectal discomfort (Panzarella et al. 2002). Constipation occurs in up to 10% of the healthy paediatric population and accounts for 25% of all visits to paediatric gastroenterologists (Guerrero and Cavender, 1999). In the paediatric oncology patient, the causative factors of constipation may include the following:

- Decreased gastric motility secondary to medications (especially vinca alkaloids and opioid analgesics)
- Tumour compression of the GI tract or spinal cord
- Hypokalaemia
- Hypercalcaemia
- Hypothyroidism
- Decreased mobility
- Changes in appetite
- Changes in toileting patterns secondary to hospitalisations

The incidence of constipation related to continuous infusion of vinblastine has been reported to be as high as 100% (Aitken, 1992).

15.4.2 Etiology

The exact etiology of constipation in the child with cancer is often difficult to assess. The etiology is likely multifocal in nature. Aitken (1992) has characterised constipation in the paediatric oncology as iatrogenic, primary, or secondary.

15.4.2.1 Iatrogenic

The most common iatrogenic agents responsible for constipation in the paediatric oncology patient are opioid analgesics and vinca alkaloids. Opioids inhibit intestinal smooth muscle motility. Decreased peristalsis of the small and large intestine and increased tone in the ileocaecal valve and pyloric and anal sphincters result in the unfortunate side effect of constipation (Yaster and Maxwell, 1993). The vinca alkaloids such as vincristine and vinblastine have a neurotoxic effect on the smooth muscle of the GI tract, resulting in decreased peristaltic activity. This results in increased transit time for the stool to pass, increased absorption of water in the bowel, and the formation of hard, dry stools. Other iatrogenic causes of constipation include decreased peristaltic bowel activity following abdominal and pelvic surgery and decreased oral intake secondary to chemotherapy-induced nausea and vomiting.

15.4.2.2 Primary Constipation

Primary constipation results from external factors such as

- Diet
- Decreased mobility
- An interruption in normal patterns of defaecation

Children with cancer experience alterations in nutrition secondary to their illness; nausea and vomiting may result in decreased oral intake; chemotherapy may result in alterations in taste; and generalised malaise may result in deficits in healthy food choices, especially fibre intake. Because hospitalised patients have their usual routine severely disrupted, periods of privacy for toileting may predispose them to constipation.

15.4.2.3 Secondary Constipation

Secondary constipation in the child with cancer results from the pathology of the disease itself. Abdominal tumours can cause partial or complete obstruction of the GI tract. Tumour growth along the spinal column can result in cord compression and decreased innervation of the bowel. Metabolic alterations such as hypercalcaemia, hypokalaemia, or hypothyroidism may predispose the patient to constipation (Panzarella et al., 2002)

15.4.3 Prevention

Prevention is crucial in managing constipation. Families should receive anticipatory education regarding the potential for and treatment of constipation. Patients on opioid therapy should be empirically started on a bowel regimen. Careful assessment for constipation should be undertaken before vincristine or vinblastine therapy; these patients may benefit from prophylactic stool softeners.

15.4.4 Treatment

A detailed physical examination and history that includes dietary and defaecation habits should be assessed in all patients. Children with constipation may present with the following:

- Decline in stool production
- Change in the characteristics of stool (hard, dry, and possibly blood-streaked)
- Hypoactive bowel sounds
- Distended or firm abdomen (a mass may be noted in the left lower quadrant)
- Diffuse abdominal tenderness
- Decreased appetite
- Feeling of satiety and nausea
- Straining with attempts to have bowel movements
- Pain associated with defaecation (Panzarella et al., 2002)

Underlying causes of constipation should be identified and treated.

Dietary interventions include maximising oral fluid intake and dietary fibre. A dietary consult may be helpful in identifying foods that may predispose patients to constipation and those that may help prevent this condition. Other nonpharmacological interventions include encouraging physical activity, maintaining normal toileting routines, and providing privacy for defaecation.

Pharmacologic interventions can be divided into two phases:

- Disimpaction
- Maintenance

In neutropenic patients, the rectal route for disimpaction must be avoided because of the risk of injury to the rectal mucosal and the potential for perirectal infection. Disimpaction is necessary before beginning maintenance therapy. In controlled clinical trials, disimpaction by the oral route, the rectal route, or a combination of the two has been found to be effective (Baker et al., 1999). A medical position statement by the North American Society for Pediatric Gastroenterology and Nutrition recommends the oral route for initiating disimpaction (Baker et al., 1999). This paper states that high doses of mineral oil and/or polyethylene glycol electrolyte solutions are highly effective. Their recommended dosage of mineral oil for disimpaction is 15–30 ml/year of age, up to 240 ml/day. Mineral oil is associated with lipoid pneumonia if aspirated and is not recommended in children under 1 year of age or those with impaired swallowing reflexes. Polyethylene glycol electrolyte solution is recommended at a dosage of 25 ml/kg/hr by nasogastric tube until clear, up to a maximum dosage of 1,000 ml/hr. It has been associated with nausea, bloating, abdominal cramps, and anal irritation. Baker et al. (1999) go on to add that high-dose magnesium hydroxide, magnesium citrate, lactulose, sorbitol, senna, or bisacodyl have all been successfully used for disimpaction, although no clinical trails have been done to document their effectiveness. Once the faecal mass has been disimpacted, maintenance of regular stooling must be achieved.

The pharmacologic management of constipation includes a combination of "motivator" laxatives and stool softeners to achieve a regular stooling pattern. Common medications used in treating constipation are listed in Table 15.7. Stool softeners include mineral oil at a dose of 1–3 ml/kg/day or docusate sodium 20–60 mg/day. Both of these preparations can be given as a divided dose one to four times a day titrated to maintain soft stools. The maintenance of soft stool ensures that the child will not have painful bowel movements that may lead to stool withholding and result in a stool impaction. Liquid docusate and mineral oil can be mixed in a variety of fluids and foods to aid in their palpability.

Motivator laxatives are also used. Magnesium hydroxide, lactulose, and sorbitol have extensive track records, and long-term studies show that these therapies are safe and effective. Because magnesium hydroxide, lactulose, and sorbitol seem to be equally effective, the choice of which laxative to use can be based on cost and the child's preference (Baker et al., 1999). Stimulant laxatives such as senna and bisacodyl are not recommended as daily therapy; they should be reserved for intermittent therapy as a rescue to prevent recurrence of the impaction (Baker et al., 1999).

Table 15.7. Medications used for treating constipation

Drug	Dose	Comments
Osmotic		
Lactulose	5–10 ml PO daily initially	Adult dose 30 ml/day; increase dose daily until stool is produced. Well tolerated. Side effects include abdominal cramps
Magnesium citrate	4 ml/kg/day Maximum dose 300 ml/day	Cathartic: Use for oral disimpaction. Monitor electrolytes
Lavage		
Polyethylene glycol-electrolyte solution	In severe impaction 25 ml/kg/hr until clear Maximum dose 1,000 ml	Most children will require a nasogastric tube because solution not well tolerated. Side effects nausea vomiting and cramps
Lubricant		
Mineral oil	Maintenance 1–3 ml/kg/day Disimpaction 15–30 ml/year up to 240 ml/day	Stool softener decreases water reabsorption; risk of lipoid pneumonia if aspirated; not to be used with infants or with children who have neurological deficits
Stimulants		
Senna	*Syrup* 2–6 years: 3–5 ml/day 6–12 years: 5–10 ml/day	Stimulant laxatives should be used for short-term use only, not daily therapy
	Granules 2– 5 years: 2.5 ml/day 6 –12 years: 5 ml/day	
	Tablet 6–12 years: 1–2 tabs/day	
Bisacodyl	5 mg tabs 1–3 tabs daily prn	Not for daily use Severe abdominal cramps

15.4.5 Prognosis

Once a patient has been identified as having had altered bowel elimination, careful attention should be given to preventing this condition in the future. Constipation is seldom a long-term sequela of cancer and its therapy. Once the causative agents are removed, patients will usually return to their previous bowel patterns.

15.5 Diarrhoea

15.5.1 Incidence

Diarrhoea is defined as an abnormal increase in the quantity, frequency, or liquidity of stool (Panzarella et al., 2002). This condition can predispose the patient to fluid and electrolyte imbalances, dehydration, renal failure, and impaired skin integrity. In the paediatric oncology patient, diarrhoea can be a potentially lethal sequela of therapy or can be secondary to the disease process itself. Diarrhoea may result in extra hospitalisations secondary to dehydration and in severe cases may result in delay of therapy. The most frequent cause of acute diarrhoea is an infectious process. Other aetiologies of diarrhoea include drug reactions, dietary alterations, inflammatory bowel diseases, intestinal ischaemia, graft versus host (GvHD) disease, or faecal impaction. Chronic diarrhoea can be complex and be caused by infections, inflammatory bowel diseases, irritable bowel syndrome, dietary alterations, surgeries, endocrine disorders, neoplasms, or radiation colitis (Cope, 2001). Chemotherapy-induced diarrhoea, a well-recognised entity in paediatric oncology, can vary in intensity from mild and self-limiting to severe and requiring aggressive medical management. The exact incidence of chemotherapy-induced diarrhoea is unknown; however, in the adult population estimates suggest that 10 % of patients with advanced cancer will experience acute or chronic diarrhoea at some time during their illnesses. Chemotherapeutic regimens that contain fluoropyrimidines and irinotecan (CPT-11) have reported incidences as high as 50–80 % (Cope, 2001).

15.5.2 Etiology

15.5.2.1 Iatrogenic

Chemotherapy

Chemotherapy-induced diarrhoea is a well-recognised side effect of a number of chemotherapeutic agents. The mechanism of this side effect is not fully understood but is thought to result from the interference of certain chemotherapy agents in the division of intestinal cells, producing acute damage to the intestinal mucosa and thereby resulting in a shortening of the intestinal villi and a shift in the balance of the numbers of absorptive and secretory cells (Panzarella et al., 2002). As a result of acute damage to the intestinal mucosa, a loss of intestinal epithelium, inflammation, and superficial necrosis of the bowel occur. This inflammatory process and necrosis can stimulate secretion of fluids and electrolytes directly. Destruction of the terminal carbohydrate and protein digestive enzymes also may lead to increased secretion of fluids and electrolytes. Thus, the intestinal absorptive cells are unable to manage the large volume of fluid and electrolytes that are produced, and diarrhoea occurs (Cope, 2001). The most common chemotherapeutic agents associated with diarrhoea are listed in Table 15.8.

Radiation

Radiation therapy to the abdomen and pelvis is one of the major causes of chronic diarrhoea in the child with cancer. The direct effect of digestive tract irradiation is the loss of regenerating cells that line the gut. Radiation damage of the fine vasculature of

Table 15.8. Chemotherapeutic agents associated with diarrhoea (adapted from Panzarella et al., 2002)

Cisplatin	Cyclophosphamide	Cytarabine
Daunorubicin	Doxorubicin	Fluorouracil
Hydroxyurea	Interferon	Interleukin-2
Irinotecan	Methotrexate	Thioguanine
Topotecan		

the digestive tract may progress to obliterative vasculitis with ultimate development of ischaemia. Acute radiation injury results from the depletion of normally proliferating cells, mucosal sloughing, villi shortening, and subsequent inflammatory infiltration and oedema. The patient may suffer from odynophagia, dysphagia, abdominal pain, and/or diarrhoea, depending on the radiation site (Halperin et al., 1999).

Other Iatrogenic Cause of Diarrhoea

Medications used in the supportive care of children with cancer may also play a role in the development of diarrhoea. Antibiotics may cause alterations in the normal flora of the GI tract, resulting in diarrhoea. Other supportive care medications such as antacids, antihypertensives, antiemetics, and, especially, electrolyte supplements are associated with the condition. Frequent hospitalisation places the paediatric oncology patient at risk for institution-acquired infectious diarrhoea.

15.5.2.2 Fungal

A fungal infection is rarely the causative agent for diarrhoea.

15.5.2.3 Viral

Viruses are the most common cause of infectious diarrhoea in developing countries. Common viral aetiologies of diarrhoea include rotavirus, adenovirus, and astroviruses.

15.5.2.4 Bacterial

Bacterial aetiologies for diarrhoea in the immuno-compromised host include *Salmonella, Campylobacter, Shigella, Yersinia, Aeromonas,* and *Plesiomonas*. Children with a recent history of antibiotic therapy are at increased risk of developing pseudo-membranous colitis caused by the toxins produced by *Clostridium difficile*. This condition occurs in 0.2–10% of patients taking antibiotics (Sondeimer, 2003)

15.5.2.5 Other Infectious Aetiologies of Diarrhoea

Diarrhoea may also be secondary to a variety of parasitic infections including *Giardia, Entamoeba,* and the various tapeworm species.

15.5.3 Prevention

In the hospital setting, strict adherence to infection control practices is the most important mechanism for preventing the spread of infectious diarrhoea to the immunocompromised patient. Good handwashing techniques must be observed by all staff and families. Parent and patient education emphasising good hygiene and strategies for preventing faecal-oral contamination are critical. Safe food handling practices should be reviewed with families, including food preparation and storage. Patients should avoid contact with others suffering from gastroenteritis.

Prevention of iatrogenic causes of diarrhoea starts with patient education regarding the early detection of chemotherapy-induced diarrhoea. In regimens associated with a high incidence of chemotherapy-induced diarrhoea, families should be instructed to promptly treat diarrhoeic episodes with the prescribed antidiarrhoeal agent.

15.5.4 Treatment

The effective management of diarrhoea is directly related to its etiology. Therefore, establishing the underlying cause is the first step in effective treatment. The nurse should obtain a detailed history including stooling patterns, volume and consistency of the stools, dietary practices, medication history, travel history, and exposure to potentially infectious persons. Physical examination should focus on potential sequelae of diarrhoea, including dehydration and skin breakdown. Infectious aetiologies are investigated by sending diarrhoeic stools for bacterial, viral, and *Clostridium difficile* toxin cultures. Stools should be examined for ova and parasites.

C. difficile infections are common in the paediatric oncology patient due to the frequent use of antibiotic therapy in this patient group (Panzarella et al., 2002). Once identified, *C. difficile* is treated with oral metronidazole or vancomycin. The use of vancomycin as frontline therapy is discouraged because of concern of drug-resistant Gram-positive organisms. There is a 10–20% rate of relapse, although most patients respond to a second course with the same or alternative therapy (Alexander et al., 2002).

The treatment of viral diarrhoea is largely supportive care for the patient. Viral diarrhoea is typically a self-limiting process. *Medications directed at slowing bowel motility are contraindicated in infectious diarrhoea because they would slow the elimination of infectious pathogens.* Hospitalised patients with diarrhoea must be assumed infectious until proven otherwise and be placed under appropriate isolation practices.

Chemotherapy-related diarrhoea is most dramatically seen with the administration of irinotecan (CPT-11), a topoisomerase I inhibitor that is currently being investigated in phase 2 studies for refractory solid tumours. Diarrhoea is the major dose-limiting toxicity for this drug. (Xie et al., 2002). Prompt management of acute diarrhoea during administration of this drug is achieved with IV atropine, and loperamide is given orally for delayed diarrhoea (Ettinger et al., 2002). Irinotecan-induced diarrhoea can be very acute and result in life-threatening fluid and electrolyte imbalances. Patient education regarding loperamide administration and signs of dehydration is critical.

Management of the patient with diarrhoea focuses on preventing dehydration and electrolyte imbalances. Frequent assessment of fluid and electrolyte status and the prompt correction of alterations are necessary. In severe cases hospitalisation and intravenous rehydration are required. Families should be taught to assess for dehydration: decreased skin turgor, decreased urine output, dry mucus membranes, sunken fontanels, and alterations in activity. Careful assessment of the perianal area is indicated because diarrhoea can lead to skin breakdown and provide a portal for infection. Hygiene must be emphasised; sitz baths are good hygienic practices and can be very soothing. Barrier creams to protect the perianal area are indicated.

Nutritional support is addressed by increasing oral hydration to correct for fluid losses in the stool. Oral rehydrating solutions can help replace lost salts. Age-appropriate feedings are continued, and foods high in fat and simple sugars should be avoided.

15.5.5 Prognosis

Typically, diarrhoea will resolve with appropriate treatment where indicated and when completed in cases such as *C. difficile*. Diarrhoea of viral aetiologies is largely self-limiting. Iatrogenic causes of diarrhoea usually resolve once a sufficient interval has passed to allow the GI tract to heal. Unfortunately, chronic diarrhoea associated with pelvic and abdominal radiation or with GvHD following stem cell transplant may have a lengthy recovery process.

15.6 Typhlitis

15.6.1 Incidence

Typhlitis, or neutropenic enterocolitis, is a necrotising inflammation of the caecum and often the surrounding tissues. This life-threatening condition is seen only in the setting of neutropenia related to severe underlying disease or treatment (Sloas et al., 1993). Typhlitis is more common in leukaemia patients and is associated with high-dose steroids. Common symptoms include diarrhoea and pain in the right lower quadrant. Clinically, the patient is toxic with fever (Kamal et al., 1997). Pathologically, the process is inflammation that is usually localised to the caecum and ascending colon although the appendix may be involved. Mucosal oedema and ulceration

are present, and inflammation changes extend throughout the bowel wall, with necrosis and perforation (Kamal et al., 1997).

The incidence of clinical typhlitis varies with the type of oncology population, the aggressiveness of chemotherapy, and the prophylactic antibiotics used; however, in autopsy-based descriptive series, an incidence of up to 32% among treated leukaemics has been reported (Otaibi et al., 2002). Historically seen in patients with leukaemia and lymphoma, there is now increasing incidence in patients with solid tumours and those undergoing bone marrow transplant (King, 2002).

15.6.2 Etiology

15.6.2.1 Iatrogenic

The exact etiology of typhlitis remains uncertain, but several mechanisms have been proposed. Cytotoxic agent-induced mucosal epithelial cell necrosis and prolonged neutropenia appear to be predisposing factors (Shamberger et al., 1985). Steroids, common to many leukaemia protocols and supportive care regimens, have long been associated with typhlitis. Neutropenia acquired secondary to cancer therapy or as part of the disease process is a prerequisite for the diagnosis of typhlitis.

15.6.2.2 Fungal

Kamal et al. (1997) reported a case study of a child on antileukaemia therapy who developed typhlitis associated with a *Candida* intraluminal mass. Other fungal isolates reported include *Candida* and *Aspergillus* in 53% of post-mortem cases (Avigan et al., 1998).

15.6.2.3 Viral

In a review of the literature, a viral etiology is not described in typhlitis. Given that the treatment of viral gastrointestinal pathogens is largely supportive care, the identification of viral pathogens would not alter the management of the patient with typhlitis.

15.6.2.4 Bacterial

A bacterial infectious etiology is most common in typhlitis. In one series, *Pseudomonas* was the most common isolated species; other common isolates include *Escherichia coli, Staphylococcus aureus,* and species of *clostridia* and *Klebsiella* (Avigan et al., 1998).

15.6.3 Prevention

Typhlitis is an expected and unavoidable sequela of high-dose chemotherapy. Prevention of the morbidity secondary to this condition is directed at early detection and prompt treatment.

15.6.4 Treatment

The assessment of the patient with suspected typhlitis should include a careful history and physical examination. Blood cultures, baseline CBC, and chemistries should be obtained. Frequent nursing assessments are vital to promptly identify life-threatening complications. Careful attention must be placed on assessment for shock: frequent vital signs and attention to fluid balance and urine output. Abdominal assessment should include inspection, palpation, auscultation, and measurement of girth. Pain should be frequently assessed with a consistent age-appropriate tool. Changes in the intensity and quality of pain may be early indicators of deterioration in the patient's condition (King, 2002)

Plain film x-rays are the least sensitive tool in diagnosing neutropenic enterocolitis but may be helpful in excluding other bowel disorders such as intussusception. Perforation, obstruction, and pneumatosis can easily be seen on plain film. Ultrasound is an easy and noninvasive technique for identifying changes in caecal mucosa and can be used safely for frequent monitoring of the child with typhlitis, as radiation is not involved. CT scan is the most sensitive modality to assess caecal wall thickening (King, 2002).

The management of the patient with typhlitis is largely supportive in nature. Bowel rest, parenteral nutrition, and broad-spectrum antibiotic coverage, including coverage against anaerobes, along with continuous and careful patient assessment are generally accepted to be the standard of care. The aggressive management of cytopenias and coagulopathies is essential. Granulocyte colony stimulating factor (GCSF) may be indicated to help decrease the period of neutropenia. Surgical intervention is rarely required except in the case of intestinal perforation or clinical deterioration despite appropriate medical management (Schlatter et al., 2002)

15.6.5 Prognosis

Typhlitis was once a very grim diagnosis in the paediatric oncology patient. Fortunately, with the early detection of the condition and aggressive supportive treatment, most children survive this potentially life-threatening condition.

15.7 Perirectal Cellulitis

15.7.1 Incidence

Perirectal cellulitis involves inflammation and oedema of the perineal and rectal area. Rectal tears or fissures can lead to perirectal cellulitis in the immunocompromised patient. Perianal breakdown, constipation and the traumatic passage of hard stools, the taking of rectal temperatures, and the administration of enemas or suppositories are predisposing factors to perirectal cellulitis and must be avoided. The incidence of anorectal infections has been reported to be as high as 5% in patients receiving myeloablative chemotherapy (Segal et al., 2001). The overall incidence of perianal cellulitis has decreased in recent years because of the early use of empiric antibiotics in febrile neutropenic patients. Nonetheless, the risk for perianal cellulitis remains, especially for high-risk patients with chronic (more than 7 days) and profound (<100 cells/mm^3) granulocytopenia (Alexander et al., 2002)

15.7.2 Etiology

15.7.2.1 Iatrogenic

Iatrogenic aetiologies of perirectal cellulitis include neutropenia secondary to chemotherapy and tissue breakdown secondary to local radiation therapy. Rectal digital examination and rectal temperatures or medications are well established as predisposing factors to this condition. Constipation and the passage of hard stools may predispose the patient to rectal tears and fistulae, which can become portals of infection.

15.7.2.2 Bacterial

The most common pathogen in perianal cellulitis are aerobic Gram-negative bacilli (e.g. *P. aeruginosa, K. pneumoniae, E. coli*), enterococci, and bowel anaerobes (Alexander et al., 2002).

15.7.3 Prevention

Prompt recognition of the signs of perirectal cellulitis and prompt initiation of appropriate therapy are critical in minimising the potentially lethal sequelae of this infection. Measures to maintain the skin and tissue integrity of the perianal area may minimise the chances of infection developing. These measures include excellent hygienic practices, maintenance of soft daily bowel movements, and the avoidance of rectal manipulation (rectal temperatures, suppositories, and enemas).

15.7.4 Treatment

Patients with perirectal cellulitis may present with fever, perianal pain, painful defaecation, or constipation. On examination the perianal area is red, irritated, and inflamed, and swelling and fissures may be present. In the very neutropenic patient, localised reaction may be minimal. In fact, the area may develop increasing inflammation and pain as counts recover, representing a localised granulocyte response. Daily assessment of the perianal area is mandatory when treating neutropenic patients. Radiologic imaging of the retroperitoneum with CT scan is required if abscess is suspected.

Treatment involves broad-spectrum antibiotics to cover Gram-negative organisms and anaerobes. GCSF may be indicated to help shorten the length of the neutropenia. Intravenous pain medication may be required. Hygiene must be meticulous, and the area must be assessed frequently. Digital rectal examination must be avoided due to the risk of infection and bleeding. Sitz baths are often effective and soothing. Barrier creams should be applied to protect this area, and stool softeners must be started to help prevent constipation. Surgical consultant may be required to have an abscess drained in severe cases that fail to resolve with medical management.

15.7.5 Prognosis

With prompt diagnosis and appropriate medical management, the outcome for children with perianal cellulitis is generally good. Recovery from neutropenia is the most important prognostic indicator for a positive outcome (Segal et al., 2001).

15.8 Acute Gastrointestinal Graft Versus Host Disease

15.8.1 Incidence

Graft versus host disease (GvHD), a sequela of allogeneic stem cell transplantation, is an immune-mediated response that occurs between the donor's immunocompetent cells and the patient's immunosuppressed cells. Acute GvHD primarily involves three organ systems: the skin, the GI tract, and the liver. Acute skin GvHD is characterised by a maculopapular eruption that may range in stage 1 from a mild rash on the soles of the feet and palms of the hands to, in stage 4, a generalised rash involving over 50% of the body, with bullae formation and desquamation (Cairo, 1994). Acute liver GvHD is characterised and staged by elevations in liver functions. Acute gut GvHD is characterised by copious diarrhoea, abdominal cramping, and nausea and vomiting, and is staged by the volume of stools passed in a day. Staging and grading of gut and liver GvHD are shown in

Table 15.9. Gastrointestinal GvHD stage and grading (adapted from Gonzalez-Ryan et al., 2002)

Organ	Stage	Description
Liver	1	Bilirubin 2.0–3.0 mg/dl
	2	Bilirubin 3.1–6.0 mg/dl
	3	Bilirubin 6.1–15.0 mg/dl
	4	Bilirubin >15.1 mg/dl
Gut	1	Diarrhoea >30 ml/kg or >500 ml/day
	2	Diarrhoea >60 ml/kg or >1,000 ml/day
	3	Diarrhoea >90 ml/kg or >1,500ml/day
	4	Diarrhoea >90 ml/kg or >2,000 ml/day or severe abdominal pain and bleeding with or without ileus

Table 15.9. The diarrhoea associated with GvHD can vary from mild to copious volumes of several litres of bloody stool per day. In severe gut GvHD, whole areas of the GI tract may be denuded, with loss of epithelium similar to that observed in the skin (Gonzales-Ryan et al., 2002). The incidence of acute GvHD following allogeneic bone marrow transplant varies with the specific disease entity being treated and the degree of genetic disparity between the donor and recipient. For most diseases, including acute lymphoblastic leukaemia, acute myeloid leukaemia, chronic myeloid leukaemia, and aplastic anaemia, the incidence of GvHD is 42–53%. These incidence rates represent patients who had HLA-matched allogeneic transplants from siblings (Cairo, 1994).

Acute GvHD is a clinicopathologic syndrome of enteritis, hepatitis, and dermatitis that develops within 100 days of allogeneic haematopoietic stem cell transplant (HSCT). The effector cells are thought to be donor T-lymphocytes that recognise antigenic disparities between donor and recipient. In addition, the altered host milieu promotes the activation and proliferation of inflammatory cells, with resulting dysregulated production of inflammatory cytokines secreted by many cell types in addition to T-cells. This cytokine network may be the final common pathway for the tissue damage associated with GvHD, and this entire cascade has been described as a "cytokine storm" (Guinan et al., 2002). By definition, GvHD has an iatrogenic etiology – HSCT. However, other causes of liver or gut dysfunction/infection are common and must be ruled out in the acute transplant setting. A definitive diagnosis of GvHD can be made only by either liver or gut biopsy.

15.8.2 Prevention

Prevention is the most important part of acute GvHD treatment. Combination immunosuppressive prophylaxis with cyclosporine as the backbone of therapy has decreased the risk of acute GvHD. Other agents commonly used include tacrolimus, methotrexate, steroids, antithymocyte globulin, and mycophenolate mofetil. Regimens for GvHD prevention vary among transplant centres (Gonzalez-Ryan et al., 2002).

15.8.3 Treatment

Meticulous ongoing assessment of the patient with gut GvHD is critical, and precise measurement of stool losses and fluid balances is required. Supportive care in the acute transplant period includes fluid and electrolyte replacement of losses secondary to the diarrhoea associated with GvHD. Patients with copious diarrhoea are prone to perianal skin breakdown. Frequent assessment of skin integrity and attention to good hygiene are essential in the nursing care of these patients. Transfusion of red blood cells is often required to replace gastric blood losses. These patients will require aggressive nutritional support and pain control. The mainstay of pharmacologic management of acute GvHD is most commonly the addition of steroids (Veys, 1997).

15.8.4 Prognosis

GvHD limited to grade 1 or 2 has a 6-month post-transplant-related mortality that is equal to that of patients without GvHD. However, patients with grade 3 GvHD have a 6-month mortality of 60%, and grade 4 GvHD is almost uniformly fatal (Veys, 1997).

15.9 Chemical Hepatitis

15.9.1 Incidence

Chemical hepatitis, or reactive hepatitis, is a nonviral inflammation of the liver caused by exposure to chemical or other environmental toxins, such as chemotherapy, biotherapy, and radiation (Kemp and Witherow, 1998). The incidence of drug-induced liver disease appears to be escalating, reflecting the increasing number of new agents that have been introduced into anticancer therapy over the past several decades (Panzarella et al., 2002). Anti-inflammatory agents, antimicrobials, anticonvulsants, and other drugs used in supportive care of children with cancer may contribute to drug-induced hepatitis (see Table 15.10). The exact incidence of treatment-induced hepatotoxicity varies depending on the therapeutic and supportive care regimens used.

Typically, chemical hepatitis is identified in the routine prechemotherapy screening of the liver function enzymes alanine transaminase (ALT) and aspartate transaminase (AST). The patient may also exhibit clinical signs and symptoms of hepatitis, including jaundice, pain, fever, diaphoresis, malaise, flu-like symptoms, nausea, vomiting, anorexia, and bruising or bleeding (Panzarella et al., 2002).

15.9.2 Etiology

Other potential disorders, including infectious hepatitis and hepatic metastasis, must be excluded in order to confirm the diagnosis of chemical hepatitis. Hepatocellular dysfunction is usually caused by a direct effect of either the parent drug or a metabolite and is an acute event. Serum hepatic enzymes rise as cellular damage occurs. Fatty infiltration and cholestasis may occur as the toxic effect progresses

Table 15.10. Medications used in paediatric oncology that are associated with hepatotoxicity

Asparaginase
Methotrexate
Carmustine
Anticonvulsants
NSAIDs
Mercaptopurine
Lomustine
Vincristine
Dactinomycin
Antimicrobials
Thioguanine
Vinblastine
Doxorubicin
Idarubicin

(Weiss, 2001). There is no histological or biochemical feature that is specific to drug-induced hepatotoxicity, and no simple and safe method for diagnosing this condition.

15.9.3 Prevention

Prevention of this condition is limited to identifying and avoiding, if possible, hepatotoxic therapies. Hepatic function can affect the pharmacokinetics of antineoplastic agents and other medications and should be assessed when dosing drugs (Alexander et al., 2002)

15.9.4 Treatment

Treatment of chemical hepatitis is largely supportive in nature. Removing the causative factors of this condition is the initial step. Hepatotoxic chemotherapy and other drugs should be reduced or discontinued if possible. Total parenteral nutrition should be avoided if possible because of its potential for liver damage. Careful monitoring of liver function studies and coagulation functions is critical. Supportive care for the physical symptoms of hepatitis should be initiated. Nursing interventions include cool baths, the application of lotions, and measures to minimise pruritus. Dietary management includes a low-fat and high-carbohydrate diet.

15.9.5 Prognosis

Chemical hepatitis can be self-limiting, with liver functions returning to normal parameters once the causative agent has been removed and the liver has had a chance to heal. Unfortunately, the complications of chemical hepatitis can sometimes be chronic and can include chronic active hepatitis, cirrhosis, and a range of extrahepatic syndromes, including associated pulmonary injury and marrow compromise (Panzarella et al., 2002).

References

Aitken, T. (1992) Gastrointestinal manifestations in the child with cancer. Journal of Pediatric Oncology Nursing 9: 99–109

Alexander S, Walsh Y, Freifeld A, Pizzo P (2002) Infectious complications in pediatric cancer patients. In Pizzo P., Pollack D. (eds) Principles and Practice of Pediatric Oncology 4th edn. Lippincott Williams & Wilkins, Philadelphia, pp 1239–1284

Avigan, D., Richardson, P., Elias, A., Demetri, G., Shapriro, M., Schnippper, L. Wheller, C. (1998) Neutropenic enterocolitis as an complication of high dose chemotherapy with stem cell rescue in patients with solid tumors. Cancer 83:409–414

Baker S, Liptak G, Colletti R, Croffie J, Di Lorenzo C, Ector W, Nurko S (1999) Constipation in infants and children: Evaluation and treatment: A medical position statement of the North American Society for Pediatric Gastroenterology and Nutrition. Journal of Pediatric Gastroenterology and Nutrition 29: 612–625

Berde C, Billett A, Collins J (2002) Symptom management in supportive care In Pizzo P., Pollack D. (eds) Principles and Practice of Pediatric Oncology 4th edn. Lippincott Williams & Wilkins, Philadelphia, pp 1301–1332

Berger A, Kilroy T (2001) Oral complications. In DeVita V, Hellman S, Rosenberg S (eds) Cancer Principles & Practice of Oncology, 6th edn. Lippincott Williams & Wilkins, Philadelphia, pp 2881–2893

Cairo, M. (1994). Graft-vs-host disease: Pathophysiology and therapy. In C Pochedly (ed) Neoplastic Diseases of Childhood. Harwood; Churchill, pp. 331-346

Cheng, K., Molassiotis, A., Chang, A., Wai, W., Cheung, S. (2001). Evaluation of an oral care protocol intervention in the prevention of chemotherapy-induced oral mucositis in pediatric cancer patients. European Journal of Cancer 37(16): 2056–2063

Chin, E. (1998). A brief overview of the oral complications in pediatric oncology patients and suggested management strategies. Journal of Dentistry for Children 65(6): 468–473

Clarkson JE, Worthington HV, Eden OB (2000). Prevention of oral mucositis or oral candidiasis for patients with cancer receiving chemotherapy (excluding head and neck cancer). Cochrane Database System Review (2): CD000978

Cope D (2001) Management of chemotherapy-induced diarrhea and constipation. Nursing Clinics of North America 36 (4): 695–708

de Wit R, de Boer G, Linden G, Stoter G, Sparreboom A, Verweij J (2001) Effective cross-over to granisetron after failure to ondansetron, a randomised double blind study in patients failing ondansetron plus dexamethasone during the first 24 hours following highly emetogenic chemotherapy. British Journal of Cancer 85: 1099–1101

Dupuis L, Lau R Greenberg M (2001) Delayed nausea and vomiting in children receiving antineoplastics. Medical and Pediatric Oncology 37(1): 115–121

Ettinger A, Bond D, Sievers T (2002) Chemotherapy C. Rasco Baggott, K Patterson, D. Fochtman (eds) Nursing Care of Children and Adolescents with Cancer, 3rd edn. Saunders, Philadelphia, pp 136–173

Gonzalez-Ryan L, Kristovich K, Haugen M, Coyne K, Hubbell M (2002) Hematopoietic stem cell transplant. In Rasco-Baggott C, Patterson K, Fochtman D (eds) Nursing Care of Children and Adolescents with Cancer, 3rd edn. Philadelphia, Saunders, pp 212–256

Gralla RJ, Osoba D, Kris MG, Kirkbride P, Hesketh PJ, Chinnery LW, Clark-Snow R, Gill DP, Groshen S, Grunberg S, Koeller JM, Morrow GR, Perez EA, Silber JH, Pfister DG (1999) Recommendations for the use of antiemetics: Evidence-based, clinical practice guidelines. Journal of Clinical Oncology 17(9): 2971–2994

Guerrero R, Cavender C (1999) Constipation: physical and psychological sequelae. Pediatric Annals 28: 312–316

Guinan E, Krance R, Lehmann L (2002) Stem cell transplantation in pediatric oncology. In Pizzo P., Pollack D. (eds) Principles and Practice of Pediatric Oncology, 4th edn. Lippincott Williams & Wilkins, Philadelphia, pp 429–452

Halperin E, Constine L, Tarbell N, Kun L (1999) Late effects of cancer treatment. In Halperin E, Constine L., Tarbell N, Kun L. Kun (eds) Pediatric Radiation Oncology, 3rd edn. Lippincott, Philadelphia, pp 457–537

Kamal M, Wilkinson A, Gibson B. (1997) Radiological features of fungal typhlitis complicating acute lymphoblastic leukaemia. Pediatric Radiology 27:18–19

Kemp R, Witherow P (1998) Gastrointestinal complications. In Hockenberry-Eaton M. (ed) Essentials of Pediatric Oncology Nursing A Core Curriculum. Association of Pediatric Oncology Nurses, Glenview, IL, pp 130–138

Kennedy HF, Morrison D, Tomlinson D, Gibson BE, Bagg J, Gemmell C (2003) Gingivitis and toothbrushes: Potential roles in viridans streptococcal bacteraemia. Journal of Infection 46(1): 67–69

King N (2002) Nursing care of the child with neutropenic enterocolitis. Journal of Pediatric Oncology Nursing 19: 198–204

Kris M, Pizzo B (1997) Chemotherapy induced nausea and vomiting In Holland J., Frei E., Blast R., Kufe D., Morton D., Weichselbaum R. (eds) Cancer Medicine, 4th edn. Williams & Wilkins, Baltimore, pp 3111–3116

Minicucci E, Lopez L, Crocci A (2002) Dental abnormalities in children after chemotherapy treatment for acute lymphoid leukemia. Leukemia Research 27: 45–50

Otaibi, A., Barker, C., Anderson, R., Sigalet, D. (2002) Neutropenic enterocolitis after pediatric bone marrow transplant. Journal of Pediatric Surgery 37:770–772

Panzarella C, Rasco Baggott C, Cameau M, Duncan J, Groben V, Woods D, Stewart J (2002) Management of disease and treatment related complication. In Baggott C. Rasco, Patterson K, Fochtman D. (eds) Nursing Care of Children and Adolescents with Cancer. Saunders, Philadelphia, pp 279–318

Rogers B (2001) Mucositis in the oncology patient. Nursing Clinics of North America 36: 745–760

Roy R, Griffiths K (eds) The 2003–2004 Formulary of Drugs: The Hospital for Sick Children, 22nd edn. The Hospital for Sick Children, Toronto, pp 240–245

Schlatter M, Synder K, Freyer D (2002) Successful management of typhlitis in pediatric oncology patients. Journal of Pediatric Surgery 37(8): 1151–1155

Segal B, Walsh T, Holland S (2001) Infection in the cancer patient. In DeVita V, Hellman S, Rosenberg S (eds) Cancer Principles & Practice of Oncology, 6th edn. Lippincott Williams & Wilkins, Philadelphia, pp 2815–2868

Shamberger R, Weinstein H, Delorey M, Levey H (1985) The medical and surgical management of typhlitis in children with acute nonlymphocytic (myelogenous) leukemia. Cancer 57: 603–609

Shaw M, Kumar D, Duggal M, Fiske J, Kinsella T, Nisbet T (2000) Oral management of patients following oncology treatment: literature review. British Journal of Oral & Maxillofacial Surgery 38: 591–524

Sloas M, Flynn P, Kaste S, Patrick C (1993) Typhlitis in children with cancer: A 30-year experience. Clinical Infectious Diseases 17: 484–490

Sondheimer, J.(2003) Gastrointestinal tract. In Hay W. (ed) Current Pediatric Diagnosis and Treatment, 16th edn. McGraw-Hill Companies Stat-Ref Online Electronic Medical Library

Steinle C, Dock M (1994) Oral complications associated with chemotherapy and radiation therapy. In Pochedly C. (ed) Neoplastic Diseases of Childhood. Harwood, Churchill, pp 1303–1316

Veys P (1997) Biology and practical aspects of stem cell transplant. In Pinkerton C, Plowman P. Paediatric Oncology: Clinical Practice and Controversies, 2nd edn. Chapman & Hall Medical, London, pp 617–627

Weiss R (2001) Miscellaneous Toxicities. In DeVita V, Hellman S, S Rosenberg (eds) Cancer Principles & Practice of Oncology, 6th edn. Lippincott Williams & Wilkins, Philadelphia, pp 2970–2971

Woo S, Treister N (2001). Chemotherapy-induced oral mucositis. www.emedicine.com

Xie R, Mathijssen R, Sparreeboom A, Verweij J, Karlsson M (2002) Clinical pharmacokinetics of irinotecan and its metabolites in relation with diarrhoea. Clinical Pharmacology & Therapeutics 72: 265–275

Yaster M, Maxwell L(1993) Opioid agonists and antagonist. In Schechter N, Berde C, Yaster M (eds) Pain in infants, children and adolescents Williams & Williams, Baltimore, pp 145–172

Bone Marrow

Sandra Doyle

Contents

Table 16.1. Normal blood values (data from Lodha, 2003)

Component of blood	Lifespan	Age	Reference interval
White blood cell count (×10^9/l)	Hours to 300 days	6 days	9.0–30.0
		7–13 days	5.0–21.0
		14 days–2 months	5.0–20.0
		3–11 months	5.0–15.0
		1–4 years	5.0–12.0
		>5 years	4.0–10.0
Neutrophils (×10^9/l)	6–8 hours	1 week	1.5–10.0
		2 weeks	1.0–9.5
		3 weeks–5 years	1.5–8.5
		6–10 years	1.5–8.0
		>10 years	2.0–7.5
Hemoglobin (g/l)	120 days	6 days	150–220
		7–30 days	140–200
		1 month	115–180
		2 months	90–135
		3–11 months	100–140
		1–4 years	110–140
		5–13 years	120–160
		Female, ≥14 years	120–153
		Male, ≥14 years	140–175
Platelet cell count (×10^9/l)	7–10 days		150–400 (prevent bleeding and promote clotting)

Bone marrow suppression may occur as a result of a child's disease or treatment of the disease process. Bone marrow suppression can result in a decrease in all areas of hematopoiesis and is one of the most common dose-limiting toxicities of chemotherapy. There can be a decrease in red blood cells (RBCs), white blood cells (WBCs), and platelets. The time of most profound bone marrow suppression (nadir) occurs approximately 10–14 days after myelosuppressive treatment. Previous chemotherapy and radiation therapy can also prolong the recovery time and nadir. Table 16.1 summarizes normal values and lifespans for hemoglobin, white cells, and platelets.

16.1 Anemia

16.1.1 Incidence and Etiology

Anemia is commonly encountered in pediatric oncology patients. This is usually due to chemotherapy-related myelosuppression but can also be related to malignant infiltration of bone marrow, radiation, viral suppression, blood loss, and nonspecific processes (inhibitory effect of tumor necrosis factor, iron deficiency, or low endogenous erythropoietin) (Rizzo et al., 2003). Chemotherapy-associated anemia is characteristically an insidious and delayed complication of treatment.

16.1.2 Treatment

16.1.2.1 Transfusion

Transfusion was the traditional means of therapy into the 1990s. The usual recommended triggers for transfusion are a hemoglobin of 60–70 g/l and no signs of imminent marrow recovery, or if hemoglobin >70 g/l and the child is symptomatic (i.e., decreased energy, fatigue, pallor, headache, tachypnea, tachycardia and/or gallop, failure to take part in normal activities of daily living) (Steele, 2003). Many radiotherapists request that transfusions be given to children receiving radiation therapy to maintain hemoglobin levels >100 g/l. This is to ensure well-oxygenated cells that can best respond to radiotherapy (Panzarella et al., 2002). Transfusions normally consist of 5–15 ml/kg of packed red blood cells (PRBC), leukocyte-filtered, irradiated, and cytomegalovirus (CMV)-negative if applicable (see 16.4 Transfusion Issues) (Steele, 2003). In an emergency, whatever blood is available can be used, with blood group O rhesus-negative being the universal donor. Nursing care includes the following:

- Being vigilant to the child's need for transfusion, assessing for increasing fatigue, headache, pallor, and a decrease in normal activity level
- Communicating with healthcare team members about pertinent laboratory values and the needs for transfusion
- Monitoring the child for transfusion reactions during blood administration
- Educating family members to recognize signs and symptoms of anemia

16.1.2.2 Use of Recombinant Human Erythropoietin

Studies have explored the use of erythropoietin in a variety of oncology settings with small samples of predominantly adult patients (Rizzo et al., 2002). Before embarking on a trial of erythropoietin in children, it is important to correct other causes of anemia. Healthcare team members should take a thorough drug history; consider iron, folate, and B12 deficiency; and access for occult blood losses (i.e., collection of stool specimens). The use of erythropoietin for children, particularly those with religious objections to blood transfusions, is a treatment option for patients with chemotherapy-associated anemia and a hemoglobin concentration >100 g/l (Rizzo et al., 2002). The recommended starting dose is 150 units/kg, subcutaneously, three times weekly for a minimum of 4 weeks. If this does not improve hemoglobin values, the dose is usually escalated to 300 units/kg, subcutaneously, three times weekly for an additional 4–8 weeks. A rise of hemoglobin of at least 2 g/l per week has been seen with this dosing

regimen (Thatcher et al., 1999). Nurses will need to assess the family's learning needs with regard to acquiring the skills necessary to administer subcutaneous injections. Involvement of community nurses is often necessary in order to support families as they develop these new skills.

16.2 Neutropenia

16.2.1 Incidence and Etiology

Leukopenia is a decrease in the absolute number of WBCs, whereas neutropenia is a decrease in the number of neutrophils that fight infection. Neutropenia is a feature of hematological and malignant diseases and arises secondary to immunological disorders, infectious diseases, and drugs. Neutrophil levels are lower in some ethnic groups including Africans, African-Americans, and Yemenite Jews (Dale, 2003). The relative risk of infection is determined by the absolute neutrophil count (ANC), calculated as total WBC count × neutrophils (% polys + % bands). Children with severe neutropenia, ANC <0.5×10^9/l, are at risk for life-threatening infections that may be bacterial, fungal, or viral (Panzarella et al., 2002).

Although bacteria account for most infections in immunocompromised children, prophylactic strategies to combat all types of infections are important. Measures such as careful handwashing before and after patient contact, vigilance in detecting potentially transmissible diseases (respiratory viruses, varicella zoster) and knowledge about the specific susceptibilities of the immunocompromised host are all important when caring for neutropenic children (Pizzo and Mueller, 1998).

16.2.1.1 Fever (Pyrexia) and Neutropenia

Fever in the neutropenic child must always be treated as an emergency, and therapy must be initiated promptly. Fever is regularly defined as temperature >38°C orally. There is a risk of morbidity with febrile neutropenia, and 10–20% of febrile neutropenic children have bacteremia on presentation. Patients who have received a bone marrow transplant within the previous 12 months should be considered neu-

Table 16.2. Common problems associated with fever and neutropenia

Source of the problem	Common infectious problem	Predominant organisms
Central venous devices, Ommaya reservoirs	Bacteremia	Gram-positive (coagulase-negative staphylococci) and enteric bacteria. *Corynebacterium jelkelum*
	Localized skin infections	*Corynebacterium spp.*, mycobacterium (*M. chelonei, M. fortuitum*), *Aspergillus spp.*
Skin or mucosa breakdown	Mucositis, esophagitis	Bacterial, viral, and fungal pathogens
	Bacteremia	α-hemolytic streptococci, gram-positive and gram-negative bacteria
	Enterocolitis	*Clostridium difficile*
Neutropenia	Bacteremia, sepsis	Coagulase-negative staphylococci, *Staph. aureus*, α-hemolytic streptococci, enterococci, *Bacillus spp.*, *Escherichia coli, Klebsiella spp., Pseudomonas spp., Enterobacter spp., Citrobacter, Serratia, Acinetobacter spp., Clostridium spp.*
	Localized fungal infections	*Candida albicans, Aspergillus spp., Mucor*
	Fungemia	*Candida spp.*

tropenic regardless of full/complete blood cell (FBC/CBC) result (Steele, 2003). Commonly associated infectious problems are listed in Table 16.2 (Hann, 1999).

16.2.2 Treatment

The management of a patient with fever and neutropenia should include the following:

- Instruct parents to monitor temperature and have a thermometer in the home
- Teach parents to understand their child's ANC and be aware of current ANC levels
- Instruct families not to give antipyretics for fever unless instructed by the treating team
- Instruct families to seek medical attention in the event of fever
- Maintain ABCs if cardiorespiratory instability is present
- Take a thorough history and do a physical examination with special attention to
  - Mucosa and perioral areas
  - Skin and indwelling catheters
  - Lungs
  - Perirectal areas
  - Any subtle sign of inflammation on the body

- Draw CBC and differential
- Draw blood cultures from periphery, and culture any indwelling catheter from each lumen of the catheter. If the child has an Ommaya reservoir and fever, obtain cerebrospinal fluid for cultures
- If ANC >500, treat with appropriate antibiotics if any infectious source is identified from history and physical
- If ANC <500, promptly start broad-spectrum antibiotics. If the child has an indwelling catheter, rotate administration of antibiotics through each lumen
- Monitor the child closely for secondary infections requiring modification of initial therapy; obtain cultures daily as long as the child is febrile and if newly febrile. If the child has a positive blood culture, cultures should be repeated daily until results are negative
- Avoid rectal temperatures, enemas, and suppositories while the patient is profoundly neutropenic

(Steele, 2003; Pizzo and Mueller, 1998; Kline, 2002; Panzarella et al., 2002)

16.2.2.1 Antibiotic Management

The standard approach to managing febrile neutropenia has been a combination antibiotic regimen. Practitioners should be aware of local bacterial organisms' susceptibilities and their institution's guidelines regarding appropriate drug coverage, toxicities of therapies, and cost differences. The first regimens with acceptable efficacy included aminoglycoside/alpha-lactam combinations. The advent of broad-spectrum alpha-lactam antibiotics with a wide spectrum of bactericidal activity have made monotherapies another option for treating febrile neutropenic children. Third-generation cephalosporins (ceftazidime) and carbapenems (imipenem) have excellent activity against *Pneumocystis aeruginosa* and are also effective for the initial management of febrile children (Pizzo, 1993; Hughes et al., 1990).

An example of an antibiotic regimen for febrile neutropenic children follows:

- Broad-spectrum coverage: piperacillin/tazobactam 80 mg/k/dose intravenously (IV) every 8 hours (maximum 4-g single dose) and gentamicin 2.5 mg/k dose IV every 8 hours (maximum 20 mg/dose before serum monitoring)
- Children with piperacillin allergy have a limited choice of antibiotics for treatment of fever and may require consultation with a specialist in infectious diseases
  - Because there is an incidence of cross-reactivity between penicillins and cephalosporins, one treatment regimen is ciprofloxacin 10 mg/kg/dose IV every 12 hours (maximum 400 mg/dose) and tobramycin and clindamycin 8 mg/kg/dose every 8 hours (maximum 600 mg/dose)
- Antibiotics specifically directed toward identified organisms should be added to broad-spectrum coverage, but broad-spectrum coverage should not be replaced by specific antibiotics alone in neutropenic patients
- Antibiotic therapeutic drug level monitoring should be done as appropriate, especially if the child is receiving other concurrent nephrotoxic drugs (amphotericin, acyclovir); follow renal function closely

- Children who deteriorate clinically should be switched to meropenem 20 mg/kg/dose IV (maximum 1 g/dose) and tobramycin and vancomycin 15 mg/kg/dose IV every 6 hours (maximum 1 g/dose)
- Persistent fever or recurrent fever without other signs of clinical deterioration is not a reason to change initial broad-spectrum therapy
- Consider adding amphotericin after 5–7 days of persistent fever after a fungal work-up has been initiated (sinus, chest, and abdominal CT scan)
- Duration of therapy:
  - Afebrile, ANC >500, cultures negative at 48 hours: discontinue antibiotics
  - Afebrile, ANC <500, cultures negative at 48 hours, IV antibiotics >48 hours: consider discontinuing antibiotics
  - Afebrile, ANC >500, cultures positive: consider discontinuing broad-spectrum antibiotics but continue with specific therapy
- Discharge management:
  - No antibiotic therapy is recommended on discharge for those who meet the following criteria:
    1. Negative blood cultures
    2. Afebrile for a minimum of 24 hours
    3. Fever no longer than 96 hours
    4. Clinically well
    5. Evidence of marrow recovery with increasing monocytes, neutrophils, or platelet count
  - Avoid routine use of oral antibiotics when discharging children unless there is a localized site of infection that may require specific therapy
  - Those who should remain in the hospital for IV therapy include
    1. Children on induction therapy for malignancy known to significantly involve the bone marrow
    2. Those with known or suspected noncompliance
    3. Those with clinical sepsis at presentation
  - Encourage families to strictly adhere to follow-up
  - Recurrence of fever should be approached as a new fever in neutropenic hosts and requires immediate reevaluation (Steele, 2006)

16.2.2.2 Special Consideration for the Management of Indwelling Intravenous Catheters

Gram-positive bacterial infections, especially staphylococci, are the most frequent cause of catheter-related infection (Ingram et al., 1991; Riikonen, 1993). It is important to culture all lumina of an intravascular device and to administer antibiotic therapy through all lumina as well. Most simple catheter-related bacteremia and exit-site infections can be cleared by appropriate antibiotic therapy and do not require removal of the device. However, should bacteremia persist after 48 hours of appropriate therapy or if the child shows signs of a tunnel infection, consideration should be given to removing the device. Failure of therapy is most common when infections are due to organisms such as *Candida albicans* and *Bacillus* species (Pizzo and Mueller, 1998).

16.2.2.3 Management of Candidiasis (Oropharyngeal Candidiasis and Candida Esophagitis)

Neutropenic children are prone to developing oropharyngeal or esophageal candidiasis, or thrush (Walsh and Pizzo, 1988). Thorough mouth care can be a challenge in the pediatric population. Encourage use of soft toothbrushes and frequent mouth rinses, and inspect the oral cavity for signs of infection. Creamy white patches on the mucosal surfaces, which may be friable and bleed easily when scratched, are typical for thrush. It can be hard to distinguish between mucositis caused by chemotherapy and *Candida albicans*. *Candida albicans* causes most of the infections (50–60%) (American Academy of Pediatrics, 2003).

Antifungal agents for the treatment of oropharyngeal or esophageal candidiasis include oral nonabsorbent agents such as nystatin or clotrimazole; oral systemic absorbable agents such as ketoconazole, itraconazole; and fluconazole; and intravenous fluconazole or amphotericin B (Walsh, 1993). Intravenous agents are often used when the neutropenic child is unable to swallow. Amphotericin B is administered for a minimum of 5 days in the neutropenic child and preferably until neutropenia is resolved. Prophylaxis is not recommended routinely for immunocompromised children (American Academy of Pediatrics, 2003).

16.2.2.4 Infections Due to *Aspergillus* Species

Invasive aspergillosis occurs almost exclusively in immunocompromised children with prolonged neutropenia induced by cytotoxic chemotherapy. These infections usually involve pulmonary, sinus, cerebral, or cutaneous sites. The hallmark of invasive aspergillosis is angioinvasion with resulting thrombosis, dissemination to other organs, and occasionally erosion of the blood vessel wall with hemorrhage (American Academy of Pediatrics, 2003). *Aspergillus* species are ubiquitous molds that grow on decaying vegetation and in the soil. The principle route of transmission is by inhalation, and nosocomial outbreaks can occur in susceptible hosts where exposure to a probable source of fungus has occurred, such as a nearby construction site or faulty ventilation. *Aspergillus* is diagnosed from biopsy specimens of a variety of body tissues and is rarely diagnosed from the blood (American Academy of Pediatrics, 2003).

Treatment of choice is amphotericin B in high doses (1.0–1.5 mg/kg/day). Therapy is continued for 4–12 weeks or longer. Lipid formulations of amphotericin B should be considered in children who cannot tolerate conventional amphotericin B due to renal toxicities or severe reaction. Voriconazole has been licensed for treatment of invasive aspergillosis in adults, but its safety and efficacy have not been established in children (American Academy of Pediatrics, 2003).

16.2.2.5 Management of Viral Infections

Herpes simplex, varicella-zoster, and cytomegaloviruses are the most commonly occurring viral infections in immunocompromised children. Table 16.3 outlines the clinical manifestations, etiology, diagnostic tests, and treatments for these viral diseases.

Table 16.3. Typical viral infections and suggested management (data from American Academy of Pediatrics, 2003; Pizzo and Mueller, 1998)

Viral infection	Clinical manifestations	Etiology	Diagnostic tests	Treatments
Herpes simplex (HSV)	Severe local lesions, disseminated HSV infection with generalized vesicular skin lesions and visceral involvement	Double-stranded DNA virus, transmitted from people who are symptomatic or asymptomatic through direct contact with infected lesions or secretions	Readily grown in culture obtained from skin vesicles, mouth, or nasopharynx, eyes, urine, blood, or stool	IV acyclovir for treatment and prevention of mucocutaneous infections; topical acyclovir may also accelerate healing; contact precautions are advised
Varicella-zoster	Generalized, pruritic, vesicular rash with mild fever; progressive severe varicella with encephalitis, hepatitis; pneumonia can develop; incidence of pneumonitis is up to 30% with mortality in nearly 1/3 of these children	Member of herpes virus family; highly contagious and spread through contact with mucosa of the upper respiratory tract; person-to-person transmission by airborne spread from respiratory secretions; incubation period is 10–21 days after contact	Vesicular scraping and fluid from lesions	IV antiviral therapy with acyclovir within 24 hours or onset of rash; utilize standard airborne isolation precautions; post-exposure immunization of VZIG within 96 hours; dose 125 units/10 kg body wt to a maximum of 625 units IM
Cytomegalo-viruses (CMV)	Interstitial pneumonitis, gastrointestinal infections such as mouth sores, esophagitis, colitis, and retinitis	Transmitted by person-to-person contact with secretions and via transfusions of blood, platelets, and WBCs from previously infected people; virus persists in latent form after primary infection and reactivates particularly under conditions of immunosuppression	Development of serum immunoglobulin IgM CMV-specific antibody; virus can also be isolated in cell cultures from areas of CMV infection	Ganciclovir and CMV-immune globulin IV has been used to treat retinitis caused by CMV infections; foscarnet and valganciclovir have been used in adult patients but have not been studied in children; good hand hygiene for prevention of spread; CMV antibody-negative donor blood and platelets, removal of buffy coat or filtration to remove WBCs

16.2.2.6 Infections Due to *Pneumocystis jiroveci* (Formerly *Pneumocystis carinii*)

Pulmonary infections with *Pneumocystis jiroveci* have in the past been a major problem in children with malignancies (Leibovitz et al., 1990). Infants and children develop a characteristic diffuse pneumonitis with dyspnea at rest, tachypnea, oxygen desaturation, nonproductive cough, and fever. Intensity of symptoms may vary, and in some immunocompromised children the onset can be acute and fulminant. Chest x-rays often show bilateral diffuse interstitial or alveolar disease. The mortality rate in immunocompromised children ranges from 5% to 40% if treated and approaches 100% if untreated (American Academy of Pediatrics, 2003). Diagnostic tests in children include bronchoscopy with broncheoalveolar lavage, sputum samples in older children, intubation with deep endotracheal aspiration, and open lung or transbronchial biopsies.

The drug of choice for treatment is intravenous trimethoprim-sulfamethoxazole (trimethoprim 15–20 mg/kg/day and sulfamethoxazole 75–100 mg/kg/daily every 6 hours). Intravenous pentamidine (4 mg/kg/day once daily) is an alternative for children who cannot tolerate or do not respond to trimethoprim-sulfamethoxazole. A minimum duration of 2 weeks of therapy is recommended (American Academy of Pediatrics, 2003: 501).

Prophylaxis for *Pneumocystis* includes

- Trimethoprim-sulfamethoxazole (trimethoprim 150 mg/m^2 per day, sulfamethoxazole 750 mg/m^2 per day) orally in divided doses twice a day, three times per week on consecutive days
- Alternatives include the following:
  - Trimethoprim 150 mg/m^2 per day, sulfamethoxazole 750 mg/m^2 per day orally as a single daily dose, three times per week on consecutive days
  - Trimethoprim 150 mg/m^2 per day, sulfamethoxazole 750 mg/ m^2 per day orally in divided doses, 7 days of the week
- Alternative regimens if trimethoprim-sulfamethoxazole is not tolerated:
  - Dapsone (children ≥1 month of age) 2 mg/kg orally once a day

- Aerosolized pentamidine (children ≥5 years of age) 300 mg administered via inhaler (American Academy of Pediatrics, 2003).

16.2.2.7 Use of Colony Stimulating Factors (CSF) in Children with Neutropenia

Most children treated for cancer are treated on clinical research protocols. Chemotherapy for pediatric patients tends to be more intensive, and myelosuppression is more frequent and severe in the pediatric population. Infants receiving chemotherapy are at a particular risk for neutropenic morbidity because of the immaturity of their hematopoietic and immune systems. These factors combine to increase the incidence of febrile neutropenia in children and the potential for life-threatening infections. The use of CSFs in the pediatric population is largely determined by the requirements of research protocols (Ozer et al., 2000). A recent review of practices by the Pediatric Oncology Group (Parsons et al., 2000) revealed that

- Primary prophylaxis with CSFs was common and guided by the anticipated duration of neutropenia (>7 days)
- Primary prophylaxis is not uniform across protocols or diseases
- Practices are influenced by physician preference
- Reduction in chemotherapy dosage is rarely selected as an alternative to the use of CSFs
- The majority of pediatric oncologists used CSFs in children who had complicated illnesses with frequent febrile neutropenia; however, they would not use CSFs in uncomplicated fever and neutropenia
- CSF doses are 5 mcg/kg/day for G-CSF (filgrastim) and 250 mcg/m^2 for GM-CSF (sargramostim) subcutaneously.

16.2.2.8 Isolation

Reverse isolation (i.e., placing the patient in a single room and requiring healthcare personnel to wear gowns, masks, and gloves) after the onset of neutropenia will not necessarily prevent infection. This is because most of the organisms that infect patients arise from the patient's endogenous flora (Pizzo, 1989). However, the use of total protective environments can reduce infection in the profoundly neutropenic child, such as one who has just received a bone marrow transplant (Pizzo and Mueller, 1998). These protective measures include a high-efficiency particulate air (HEPA)-filtered laminar air flow room; an aggressive program of surface cleaning; use of sterile objects within the patient room; and a bacterially-reduced diet (no fresh fruits or vegetables, no fast or restaurant foods, completely and thoroughly cooked foods).

16.3 Thrombocytopenia

16.3.1 Incidence and Etiology

Thrombocytopenia in children is usually due to myelosuppression from chemotherapy or malignancy. The risk of spontaneous hemorrhage increases when platelets fall below $10\times10^9/l$ (Steele, 2003).

16.3.2 Treatment

Prophylactic platelet transfusions are administered to children with thrombocytopenia resulting from impaired bone marrow function to reduce the risk of hemorrhage when platelets fall below a predefined level, such as $10\times10^9/l$. This threshold can vary according to the child's diagnosis, clinical condition, and treatment modality. Platelets for transfusion can be prepared either by separation of units of platelet concentrations from whole blood, which is pooled before administration, or by aphaeresis from single donors. Studies have shown that the post-transfusion increments, hemostatic benefits, and side effects are similar with either product. In most centers pooled platelets are less costly to obtain (Schiffer et al., 2000). Single donor platelets from selected donors are reserved for histocompatible platelet transfusions (see 16.4.4 Platelet Refractoriness).Transfusions may be necessary at higher levels in

- Newborns
- Patients with signs of hemorrhage, high fever, hyperleukocytosis, rapid fall of platelet count, or coagulation abnormalities

- Patients undergoing invasive procedures – ensure that the platelet count $>50\times10^9/l$ for minimally invasive procedures such as lumbar puncture and $80–100\times10^9/l$ for surgery (Schiffer et al., 2000)

When platelet transfusion is necessary, 1 unit/5 kg of pooled platelets to a maximum of 5–6 units is normally prescribed

Patient safety should be ensured when platelets are low. Instruction should include avoiding activities that can cause injury when platelet counts fall below 50×10^9, cleaning teeth with a soft toothbrush; wearing protective equipment such as a bike helmet, and avoiding contact sports, diving, horseback riding, and other activities that could potentially lead to serious injury. Families should be educated in the proper method to stop nosebleeds or other profuse bleeding. Maintaining soft stools and avoiding rectal temperatures, enemas, or suppositories when platelet counts are low should prevent perirectal injury. Advice should include avoiding over-the-counter medications containing ibuprofen or aspirin, as well as Pepto-Bismol and Alka-Seltzer (Panzarella et al., 2002).

16.4 Transfusion Issues

16.4.1 Granulocyte Transfusions

In the 1970s and 1980s, several studies investigated the use of granulocyte transfusions in neutropenic patients. A comprehensive review by Strauss (1994) demonstrated that there is no benefit in the prophylactic administration of granulocyte transfusions. Enthusiasm for the use of granulocyte transfusions has decreased for the following reasons:

- Granulocyte preparations are difficult to prepare and cannot be stored
- Infusions have been associated with severe pulmonary reactions, especially in patients concurrently receiving amphotericin B
- Survival from septic episodes is much improved with early introduction of antibiotic treatment and the availability of better antibiotics

- Use of GSFs to prevent prolonged periods of neu-tropenia (Hume, 1999). Currently, granulocyte transfusions are reserved for patients with profound neutropenia not expected to recover, in whom severe bacterial infection has been documented and who are clinically deteriorating despite optimal antibiotic therapies (Strauss, 1994; Chanock and Gorlin, 1996).

16.4.2 Transfusion-associated Graft-Verses-Host Disease

Graft versus host disease (GvHD), which results from the engraftment of immunocompetent donor T-lymphocytes into a recipient whose immune system is unable to reject them, is a recognized risk of blood transfusions. Almost all cellular blood components have been implicated in reported cases of transfusion-associated (TA)-GvHD. The threshold of number of viable cells necessary to produce a graft-versus-host reaction will vary depending upon the host's immune status as well as the antigenic similarity or disparity between donor and host histocompatibility antigens (Luban et al., 1999).

GvHD following blood transfusions generally manifests as an acute syndrome, the onset typically occurring within 4–30 days of transfusion. The initial clinical symptoms include a high fever occurring 8–10 days after the transfusion, appearance of a central maculopapular rash that follows the fever by 24–48 hours, the rash's spread to the extremities, and in severe cases, the rash's progression to a generalized desquamation (Vogelsang and Hess, 1994). Diagnosis of TA-GvHD is usually based on the clinical presentation and histological findings on skin biopsy. TA-GvHD has been reported in children with hematological malignancies and solid tumors who have received cytotoxic chemotherapy, radiation treatment, or both (Greenbaum, 1991).

Because the treatment of TA-GvHD is almost always ineffective, efforts have focused on preventing and minimizing the risks by reducing or inactivating transfused donor lymphocytes. The methods available in blood banks to physically remove T-lymphocytes include washing or filtering blood products (Vogelsang and Hess, 1994). Current leukocyte reduc-tion filters can achieve a three-log reduction in leukocyte contents of blood components. This reduction is not sufficient to prevent TA-GvHD. Inactivation of transfused lymphocytes by alpha-irradiation of blood components remains the most effective method for prevention of TA-GvHD. The current dose of irradiation is 25 Gy, and the effects of this dose on platelet and other cell viability are not clinically significant (Luban et al., 1999).

16.4.3 Cytomegalovirus and Transfusions

Cytomegalovirus (CMV) belongs to the herpes family and is harbored in WBCs. From 30–70% of blood donors are CMV-seropositive, although there can be a great deal of regional differences due to donor demographics such as age, sex, race, and socioeconomic status (Luban et al., 1999). Primary infections occur in a seronegative recipient of blood products from a donor who is actively or latently infected (Gunter and Luban, 1996). There is a wide clinical spectrum associated with post-transfusion CMV. CMV infections may be asymptomatic and discovered by serologic tests, or they may produce significant morbidity and mortality (Sayer et al., 1992).

16.4.3.1 Treatment

The use of IgG-seronegative blood products is considered to be the gold standard. The availability of these products, however, is dependent upon the characteristics of the donor pool and may not be available in some areas (Luban et al., 1999). Because the virus is carried in WBCs, manipulation that can reduce or attenuate leukocyte cell numbers should reduce the risk of transmission. These methods include washing, freezing followed by washing, and filtration with third-generation leukocyte-depletion filters (Przepiorka et al., 1996). Recommendations based on the American Association of Blood Banks (1997, Bulletin 97–2) are included in Table 16.4.

Table 16.4. CMV prophylaxis and transfusion therapy (*LR* leukocyte-reduced; data from Chalmers and Gibson, 1999; Hambleton and George, 2003)

Type of patient	Clinical circumstance	CMV-seronegative blood	LR blood; CMV unscreened
Patients who receive chemotherapy that produces severe immunosuppression	CMV-positive patient	Not indicated	LR blood to prevent viral reactivation
	CMV-negative patient	Either CMV-negative or LR blood	Either CMV-negative or LR blood
Patients receiving allogeneic or auto-logous progenitor cell transplants	CVM-positive recipient	Not indicated	LR blood to prevent viral reactivation
	CMV-negative recipient of a CVM-positive donor	Either CMV-negative or LR blood	Either CMV-negative or LR blood

16.4.4 Platelet Refractoriness

The response to a platelet transfusion, known as the corrected platelet count increment (CCI), is determined by using the following formula:

$$CCI = \frac{\left[\left(\text{Post transfusion - pretransfusion}\right)\text{platelet count}\left(\times 10^9\right)\right]}{\text{Number of platelets transfused}\left(\times 10^9\right)}$$

In general, a platelet transfusion is considered successful if the CCI is $>7.5\times 10^9$ within 10–60 minutes of a transfusion and $>5.0\times 10^9$ if measured 18–24 hours after transfusion (Hume, 1999). Because most centers do not routinely obtain platelet counts of the infused product, a rough estimate of an absolute platelet increment is 3,500/m²/unit for children. Refractoriness to platelet transfusion is defined as a consistently inadequate response to platelet transfusion on two separate transfusions of adequate numbers of platelets. Refractoriness can be due to immune (presence in the recipient of HLA- or platelet-specific alloantibodies) or nonimmune causes (treatment with amphotericin B, vancomycin, or ciprofloxacillin, fever, splenomegaly, disseminated intravascular coagulation, and bone marrow transplant) (Alcorta et al., 1996).

16.4.4.1 Treatment

Management of a child who is refractory to random donor platelet transfusions includes first obtaining ABO-identical platelets for the child. Second, platelets should be as fresh as possible. When HLA alloimmunization is the cause of refractoriness, HLA-matched platelets should be used (Slichter, 1990; Engelfriet et al., 1997).

It is important to note that some children may lose their antibodies over time and can again become responsive to random donor platelet transfusions (Murphy et al., 1987). The management of alloimmunized children who do not respond to interventions can be difficult. It is likely to be of no benefit to administer prophylactic platelets and instead one should administer platelets only in the presence of clinically significant bleeding (Hume, 1999). The administration of intravenous immunoglobulin may improve post-transfusion platelet increments but does not increase platelet survival (Kicker, 1990).

16.5 Disseminated Intravascular Coagulation

Disseminated intravascular coagulation (DIC) is a common acquired coagulopathy that is almost always acute and related to a generalized disorder in children. It results from disordered regulation of normal coagulation and is characterized by excess thrombin generation with secondary activation of the fibrinolytic system (Chalmers and Gibson, 1999).

Table 16.5. Conditions associated with disseminated intravascular coagulation

Infections	Metabolic disorders	Tumors	Others
Bacteremia (meningococcus, streptococcus) Viremia (varicella, CMV) Fungemia	Hypotension Hypoxia Hyper/hypothermia	Tumor lysis syndrome Acute promyelocytic, myelomonocytic, or monocytic leukemias	Liver diseases Intravascular hemolysis (ABO incompatibility)

16.5.1 Etiology and Manifestation

Infection is the most common cause of DIC in children. Bacterial infections predominate, but viruses, systemic fungal infections, malaria, and the viral hemorrhagic fevers can trigger DIC. Many bacterial agents can trigger a consumptive coagulopathy; however, meningococcal meningitis remains one of the most frequent causes of severe DIC in children (Chalmers and Gibson, 1999). Table 16.5 outlines common causes of DIC.

Any of these diverse diseases can lead to pathological activation of the coagulation system via the contact system, which follows endothelial injury, or via the tissue factor pathway following release of tissue factor. Figure 16.1 outlines a simplified pathway of blood coagulation

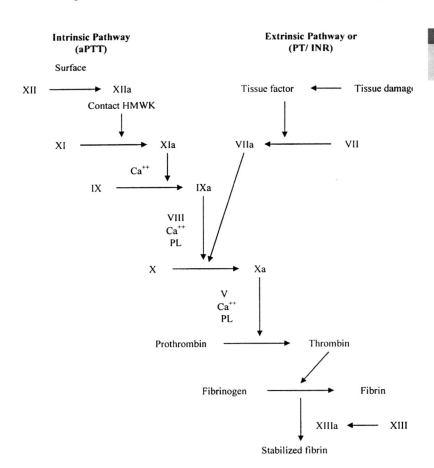

Figure 16.1

The pathway of blood coagulation (data from Shamsah, 2003)

Once the coagulation system has been activated and DIC is triggered, the pathophysiology is basically the same regardless of the underlying etiology. Following activation, both thrombin and plasmin circulate systemically. Thrombin converts fibrinogen to fibrin, which then polymerizes. This is associated with the consumptions of procoagulant proteins and platelets. Fibrin deposits lead to microvascular and sometimes large vessel thrombosis, with impaired perfusion and subsequent organ damage. Coagulation inhibitors also become depleted as thrombin continues to be generated. Circulating plasmin results in the generation of fibrin deregulation products, which interfere with fibrin polymerization and platelet function, leading to hemorrhagic problems (Bick, 1994; Bick, 1996).

Hemorrhage is the most obvious manifestation of DIC, although spontaneous bruising, purpura, oozing from venipunctures, and bleeding from surgical wounds or trauma sites are all common (Chalmers and Gibson, 1999).

16.5.1.1 Diagnosis

The diagnosis of DIC is based on both procoagulant and fibrinolytic activation with concomitant inhibitor consumption (Chuansumrit et al., 1993). Fulminant DIC is characterized by prolonged prothrombin time, activated partial thromboplastin time, and thrombin clotting time, combined with thrombocytopenia and increased fibrin regulatory products (Chalmers and Gibson, 1999).

16.5.2 Treatment

Because DIC is always a secondary phenomenon, the most important aspect of management is treating the underlying cause. Almost all aspects of DIC management are controversial, and there has been no clear evidence supporting how to best manage this event (Chalmers and Gibson, 1999). Blood product replacement is still a major component of most treatment strategies. The choice of product – fresh frozen plasma (10–15 mg/kg body weight every 8 hours), cryoprecipitate, platelets (1 unit/5 kg body weight), or fibrinogen concentrate (1 bag/5 kg body weight), and

PRBCs as required – the timing of administration, and the efficacy of treatment are unclear (Shamsah, 2003).

Nursing interventions include

- Monitoring the patient for bleeding (observe skin for color and petechiae, monitoring potential sites of bleeding including mucosa, sclera, esophagus, joints, and intestine) and assessing tissue perfusion
- Ensuring adequate circulation and oxygenation
- Evaluating mental status to monitor for intracranial bleeding (Wilson, 2002)

Prognosis has improved over the last 20 years because of advances in supportive care, including improved antibiotics, antifibrinolytic therapy, and platelet transfusions (Kitchens, 1995).

16.6 Septic Shock

Septic shock is a systematic response to pathogenic microorganisms in the blood (Brown, 1994). Children who have a compromised immune system from diseases such as human immunodeficiency virus (HIV), asplenia, or cancer chemotherapy have the greatest risk of developing septic shock. Fever is the first symptom of possible sepsis; however, the febrile neutropenic child will frequently not demonstrate clinical symptoms of sepsis until after the initiation of antibiotic therapy (Bruce and Grove, 1992).

16.6.1 Etiology

As bacteria die they release endotoxins into the bloodstream that interfere with the uptake and transportation of oxygen, leading to decreased tissue perfusion, cellular hypoxia, and cell death (Ackerman, 1994). Sixty percent of all septic episodes in neutropenic cancer patients are from gram-positive organisms; however, the organisms involved in septic shock are usually gram-negative and often arise from endogenous flora (Lange et al., 1997; Rubin and Ferraro, 1993). Septic shock can be defined as circulatory dysfunction, or a(reduction of 40 mmHg from baseline systolic blood pressure despite fluid resuscitation, leading to insufficient delivery of oxygen and nutrients to meet tissue needs. Compensated shock occurs when vital organ perfusion is maintained via endogenous compensatory mechanisms, whereas decompensated shock occurs when compensatory mechanisms have failed, and it results in hypotension and impaired tissue perfusion (Metha and MacPhee, 2003). Risk factors include age (infants are at greater risk due to decreased production of T-lymphocytes), ANC <0.1×10^9/l, prolonged neutropenia, breaks in the integrity of the skin and mucous membranes, invasive devices such as central venous lines and Ommaya reservoirs, malnutrition, and asplenism (Ackerman et al., 1994; Ellerhost-Ryan, 1993).

16.6.2 Treatment

Treatment initially focuses on maintaining cardiovascular volume and blood pressure by administering hyperhydration, vasopressors, and blood and coagulation products. Interventions to support the respiratory system include keeping O_2 saturation >90% or PaO_2 >60 mmHg. Hemodynamic support interventions include

- Isotonic crystalloid (0.9% saline or Ringer's lactate) 20 ml/kg bolus, then assess for response (heart and respiratory rate, capillary refill, sensorium, urine output); may repeat once or twice
- If not simple hypovolemia, consider early use of inotropes such as dopamine or epinephrine
- If hypovolemic and some response to fluids has occurred, consider isotonic colloid (5% or 25% albumin, dextran) or blood products
- Further boluses of 20 ml/kg as needed; central venous pressure monitoring
- May need to increase contractility and afterload, avoiding the use of large amounts of fluids in distributive or cardiogenic shock
  - Correct pH and other substrate abnormalities
  - NAHCO$_3$ (sodium bicarbonate) if pH still <7.2
  - Glucose infusions; ensure that calcium and other electrolytes are normal (Metha and MacPhee, 2003)

Investigations include full/complete blood count, platelets, coagulation screen, arterial blood gas (ABG), electrolytes, glucose, urea, creatinine, calcium, lactate, and liver functions. Blood cultures should be drawn followed by immediate administration of IV antibiotics; cross-match should be drawn if needed; and chest radiography and a septic work-up should be done if needed. Vital signs should be completed at least every 5–15 minutes, including blood pressures, pulse oximetry for O_2 saturation monitoring, and continuous cardiac monitoring. Bladder catheterization for urine output monitoring should be completed as well as an ABG if oximetry is unavailable (Metha and MacPhee, 2003; Wilson, 2002).

16.6.3 Prognosis

Prognosis depends on the nature of the infectious organism, timely initiation of treatments, and the individual's response to the therapy. In the past 2 decades, the mortality for infections from gram-negative organisms in the profoundly neutropenic child has dropped from 80% to 40% with the prompt initiation of empiric antibiotics in the event of fever (Lange et al., 1997).

16.7 Immune Suppression

The effector cells of the immune response include polymorphonuclear leukocytes (PMN), T-lymphocytes, B-lymphocytes, natural killer cells, peripheral blood monocytes, and fixed tissue macrophages including the cells of the spleen and reticuloendothelial system. Cancer or therapy-mediated immune dysfunction most severely affects PMPs, monocytes, and lymphocytes, whereas the cells of the reticuloendothelial system are relatively less sensitive to the effects of antineoplastic therapy (Alexander et al., 2002).

16.7.1 Polymorphonuclear Leukocytes

Susceptibility to infections in children receiving chemotherapy is related to the number of circulating neutrophils. The more profound and protracted the neutropenia, the greater the likelihood of a serious infection. Persistent neutropenia lasting more than 1 week is associated with increasing risk for recurrent or new infections (Bodey et al, 1966). Neutropenia can be secondary to a child's disease (acute leukemia or aplastic anemia) but is more commonly a consequence of cytotoxic chemotherapy or radiotherapy. Most bacteremias occur when the absolute neutrophil count is <0.1×10^9/l (Alexander et al., 2002).

Qualitative abnormalities of neutrophil function may occur as a result of underlying diseases (acute leukemias) or be secondary to antineoplastic therapy. Neutrophils from patients with leukemia have suboptimal chemo-attractant responsiveness, bactericidal activity, and superoxide production (Baehner et al., 1973). Radiation may cause myelosuppression if a large amount of bone marrow is radiated. Radiation to the pelvis, spine, and long bones can cause neutropenia to develop. Medications commonly used in treating children, such as opiates, corticosteroids, and antibiotics, may have a detrimental effect on neutrophil function (Dale and Peterdorf, 1973). Patients with qualitative or quantitative defects in their PMPs are subject to bacterial infections from gram-positive or gram-negative bacteria and invasive fungi such as *Candida* and *Aspergillus* (Alexander et al., 2002: 1241).

16.7.2 Lymphocytes

Cancer and the treatments involved in a child's care create abnormalities of lymphocytes that affect both the humoral (B-cell-mediated) and the cellular (T-cell-mediated) immune response. A significant alteration in the humoral immune response (alteration in the ability to generate antigen-specific neutralizing antibodies) occurs in persons with chronic lymphocytic leukemia. These patients are susceptible to infections by encapsulated bacteria, especially *Streptococcus pneumoniae*, *Haemophilus influenzae*, and *Neisseria meningitidis* (Hersh et al., 1976).

Children with Hodgkin's and non-Hodgkin's lymphoma have impaired cellular immune responses. Corticosteroids and radiotherapy can also contribute to lymphocyte dysfunction (Fisher et al., 1980). Children who receive T-cell-depleted bone marrow transplants are more susceptible to viral pathogens and especially CMV. CMV can also act to further suppress the host's defenses (Rouse and Horohov, 1986). Chil-

dren with deficiencies of cellular immunity are more prone to fungal, viral, and bacterial infection that replicates within the cells such as *Listeria monocytogenes* and *Salmonella* species (Alexander et al., 2002).

Depletion of helper T-cells occurs as a result of cytotoxic chemotherapy. Studies have shown that lymphocyte numbers do not promptly recover after chemotherapy ends. Lymphopenia may persist for many months, while neutrophil, monocyte, and platelet numbers recover to 50% of pretreatment values between cycles of chemotherapy (Mackall et al., 1995). The capacity for T-cell regeneration after chemotherapy seems to decrease with age, so that younger children have a significantly greater recovery of T-cells 6 months after chemotherapy compared with young adults, who have persistent, markedly low levels of T-cells after completion of therapy. It is postulated that the thymus-dependent regeneration of T-cells plays a larger role in younger children, whereas in older children and adults the normal thymic involution that occurs with age results in dramatically less thymus-dependent generation (Mackall et al., 1995). Prolonged T-cell depletion contributes to the development of opportunistic infections such as herpes zoster or *Pneumocystis* pneumonia (Alexander et al., 2002).

16.7.3 Spleen and Reticuloendothelial System

The spleen and the fixed tissue cells of the reticuloendothelial system act as a mechanical filter and as an immune effector organ. The spleen is involved in the production of antibodies and acts as a filter to remove damaged cells and opsonin-coated organisms from the circulation (Rosse, 1987). Children who have had a splenectomy are: deficient in antibody production, especially to particulate type of antigens; have decreased levels of immunoglobulin M (IgM) and properdin (a component of the alternate complement pathway); and are deficient in the phagocytosis-promoting peptides (Spirer et al., 1977). Thus, these children are at increased risk for developing septicemias from encapsulated bacterial organisms such as *Streptococcus pneumoniae*, *Haemophilus influenzae*, and *Neisseria meningitidis* (Eraklis et al., 1967).

16.7.4 Other Factors Contributing to Immunocompromised States

Several other factors can exacerbate the immuno-compromised state of children with cancer. Malnutrition has a documented effect on immune function. Nutritional deficiencies in children affect B- and T-lymphocytes, polymorphonuclear leukocytes, mononuclear phagocytes, and the complement system functioning (Santos, 1994). Chemotherapy and radiation therapy can cause decreased immunoglobulin concentration, deficient agglutination and lysis of bacteria, inadequate neutralization of bacterial toxins, and diminished opsonic activities, which inhibits phagocytosis of bacteria (Groll et al., 2001).

Tumor masses, either primary or metastatic, can promote infection by organisms that colonize sites of tumor mass obstruction in the biliary tree, gastrointestinal or genitourinary tracts, or respiratory passages. Children with central nervous system tumors may be at increased risk of aspiration pneumonias related to a diminished or absent gag reflex or a decreased level of consciousness. Aspiration pneumonias and subsequent infections that develop can be exacerbated by decreased mucosal clearance mechanisms damaged as a result of antineoplastic therapies (Alexander et al., 2002).

References

Ackerman, M.H. (1994). The systemic inflammatory response, sepsis, and multiple organ dysfunction: New definitions for an old problem. Critical Care Nursing Clinics of North American, 6:243–250

Ackerman, M.H., Evans, N.J., Ecklund, M.M. (1994). Systemic inflammatory response syndrome, sepsis, and nutritional support. Critical Care Nursing Clinics of North America, 6:321–340

Alcorta, I, Perira, A., Ordinas, A. (1996). Clinical and laboratory factors associated with platelet transfusion refractoriness: a case control study. British Journal of Haematology, 93: 220–224

Alexander, S.A., Walsh, T.J., Freifeld, A.G, et al. (2002). Infectious complications in pediatric cancer patients. In Pizzo P.A., Poplack D.G. (eds), Principles and Practices of Pediatric Oncology, 4th edn., pp. 1239–1283. Philadelphia: Lippincott Williams & Wilkins

American Academy of Pediatrics. (2003). Summary of infectious diseases. In Pickering, L.K. (ed.). Red Book: 2003 Report of the Committee on Infectious Diseases, 26th edn. pp. 189–690. Elk Grove Village, IL: American Academy of Pediatrics

American Association of Blood Banks. (1997). Recommendations of AABB on use of CMV safe blood. Association Bulletin 97–2, April

Baehner, R.L., Neiberger, R.G., Johnson, D.G., et al. (1973). Transient bacterial defect of peripheral blood phagocytes form children with acute lymphoblastic leukemia receiving craniospinal irradiation. New England Journal of Medicine, 289:1209–1219

Bick, R.L. (1994). Disseminated intravascular coagulation. Objective criteria for the diagnosis and management. Medical Clinics of North America, 578:511–543

Bick, R.L. (1996). Disseminated intravascular coagulation: objective clinical and laboratory diagnosis, treatment and assessment of therapeutic response. Seminars in Thrombosis and Hemostasis, 22:69–88

Bodey, G.P., Buckley, M., Sate, Y.S., et al. (1966). Quantitative relationship between circulating lymphocytes and infection in patients with acute leukemia. Annals of Internal Medicine, 64:328–30

Brown, K.K.(1994). Septic shock. American Journal of Nursing, 94, 94(10):21–22

Bruce, J.L., Grove, S.K. (1992). Fever: pathology and treatment. Critical Care Nurse, 12(1):40–49

Chalmers, E., Gibson, B. E. (1999). Acquired disorder of hemostasis during childhood. In Lilleyman J.S., Hann I.M., Blanchette V.S. (eds) Pediatric Hematology, 2nd edn., pp. 629–649. London: Churchill Livingstone

Chanock, S.J., Gorlin, J.B. (1996). Granulocyte transfusions. Time for a second look. Infectious Diseases Clinics of North America, 10:327–343

Chuansumrit, A., Hotrakitay, S., Hathirat, P., et al. (1993). Disseminated intravascular coagulation in children: diagnosis, management and outcome. Southeast Asian Journal of Tropical Medicine and Public Health, 24:229–233

Dale, D. (2003). Myeloid disorders. In George J. N., Williams M. E. (eds) ASH-SAP American Society of Hematology Self Assessment Program, pp.116–128. Massachusetts: Blackwell

Dale, D.C., Peterdorf, R.G.(1973). Corticosteroids and infectious disease. Medical Clinics of North America, 57:1277–90

Dipchand, A., Ellis, G., Petric, M., Poon, A.O. (1997). Laboratory Reference Values. In Dipchand A. (ed.) The HSC Handbook of Pediatrics, 9th edn. pp. 507–556. Toronto: Mosby

Ellerhost-Ryan, J.M. (1993). Infection. In Groenwail S. L., Frogge M.H., Goodman M. (eds) Cancer Nursing: Principles and Practices, pp. 557–554. Boston: Jones and Bartlett

Engelfriet, C.P., Resink, H.W., Aster, R.H, et al. (1997). Management of alloimmunized refractory patients in need of platelet transfusions. Vox Sang, 73:191–198

Eraklis, A.J., Kevy, S.V., Diamond, L.K., et al. (1967). Hazard of overwhelming infection after splenectomy in childhood. New England Journal of Medicine, 276:1225–30

Fisher, R.J., DeVita, V.T., Bostick, F. (1980). Persistent immunological abnormalities in long term survivors of advanced Hodgkin's disease. Annals of Internal Medicine, 92:595–598

Greenbaum, B.H. (1991). Transfusion associated graft-verses-host disease: historical perspectives, incidence, and current use of irradiated blood products. Journal of Clinical Oncology, 9:1889–1902

Groll, A.H., Irvin, R.S., Lee, J.W., et al. (2001). Management of specific infectious complications in children with leukemias and lymphomas. In Patrick C.C. (ed) Clinical Management of Infections in Immunocompromised Infants and Children, pp. 111–143. Philadelphia: Lippincott Williams & Wilkins

Gunter, K.C., Luban, N.L. (1996). Transfusion transmitted cytomegalovirus. In Rossi E.C., Simm T.L., Moss G.S., Gould S.A. (ed.) Principles of Transfusion Medicine, pp. 717–73). Baltimore: Williams & Wilkins.

Hambleton, J., George, J. (2003). Hemostasis and thrombosis. In George J. N., Williams M. E. (eds) ASH-SAP American Society of Hematology Self Assessment Program, pp. 249–288. Massachusetts: Blackwell

Hann, I. (1999). Management of infection in children with bone marrow failure. In. Lilleyman J.S., Hann I.M., Blanchette V.S. (eds) Pediatric Hematology, 2nd edn., pp. 759–767. London: Churchill Livingstone

Hersh, E., Gutterman, J., Mavligit, G.M. (1976). Effect of haematologic malignancies and their treatment on host defense factors. Clinical Haematology, 5:425–30

Hughes, B.S., Armstrong, D., et al. (1990). Guidelines for the use of antimicrobial agents in neutropenic patients with unexplained fever. Journal of infectious Diseases, 161:381–383

Hume, H.A. (1999). Blood components: preparation, indications and administration. In Lilleyman J.S., Hann I.M., Blanchette V.S. (eds) Pediatric Hematology, 2nd edn., pp. 629–649. London: Churchill Livingstone

Ingram, J., Weitzman, S., et al. (1991). Complications of indwelling venous access lines in pediatric hematology patients: a prospective comparison of external venous catheters and subcutaneous ports. American Journal of Pediatric Hematology Oncology, 13:130–136

Kicker, T., Braine, H. G., Piantadosi, S., et al. (1990). A randomized, placebo-controlled trial of intravenous gammaglobulin in alloimmunized thrombocytopenia. Blood, 75:313–316

Kitchens, C.S. (1995). Disseminated intravascular coagulation. In Brian M.C., Carbone P.P., Kelton J.G., et al. (eds) Current Therapy in Hematology-Oncology, pp. 182–187. St. Louis: Mosby

Kline, N. E. (2002). Prevention and treatment of infections. In Baggott C. Rasco, Kelly K. Patterson, Fochtman D., Foley G.V. (eds) Nursing Care of Children and Adolescents with Cancer, 3rd edn., pp. 266–278. Philadelphia: W.B. Saunders

Lange, B., O'Neill, J., Goldwein., J., et al. (1997). Oncologic emergencies. In Pizzo P.A., Poplack D.G. (eds) Principles and Practices of Pediatric Oncology, 3rd edn., pp. 1025–1049. Philadelphia: Lippincott-Raven

Leibovitz, E, Rigaud, M., et al. (1990). *Pneumocystis carinii* pneumonia in infants infected with the HIV virus with more than 450 CD4 t lymphocytes per cubic millimeter. New England Journal of Medicine, 333:531–533

Lodha, A. (2003). Laboratory reference values. In Cheng A., Williams B.A., Sivarajan V.B. (eds) The HSC Handbook for Pediatrics, 10th edn. pp. 813–898. Toronto: Elsevier Canada

Luban, A.L., Pisciotta, A., Manno, C. (1999). Hazards of transfusion. In Lilleyman J.S., Hann I.M., Blanchette V.S. (eds) Pediatric Hematology, 2nd edn., pp. 741–757. London: Churchill Livingstone

Mackall, C.L., Fleissher, T.A., Brown, M.R., et al. (1995). Age, thymopoiesis and CD4+ T-lymphocyte regeneration after intensive chemotherapy. New England Journal of Medicine, 332:143–149

Metha, S., MacPhee, S. (2003). Emergencies. In Cheng A., Williams B.A., Sivarajan V.B. (eds) The HSC Handbook for Pediatrics, 10th edn. pp. 1–38. Toronto: Elsevier Canada

Murphy, M.F, Metcalfe, P., Ord, J., et al. (1987). Disappearance of HLA and platelet-specific antibodies in acute leukemia patients alloimmunized by multiple transfusions. British Journal of Haematology, 67:255–260

Ozer, H., Armitage, J.O., Bennett, C.L., et al. (2000). 2002 Update of recommendations for the use of hematopoietic colony-stimulation factors: evidence-based, clinical practice guideline. Journal of Clinical Oncology, 18:3558–3585

Panzarella, C., Rasco Baggott, C., Comeau, M, et al. (2002). Management of Disease and treatment-related complications. In Baggott C. Rasco, Kelly K. Patterson, Fochtman D., Foley G.V. (Eds), Nursing Care of Children and Adolescents with Cancer, 3rd edn., pp. 279–318. Philadelphia: W.B.Saunders

Parsons, S.K., Mayer, D.K., Alexander, S.W. et al. (2000). Growth factor practice patterns among pediatric oncologist; results of a 1998 Pediatric Oncology Group survey: Economic evaluation working group the Pediatric Oncology Group. Journal of Pediatric Hematology Oncology, 22:227–241

Pizzo, P.A. (1989). Considerations for the prevention of infectious complications in patients with cancer. Review of Infectious Disease, 11(Suppl. 7):S1551

Pizzo, P.A. (1993). Management of fever in patients with cancer and treatment induced neutropenia. New England Journal of Medicine, 328:1323–1332

Pizzo, P.A., Mueller, B.U. (1998). Infectious complications in children with hematologic disorders. In Nathan D.A., Orkin S. H. (eds) Nathan and Oski's Hematology of Infancy and Childhood, 5th edn., pp. 1738–1759. Philadelphia: W.B. Saunders

Przepiorka, D., LeParc, G. F., Werch, J., et al. (1996). Prevention of transfusion associated cytomegalovirus infection: practice parameter. American Journal of Clinical Pathology, 106:163–169

Riikonen, P, Saarinen, N.M., et al. Management of indwelling venous catheters in pediatric cancer patients with fever and neutropenia. Scandinavian Journal of Infectious Disease, 25:357–360

Rizzo, J.D, Lichtin, A.L., Woolf, S.H., et al. (2002). Use of Epoetin in patients with cancer: evidence-based clinical practice guidelines of the American Society of Clinical Oncology and the American Society of Hematology. Journal of Clinical Oncology, 20:4083–4107

Rosse (1987). The spleen as a filter. New England Journal of Medicine, 317:705–706

Rouse, B.T., Horohov, D.H. (1986). Immunosuppression in viral infections. Review of Infectious Disease, 8:850–855

Rubin, R.H., Ferraro, M.J. (1993). Understanding and diagnosing infectious complications in the immunocompromised host: Current issues and trends. Hematology/Oncology Clinics of North America, 7:795–811

Santos, J.I. (1994). Nutrition, infection and immunocompetence. Infectious Disease. Clinics of North America, 8:243–50

Sayer, M.H., Anderson, K. C., Goodnough, L.T., et al. (1992). Reducing the risk for transfusion-transmitted cytomegalovirus. Annals of Internal Medicine, 116:55–62

Schiffer, C.A., Anderson, K.C., Bennett, C.L., et al. (2003). Platelet transfusion for patients with cancer: clinical practice guidelines of the American Society of Clinical Oncology. Journal of Clinical Oncology, 19:1519–1538)

Shamsah, A. (2003). Hematology. In Cheng A., Williams B.A., Sivarajan V.B. (eds) The HSC Handbook for Pediatrics, 10th edn., pp.350–378. Toronto: Elsevier Canada

Slichter, S.J. (1990). Mechanisms and management of platelet refractoriness. In Nance S.T. (ed) Transfusion Medicine in the 1990s, pp. 95–179. Arlington: American Association of Blood Bank

Spirer, Z., Zakuth, V, Diamant, S., et al. (1977). Decreased tuftsin concentration in patients who have undergone splenectomy. British Medical Journal, 2:1574–1576

Steele, M. (2003). Oncology. In Cheng A., Williams B.A., Sivarajan V.B. (eds) The HSC Handbook for Pediatrics, 10th edn., pp. 609–639. Toronto: Elsevier Canada

Strauss, R.G. (1994). Granulocyte transfusion therapy. In Mintz P.D. (ed). Transfusion medicine 1. Hematology Oncology Clinics of North America, 8:1159–1166

Thatcher, N., DeCampos, E.S., Bell, D.R., et al. (1999). Epoetin alpha prevents anaemia and reduces transfusion requirements in patients undergoing primarily platinum based chemotherapy for small cell lung cancer. British Journal of Cancer, 80:396–402

Vogelsang, G.B, Hess, A.D. (1994). Graft-versus-host disease: new directions for a persistent problem. Blood, 84:2061–2067

Walsh, T.J. (1993). Management of immunocompromised patients with evidence of invasive mycosis. Hematology Oncology Clinics of North America, 7:1003-1008

Walsh TJ, Pizzo PA (1988) Nosocomial fungal infections: a classification for hospital-acquired fungal infections and mycoses arising from endogenous flora or reactivation. Annual Review of Microbiology 42:517-45

Wilson, K.D. (2002). Oncologic emergencies. In Baggott C. Rasco, Kelly K. Patterson, Fochtman D., Foley G.V. (eds) Nursing Care of Children and Adolescents with Cancer, 3rd edn., pp.334–346. Philadelphia: W.B. Saunders

Respiratory System

Margaret Parr

Contents

17.1 *Pneumocystis* Pneumonia

Note: The *Pneumocystis* infecting humans, once called *Pneumocystis carinii*, should now be called *Pneumocystis jiroveci*. *Pneumocystis carinii* now refers to *Pneumocystis* from other host species. It is now clear that *Pneumocystis* from humans and other animals are quite different and that there are multiple species in the genus. Analysis of protein sizes has shown that the organism tends to be host-specific (Stringer et al., 2002). Changing the organism's name does not preclude using the acronym PCP, as it can be read "*Pneumocystis pneumonia*".

17.1.1 Incidence

Pneumocystis jiroveci pneumonia (PCP) caused by the pathogen *Pneumocystis jiroveci* occurs in immunocompromised individuals including children and adolescents undergoing treatment for cancer. Now rarely seen in the child and adolescent cancer population, PCP was once common in patients who were treated on immunosuppressive regimes. The use of sulphamethoxazole-trimethoprim (co-trimoxazole) given prophylactically to these patients alongside their chemotherapy treatment regimes has greatly reduced the incidence of PCP in this patient population. The highest incidence of PCP is now seen in patients who have HIV infection (Wakefield, 2002).

17.1.2 Etiology

PCP is caused by the pathogen *Pneumocystis jiroveci*. Once thought to be a protozoon, it is now considered to be fungal in origin (Wakefield, 2002). PCP in the immunocompromised child is thought to most likely result from latent cysts being reactivated, because children who are not immunocompromised are found to carry the antibody to *Pneumocystis carinii* (*jiroveci*) (Freifield et al., 2002; Wakefield, 2002). It is thought that as the child becomes immunocompromised during treatment, the latent cysts reactivate. Patient-to-patient transmission has also been suggested. Clusters have been described in the paediatric oncology population and in transplant patients (Wakefield, 2002). The children considered to be most at risk for PCP are

— Children with lymphomas
— Children on maintenance chemotherapy for acute lymphoblastic leukaemia; the prolonged immunosuppressive effect of 6-mercaptopurine is directly responsible for a predisposition to *Pneumocystis carinii* (*jiroveci*) (Pinkerton et al., 1994)
— Children who have undergone a bone marrow transplant (BMT)

17.1.3 Prevention

Children receiving chemotherapy for acute lymphoblastic leukaemia (ALL), particularly those in the maintenance phase of chemotherapy, are considered most susceptible to PCP due to the immunosuppressive properties of 6-mercaptopurine. Sulphamethoxazole-trimethoprim is routinely used with the ALL protocol as prophylactic treatment against *Pneumocystis jiroveci*.

Sulphamethoxazole-trimethoprim has several side effects: fever, rash, pruritus, vomiting, headaches, and bone marrow suppression. If children are experiencing any of the side effects, it may not be advisable to use sulphamethazole-trimethoprim. Indeed, prolonged bone marrow suppression is the most common reason to discontinue the prophylactic dose of sulphamethoxazole-trimethoprim. If the child shows intolerance to the drug, pentamidine may be chosen as a substitute in order to maintain the prophylactic treatment with minimal disruption to the child. (Other alternatives include oral dapsone and oral atovaquone.) It is recognised that pentamidine has been linked to a number of toxicities, including metabolic and haematological abnormalities, pancreatitis, hypotension, and nausea and vomiting (Freifield et al., 2002). Walzer (1994, in Bastow, 2000) reports minor adverse reactions in most patients when pentamidine is administered intravenously (IV) or intramuscularly (IM), with serious toxicity in 47 % of patients. Administering pentamidine via the nebulised route seems to reduce the toxicity risk. It is important to note that the effect that nebulised pentamidine may have on the staff administering the drug is largely unknown; therefore, care must be taken. Although administration usually requires a visit to the hospital or clinic, nebulised pentamidine is administered monthly, and it can usually be planned to coincide with a routine clinic visit. It is recommended that the patients receive the treatment in a single patient room and, if possible, some method of extraction or ventilation should be used to enable removal of the airborne particles produced during the drug's nebulisation. Access to the room should be limited during the administration.

Bronchospasm is a recognised side effect that may occur at the time of administration. Nebulised bronchodilators may be prescribed routinely to prevent this from occurring.

17.1.4 Treatment

A child presenting with a suspected diagnosis of PCP would most commonly present with pyrexia, cough, dyspnoea, tachypnoea, a characteristic x-ray, and possibly intercostal recession (Bastow, 2000). The chest x-ray would normally show a bilateral, diffuse interstitial infiltrate (Bastow, 2000; Freifield et al., 2002). PCP in the paediatric oncology patient can be diagnosed by the monoclonal staining of induced sputum, a specimen that is recommended as the first approach to assist diagnosis (Freifield et al., 2002). However, obtaining sputum specimens from children can be difficult, particularly because a presenting feature of the disease is an unproductive cough. Induced sputum specimens involve administering nebulised hypertonic saline. This method enables the particles to penetrate smaller airways. The hyperosmolality of the saline causes fluid to be drawn into the lung interstitiam; this washes the cysts and debris into the

Table 17.1. Common drugs used for prophylaxis and treatment of *Pneumocystis* pneumonia

Drug	Use	Route	Dose	Administration
Pentamidine	Prophylaxis	Inhalation	300 mg inhaled once per month	Continue monthly throughout duration of cancer treatment (consult product literature for method of administration)
	Treatment	Intravenous	4 mg/kg/day	Infuse in glucose 5% or sodium chloride 0.9% for 14–21 days. Dilute (once dissolved in water for injection) in 50–250 ml. Infuse over at least 60 minutes.
		Inhaled	600 mg/day	For 14–21 days
Sulphamethoxa-zole-trimethoprim-(co-trimoxazole)	Prophylaxis	Oral	Surface area (SA) 0.5–0.75 m² = 480 mg/day	Given in two divided doses on two or three per week
			SA 0.76–1.0 m² =720 mg/day	
			SA >1.0 m² = 960 mg/day	
	Treatment	Intravenous	120 mg/kg/day	Two to four divided doses for 14 days as infusion in glucose 5% or 10%, or sodium chloride 0.9%
				Dilute 5 ml to 125 ml (or to 75 ml if fluid restrictions apply)
				Infuse over 60–90 minutes

larger airways from where they can be expectorated (Bastow, 2000). The use of the physiotherapist and the play specialist to work with the child may reduce the difficulty and help to ease the distress of the procedure.

If obtaining a sputum specimen is not possible, or the result is negative, then broncheoalveolar lavage or open biopsy may need to be considered (Freifield et al., 2002). Not all centres treating oncology patients will have the facilities for these diagnostic tests, or the child's condition may render him or her too ill for the procedure. If this is the case, then the health care practitioner can and should proceed directly to treatment. The first-line treatment for a suspected or confirmed diagnosis of PCP is high-dose oral or IV sulphamethoxazole-trimethoprim (see Table 17.1), with IV being the primary route of choice. Although central venous catheters (CVC) are the most commonly used method of venous access in the paediatric cancer patient, some children may still receive treatment via peripheral veins. If the drug is administered through a peripheral vein, nurses should note that there is a risk of abscess formation and necrosis of the injection site. Staff should regularly observe the site for patency, flashback, pain, redness, or swelling.

If the diagnosis has not been confirmed, then erythromycin may be prescribed alongside the sulphamethoxazole-trimethoprim to include treatment for *Mycoplasma*, as PCP and *Mycoplasma* are the two most common pathogens to cause the diffuse pulmonary infiltrate (Pinkerton et al., 1994). The use of steroids in combination with sulphamethoxazole-trimethoprim has been found to improve outcomes of adult AIDS patients with moderate or severe PCP (Freifield et al., 2002). In response to this finding, some paediatricians are prescribing an adjuvant short course of steroids to patients diagnosed with PCP.

Nurses must also consider the supportive care required by a child with a suspected or confirmed diagnosis of PCP. Oxygen therapy may be required to maintain oxygen saturation, and the child's condition may deteriorate to the stage where mechanical ventilation may need to be considered. The team managing the child with PCP must also consider maintenance of nutrition and fluid, electrolyte, and acid-base balance; the child may require total parenteral nutrition. The child will require antipyrexial medication for comfort and will also need psychological support, which will be particularly important if he or she is isolated due to the diagnosis.

Chemotherapy is most likely to be interrupted until the child's condition improves and neutropenia subsides.

17.1.5 Prognosis

PCP is now much rarer in the paediatric oncology population, and although the condition is treatable, it must still be recognised as a potentially fatal condition. It is essential that parents be taught to recognise the signs and symptoms their child may present with if *Pneumocystis* pneumonia develops: dyspnoea, tachypnoea, pyrexia, and a cough. Staff should emphasise to the parents the importance of maintaining prophylactic co-trimoxazole administration and reassure them that they can contact the hospital or clinic if they have any concerns regarding their child's condition.

17.2 Pneumonitis

17.2.1 Incidence

Pneumonitis secondary to a diagnosis of childhood cancer is very rare, but nevertheless should be considered in children presenting with a cough, dyspnoea, and fever. Children most at risk of developing pneumonitis are those who have received radiotherapy to the thoracic, mediastinal, mantle, spinal, or flank fields. Children who have received total body irradiation as conditioning for BMT may also be considered at risk.

Radiation to the thoracic area can cause oesophagitis, indigestion, nausea, and acute pneumonitis. Pneumonitis occurs in approximately 10% of pa-

tients who receive full-dose radiation in this area (McGuire, 1993).

Acute pneumonitis usually occurs between 1 and 6 months after radiotherapy treatment (McGuire, 1993; Kun, 1997). Radiotherapy in conjunction with chemotherapy (especially dactinomycin or bleomycin) increases the risk of pneumonitis from 5% at 20 Gy to 50% at 24 Gy (Kun, 1997).

17.2.2 Etiology

Radiation pneumonitis is thought to occur as the result of excess free radical generation following radiotherapy (Cottier et al., 1996). The pathophysiology of the condition is immediate injury to alveolar type II pneumocytes (Kun, 1997). Oedema and sloughing of endothelial cells in smaller vessels allows fluid to accumulate in the interstitial tissues. The cell linings of the alveoli are also affected, and the swelling and sloughing of these cells also causes excess exudate (Strohl, 1992). Pneumonitis can occur with radiation doses higher than 7.5 Gy, even as a cumulative fractionated dose (Van Dyke et al., 1981). Pneumonitis can also be related to some chemotherapy agents (see Table 17.2); those known specifically to cause pneumonitis are carmustine (BCNU), lomustine (CCNU), and bleomycin. They cause a decrease in type I pneumocytes and an increase and redistribution of type II pneumocytes into the alveolar spaces, leading to pneumonitis (Selwood et al., 2000).

Chemotherapy is also thought to accentuate the effects of radiation on the lungs. Dactinomycin is a radiation sensitiser that can enhance the local toxicity of the radiation therapy if administered concurrently. Protocols using dactinomycin advise stopping the drug during the course of radiotherapy and for a period of time after radiotherapy treatment is complete (approximately 6 weeks).

Children receiving bleomycin without radiotherapy are still at risk of interstitial pneumonitis. If this condition develops, the drug may need to be stopped. High oxygen levels may exacerbate the toxicity to the lungs; therefore, if anaesthesia is being considered, the anaesthetist should be aware that the child is or has been receiving this drug.

Table 17.2. Chemotherapy agents with the potential to cause pneumonitis (adapted from Balis et al., 2002)

Drug	Cytotoxic classification	Route	Antitumour spectrum
Lomustine	Alkylating agent	Oral	Brain tumour, lymphoma, Hodgkin's disease
Carmustine	Alkylating agent	Intravenous	Brain tumour, lymphoma, Hodgkin's disease
Busulfan	Alkylating agent	Oral	CML, leukaemias (BMT)
Bleomycin	Antitumour antibiotic	Intravenous	Lymphoma, testicular, and other germ cell tumours
		Intramuscular	
		Oral	

17.2.3 Prevention

The risk of pneumonitis is directly linked to the dose of radiotherapy the child receives. The greater the total dose of radiotherapy and the larger the dose per fraction, the greater the risk of significant lung damage. Lowering the radiation doses to 15–25 Gy has virtually eliminated the problem.

Children who are receiving bleomycin as part of their treatment regime should not be exposed to unnecessary high levels of oxygen. Anaesthetists should be made aware of the fact that these children have received bleomycin as part of their cancer treatment.

17.2.4 Treatment

A child with suspected radiation pneumonitis will present with a cough, dyspnoea, fever, and increased respiratory effort. The child may also complain of pleuritic pain. It is important that the parents be aware of the risk of pneumonitis following radiation therapy to the lungs and that they know the signs and symptoms to look for; the signs parents will notice are the cough and a reduced exercise tolerance. Parents should be given the confidence and support to contact the clinic or hospital if they become concerned that their child may be showing any indication of developing pneumonitis. The child may require hospitalisation and, in some rare but severe cases, ventilation.

If the child is admitted, he or she will require rest, oxygen therapy, oxygen saturation monitoring, observation of respiratory effort, possible treatment with corticosteroids, and psychological support. Symptoms may resolve in 2–3 months.

17.2.5 Prognosis

Reduced respiratory function increases susceptibility to infection, which will increase the risk of serious complications.

Because all children and young people who have been treated for cancer will be followed up regularly, it is important that the patient's exercise tolerance be assessed at each clinic appointment. Lung function may also be assessed but usually only if the patient is displaying symptoms such as dyspnoea or a persistent cough.

17.3 Fibrosis

As pneumonitis is the acute interstitial complication of radiotherapy and chemotherapy, fibrosis is the chronic complication, and the former often leads on to the latter.

17.3.1 Incidence

Pulmonary fibrosis as a consequence of treatment for childhood cancer is very rare. Nevertheless, it should be recognised as a possible late effect of treatment, particularly of radiotherapy to the thoracic region.

Boughton (2002) states that the Childhood Cancer Survivor Study analysed 12,390 survivors of childhood cancer and found that pulmonary complications can occur any time after treatment. The survivors were found to have a significantly higher incidence of lung fibrosis, emphysema, pneumonia, pleurisy, and need for oxygen compared with sibling controls.

17.3.2 Etiology

Rolla et al. (2000) suggest that injury to the lung from radiation does not occur just from direct damage to the cell membranes, proteins, and DNA, but also from an inflammatory syndrome. A study by Rubin et al. (1995) was able to demonstrate that there is a continuous cascade of cytokines beginning soon after radiation therapy begins and lasting until lung fibrosis develops. As the pneumonitis subsides, the exudate is absorbed, and the regeneration of the cells begins, fibrosis will occur. Fibrosis can occur in tissue as a result of scarring from previous injury. Chemotherapy can also cause fibrosis. Bleomycin may cause fibrosis, and this effect may occur for many years. Methotrexate and vinblastine have also been associated with chronic pneumonitis and fibrosis (Galvin, 1994). Fibrosis has also been reported in children who have been treated with cyclophosphamide (Chen et al., 2002). Fibrosis will cause loss of volume, loss of compliance, and reduced diffusing capacity.

17.3.3 Prevention

Survivors of childhood cancer who are thought to be at risk of developing fibrosis of the lung will be followed up appropriately in the late-effects clinics. They will require assessment of lung function, particularly if they are starting to display symptoms of dyspnoea or a dry hacking cough. However, the length of time the patients would need to be followed up would be difficult to determine, as the time period for developing fibrosis is quite varied. The Childhood Cancer Survivors Study showed people developing symptoms more than 5 years after completion of cancer treatment, and in some cases were newly present up to 20 years after treatment (Boughton, 2002).

17.3.4 Treatment

A patient presenting with fibrosis will have a dry hacking cough and dyspnoea, requiring treatment with steroids and, probably, oxygen. On admission to hospital, the patient will require a chest x-ray and a lung function test to determine the extent of damage to the lung tissue. The patient should be observed for any signs of infection, which will exacerbate the condition. Oxygen saturation should be monitored. If the condition is severe, the patient may require mechanical ventilation. Once a patient has been ventilated for fibrosis, it may be difficult to wean him or her off, and this may be a long process. Exercise tolerance may be a problem, and the patient will need a great deal of psychological support to cope with the impact of this new restriction on his or her life.

17.3.5 Prognosis

Reduced respiratory function increases susceptibility to infection, which will increase the risk of serious complications. If the patient with fibrosis goes on to require mechanical ventilation, then the prognosis is poorer than that of those patients who do not require ventilation.

17.4 Compromised Airway

17.4.1 Incidence

The incidence of compromised airway in the child with cancer is very rare but, because of anatomical differences, can occur more easily in the paediatric patient than in the adult. Any tumour occurring within the thoracic area can give rise to a compromised airway. The paediatric airway is small and compliant, making it susceptible to collapse (Jenkins, 2001). Although airway compromise is rare, when it occurs it can rapidly become an oncological emergency (Fig. 17.1).

17.4.2 Etiology

There are several possible causes of compromised airway in the child with cancer. Any tumour developing in the thorax could compromise the airway due to compression. The anterior mediastinum is the area most commonly involved in malignant disease (Braverman and Parker, 2002). Tumours commonly found in the anterior mediastinum are non-Hodgkin's lymphoma (NHL), Hodgkin's lymphoma, and leukaemia. Tumours that can be found in the posterior mediastinum are neuroblastomas, malig-

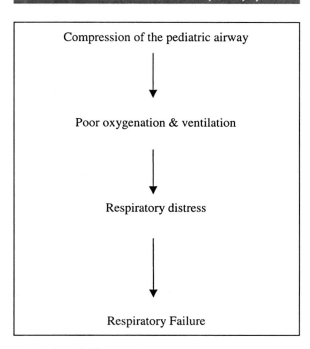

Compression of the pediatric airway

↓

Poor oxygenation & ventilation

↓

Respiratory distress

↓

Respiratory Failure

Figure 17.1

The pathway to oncological emergency

nant germ cell tumours, and primitive neuroectodermal tumours (PNETs). Ginsberg et al. (2002) reported that the data from 18 studies from Europe, the United States, and Japan over a 10-year period showed that 74% of peripheral PNETs occurred in the central axis and 60% occurred in the chest. Rhabdomyosarcoma, Ewing's sarcoma, and PNET may also occur in the chest wall. Children with mediastinal masses may present with superior vena cava syndrome (SVCS) or superior mediastinal syndrome (SMS). SVCS is the term used when a child presents with symptoms of compression, obstruction, or thrombosis of the superior vena cava; if the trachea is also compressed, then the term SMS is used (Rheingold and Lange, 2002). SVCS and SMS most commonly occur with lymphoma and leukaemia.

Laryngeal tumours may also cause an airway obstruction, with rhabdomyosarcoma being the most common of the malignant laryngeal tumours (Ferlito et al., 1999).

Some tumours – for example, osteosarcoma and Wilms' tumour – commonly metastasise to the lungs and can increase the risk of compromised airway in that patient.

Mucositis in the immunocompromised patient can also be a cause of compromised airway, and thrombocytopenia will create a risk of bleeding into the airway.

17.4.3 Prevention

Preventing a compromised airway from a tumour would be difficult, and efforts must be concentrated on preparing general practitioners and paediatricians to consider the possibility of a malignant diagnosis in children presenting to them with the signs and symptoms discussed above. This could then prevent wrong diagnoses, wrong treatment, and deterioration in the child's condition.

17.4.4 Treatment

The signs and symptoms that the child may present with depend on the speed at which the condition arises. If the onset is slow and insidious, the child may present with cough, wheeze, tachypnoea, and possible stridor. If the onset is acute, then the child may present with fever, cough, and mild shortness of breath, but may progress quickly to signs and symptoms of respiratory distress (Jenkins, 2001) The child may also show signs of dyspnoea, orthopnoea, chest pain, jugular venous obstruction, and hoarseness. This condition can rapidly become an oncological emergency and must be managed promptly. If it is possible and time allows, then a biopsy for diagnosis would be the best option. However, several things must be taken into consideration: This group of patients is at high risk of respiratory or cardiac arrest if put in the supine position due to impedance of venous return and airflow. Needle biopsy should only be considered if it can be undertaken under local anaesthesia, as there is a high risk of arrest with either general anaesthesia or sedation. A simple blood test could indicate whether leukaemia is the underlying diagnosis. One could also take a blood sample for alpha-fetoprotein if a germ cell tumour is being considered, and a urine sample for catecholamines could be obtained if neuroblastoma were being considered.

This is one of the few occasions when medical staff may choose to start treatment without a definite diagnosis, and it would be advisable to nurse these patients within the intensive care unit until the acute phase has settled. To protect the child from obstruction, he or she may need ventilation until the tumour bulk has decreased. Neuromuscular blockade agents should be avoided during intubation because if the health care practitioner were unable to intubate past the obstruction, the child would be unable to breathe spontaneously (Jenkins, 2001).

The team may choose to give chemotherapy and assess the situation; if the child's condition improves, they may then carry out the diagnostic tests. If the diagnosis is NHL, corticosteroids and possibly vincristine may be enough to improve the child's airway obstruction. It is important to note, however, that a child with mediastinal NHL is at high risk of tumour lysis syndrome.

If the chemotherapy does not improve the child's condition, the team may choose to give radiotherapy. There is a risk of the child deteriorating after radiotherapy, thought to be due to tracheal swelling post-radiotherapy (Rheingold and Lange, 2002). There is also the chance that the child may suffer the risks of radiotherapy, i.e. pneumonitis, without seeing a benefit. NHL is both chemosensitive and radiosensitive, making biopsy and diagnosis difficult after treatment has already begun. (With most of the other tumours, biopsy will still be possible.) This will be a very frightening time for both the child and the family, and they will require a great deal of psychological care.

17.4.5 Prognosis

The prognosis for recovering from compromised airway if due to tumour mass is very good. In their review of oncology patients requiring paediatric intensive care treatment, Keengwe et al. (1999) showed that four patients with tumour mass effect that resulted in respiratory compromise were admitted and ventilated, and all four survived.

References

Balis FM, Holcenberg JS, Blaney SM (2002) General principles of chemotherapy. In Pizzo PA, Poplack DG (eds) Principles and Practice of Pediatric Oncology, 4th edn. Philadelphia: Lippincott Williams & Wilkins, pp 237–308

Bastow V (2000) Identifying and treating PC.P. Nursing Times l96(37):19

Boughton B (2002) Childhood cancer treatment causes complications later in life. Lancet Oncology 3(7):390

Braverman RM, Parker BR (2002) Imaging studies in the diagnosis and management of paediatric malignancies. In Pizzo PA, Poplack DG (eds) Principles and Practice of Pediatric Oncology, 4th edn. Philadelphia: Lippincott Williams & Wilkins, pp 205–236

Chen J, Wang PJ, Hsu YH, Chang PY, Fang JS (2002) Severe lung fibrosis after chemotherapy in a child with ataxia-telangectasia. Journal of Pediatric Hematology and Oncology 24(1):77–79

Cottier B, Cassapi L, Jack CIA, Jackson MJ, Fraser WD, Hind CRK (1996) Indicators of free radical activity in patients developing radiation pneumonitis. International Journal of Radiation Oncology, Biology and Physics 34(1):149–154

Ferlito A, Rinaldo A, Marioni G (1999) Laryngeal malignant neoplasms in children and adolescents. International Journal of Pediatric Otorhinolaryngology 49(1):1–14

Freifield AG, Walsh TJ, Alexander SW, Pizzo PA (2002) Infectious complications of in the pediatric cancer patient. In Pizzo PA, Poplack DG (eds) Principles and Practice of Pediatric Oncology, 4th edn. Philadelphia: Lippincott Williams & Wilkins

Galvin H (1994) The late effects of treatment of childhood cancer survivors. Journal of Cancer Care 3(2):128–133

Ginsberg JP, Woo Sy, Johnson ME, Hicks MJ, Horowitz ME (2002) Ewing's sarcoma family of tumors: Ewing's sarcoma of bone and soft tissue and the peripheral primitive neuroectodermal tumours. In Pizzo PA, Poplack DG (eds) Principles and Practice of Pediatric Oncology, 4th edn. Philadelphia: Lippincott Williams & Wilkins, pp 973–1016

Jenkins TL (2001) Oncological critical care problems. In Curley MAQ, Moloney-Harmon PA (eds) Critical Care Nursing of Infants and Children, 2nd edn. Philadelphia: WB Saunders, pp 853–874

Keengwe IN, Nelhans ND, Stansfield F, Eden OB, Dearlove OR, Sharples A (1999) Paediatric oncology and intensive care treatments: changing trends. Archives of Disease in Childhood 80(6):553–555

Kun LE (1997) General principles of radiotherapy. In Pizzo PA, Poplack DG (eds) Principles and Practices of Pediatric Oncology, 3rd edn. Philadelphia: Lippincott Williams & Wilkins

McGuire P (1993) Radiation therapy. In Foley G.V, Fochtman D, Hardin Mooney K (eds) Nursing Care of the Child with Cancer, 2nd edn. Philadelphia: WB Saunders

Pinkerton CR, Cushing P, Sepion B (1994) Childhood Cancer Management: A Practical Handbook. London: Chapman & Hall

Rheingold SR, Lange BJ (2002) Oncologic emergencies. In Pizzo PA, Poplack DG (eds) Principles and Practice of Pediatric Oncology, 4th edn. Philadelphia: Lippincott Williams & Wilkins, pp 1177–1204

Rolla G, Ricardi U, Colagrande P, Nassisi D, Dutto L, Chiavassa G, Bucca C (2000) Changes in airway responsiveness following mantle radiotherapy for Hodgkin's disease. Chest 117(6):1590–1596

Rubin P, Johnston CJ, Williams JP, McDonald S, Finkelstein JN (1995) A perpetual cascade of cytokines postirradiation leads to pulmonary fibrosis. International Journal of Radiation, Biology and Physics 33(1):99–109

Selwood K, Gibson F, Evans M (2000) Side effects of chemotherapy. In Gibson F, Evans M (eds) Paediatric Oncology: Acute Nursing Care. London: Whurr

Stringer JR, Beard CB, Miller RF, Wakefield AE (2002) A new name (Pneumocystis jiroveci) for Pneumocystis from humans. Emerging Infectious Diseases 8(9):891–896

Strohl RA (1992) Ineffective breathing patterns. In Hassey-Dow K, Hilderley L (eds) Nursing Care in Radiation Oncology. Philadelphia: WB Saunders, pp 160–177

Van Dyk J, Keane TJ, Kan S, Rider WD, Fryer CJ (1981) Radiation pneumonitis following single dose irradiation: a re-evaluation based on absolute dose to lung. International Journal of Radiation Oncology, Biology and Physics 11(3): 461–467

Wakefield AE (2002) Pneumocystis carinii childhood respiratory diseases. British Medical Bulletin 61:175–188

Renal System

Fiona Reid

Contents

18.1 Nephrectomy

18.1.1 Incidence

In general, justifications for childhood nephrectomy would include trauma, nephrolithiasis, or a nonfunctioning kidney, but within the field of oncology, surgery is performed predominantly for tumor control and occasionally for severe infections.

Nephrectomy of some kind is indicated in all cases of renal tumors and in certain cases may need to be bilateral. Wilms' tumor (nephroblastoma or WT) represents 5–6% of all childhood renal cancers and is the most common primary malignant tumor of childhood (90%), with an incidence of 7.8/million. Approximately 5% involve both kidneys, possibly displaying discordant histologies. Other renal neoplasms include renal cell carcinomas (0.1/million), clear cell carcinomas (2–4%), rhabdoid tumors (<2%), congenital mesoblastic nephroma (3%), and benign angiomyolipoma.

In most oncology patients requiring nephrectomy, time is available for appropriate radiography and assessment prior to surgery; however, primary emergency nephrectomy (3%) may occur in situations of massive bleeding from tumor rupture, suspicion of "acute abdomen" or bowel occlusion.

18.1.2 Etiology

18.1.2.1 Neoplasms

Wilms' tumor has a peak incidence in children at 2–4 years of age. Few are seen after 7 years of age and rarely after 15 years of age; in bilateral cases the child tends to be younger. In most cases WT is sporadic, but it is thought to have an inheritable link in 15–20% (see Chapter 2 on Solid Tumors).

There are also increased frequencies of associated congenital urological abnormalities (1%), in particular hypospadias, cryptorchidism, and renal function anomalies. These may be associated with

- Beckwith-Wiedemann syndrome (BW) with a 25% increased risk of WT

- Denys-Drash syndrome (DD), displaying pseudohermaphroditism, WT, and glomerulonephritis, or nephrotic syndrome leading to progressive renal failure

The latter almost always results in renal failure requiring dialysis and then renal transplantation following surgery for tumor removal (Ebb et al., 2001).

18.1.2.2 Bacterial

Some renal infections leading to xanthogranulomatosis pyelonephritis are characterized by persistent chronic bacteruria and renal mass associated with renal pelvis calcification for which simple nephrectomy is the remaining option after failure to resolve with antibiotic treatment (Sanders and Anderson, 1988).

18.1.3 Treatment

18.1.3.1 Preoperative

The aims of preoperative evaluation are to

1. Attempt to assess the function of both kidneys
2. Locate tumor origin (WT is intrinsic to the kidney; neuroblastoma is adrenal in origin)
3. Exclude intracaval tumor extension (seen in 4% of WT patients)
4. Exclude ureteral invasion
5. Determine the relationship of the tumor to adjacent structures including lymph nodes
6. Assess renal vasculature (e.g., up to 30% may involve more than one renal artery)

Hypertension is present in 25% of WT patients due to raised renin levels as a result of renal artery compression. Hematuria is seen in 25%, but gross hematuria should lead to a suspicion of extension into the renal collecting system. Examination is needed to eliminate associated syndromes (DD, BW, or congenital uro-anomalies). Laboratory investigations include complete/full blood count, blood urea nitrogen and electrolytes, serum creatinine, serum calcium, clotting studies, renal and liver function, and urinalysis. Acquired von Willebrand's disease has been found in

8% of newly diagnosed WT patients (Coppes et al., 1993), and serum calcium has been found elevated in rhabdoid tumors and congenital mesoblastic nephroma. Intravenous pyelograms have been superseded by ultrasound, which is particularly useful in differentiating solid and cystic lesions, venous tumor thrombosis, and extension into the renal pelvis. Computerized tomography (CT) scan, the spiral form of which is particularly valuable when partial nephrectomy and delineation for maximal parenchymal sparing needs evaluating, may be confusing because tumors thought to be invasive of adjacent structures at scan may be found to be only compressive at the time of surgery.

Figure 18.1 shows a CT scan image using oral and intravenous contrast to demonstrate a large mass (WT) arising from the left kidney.

Preoperative imaging is necessary to establish both the presence and function of the contralateral kidney as well as synchronous bilateral tumors; however, up to 7% of contralateral tumors may be missed by diagnostic imaging, especially those <1 cm (Ritchey et al., 1992). Chest radiographs are required to detect pulmonary metastases.

Preoperative chemotherapy has been shown to reduce both the chances of tumor rupture, small bowel occlusions (Godzinski et al., 2001), and tumor embolism but with implications for altering tumor histology, downstaging tumor diagnosis, and risking inappropriate treatment with increased relapse rate (Capra et al., 1999). Presurgical chemotherapy treatment with initial percutaneous needle biopsy is generally accepted in the following situations:

- For solitary kidneys
- For bilateral renal tumors
- For tumors in a horseshoe kidney
- When there is high inferior vena cava tumor extension
- In cases of respiratory distress from extensive pulmonary metastases
- When otherwise radical organ resection (which carries high morbidity and mortality rates) would be indicated

18.1.3.2 Surgery

Simple nephrectomy, involving the removal of the kidney from within Gerota's fascia, is usually performed for non-neoplastic disease states. In most renal tumors, radical nephrectomy (in which the entire contents of Gerota's fascia, including the kidney, perinephric fat, lymphatics, and ipsilateral adrenal gland, are removed to leave negative margins) is the ideal mode of choice, but only after a normal contralateral kidney has been established. Partial nephrectomy entails local tumor resection with least positive margins and leaving maximal normally functioning parenchyma. It is reserved for situations of bilateral tumor or when radical nephrectomy would leave the patient either anephric or in renal failure. In these cases prior chemotherapy is given to reduce tumor size and increase potential nephron sparing. Histopathology and tumor stage are the key determinants of prognosis and subsequent therapy in WT patients; therefore, surgical staging and careful technique are essential. A large transperitoneal approach is recommended to enable full visualization of the contralateral kidney, with palpation for small bilateral tumors, assessment of other organs, lymph node involvement and biopsy, and careful manipulation and removal of tumor. Large necrotic, cystic, fluid-filled tumors, especially WT, are extremely friable and need to be removed en bloc.

Figure 18.2 shows an image of the removal of a Wilms' tumor by radical nephrectomy.

Tumor spillage significantly increases local recurrence; therefore, its existence, local or diffuse, elevates staging and has repercussions for treatment intensification. The renal artery and vein are palpated and ligated early, as close to the aorta as possible, to detect thrombus and prevent tumor embolization, bearing in mind that renal vasculature anomalies are frequent. The ureter is divided as low as possible, again after palpation, to rule out intraureteral extension. Any residual tumor may be marked with titanium clips to define areas needing future management.

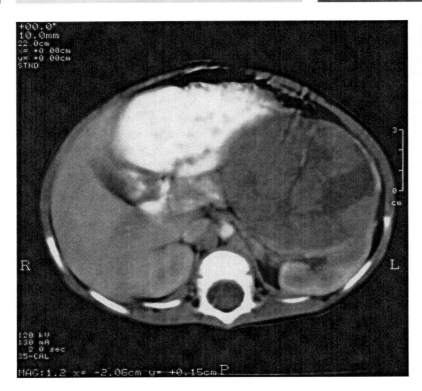

Figure 18.1

CT scan using oral and intravenous contrast demonstrating a large mass arising from the left kidney (Wilms' tumor). Image courtesy of Dr Sandra Butler, Consultant Radiologist, RHSC, Glasgow, Scotland

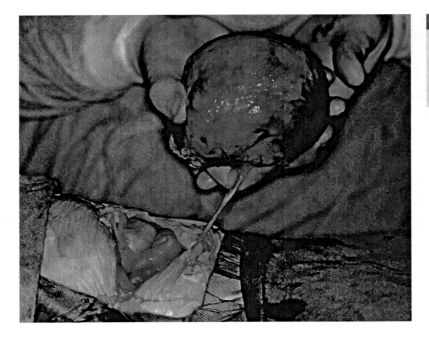

Figure 18.2

Image of removal of a Wilms' tumor by radical nephrectomy. Image courtesy of Dr Sandra Butler, Consultant Radiologist, RHSC, Glasgow, Scotland

18.1.3.3 Postoperative Care

Complications of postnephrectomy may well be related to the type of excision, tumor histology and stage, place of incision, and intravascular tumor extension. High thoracoabdominal or flank incisions may result in pleural lacerations or pneumothorax requiring chest drain insertion. Pain related to the posture required during surgery and to the incision site predisposes to chest infections. Significant intraoperative hemorrhage is documented (6%) from tumor vessels (especially during partial nephrectomy) and adrenal glands and adjacent structures (particularly the liver and duodenum during right and the spleen during left radical nephrectomy). Distorted vascular anatomy increases the risks for iatrogenic injury to or incorrect ligation of the aortic arterial branches during surgery (Ritchey et al., 1992). Tumor rupture from friable Wilms' or highly vascular angiomyolipomas may lead to extensive hemorrhage. Bleeding may be exacerbated by preexisting coagulation disorders from neochemotherapy. Small bowel occlusions (SBO) that can cause intestinal obstructions through adhesions or intussusception are the most common postoperative complication (7%) and may be exacerbated by edematous pressure necrosis of the bowel, which may lead to perforation and infection. Recognition of SBO may be difficult in the immediate postoperative period due to the relative frequency of paralytic ileus as a result of extensive bowel handling. This may be accentuated if vincristine has been part of the preoperative chemotherapy regime. Intravascular extension of the tumor and subsequent risks of embolization on mobilization can be reduced by early renal vessel ligation and palpation; however, this may risk tumor rupture and spillage. Other problems that may arise following partial nephrectomy include the following:

- Blockage from postoperative bleeding into the ureter, with clot obstruction or persistent urinary flank drainage that may suggest urinary fistula formation (Campbell et al., 1994).
- Impaired wound healing and loss of host defense mechanisms as a result of chemotherapy and poor nutritional status, leading to increased risk of infection and delayed recovery

- Ureteral obstruction and varying degrees of renal insufficiency, which may require temporary dialysis

Table 18.1 summarizes the postoperative nursing management required following nephrectomy.

After the patient has recovered from surgery, both chemotherapy and occasionally radiation are often prescribed. Appropriate radiographic follow-up is required because clear cell carcinomas and renal cell carcinomas may metastasize to bone, rhabdoid tumors and clear cell carcinomas to the brain, and in particular WT to the lungs, with a potential for contralateral kidney tumor development.

18.1.4 Prognosis

Overall survival with multimodal therapy for WT of favorable histology is high – 95%. Follow-up for pulmonary metastatic recurrence and appearance of a second WT in the remaining kidney is mandatory, alongside assessment of renal function and control of any presenting hypertension. Renal prognosis is also poorer with subsequent cytotoxic therapy.

Renal hyperperfusion syndrome can follow unilateral nephrectomy, with focal glomerulonephritis and a deterioration in renal function leading to the need for dialysis and transplantation.

Congenital mesoblastic nephroma presenting in neonates has survival figures nearing 100% cure after complete excision. However, 4-year survival for clear cell sarcoma and rhabdoid tumors is less encouraging, with high rates of cerebral metastatic disease.

Patients with bilateral disease responsive to chemotherapy may require unilateral nephrectomy with partial nephrectomy on the contralateral side that is least affected and/or with better histology with maximal parenchymal sparing (of more than 50%) and removal of positive margins. Dialysis may be needed to supplement renal function when the complexity of simultaneous chemotherapy temporarily reduces renal performance.

Survival rates for patients with bilateral nephrectomy and transplantation are dismal in the early stages due to sepsis from chemotherapy and immunosuppression. However, delaying the transplan-

Table 18.1. Postoperative nephrectomy nursing management

Nursing action	Rationale	Potential problems detected
1. Vital signs, TPR, BP, SaO₂, air entry, abdominal distension	Signs of shock, infection, hypovolemia, respiratory depression, hypoxia, poor chest expansion	Hemorrhage, wound or chest infection, pneumothorax, thrombocytopenia, bowel obstruction, opiate-induced respiratory depression
2. Accurate fluid balance intake vs. urine and bowel output, care of urinary catheter	Assess renal function, urinary flow, vomiting, and bowel activity	Ureteral obstruction, renal insufficiency, edema, dehydration, bowel obstruction, paralytic ileus
3. Pain management, use of patient-controlled analgesia and pain tool, good postural support	Postural and procedural pain control aids mobility, well-being; and cooperation	Inadequate chest expansion leads to chest infections, delayed return of bowel activity due to immobility
4. Management of IV fluid and blood product replacement, introduction of oral fluids, diet, antiemetics	NPO for 1st 24 hours or until bowel activity begins; nausea reduces oral intake; promote renal flow	Paralytic ileus, bowel obstruction, renal function reduced with dehydration, hypovolemia, anemia
5. Observation of wound site and any drainage systems	Ensure good healing, detect infection, assess bleeding/serous fluid loss. May be of poor nutritional status and immunocompromised	Wound infection, abscess formation, hematoma, urinary flank drainage, fistula formation
6. Laboratory investigations: urine and blood	Full/complete blood count, BUN, creatinine, electrolytes, osmolality, clotting, calcium, magnesium, renal and liver function, phosphate	Renal insufficiency, dehydration, fluid overload, electrolyte imbalance, infection, thrombocytopenia

tation procedure with dialysis in the interim for approximately 2 years also allows for likely metastatic recurrence.

Wilms' tumorigenesis is due to local rather than systemic factors, so recurrence in the transplanted kidney is unlikely (Mitchell, 1997). Children with acquired solitary kidney are at risk of hypertension, proteinuria, Fanconi's syndrome, and renal insufficiency with compensatory renal hypertrophy.

After nephrectomy, patient education is of great importance regarding follow-up, hypertension management, any dietary restrictions, and awareness of the risk of urinary infections and trauma to the remaining kidney, and the patient should wear Medic Alert discs.

18.2 Cytotoxic Drug Excretion

The mechanisms involved in effective drug administration are intricate on all occasions, but even more so when a variety of cytotoxic drugs (whose primary aim of cell kill provides for multiorgan impact), with their possibility of drug interactions, is used.

Without careful control and intervention, a perpetuating cycle of increasing toxicity, organ failure, morbidity, and mortality may occur. Absorption and metabolic and excretory patterns of antineoplastic agents are important determinants of therapeutic index, mechanisms of delivery, and drug modification.

18.2.1 Pharmacokinetics/Dynamics

The bioavailability of a drug depends on absorption, distribution, biotransformation (metabolism), and excretion, and reflects total exposure of that drug, time versus concentration, half-lives, and clearance, which are significant in predicting cytotoxicity and optimizing scheduling and methods of administration. Knowledge of half-lives can be important when estimating the lowest plasma cytotoxic activity for planning peripheral stem cell transfusion or granulocyte colony stimulating factor (GCSF) dosing. Third-space fluid collections, such as ascites or pleural effusions, can substantially alter pharmacokinetics, with important ramifications for highly scheduled agents (e.g., methotrexate) and may require evacuation before therapy begins.

Pathways of drug clearance can be affected by

- The patient's physiological state
- Genetic individuality
- The patient's prior exposure to the drug
- Drug interactions
- The patient's age

Pharmacodynamic variation between children and adults have led to different toxicities and altered outcomes of therapy. At times of major physiological change, such as infancy and puberty, pharmacokinetic variations also occur (see Fig. 18.3), making therapeutic drug monitoring and dose adjustment critical for safe, effective delivery in children. For example, methotrexate appears to have faster clearance in younger children (Borsi, 1994a). There is a concept that drug clearance, and hence exposure, is based on body size. However, infants weighing <10 kg conventionally have their doses based on weight rather than surface area, with some protocols reducing doses further on the basis of tissue tolerance in infants being lower than in older children.

Dietary intake, nutritional status, gut motility, mucosal changes, and surgery may affect oral absorption.

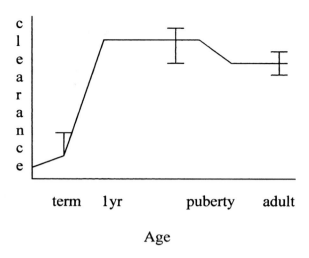

Figure 18.3

Representative developmental changes in drug clearance (Nies and Spielberg, 1996) Copyright McGraw-Hill; reproduced with permission

18.2.2 Metabolism

The metabolic activation and inactivation of drugs is carried out primarily by the liver, although enzymes are present in the small bowel that may be influenced by gut bacteria (and consequent antibiotic therapy) and deaminases in plasma and other normal tissues. Hepatic dysfunction, malnutrition, or genetic predisposition can affect metabolic capacity. Evidence of liver failure will mean that some cytotoxics will require dose modification (Table 18.2).

Circadian timing of anticancer drugs (e.g., cisplatin) and biologic agents can result in altered metabolism, with improved toxicity profiles and enhanced tumor control (Wood and Hrushesky, 1996).

Table 18.2. Cytotoxic drug dose modification and drug interactions (Borsi, 1994b; Ignoffo et al., 1998; Neonatal and Paed. Pharm. Group, 2001; Tortorice, 1997)

Drug	Reduce dose in	Modification	Drug interactions
Amsacarine	Renal failure (RF) and liver failure (LF)	35% reduction in hepatic dysfunction; 25–50% reduction if GFR<10 ml/minute	
Asparaginase	RF and LF		Methotrexate reduces toxicity; increases vincristine-associated peripheral neuropathy
Bleomycin	RF	Creatinine clearance 20–30 ml/min = 50% of dose <20 ml/min = 40% of dose	Half-life increased with cisplatin
Busulfan	RF and LF		Phenytoin increases clearance
Carboplatin	RF	Specific formulas	Acute reduction in GFR with other nephrotoxics
Cisplatin	RF	Creatinine clearance >60 ml/min = 100% dose 30–60 ml/min = 50% of dose <30: avoid	Toxicity increased by ifosfamide, amino glycosides, and amphotericin Enhances cytotoxicity of etoposide; reduces anticonvulsant absorption; inactivated by mesna
Cyclophosphamide	RF	Creatinine clearance <10 ml/min = 50% of dose Mesna + hyperhydration	Allopurinol prolongs half-life Dexamethasone shortens half-life Barbiturates may enhance cytotoxic activity Reduces oral digoxin absorption
Cytarabine	RF	Creatinine clearance <60 ml/min = 50% of dose	Inhibits methotrexate
Dacarbazine	RF and LF		
Dactinomycin	RF and LF		Reactivation of radiation reactions
Daunorubicin	LF		
Doxorubicin	LF	Bilirubin level: 1.2–3 mg/dl = 50% of dose >3 mg/dl = 25% of dose	Increases cyclosporine levels
Etoposide	RF	Creatinine clearance >50 ml/min = 100% dose 10–50 ml/min = 75% of dose <10 = 50% of dose	Metabolic clearance raised by corticosteroids, cyclophosphamide, ifosfamide, phenobarbital, phenytoin Clearance decreased by erythromycin and clarithromycin Cytotoxicity enhanced by cisplatin Increases cyclosporine levels
Ifosfamide	RF	Creatinine clearance >50 ml/min = 100% dose 10–50 ml/min = 75% of dose <10 ml/min = 50% of dose	Activation decreased by erythromycin/ clarithromycin Metabolism increased by phenobarbital Prolongs warfarin prothrombin time (PT) Raises cisplatin nephrotoxicity
Melphalan	RF		
Mercaptopurine	LF	Reduce by third to quarter of dose with allopurinol administration	Metabolic activity decreased by co-trimoxazole Shortens warfarin PT Allopurinol reduces metabolic clearance

Table 18.2. (Continued)

Drug	Reduce dose in	Modification	Drug interactions
Methotrexate	RF and LF	Calcium leucovorin administration in high dose or with creatinine clearance of <60 ml/min Creatinine clearance 10–50 ml/min =25–50% of dose <10 ml/min: avoid Urinary pH must be >7	Competition for tubular secretion by salicylates, NSAIDs, aminoglycoside, penicillins, cisplatin, cephalosporins. Uptake inhibited by cytarabine Increased toxicity by co-trimoxazole *(stop 1/52 before infusions)*
Procarbazine	RF and LF		Additive CNS depression with narcotics, barbiturates, and phenothiazines
Thioguanine	LF		With busulfan can cause hepatic hyperplasia and portal hypertension
Vinblastine	LF (especially infants)	Bilirubin level: 1.2–3 mg/dl = 50% dose >3 mg/dl = 25%	Increased clearance by corticosteroids, cyclophosphamide, ifosfamide Clarithromycin and erythromycin increase toxicity Acute pulmonary reaction with mitomycin C Decreases phenytoin blood levels
Vincristine	LF	Bilirubin level: 1.2–3mg/dl = 50% dose >3 mg/dl = 25%	Increases asparaginase peripheral neuropathy Erythromycin, phenytoin, and clarithromycin interactions as for vinblastine

Cyclosporine levels are reduced with phenytoin and barbiturates and increased with erythromycin, doxorubicin, and etoposide. Nephrotoxicity is increased after melphalan, cisplatin, carboplatin, vancomycin, amphotericin B, and aminoglycosides

18.2.3 Excretion

The kidneys are responsible for the majority of elimination of exogenously administered drugs, their metabolites, and potentially dangerous endogenous compounds. Any significant decrease in renal function will be reflected by an increase in all body toxicities of anticancer drugs dependant on this route, some of which are, themselves, nephrotoxic.

To recall:

Renal excretion = (Glomerular filtration
+ tubular secretion) – tubular reabsorption

The main impediments to solute passage through glomerular capillary walls are particle size and charge (i.e., positive or negative). Serum proteins do not filtrate; therefore, drug protein binding affects the efficiency of excretion. Renal blood flow remains constant through a wide range of perfusion pressures, but autoregulation may be impaired by ischemic injury, furosemide/frusemide use, or extracellular fluid depletion. Renal clearance of many acid/base drugs varies over the pH range. Alkalinization of tubular urine means that weak acids are excreted more rapidly. This is particularly relevant with methotrexate use, where co-administration of acids competing for excretion in the renal tubules or alkalinization with allopurinol can have potentially disastrous consequences (Tables 18.2 and 18.3). Biliary excretion is secondary but forms the primary elimination pathway for the vinca alkaloids. It involves a number of transport mechanisms that can be inhibited by a variety of drugs and disease processes. After excretion some may be broken down in the gut by bacterial enzymes and reabsorbed in the small bowel, leading to an enterohepatic circulation. The respiratory system and skin are lesser-documented pathways of excretion.

Table 18.3. Excretory pathways of cytotoxic drugs (Borsi, 1994b; Ignoffo et al., 1998; Neonatal and Paed. Pharm. Group, 2001; Tortorice, 1997)

Drugs	Pediatric use	Excretory pathway	Comments
Asparaginase	ALL, AML, CML	Biliary, minimal renal	May cause anaphylaxis, coagulopathies, hyperammonemia
Bleomycin	Lymphoma; Hodgkin's disease	50% renal (40% as active drug)	Children <3 years have a faster clearance; prior cisplatin therapy may reduce clearance
Busulfan	BMT	Metabolites renally	Requires hydration and allopurinol
Carboplatin	Solid tumors; BMT	Extensive hepatic metabolism 70% renal excretion	Abnormal LFTs reported, renal toxicity increased with prior impairment; removed by hemo-dialysis in overdosage
Carmustine	Hodgkin's disease, NHL, brain tumors	80% renal excretion	
Cisplatin	Solid tumors, osteosarcoma, neuroblastoma	90% renal, <10% biliary	Acute/chronic renal insufficiency; magnesium wasting
Cyclophos-phamide	ALL, AML, NHL, Ewing's sarcoma, rhabdomyosarcoma, neuroblastoma, BMT	Liver-activated, exclusively renal elimination	Hemorrhagic cystitis, antidiuretic effect (SIADH); avoid low-sodium-containing solutions; care with furosemide; use of mesna
Cytarabine	AML, ALL, lymphoma	90% renal excretion	May cause hyperuricemia
Dacarbazine	Neuroblastoma, Hodgkin's, sarcomas	Renal, some biliary	Hepatotoxic
Dactinomycin	Wilms' tumor, Ewing's sarcoma, rhabdomyo-sarcoma, Hodgkin's, NHL	50% biliary, 10% renal	Hepatoveno-occlusive toxicity
Daunorubicin	AML, ALL	20% renal, mainly biliary	Turns urine red/orange
Doxorubicin	ALL, neuroblastoma, Hodgkin's, osteosarcoma	5–10% renal, 40–80% biliary	Turns urine red/orange; may enhance cyclophosphamide chronic hemorrhagic cystitis
Etoposide	ALL, AML, BMT, Ewing's sarcoma, neuroblastoma	Minimal biliary, mainly urinary	
Ifosfamide	Solid tumors	70–80% urinary	Hemorrhagic cystitis requiring concurrent mesna
Melphalan	BMT	30% renal, 30% fecal	Ensure GFR>30 ml/min with prior established hydration
Mercaptopurine	ALL	50% renal	Drug accumulation in renal failure
Methotrexate	ALL, BMT, osteosarcoma	60–90% unchanged renal excretion, 10% biliary	Increase hydration, urinary alkalization >pH 7, folinic acid rescue in high dose; 3rd-space fluid collections alter clearance times; renal dys-function results in increased biliary excretion
Procarbazine	Hodgkin's	25–70% renal as metabolites	

Table 18.3. (Continued)

Drugs	Pediatric use	Excretory pathway	Comments
Thioguanine	AML, ALL (pre-2003)	40–80% renal, some fecal	Can cause hepatic dysfunction, veno-occlusive disease
Thiopeta	BMT	60% renal as metabolites	
Vinblastine	Lymphoma, Hodgkin's, histiocytosis	35% renal, 20% biliary (70% retained for 7 days)	Risk of urinary retention due to bladder atony
Vincristine	ALL, many cancers	10–20% urinary, 70% biliary	Dysuria; polyuria (SIADH), urinary retention due to bladder atony. Plasmapheresis and pheno-barbitone required in overdose
Mesna	With ifosfamide and cyclophosphamide	Rapid urinary excretion	Delayed excretion in even mild renal failure means lengthening delivery times

18.2.4 Drug Interactions

Given the complexity of most treatment regimens using multiple cytotoxics, analgesics, anticonvulsants, antiemetics, and steroids, relatively little specific data are available. Interactions may result in beneficial effect, improving therapeutic response or lessening toxicity. But in most cases the reverse is true, with some drugs indirectly altering the eliminating function of end organs and so resulting in delayed clearance. Some patients may feel the need to complement treatment with homeopathic remedies that can enhance or decrease both effect and toxicity.

Selected drugs are known to enhance hepatic microsomal metabolism (cyclophosphamide, phenobarbital, phenytoin, rifampicin), whereas others inhibit (cimetide, alpha-interferon). Trimethoprim-sulfamethoxazole (co-trimoxazole) can decrease protein binding of methotrexate and increase systemic exposure.

Asparaginase may reduce hepatic clearance of vinca alkaloids.

Unfortunately, many of the drug interactions involve other medications commonly used in the oncology setting, and the potential increases with the number of drugs received.

18.2.5 Dose Modification

Understanding pharmacokinetics, pharmacodynamics, and drug interactions means that adaptive control and, in some circumstances, individualization can be used to maximize the therapeutic effect within acceptable toxicity ranges. Dose modification due to impaired clearance or altered pharmacodynamics, use of modulating drugs (e.g., folinic acid given as calcium folinate/leucovorin) and careful monitoring of end-organ function form essential components of cancer chemotherapy management (see Table 18.2).

Methotrexate is an example where there is known faster clearance in younger children. Many acid-based drugs compete for tubular secretion, determining the need for accurate urinary pH regulation and good hydration/diuresis; consequently, creatinine clearance does not reflect methotrexate elimination. Folinic acid, a drug modulator, is used as "rescue" in high-dose regimens or in renal failure. Accurate measuring of plasma concentrations of methotrexate is available and should be implemented, particularly in high methotrexate dosages or when there is evidence of fluid collections. Such measuring can prevent the bone marrow, hepatic, nephrological, and, less commonly, neurological toxicities that can occur and can allow folinic acid treatment to be tailored appropriately.

Carboplatin clearance is closely correlated with glomerular filtration rate (GFR). If the dose is based on body surface area (BSA) and GFR is high, there is a risk of underdosing, whereas a low GFR risks unacceptable toxicity. Hence, dosing formulas have been developed based on an individual's GFR and have been further adapted for pediatric use (Newell et al., 1993). It is important to remember that GFR is correlated with BSA, and smaller patients will appear to have poorer renal function unless the GFR is adjusted for the BSA (ml/min/m^2).

In view of enterohepatic circulation, serum bilirubin, although representative of hepatic function, may not reflect clearance of drugs that are primarily excreted through this route and should be complemented with a measurement of function, such as albumin.

Useful agents should not be withheld because of potential toxicities, but preventative measures may reduce the risks. Preventative measures include

- Assessment of preexisting renal disease
- Use of ultrasound or isotope scans
- Dose modification
- Hydration, diuresis, and urinary pH adjustment
- Substitution with agents that have less similar/synergistic end-organ toxicity
- Monitoring of drug levels, creatinine clearance, uric acid, GFR, electrolytes, BUN (urea), complete/full blood count, calcium, phosphate, magnesium, serum albumin, osmolality, liver function tests, and bilirubin
- Monitoring of urinary pH and urinary morphology, proteinuria, level of hydration, and volume of urinary output

Certain drugs are incompatible and may have their pharmacokinetic/dynamic properties altered if delivered concurrently or within the same infusion devices.

18.2.6 Safe Handling of Cytotoxic Excreta

Anticancer drugs are well documented as being irritative, carcinogenic, mutagenic, and teratogenic. They can also have many side effects, such as skin rashes, scarring, dizziness, and blurred vision. Safety measures regarding preparation, administration, and disposal of cytotoxically contaminated material are vital to protect health care professionals, patients, and their families. Pregnant women, whether they are medical personnel or, as is likely in the pediatric setting, mothers, particular need education about the meticulous care required for both self- and fetal protection. Avoidance of pregnancy is preferable but may be unrealistic. Contraceptive advice should be given.

Preparation and administration of cytotoxics is rapidly becoming more controlled as evidence becomes available about the potentially long-term damaging effects to all concerned. It is, however, understandable that many falsely view the less-invasive methods of administration (i.e., oral) to be less significant, and lapses in safeguards can occur. Suitability of protective clothing is a key factor in affecting permeation of cytotoxics (Allwood et al., 1997), with glove thickness and material (latex is better than vinyl) and completely absorbent disposable isolation gowns playing a role in preventing contamination. Awareness and staff attitude vary among different professional areas, with pharmacists showing the most, and doctors the least, awareness regarding the significance of

- eye protection
- inhalation from aerosolization
- risks of skin contamination directly via drugs/excreta
- contamination indirectly from contact during poor removal techniques of infected gloves, gowns, or aprons (Labuhn et al., 1998)

Healthcare workers should remember that all patient excreta should be considered potentially cytotoxic:

- Urine
- Skin
- Sweat
- Feces
- Blood
- Vomitus
- Breast milk
- Dressings/wounds/drains

Table 18.4. Classification and causes of oncological-related renal failure

Classification	Factors	Causes
Prerenal	Hypovolemia	Hemorrhage, hypoproteinemia
	Hypotension	Septicemia, hemorrhage, disseminated intravascular coagulation
Renal	Localized intravascular coagulation	Renal vein thrombosis, cortical necrosis, hemolytic uremic syndrome (HUS)
	Acute tubular necrosis	Chemicals, drugs, heavy metals, hemoglobin, shock, ischemia
	Acute interstitial nephritis	Infection, drugs
	Tumors	Renal parenchymal infiltration, uric acid nephropathy
Postrenal	Obstructive nephropathy	Tumor, *Aspergillus* spores, blood clots, stones (uric acid)

Certain measures effective in reducing risks of exposure to staff and families include wearing gloves whenever handling excreta and washing hands thoroughly after removing them. Males should be encouraged to sit to pass urine, and toilets should be double-flushed with lids closed to avoid aerosolization. Vomitus may contain high concentrations of chemotherapy for 2 hours after oral administration. There is vast variation in clearance from urine and feces, but contact should generally be considered hazardous for up to 7 days after cytotoxic treatment.

Until recent years the dangers of poor handling and disposal of cytotoxic drugs and excreta have been underestimated, and staff education in this area must be reinforced to protect all involved.

18.3 Nephrotoxicity

18.3.1 Incidence

The kidneys form the elimination pathway for many drugs used in the oncological setting and are particularly vulnerable to toxicity because of their

- Vascular supply
- Large endothelial surface area
- High metabolic activity
- Potential for accumulation/precipitation of drugs and their breakdown products within the glomerulus and tubular cells

The entire anatomical system, from glomerulus through distal tubule to ureter, is at risk. Nephrotoxicity is a dose-limiting side effect of some chemotherapeutic agents, and its presence will potentiate overall toxicities of many other drugs that depend on this excretory pathway (see 18.2 Cytotoxic Drug Excretion). Acute renal failure with sudden loss of renal function will cause serious fluid and electrolyte imbalances and, without prompt action, result in severe short- and long-term morbidity and death. Nephrotoxicity leading to renal failure can be classified as prerenal, renal, or postrenal (see Table 18.4). Additional risk factors include the patient's nutritional status, hydration, radiation, unilateral or partial nephrectomy, duration of cancer therapy, large tumor bulk, preexisting renal disease, infection, and age.

Aminoglycoside antibiotics are thought to cause transient nonoliguric renal failure in 10–30% of patients and are one of the greatest causes of drug-induced acute nephrotoxicities.

Renal toxicity from ifosfamide treatment ranges from 5–40%, with children under 5 years being at greatest risk. Some studies show the risk of dysfunction being as high as 9% for moderate and 9% for severe in the acute phase, leading to chronic tubular damage over a 5-year-period of 25–44% (Loebstein et al., 1999). This underlines the need to balance toxicity with efficacy.

Late onset renal failure has occurred in up to 20% of bone marrow transplant (BMT) survivors, with total body irradiation (TBI) being a major factor, potentiated by chemotherapy (Cohen et al., 1995)

18.3.2 Etiology

18.3.2.1 Iatrogenic

Radiation

Fortunately, with the rise in neochemotherapy and surgery, the role of irradiation of renal structures has decreased; consequently, less radiation nephritis is seen. Dosages of >2,300 cGy are a cause of damage to the epithelial lining in the acute phases and of chronic nephritis – which may have a delayed onset of 3–13 years – as a result of arterionephrosclerosis and vascular occlusion. Pediatric renal tolerance is lower than in adults; the National Wilms' Study Group (NWSG) showed a threshold of around 14 Gy (Cassady, 1995). Conditioning regimens for BMT are near this dosage. In addition, nephrotoxic chemotherapy, aminoglycosides, antifungals, and immunosuppressants are prescribed; therefore, late chemoradiation marrow transplant renal dysfunction occurs. Thrombomicroangiopathy and hemolytic uremic syndrome (HUS) with hemoglobinuria can develop after BMT, resulting in renal insufficiency due to a combination of TBI, graft versus host disease (GvHD), and cyclosporine.

Chemicals

Treatment of large bulk, chemosensitive tumors in the initial phase leads to massive toxic breakdown of nucleic acid from tumor cells within 1–5 days, resulting in tumor lysis syndrome. Liberation of vast quantities of urate, phosphate, and potassium overwhelms the excretory capacity of the kidneys, causing hyperkalemia, hyperuricemia, and hyperphosphatemia (with secondary hypocalcemia). Precipitation of urate or calcium phosphate crystals in renal tubules causes acute renal failure and worsening metabolic dysfunction, so even with prophylaxis, as many as 10% will experience some degree of renal deterioration.

Malignant infiltration of parenchymal tissue and ureters will only manifest loss of renal function if both kidneys are affected; however, surgical release can lead to brisk diuresis, hypovolemia, shock, and reduced renal perfusion.

Nephrotoxic compounds may alter the kidneys either directly by reducing renal blood flow (causing obstruction during urine production) or through tubular necrosis, or indirectly through hypersensitivity reactions. Many chemotherapy agents are metabolized with the drug and/or metabolites being excreted by the kidneys (see 18.2, Cytotoxic Drug Excretion), and notably cisplatin, carboplatin, ifosfamide, cyclophosphamide, and methotrexate are the instigators of most toxicities (see Table 18.5 for details of nephrotoxic drugs). Pediatric patients are particularly sensitive and can demonstrate subclinical glomerular dysfunction and tubular toxicity (Cachat and Guignard, 1996). Fanconi's syndrome, caused by a number of medications, is demonstrated by renal phosphate and amino acid loss, which results in bone mineralization interference and renal rickets, growth failure, and decompensated renal tubular injury.

Hypotension can occur if drugs are given too rapidly (carmustine, etoposide) or as a result of anaphylaxis (asparaginase, cisplatin, amphotericin). Many of the supportive drugs used in oncology, such as salicylates, nonsteroidal anti-inflammatory medications, and medications used for immunosuppression and treatment of infection, are also nephrotoxic and additionally cause or potentiate damage to the already vulnerable renal system.

18.3.2.2 Fungal

The two most common opportunistic fungal infections seen in oncology patients are *Candida* and *Aspergillus*. Systemic invasion of these requires aggressive therapy in the immunocompromised patient. On rare occasions, *Aspergillus* spores have been known to invade renal vasculature, leading to medullary and cortical microabscesses and renal infarction, or spores may lodge in the filtration pathways and lead to an obstructive nephropathy that requires surgery. It is, however, the antifungal agents themselves, particularly conventional as opposed to lipid amphotericin B, that cause substantial nephrotoxicity, especially in conjunction with cyclosporine or aminoglycoside use.

Table 18.5. Nephrotoxic drugs in pediatric oncology

Drug	Mechanism of damage	Synergistic drugs	Risk factor	Other comments
BCNU/CCNU	Direct glomerular damage, tubular atrophy, interstitial nephritis		Cumulative dose of 1,200 mg/m²	
Carboplatin	Interstitial nephritis, renal tubule damage, HUS (<cisplatin)	Prior use of nephrotoxics	High doses for stem cell transplant	Transient, use pediatric GFR-based dose formula
Cisplatin	Platinum metal chelates in renal tubules, electrolyte imbalance, HUS; tubular nephritis, necrosis, atrophy	Ifosfamide Amphotericin Aminoglycosides, vancomycin	Multidoses >50 mg/m² Damage dose-related and cumulative	Renal tubular injury causes salt-losing syndrome and hypomagnesemia
Cyclophos-phamide	Rarely, renal tubular necrosis	Cisplatin Vincristine		Rarely, inappropriate ADH
Ifosfamide	Glomerular and tubular toxicity, proteinuria, Fanconi's syndrome	Prior use of nephrotoxics Cisplatin Radiotherapy	>119 g/m²: very high risk >84 g/m²: moderate risk Children <3 years: high risk	Renal deterioration after cessation of treatment; toxicity cumulative
Methotrexate	Obstructive tubular precipitation of drug and metabolites, tubular necrosis	Other acids Cephalosporins Cisplatin Co-trimoxazole NSAIDs	High dose >1gm/m² (plus leucovorin)	Renal swelling, oliguria, anuria (plus with hydration)
Mitomycin	Glomerular cell damage, deposition of platelets and fibrin, rise in creatinine	Vincristine	Risks increase with cumulative doses	Microangiopathic hemolytic anemia can develop later
Thioguanine	Crystallization of 6-thiouric acid causes hematuria	Allopurinol	Massive intravenous doses of 6TG	Clears with drug cessation
Amino-glycosides	Proximal tubule necrosis, proteinuria, loss of protein concentration ability	Amphotericin, vancomycin Piperacillin Cephalosporin.	Cumulative risk	Nonoliguric renal failure, hypomagnesemia, Fanconi's
Amphotericin	Tubular transport defects and vasoconstriction, tubular acidosis	Aminoglycosides	Lipid form is less toxic	Salt-loading ameliorates toxicity, hypomagnesemia, hyponatremia
Cyclosporin	Increased renal vascular resistance, renal dysfunction, hypertension	Aminoglycosides Carboplatinum Cisplatin Amphotericin		Renal damage usually reversible, hypomagnesemia
Others:				
NSAIDs	Interstitial nephritis, nephrotic syndrome			
Penicillamines	Interstitial nephritis, nephrotic syndrome			
Pentamidine	Hypomagnesemia			
Salicylates	Interstitial nephritis, Fanconi's syndrome			
Sulfonamides	Interstitial nephritis, renal vasculitis			

18.3.2.3 Viral

Although a number of viruses are known to damage the epithelial lining of the bladder, little is documented with regard to kidney involvement. It should be noted, though, that renal manifestations of injury can be seen with acyclovir use (Bergstein, 1996).

18.3.2.4 Bacterial

Renal infections and generalized septicemia can result in shock, hypovolemia, hypotension, and decreased renal perfusion, which will lead to a reduced GFR and acute renal failure. Aminoglycosides and vancomycin form the mainstay of gram-negative organism treatment but, unfortunately, are nephrotoxic, necessitating careful serum concentration measurement.

18.3.3 Prevention

Balancing the efficacy of chemotherapy and radiotherapy against possible side effects and short- and long-term morbidity makes for challenging sequencing of treatment. Risks should be reduced by

- Substitution with nonnephrotoxic compounds
- Careful drug, blood, and urine monitoring
- Dose modification/withdrawal
- Avoidance of simultaneous and/or synergistic therapies

The main protective measure used in *all* cytotoxic drug administration emphasizes establishing hydration and good diuresis (in some cases with diuretics) prior to, during, and after their delivery.

Preventative measures include the following:

- Prior hydration and allopurinol with urinary alkalinization when tumor lysis and urate production are anticipated
- Consideration of the elimination pathways and optimal conditions for excretion; e.g., alkalinization, avoidance of acid drugs, and leucovorin prophylaxis with methotrexate
- Awareness of cumulative dose effects

Prompt action in the event of febrile neutropenia should avoid septic shock. Increasingly, once-daily dosing with aminoglycosides given during the activity period of the day seems to reduce their nephrotoxicity (Beauchamp and Labrecque, 2001). Liposomal amphotericin B for empirical antifungal therapy has been shown to be as effective as the conventional form but is associated with less nephrotoxicity and fewer breakthrough fungal infections (Walsh et al., 1999). Nephroprotective measures, including supplementation of potassium, sodium, and magnesium ions in conjunction with hydration to replace expected kidney losses, appear to meliorate amphotericin B nephrotoxicity (Doubek et al., 2002).

18.3.4 Treatment

Signs of nephrotoxicity may initially be insidious and detectable only by blood analysis and monitoring of fluid balance. If the cause is prerenal with defective kidney perfusion and the underlying reason is anticipated and promptly corrected, then acute renal failure can be avoided.

In oliguric patients there is a need to distinguish between hypoperfusion, in which urine is concentrated (urine osmolality >500 mOsm/kg and sodium content <20 mEq/l [mmol/l]) and impending tubular necrosis, in which urine is more dilute (osmolality is <350 mOsm/kg and sodium concentration >40 mEq/l [mmol/l]).

Acute renal failure develops when renal function is diminished functionally, resulting in decreases in GFR, tubular transport of substances, urine production, and renal clearance. Oliguria (urine volume <400 ml/m²/day) is common, but nonoliguric renal failure may occur (e.g., aminoglycoside toxicity).

Signs of acute renal failure include

- Anemia
- Diminished urine output
- Peripheral edema
- Vomiting
- Lethargy
- Hypertension
- Consequent complications of congestive cardiac failure
- Pulmonary and cerebral edema and seizures

Figure 18.4

Progressive algorithm for management of acute renal failure

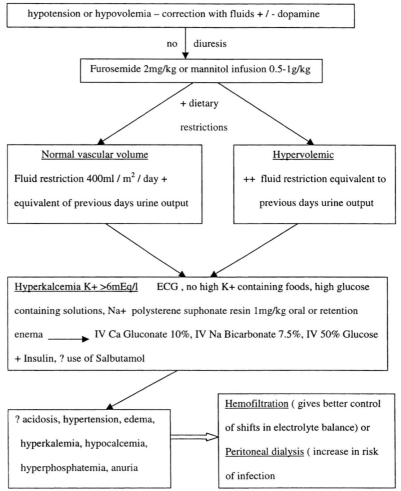

Figure 18.4

Progressive algorithm for management of acute renal failure

hypotension or hypovolemia – correction with fluids + / - dopamine

no | diuresis

Furosemide 2mg/kg or mannitol infusion 0.5-1g/kg

+ dietary

restrictions

Normal vascular volume

Fluid restriction 400ml / m^2 / day +

equivalent of previous days urine output

Hypervolemic

++ fluid restriction equivalent to

previous days urine output

Hyperkalcemia K+ >6mEq/l   ECG , no high K+ containing foods, high glucose

containing solutions, Na+ polysterene suphonate resin 1mg/kg oral or retention

enema _____→ IV Ca Gluconate 10%, IV Na Bicarbonate 7.5%, IV 50% Glucose

+ Insulin, ? use of Salbutamol

? acidosis, hypertension, edema,

hyperkalemia, hypocalcemia,

hyperphosphatemia, anuria

Hemofiltration (gives better control

of shifts in electrolyte balance) or

Peritoneal dialysis (increase in risk

of infection

Laboratory investigations:
urine – hematuria, pH, creatinine clearance, osmolality, specific gravity, casts.
blood - osmolality, protein, glucose, pH, Hb, FBC, urea, uric acid, electrolytes.

Correct precipitating disorders – infection, bleeding, anaphylaxis, drugs, obstruction.

Obstruction to the renal tract, which may be demonstrated by pain, dysuria, urinary retention, or renal dysfunction, may be excluded by radiography ± ultrasound. Intravenous contrast agents should be avoided because of increased risks of tubular necrosis. Percutaneous nephrostomy may be required to reverse a blockage.

Hypovolemia and hypotension need correction with appropriate fluids (blood products/albumen bolus/saline infusions) depending on the cause, and possibly a dopamine infusion to raise blood pressure.

If these conditions are associated with anaphylaxis, treatment will include hydrocortisone and adrenaline, or in the case of septicemia, treatment with antibiotics and/or antifungals will be required. A one-time dose of furosemide/frusemide or mannitol in the event of oliguria may be administered to attempt to effect a diuresis once hypovolemia and hypotension correction has been established. If there is no response, then fluid restriction and electrolyte balancing will need to commence. Figure 18.4 shows the algorithm for managing acute renal failure.

Table 18.6. Signs of electrolyte imbalance associated with nephrotoxicity

Electrolyte abnormality	Signs
Hypernatremia	Thirst, edema, weight gain, hypertension, tachycardia, dyspnea, CNS effects, seizures
Hyponatremia	CNS lethargy, coma, weakness, abdominal pain, muscle twitching, convulsions, nausea, vomiting, diarrhea
Hyperkalemia	Weakness, paralysis, paresthesias, nausea, diarrhea, abdominal pain, irregular pulse, muscle irritability, ECG changes, bradycardia, ventricular fibrillation, cardiac arrest
Hypokalemia	Weakness, paralysis, hypoventilation, polyuria, hypotension, paralytic ileus, nausea, vomiting, ECG changes
Hypocalcemia	Altered mental state, numbness/tingling of peripheries, muscle cramps, seizures, ECG changes, give high-calcium/low-phosphorus diet
Hypermagnesemia	Weakness, hypoventilation, hypotension, flushing, behavior changes
Hyperphosphatemia	Tetany, numbness of peripheries

When known nephrotoxic agents have been employed, monitoring of drug serum levels, dose modification relative to creatinine clearance, or drug withdrawal might be required (see 18.2 Cytotoxic Drug Excretion), and substitution with alternative non-nephrotoxic agents and avoidance of simultaneous nephrotoxics considered. In addition, certain drugs may have specific aids to reducing toxicity (see prevention) and treating a treatment overdose. For example,

Methotrexate overdose requires hemodialysis, charcoal hemofiltration, and cerebrospinal fluid exchange in the event of intrathecal overdose

Cisplatin overdose requires osmotic diuresis and plasmapheresis

Skill in accurate actual and anticipatory nursing management for acute renal failure heavily influences the ultimate outcome. Observation for fluid overload, metabolic disturbances, and electrolyte imbalance is essential.

18.3.4.1 Fluid Overload

— Weigh daily (or more often) at same time of day
— Strict fluid intake/output records
— Fluid intake restriction as per volemic status, ideally balanced throughout the 24 hours; may need reassessed hourly if patient critically imbalanced
— Vital signs of temperature, pulse, respirations, and blood pressure

— Check for dependant edema: sacral, periorbital, pedal
— Signs of respiratory edema or cardiac overload
— Urine specific gravity and urinalysis

18.3.4.2 Metabolic Acidosis

— Headache, nausea, vomiting
— Behavioral changes, lethargy, drowsiness
— Rapid, shallow respiration
— Restrict fat and protein intake to reduce acid end products
— Assist with bicarbonate dialysis if required

18.3.4.3 Electrolyte Imbalance

— Blood and urinary monitoring
— Strict dietary management
— Monitor for signs of electrolyte imbalance (see Table 18.6)
— Hemodialysis

18.3.5 Prognosis

The numbers of known adult survivors of childhood cancer have risen over the last 20 years but studies of long-term sequelae of treatment are restricted by the relatively recent development of intensive antitumoral therapy. Long-term outcomes are unknown, and careful monitoring for chronic toxicity is vital. The prognosis for recovery of renal function depends on its cause and the rapidity of response to diagnosis. Acute renal failure can be reversed if identified promptly before permanent damage occurs, which in its worst form may lead to a need for hemodialysis and transplantation. Renal tubulopathy effects are seen as metabolic acidosis, hypokalemia/magnesemia, proteinuria, Fanconi's syndrome, rickets, or a nephrogenic diabetes insipidus. Glomerular effects are demonstrated by a reduced GFR. Renal tubular dysfunction can persist for 2–4 years and may even be irreversible following cisplatin use, damage being accumulative (Skinner et al., 1998), and hypomagnesemia may be present in as many as 10 % of patients. Ifosfamide-induced problems may or may not be reversible and may progress after cessation of treatment, eventually resulting in chronic failure necessitating dialysis (Loebstein et al., 1999). The tubular toxicity from aminoglycosides is generally reversible if the response to serum concentration levels is timely.

Radiation nephropathy is seen as a result of dose-related nephroarteriosclerosis or ureteral fibrosis, causing reduced GFR, obstruction, and hypertension. Late-onset renal failure can occur in up to 20 % of BMT survivors. The bone marrow transplant nephropathy, which is mainly attributed to TBI potentiated by prior chemotherapy, eventually stabilizes, and survival becomes dependant on control of hypertension (Cohen et al., 1995; Oyama et al., 1996).

18.4 Hemorrhagic Cystitis

18.4.1 Incidence

The degree of vascularity and large surface area of the entire uroepithelium of the renal system mean that exposure to the causes of hemorrhagic cystitis (HC) can cause damage throughout the urological tract. The bladder is at particular risk because of the prolonged contact endured while storing urine that contains toxic elements, and its essential position makes it susceptible during pelvic irradiation.

Table 18.7. Grading of hemorrhagic cystitis

Grade	Hematuria present
0	None
1	Microhematuria
2	Macrohematuria (gross), no clots
3	Macrohematuria (gross), with clots
4	Severe bleeding/exsanguinating hemorrhage: transfusion required

HC can present

1. Symptomatically
   - Bladder irritation
   - Suprapubic or flank pain
   - Dysuria/frequency/urgency, hematuria of differing degrees
2. With mucosal changes
   - Inflammation
   - Edema
   - Ulceration
   - Bleeding
   - Ischemia
   - Necrosis

It is important to distinguish between red urinary discoloration caused by anthracyclines and true hematuria, which may range from minimal to life-threatening exsanguinating hemorrhage. (See Table 18.7 for grading of HC.) The incidence of HC is broad-ranging, being related to cause, co-morbidity, and synergistic effects of treatment.

Onset may be

- acute: within hours of chemotherapy/weeks of radiation
- chronic: months or years after BMT/radiation/chemotherapy

An estimated 50–80 % of patients receiving pelvic irradiation develop mild symptoms. As many as 50 % have microhematuria and 15 % have gross hematuria as a result of chemical cystitis (around 5–10 % with cyclophosphamide and 20–40 % with ifosfamide).

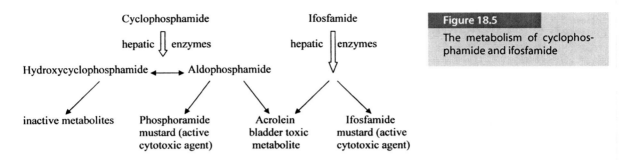

Figure 18.5

The metabolism of cyclophosphamide and ifosfamide

Late-onset HC after BMT ranges from 7–25% and can be correlated with conditioning, viral activation, and degree of graft versus host disease (GvHD) (Leung et al., 2002). The degree of myelosuppression heightens the risks and the severity as neutropenia allows for sepsis, and thrombocytopenia reduces clotting potential.

18.4.2 Etiology

18.4.2.1 Iatrogenic

Radiation and bladder-toxic chemotherapy (namely oxazophosphorine alkylating agents) are responsible for most HC cases; a minority can be attributed to coagulation disorders caused by myelosuppression, antifungals, antibiotics (penicillamines), and immunosuppressives (methotrexate and cyclosporine).

Radiation

Normal tissue tolerance of the bladder mucosa is 60–65 Gy (fractioned doses). Less radiosensitive tumors (e.g., rhabdomyosarcoma) may require 60–65 Gy to gain local control as a single form of treatment with huge morbidity; therefore, principles of management aim to reduce dosages to as low as 35 Gy using cytotoxic therapy and surgery prior to irradiation.

The acute inflammatory response, seen within 4–6 weeks, can occur years after cessation of treatment, and the time between radiation and development of symptoms is proportional to the dose received.

Simultaneous use of cyclophosphamide greatly increases the risks of radiation cystitis.

Chemical

HC is a major dose-limiting factor in the administration of cyclophosphamide and in particular ifosfamide. The drugs are metabolized through hydroxylation by microsomal hepatic enzymes to produce their inactive and active metabolites. Figure 18.5 shows the sequence of events in the metabolism of these drugs.

Urinary excretion of acrolein, which binds to the bladder mucosa, is believed to be the source of urothelial damage. The degree of the problem is

- Cumulative
- Dose-related (especially intensive regimes)
- Experienced more with ifosfamide use than with cyclophosphamide
- Seen in children despite lower doses and with shorter duration of cyclophosphamide
- Increasingly affected by similarly timed or prior use of bleomycin, carboplatin, etoposide, vincristine, cisplatin, busulfan, pelvic irradiation, and GU cancers

BMT patients using total body irradiation (TBI) and in particular busulfan in conditioning regimes are the most at risk.

18.4.2.2 Fungal

Renal aspergillosis results in renal vascular invasion, leading to cortical and medullary microabscesses and renal infarction. Dissemination of infection through the system consequently evokes cystitis, hematuria, pyuria, and proteinuria. *Candida* can also be causative. Amphotericin may potentiate renal failure and should be used cautiously.

18.4.2.3 Viral

HC in BMT patients can be classed as pre-engraftment, when hematuria is brief and not more severe than grade 2, or as post-engraftment, when HC is more protracted and often of grade ≥ 3 and associated with GvHD. Immunosuppression therapy inclusive of cyclosporine risks new viruses or reactivation of old viruses (adenovirus, polymavirus BK, cytomegalovirus [CMV], papovirus, influenza A).

18.4.2.4 Bacterial

Urosepsis is less commonly seen in children than adults and is usually associated with more intensive bone marrow suppressive schedules and episodes of urethral catheterization. Hematuria is usually mild although exacerbated by concurrent use of other known HC causative agents. The use of penicillin including methicillin, piperacillin, and penicillin G has been implicated in 4–8% of patients with no other known cause (Relling and Schunk, 1986).

18.4.3 Prevention

Prophylaxis is the primary management for HC. Preventative viral coverage post-BMT with acyclovir and ganciclovir/foscarnet and ensuring previous deliveries of CMV-negative and irradiated blood products will lessen the risks. Neoadjuvant chemotherapy and surgery prior to irradiation can help reduce exposure fields in the pelvic region.

Anticipatory administration of mesna (mercaptoethane sodium sulfonate), an organ-specific uroprotective agent, has become standard protocol with schedules involving cyclophosphamide or ifosfamide, but it only limits cystitis, not nephrotoxicity. Mesna does not compromise antitumor activity or BMT engraftment (Haselberger and Schwinghammer, 1995); it reduces the incidence of oxazophosphorine-induced bladder cancers; and it also inhibits the spontaneous breakdown of cyclophosphamide to acrolein in the urine. Cisplatin toxicity and side effects are also diminished with mesna, so it may be used as an antidote.

When absorbed, mesna undergoes oxidization to the dimerized form, dimesna. After glomerular filtration and tubular reabsorption, it is reduced back to its active form. The sulfhydryl group of mesna then complexes with acrolein to form a nontoxic thioether. Preexisting renal tubular damage leads to reduced mesna clearance and availability (Goren et al., 1987). Oral mesna tastes unpleasant, which, together with concomitant administration of emetogenic chemotherapy, makes for poor compliance. Early-morning chemotherapy allows for frequent daytime bladder emptying as opposed to nocturnal accumulation of toxic metabolites. The half-life of mesna is 35 minutes compared with 4 hours for cyclophosphamide. Any timing error in delivery affords reduced uroprotection and crucially gambles the development of HC by up to 60%. To be effective, sufficient urine concentrations of mesna (10–20 µmol/ml) must be achieved during acrolein excretion (Borsi, 1994b). A variety of protocols have been drawn up, but each adheres to these essential principles:

- Hyperhydration of $3 \, l/m^2/day \pm$ furosemide/frusemide to attain adequate diuresis
- Close blood and urine monitoring; observation for signs of syndrome of inappropriate antidiuretic hormone (SIADH)
- Oral mesna dosage is twice cyclophosphamide dose, commences 2 hours earlier, and is repeated after 2 and 6 hours
- If the daily or total cyclophosphamide dose $<300 \, mg/m^2$ then hydrate only
- If the daily or total cyclophosphamide dose is equal to $300 \, mg/m^2$, to $1 \, gm/m^2$, then hydrate at $3 \, l/m^2/day$, continuing for at least 6 hours after cessation of chemotherapy
- If the daily or total cyclophosphamide dose $>1 \, gm/m^2$ or any ifosfamide administration, then hydrate at $3 \, l/m^2/day$ plus mesna via either regime (A) or (B):
  - (A) Intravenous (IV) loading dose of mesna 15 minutes precytotoxic delivery of 20–25% ifosfamide or 60–120% cyclophosphamide (mg:mg) dose and repeat every 4 hours for three to five doses

Table 18.8. Nursing interventions in the management of hemorrhagic cystitis

1. Vital signs: temperature(T), pulse(P), respirations (R), blood pressure(BP)	T raised, P and BP up/down with infection, hypovolemia, or transfusion reaction
2. Monitor intake and output, check weight	Assess diuresis, need for furosemide. Signs of ifosfamide-induced renal tubular dysfunction (SIADH)
3. Maintain hydration (3 l/m²/day)	Encourage diuresis, bladder voiding
4. Administer mesna as per protocol	Correct timing with antineoplastics influences amelioration of HC
5. Urinalysis qid	Degree of hematuria affects management
6. Encourage frequent voiding, maintain continuous bladder irrigation	Reduces clot production/retention and acrolein accumulation in urine
7. Administer anticipatory antiemetics, analgesics, and antispasmodics	Reduce discomfort, promote urinary voiding compliance and hydration
8. Minimize constipation	Straining to eliminate exacerbates bleeding
9. Safe administration of blood products	Correct hypovolemia, thrombocytopenia, and PT time
10. Monitor for mesna toxicity	Headache, nausea, diarrhea, and limb pain
11. Blood sampling: urea, electrolytes, creatinine, Hb, BUN, WCC, uric acid, HCT, serum albumen, serum bilirubin, ALT[a], AST[b]	Effects of hemodilution, hypovolemia, furosemide, obstructive nephropathy nephrotoxicity, toxic hepatitis, blood clotting disorders, SIADH

[a] ALT (serum alanine aminotransferase) = SGOT(serum glutamic oxaloacetic transaminase)
[b] AST (serum aspartate aminotransaminase) = SGPT (serum glutamic pyruvic transaminase)

– (B) Continuous IV infusion of mesna beginning 3 hours before chemotherapy and continuing for at least 12 hours after completion, at 100–120% (mg:mg) of cyclophosphamide or ifosfamide dose

Hematuria appears to be greater in children who receive intermittent boluses, suggesting that 4 hours is too long a gap and making continuous infusion the delivery mode of choice (Magrath et al., 1986).

18.4.4 Treatment

Prediction of risk and initiation of prophylactic measures is paramount in limiting oxazophosphorine-induced HC. Once severe bleeding has started, management becomes complex and morbidity high. Table 18.8 highlights the initial nursing interventions that are necessary.

Adherence to timely administration of mesna should prevent most cases of gross hematuria; those that do occur are often related to BMT in which

conditioning included busulfan. Usually, escalation of hydration and mesna ± forced diuresis and furosemide/frusemide are sufficient, but more invasive measures are occasionally required. See Fig. 18.6 for the treatment pathway of hemorrhagic cystitis. Bladder irrigation via a 3-way Foley suprapubic catheter to remove clots and reduce acrolein availability is effective. Bladder instillation of chemical astringents using the least toxic materials, such as silver nitrate, a cauterizing agent, and alum, will stop bleeding but are not without risking long-term complications, especially in children, and monitoring for neurotoxicity with a view to discontinuing treatment is necessary. The next stage is cystoscopy or suprapubic cystotomy to allow clot evacuation and fulguration of bleeding points and to treat bladder tamponade. Formalin 1% instillations are reserved for life-threatening HC refractory to more conservative measures, as the side effects of bladder fibrosis and contractions are severe. Prior ultrasound, cystogram, and removal of clots must be established to prevent ureteric reflux of caustic substances to the kidney. The procedure is

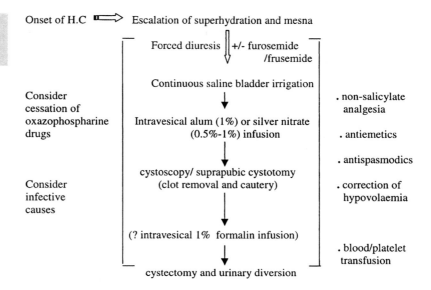

Figure 18.6

The treatment pathway for hemorrhagic cystitis

Onset of H.C ⟹ Escalation of superhydration and mesna

Forced diuresis +/- furosemide /frusemide

Continuous saline bladder irrigation

Consider cessation of oxazophospharine drugs

Intravesical alum (1%) or silver nitrate (0.5%-1%) infusion

cystoscopy/ suprapubic cystotomy (clot removal and cautery)

Consider infective causes

(? intravesical 1% formalin infusion)

cystectomy and urinary diversion

. non-salicylate analgesia

. antiemetics

. antispasmodics

. correction of hypovolaemia

. blood/platelet transfusion

painful and requires general anesthesia (Traxer et al., 2001). If all of the above fail, then arterial ligation, cystectomy, and urinary diversion are a last resort to preserve life.

Correction of thrombocytopenia, prothrombin time, and hypovolemia using blood products, together with pain management using nonsalicylate analgesics and antispasmodics, antiemetics, and sedation are also needed. Prostaglandin instillation, which inactivates acrolein, causes severe bladder spasms requiring morphine and sedation and is of impractical use in pediatrics. Because urosepsis is also causative of HC, exclusion of bacterial and, particularly post-BMT, viral etiology should be taken into account. Vidarabine, cidofovir, and ganciclovir for viral infections have been deployed successfully, the latter being superior to foscarnet, which has been suggested to be bladder-toxic (Gonzalez-Fraile et al., 2001). Consideration of alternatives to penicillin-based antibacterials may be necessary if no other reasons are found.

18.4.5 Prognosis

The consequences of hemorrhagic cystitis, including increased hospitalization and the effects on short- and long-term morbidity, cannot be underestimated.

Deaths are not exceptional. Chronic mucosal changes may be seen as pale bladder mucosa, epithelial thinning, edema, small arterioles, and telangiectasia, and calcification and sclerosing endarteritis with radiation therapy. Patients receiving cyclophosphamide require thorough evaluation because of the increased danger of malignant lesions – commonly traditional cell carcinomas, although markedly abnormal cytologies seen during treatment may be confusing. Bladder biopsies should be exercised cautiously because the mucosa heals poorly.

Frequently seen effects, often developing as many as 23 years later, are chronic cystitis ± hemorrhage or infection, bladder fibrosis /contraction, atrophy, prevention of bladder development in the young, loss of voluntary sphincter control, and ureteral/urethral strictures. The latter may lead to peri-urethral abscesses in boys as a result of high peri-urethral pressure causing extravasation of infected urine. Morbidity related to treatment for severe HC in the form of cystotomy, cystectomy with urinary diversion, exsanguinating hemorrhage, and bladder tamponade, and the effects of intravesical alum instillation leading to fibrosis, bladder rupture, and fistula can result in renal failure, mental changes, and encephalopathy (Murphy et al., 1992).

References

Allwood M, Stanley A, Wright P (1997) The Cytotoxics Handbook 3rd edn. Radcliffe Medical Press, Oxford

Beauchamp D, Labrecque G (2001) Aminoglycoside nephrotoxicity: do time and frequency of administration matter? Current Opinion in Critical Care 7(6): 401–408

Bergstein JM (1996) Toxic nephropathies: renal failure, pp 1513–1514. In Nelson W, Behrman R, Kliegman R, Arvin A (eds) Textbook of Pediatrics, 15th edn. W.B. Saunders, Philadelphia

Borsi JD (1994a) Clinical pharmacology of anticancer drugs in children I. Antimetabolites, p 186. In Pochedly C. (ed) Neoplastic Diseases of Childhood, vol.1. Harwood Academic, Switzerland

Borsi JD (1994b: Principles of administration and monitoring chemotherapy in children, pp 175–181. In Pochedly C. (ed) Neoplastic Diseases of Childhood Vol.1. Harwood Academic, Switzerland

Cachat F, Guignard JP (1996) The kidney in children under chemotherapy. Review Medicale de la Suisse Romande 116 : 985–993

Campbell SC, Novick AC, Streem SB, Klein E, Licht M (1994) Complications of nephron-sparing surgery for renal tumors. Journal of Urology 151: 1177–1180

Capra ML, Walker DA, Mohammed WM, Kapila L, Barbor PR, Sokal M, Robson K, Hewitt M, Stewart R. (1999) Wilms' tumor: a 25-year review of the role of pre-operative chemotherapy. Journal of Pediatric Surgery 34(4): 579–582

Cassady JR (1995) Clinical radiation nephropathy. International Journal of Radiation Oncology, Biology and Physics 31:1249–1256

Cohen EP, Lawton CA, Moulder JE (1995) Bone marrow transplant nephropathy: radiation nephritis revisited. Nephron 70(2): 217–222

Coppes MJ, Zandvoort SWH, Sparling CR, Poon AO, Weitzman S, Blanchette VS (1993) Acquired von Willebrand disease in Wilms' tumor patients. Journal of Clinical Oncology 10: 1–7

Doubek M, Mayer J, HorkyD (2002) Safety of long-term administration of conventional amphotericin B in oncology patients. Casopsis Lekaru Ceskych 141(5): 156–159

Ebb D, Green D, Shamberger R, Tarbell N (2001) Solid tumors of childhood, ch 44.2. In DeVita (ed) Principles and Practice of Oncology, 6th edn. Lippincott Williams & Wilkins, Philadelphia

Godzinski J, Weirich A, Tournade M-F, Gauthier F, Buerger D, Moorman-Voestermans CGM, De Kraker J, Voute P, Ludwig R, Sawicz-Birkowska K, Vujanic G, Ducourtieux M (2001) Primary nephrectomy for emergency: a rare event in the international society of paediatric oncology nephroblastoma trial and study no.9. European Journal of Pediatric Surgery 11(1): 36–39

Gonzalez-Fraile MI, Canizo C, Caballero D, Hernandez R, Vazquez L, Lopez C, Izarra A, Arroyo JL, de la Loma A, Otero MJ, San Miguel JF (2001) Cidofovir treatment of human polyomavirus-associated acute haemorrhagic cystitis. Transplant Infectious Disease 3(1):44–6

Goren MP, Wright RK, Horowitz ME, Pratt CB (1987) Ifosfamide-induced subclinical tubular nephrotoxicity despite mesna. Cancer Treat Rep. 71(2):127–30

Haselberger MB, Schwinghammer TL (1995) Efficacy of mesna for prevention of hemorrhagic cystitis after high-dose cyclophosphamide therapy. Annals of Pharmacotherapy 29(9):918–21

Ignoffo RJ, Viele CS, Dallon LE, Venook A (1998) Cancer Chemotherapy Pocket Guide. Lippincott-Raven, Philadelphia

Labuhn K, Valanis B, Schoeny R (1998) Nurses' and pharmacists' exposure to antineoplastic drugs: findings from industrial hygiene scans and urine mutagenicity tests (research on risks of handling cytotoxic drugs) Cancer Nursing 21(2): 79–89(1998)

Leung AY, Mak R, Lie AK, Yuen KY, Cheng VC, Liang R, Kwong YL (2002) Clinicopathological features and risk factors of clinically overt haemorrhagic cystitis complicating bone marrow transplantation. Bone Marrow Transplantation 29(6):509–13

Loebstein R, Atanackovic G, Bishai R, Wolpin J, Khattak S, Hashemi G, Gobrial M, Baruchel S, Ito S, Koren G (1999) Risk factors for long-term outcome of ifosfamide-induced nephrotoxicity in children. Journal of Clinical Pharmacology 39(5): 454–461

Magrath I, Sandlund J, Raynor A, Rosenberg S, Arasi V, Miser J (1986) A phase II study of ifosfamide in the treatment of recurrent sarcomas in young people. Cancer Chemotherapy and Pharmacology 18(Suppl 2):S25–8

Mitchell CD (1997)Wilms' tumor. In Pinkerton CR, Plowman PN (eds). Paediatric Oncology: Clinical Practice and Controversies. Chapman and Hall, London

Murphy CP, Cox RL, Harden EA, Stevens DA, Heye MM, Herzig RH (1992) Encephalopathy and seizures induced by intravesical alum irrigations. Bone Marrow Transplantation 10(4):383–5

Neonatal and Paediatric Pharmaceutical Group (2001) Medicines for Children RCPCH Publications, London.

Newell DR, Pearson ADJ, Balmanno K, Price L, Wyllie RA, Keir M, Calvert AH, Lewis IJ, Pinkerton CR, Stevens MC (1993) Carboplatin pharmacokinetics in children: the development of a pediatric dosing formula. The United Kingdom Children's Cancer Study Group. Journal of Clinical Oncology 11(12):2314–23

Nies A, Spielberg S (1996) Principles of Therapeutics, p. 50. In Hardman J, Limbird L, Molinoff P, Ruddon R, Goodman Gilman A: The Pharmacological Basis Of Therapeutics, 9th edn. McGraw-Hill, New York

Oyama Y, Komatsuda A, Imai H, Ohtani H, Kamai K, Wakini H, Miura AB, Nakamoto Y (1996) Late onset bone marrow transplant nephropathy Internal Medicine 35: 489–493

Relling MV, Schunk JE (1986) Drug-induced hemorrhagic cystitis. Clinical Pharmacy 5: 590

Ritchey ML, Lally KP, Haase GM, Shochat SJ, Kelalis PP (1992) Superior mesenteric artery injury during nephrectomy for Wilms' tumor. Journal of Pediatric Surgery 27(5): 612–615

Sanders WH, Anderson C (1988) A simple nephrectomy. In Glenn J and Graham S (eds) Glenn's Urologic Surgery. Lippincott-Raven, Philadelphia

Skinner R, Pearson ADJ, English MW, Price L, Wyllie RA, Coulthard MG, Craft AW (1998) Cisplatin dose rate as a factor for nephrotoxicity in children. British Journal of Cancer 77(10): 1677–1682

Tortorice PV (1997) Chemotherapy: principles of therapy, p. 299–301. In Groenwald S, Hansen Frogge M, Goodman M, Henke Yarbro C (eds). Cancer Nursing: Principles and Practice, 4th edn. Jones and Bartlett, Sudbury, MA

Traxer O, Desgrandchamps F, Sebe P, Haab F, Le Duc A, Gattegno B, Thibault P (2001) [Hemorrhagic cystitis: etiology and treatment.] [article in French] Progres en Urologie 11(4):591–601

Walsh TJ, Finberg RW, Arndt C, Hiemenz J, Schwartz C, Bodensteiner D, Pappas P, Seibel N, Greenberg RN, Dummer S, Schuster M, Holcenberg JS, Dismukes WE (1999) Liposomal amphoterecin B for empirical therapy in patients with persistent fever and neutropenia. The New England Journal of Medicine 340(10): 764–771

Wood PA, Hrushesky WJM (1996) Circadian rhythms and cancer chemotherapy. Critical Reviews in Eukaryotic Gene Expression 6(4): 299–343

Cardiovascular System

Ali Hall

Contents

19.1 Cardiotoxicity/Cardiomyopathy

More than half of all new paediatric malignancy cases in the United Kingdom (UK) will receive therapy with cardiotoxic agents. As the number of survivors increases, so does the number of survivors developing cardiomyopathy, despite efforts to limit toxicity through dose reduction (Bu Lock et al., 1996).

Cardiotoxicity occurs primarily as a result of treatment with anthracyclines. Doxorubicin and daunorubicin are cited as having the greatest cardiotoxicity, though this may be because their effects have been studied more; the cardiac effects of mitoxantrone, idarubicin, and amsacrine are less well documented. Before any anthracycline therapy, baseline cardiac function tests (normally an echocardiogram [ECG]) should be performed. Cardiotoxicity, if it occurs, can be classified according to time of onset into acute, subacute, and progressive/chronic. Abnormalities in cardiac function increase over time, and cardiotoxicity occurring early – within 1 year of completion of therapy – carries the highest risk for developing late/progressive cardiotoxicity (Grenier and Lipshultz, 1998).

19.1.1 Incidence

The incidence of cardiomyopathy in haematology/oncology patients is related to the cumulative anthracycline dose. Actual incidence figures vary, probably due to differing methods of evaluation, baselines, and doses used in the studies reported. One recent literature review of 25 published studies reported frequencies from 0–57 % (Kremer et al., 2002). The shortening fraction (SF) has been reported to decline at an

Table 19.1. Incidence of cardiomyopathy related to anthracycline dosage (from Lanzkowsky, 1999)

Cumulative anthracycline dose	% Patients affected
<400 mg/m²	11%
400–599 mg/m²	23%
600–799 mg/m²	47%
800 mg/m²	100%

Table 19.3. Criteria for progressive deterioration of cardiac function

Test	Result
ECG	SF <29% *or* decreased by absolute value of 10% from previous test
RNA/LVEF	Value <55% *or* decreased by absolute value of 10% from previous test *or* absolute value decreased with stress

Table 19.2. Diagnostic cardiac function tests

Test	Result if damage is present
ECG	Heart block, tachycardia, and possibly wave changes
ECG (the most common test)	Fractional shortening (SF) <30%
Radionuclide cardiac cineangiocardiography (RNA or MUGA) (this is rarely used in the UK, but useful in patients in whom a good ECG cannot be obtained)	A left ventricular ejection fraction (LVEF) <55% indicates abnormal systolic function

average rate of 1% per every 100 mg/m² increase in anthracycline dose (Bu Lock et al., 1996).

General incidence can be summarised as shown in Table 19.1.

Because modification therapy is possible while on treatment, children should have ongoing cardiac function tests both during and post-treatment (see Tables 19.2 and 19.3). Though dobutamine stress echocardiography has also been proposed as a more sensitive screening test (Lanzarini, 2000), conflicting information exists, and it is a difficult test to standardise, particularly in children.

19.1.1.1 On Treatment Recommendations

Due to lack of specific evidence, there is ongoing discussion within the UK as to the exact universal guidelines that should be in place for this monitoring. At present, individual guidelines are laid out in each protocol. But as a general rule, if the child's cumulative anthracycline dose will exceed 200 mg/m², he or she should be tested during treatment as well as pre-

and post-treatment. During treatment, tests vary but often increase in frequency with the higher anthracycline doses.

19.1.1.2 Modification Therapy

As with on-treatment testing, modification therapy may vary among protocols. An example of possible modifications is given in Table 19.4. However, any modifications depend on the grade of toxicity and are usually done in consultation with a cardiologist. Toxicity grading is included in many protocols; most use either the Bearman grading or the Common Terminology Criteria for Adverse Events Version 3.0 (CT-CAE) given in Tables 19.5 and 19.6, respectively.

19.1.2 Etiology

Anthracyclines are unique in their requirements for limiting the cumulative dose, and it was thought that both the cumulative and peak doses of anthracyclines (doxorubicin, daunorubicin, and epirubicin) affect the child's risk of cardiac toxicity. However, re-

Table 19.4. Modification of therapy associated with cardiotoxicity (Lanzkowsky, 1999)

Investigation	Action
Abnormal SF and RNA LVEF	Anthracycline therapy should be stopped. Restart only when both results normal in two consecutive tests 1 month apart
Abnormal SF *or* RNA LVEF	Temporary discontinuation of anthracycline therapy. Repeat both tests at 1 month. If one still abnormal but no further deterioration, resume therapy

Table 19.5. Cardiac toxicity after high-dose chemotherapy (Bearman et al., 1988)

Grade of cardiac toxicity	Presentation
Grade 1	Mild ECG abnormality not requiring medical intervention, or noted heart enlargement on chest x-ray with no clinical symptoms
Grade 2	Moderate ECG abnormalities requiring and responding to medical intervention, or requiring continuous monitoring without treatment, or congestive heart failure responsive to digitalis or diuretics
Grade 3	Severe ECG abnormalities with no or only partial response to medical intervention, or heart failure with no or only minor response to medical intervention, or decrease in voltage by >50%

cent literature has weakened the case for continuous infusions being safer (Lipshultz et al., 2002). Anthracycline-induced cardiac toxicity usually manifests as congestive heart failure. This follows permanent changes in the myocardium, most consistent with the contractile failure of cardiomyopathy (Iarussi et al., 2000). Rarely, acute cardiotoxicity may occur that is dose-independent. This manifests as transient tachycardia, nonspecific ECG changes, and atrioventricular and branch blocks (Langebrake et al., 2002).

It is thought that anthracyclines may cause multiple effects, but most evidence points to cardiotoxicity due to free-radical-mediated myocyte death that results in decreased thickness of the heart wall and interstitial fibrosis. The heart is then unable to adequately compensate to meet the demands of growth, pregnancy, or cardiac stress, thus leading to late-onset anthracycline-induced cardiac failure. Hence, this is mainly a progressive disorder that manifests itself with the symptoms highlighted in Table 19.7.

Unfortunately, there is increasing evidence that cardiac damage may only become apparent in the long term as children with late decompensation are only now becoming apparent. It appears there is an initial period during which the SF may even almost return to normal as surviving myocytes compensate, via hypertrophic changes, for acute myocyte loss (Bu Lock et al., 1996). It is thought that in these cases the loss in cardiac function only becomes apparent when the "overworked" myocytes fail and there is lack of further myocyte growth.

Certain factors also enhance the myocardial toxicity of anthracyclines:

- Exposure to other cytotoxic chemotherapy agents, e.g. high-dose cyclophosphamide[1], amsacrine, dactinomycin, mitomycin, dacarbazine, vincristine, bleomycin, and methotrexate

---

1 Cyclophosphamide: Cyclophosphamide induced cardiac effects occur primarily with high-dose bone marrow transplant (BMT) regimens and are not chronic. The drug causes intramyocardial oedema and haemorrhage, often in association with serosanguinous pericardial effusion and fibrous pericarditis.

Table 19.6. Summary of Common Terminology Criteria for Adverse Events Version 3 (CTCAE) grading of cardiac toxicity (formerly Common Toxicity Criteria [CTC]; Cancer Therapy Evaluation Program, 2003)

Grade of cardiac toxicity	Cardiac abnormality					
	Conduction abnormality/ atrioventricular heart block	Prolonged QTc interval	Ventricular arrhythmia	Cardiac ischaemia/ infarction	Hypotension	Hypertension REMARK: Use age and gender-appropriate normal values >95th percentile ULN for paediatric patients
Grade 0	Asymptomatic, intervention not indicated	QTc >0.45–0.47 second	Asymptomatic, no intervention indicated	Asymptomatic arterial narrowing without ischaemia	Changes, intervention not indicated	*Paediatric:* Asymptomatic, transient (<24 h) BP increase >ULN; intervention not indicated
Grade 1	Non-urgent medical intervention indicated	QTc >0.47–0.50 second; >0.06 second above baseline	Non-urgent medical intervention indicated	Asymptomatic and testing. Suggesting ischaemia; stable angina	Brief (<24 h) fluid replacement or other therapy; no physiologic consequences	*Paediatric:* Recurrent or persistent (>24 h) BP >ULN; monotherapy may be indicated
Grade 2	Incompletely controlled medically or controlled with device (e.g., pacemaker)	QTc >0.50 second	Symptomatic and incompletely controlled. Medically or controlled with device (e.g. defibrillator)	Symptomatic and testing consistent with ischaemia; unstable angina; intervention indicated	Sustained (>24 h) therapy, resolves without persisting physiologic consequences	Requiring more than one drug or more intensive therapy than previously
Grade 3	Life-threatening (e.g. arrhythmia associated with CHF, hypotension, syncope, shock)	QTc >0.50 second; life-threatening signs or symptoms (e.g. arrhythmia, CHF, hypotension, shock syncope)	Life-threatening (e.g. arrhythmia associated with CHF, hypotension, syncope, shock)	Acute myocardial infarction	Shock (e.g. acidaemia; impairment of vital organ function)	Life-threatening consequences (e.g., hypertensive crisis)
Grade 4	Death	Death	Death	Death	Death	Death

Table 19.7. Signs and symptoms of cardiotoxicity

Signs and symptoms of cardiotoxicity	Cause
Dyspnoea, tiredness, exercise intolerance	Incapability of heart to supply oxygen demands of the body
Peripheral oedema	Diminished blood flow and accumulation of excess blood in tissues and organs as heart is unable to adequately circulate blood volume
Pulmonary rales	
Hepatomegaly	

Table 19.8. Maximum dosing guides for cardiotoxic chemotherapeutic agents

Drug	Maximum cumulative dose per m^2
Doxorubicin	<450 mg
Daunorubicin	<450 mg
Idarubicin[a]	125 mg
Mitoxantrone[a]	160 mg[b]

[a] Maximum doses of idarubicin and mitoxantrone are not definitively known
[b] Patients who have received a cumulative dose of 450 mg/m^2 of doxorubicin should NOT receive mitoxantrone. Recommended cumulative dose of mitoxantrone for patients who have received doxorubicin is 120 mg/m^2

- Underlying cardiac abnormalities (tumour, uncontrolled hypertension)
- Mediastinal radiation[2]
- Younger age
- Female gender

Septic episodes are also known to affect cardiac function, decreasing left ventricular function, but this decrease is often subsequently recoverable.

Rapid progression of symptoms may occur in certain circumstances, e.g. with anaesthesia, pregnancy, and use of illegal and prescription drugs (such as beta-blockers) and alcohol.

19.1.3 Treatment

The optimal treatment of cardiomyopathy as yet remains unclear and should be commenced with cardiological input. Though an angiotensin-converting enzyme (ACE) inhibitor such as captopril or enalapril may demonstrate symptomatic relief (lowering sodium and water retention and decreasing afterload), any long-term benefit is yet to be proven (Jensen et al., 1996).

19.1.4 Prevention

Attempts to decrease the cardiotoxicity of anthracyclines fall into four categories:

1. Limiting the effects of myocardial concentrations of anthracyclines and their metabolites
2. Concurrent administration of cardioprotective agents
3. Developing less cardiotoxic therapies
4. Lifestyle advice

19.1.4.1 Limiting the Effects of Myocardial Concentrations of Anthracyclines and Their Metabolites

Limiting the effects of myocardial concentrations of anthracyclines and their metabolites uses the principles of maximum dosing (see Table 19.8). Lower doses of radiation with combination chemotherapy should be considered. A lower dose of anthracycline is required when radiation includes the cardiac field.

There has been much interest in the effects of length of time of anthracycline administration. Controversy surrounding this issue remains (Langebrake et al., 2002). Administration times vary between bolus, 1 hour, 6 hours, and continuous infusion over 48 hours. Recent research has indicated no benefit to date from 48-hour infusions in leukaemic children (Lipshultz et al., 2002), and the British Medical Research Council in 2003 is recommending 1-hour infusions.

---

2 Radiation: Cardiac radiation doses of up to 25 Gy are generally felt to be safe; evidence is stronger for cardiac effects in later life at doses of over 30–35 Gy

19.1.4.2 Concurrent Administration of Cardioprotective Agents

The use of many potentially cardioprotective agents has been evaluated; however, to date in preliminary studies only dexrazoxane (ICRF-187) has proven protective against acute cardiotoxicity without decreasing the antitumour effect (Langebrake et al., 2002). Long-term benefits remain to be seen. Dexrazoxane is thought to act by binding to both bound and free iron, hence reducing the formation of anthracycline-iron complexes and the free radicals that are toxic to cardiac tissues (Lopez, 1999; Speyer and Wasserheit, 1998).

19.1.4.3 Developing Less Cardiotoxic Therapies

Newer cytotoxic agents are potentially less cardiotoxic. Incorporating anthracyclines into liposomes, such as liposomal daunorubicin, appears to reduce cardiac toxicity (Speyer and Wasserheit, 1998,) though there is insufficient evidence to make recommendations, and it is too soon to assess the longer-term chronic cardiotoxicity in children treated with this drug (Langebrake et al., 2002).

19.1.4.4 Lifestyle Advice

Lifestyle and non-smoking advice should also be emphasised. Healthy nutrition and regular exercise could reduce the risk of cardiovascular disease in later life (Hrstkova et al., 2001). Young adult obesity in survivors of childhood ALL has been well documented, though the cause is not clearly solely drug or lifestyle. Childhood ALL survivors have also been shown to be at risk of hypertension, obesity, dyslipidaemia, insulin resistance, and, ultimately, cardiovascular disease (Oeffinger et al., 2001).

Survivors who wish to take part in competitive sports and those considering pregnancy should be advised to have a detailed cardiological assessment beforehand. Patients with cardiomyopathy are at risk of ventricle arrhythmias and should have 24-hour ECG monitoring on a regular basis.

Guidelines for Long-term Follow-up Post-completion of Anthracycline Therapy

All children should have an ECG, preferably within 1–3 months, and definitely by 6 months of their last anthracycline dose (which may, in the example of ALL, be much sooner than the end of their treatment). Subsequent follow-up depends on the results of this ECG. If normal, then subsequent testing may be at 1 year and then every 2–5 years. Abnormal studies at any time warrant more frequent testing.

19.1.5 Prognosis

Late-onset anthracycline-induced cardiomyopathy carries a poor prognosis, with some patients going on to die of congestive cardiac failure. Heart transplantation should be considered because a study of all British cancer survivor cardiomyopathy patients since 1970 treated with a heart transplant showed a favourable (74%) 5-year survival rate (Levitt et al., 1996).

There are, at present, many ongoing clinical trials and long-term follow-up studies to evaluate the various aspects of cardiotoxicity and the preventative treatments described above.

19.2 Veno-occlusive Disease

Veno-occlusive disease (VOD) may occur in the liver or, more rarely, the lungs.

19.2.1 Hepatic Veno-occlusive Disease

Hepatic veno-occlusive disease is thought to occur as a result of liver damage by pretransplant conditioning regimens (chemotherapy and radiation). Rarely, it has also been reported following standard cytotoxic chemotherapy treatment (Ortega et al., 1997). It is characterised by fibrous narrowing and sclerosis of the endothelial lining of both the sinusoids and terminal hepatic venules, leading to necrosis of the hepatocytes. As the hepatic veins become increasingly occluded with cellular debris and the blood flow becomes obstructed, the protein-rich fluid content of

Table 19.9. Baltimore and Seattle criteria for clinical criteria associated with venous occlusive disease

Baltimore criteria	Modified Seattle criteria
At least two of the following features within day 20: Hyperbilirubinaemia >34.2 µmol/l Hepatomegaly and upper right quadrant pain Ascites and/or unexplained weight gain >2 %	Hyperbilirubinaemia >34.2 µmol/l before day 21 and at least two of the following: Hepatomegaly and right upper quadrant pain Ascites Weight gain >5 % from baseline

the blood leaks out into the peritoneal cavity, causing ascites.

Hepatic VOD is one of the most common life-threatening regimen-related toxicities in allogeneic BMT. VOD can be mild, moderate, or severe and can last for over 100 days.

19.2.1.1 Incidence

VOD usually occurs within the first 30 days of transplant. Incidence is approximately 20 % in allogeneic transplants and 10 % in autologous, though some literature reviews report an incidence of up to 28 % in some cohorts, reflecting differing diagnostic criteria. Though incidence does not appear to have changed over the last 10 years (indicating the need for more effective prophylaxis), there has been a recent unexpected rise in the rate of VOD. This may be due, in part, to the higher number of children with advanced disease (an identified risk factor) being transplanted.

Clinical criteria vary, but those developed in Baltimore and Seattle predict VOD with great accuracy (see Table 19.9).

Other signs and symptoms include the following:

- Oedema
- Jaundice
- Refractory thrombocytopenia
- Increase in alanine-transferase (ALT)
- Hypoalbuminaemia
- Clotting abnormalities
- Abnormal renal function

In severe cases the child may require dialysis and ventilation; renal impairment expands the ascites, elevating the diaphragm and increasing respiratory impairment, which leads to a decreased conscious-

ness level. Late signs and symptoms also include encephalopathy, though this would probably be terminal. All other causes of hepatic dysfunction, such as graft versus host disease (GVHD) of the liver, infection, and chemical hepatitis, must be excluded before a diagnosis of VOD is made. Of those four, only VOD presents with fluid retention and unexplained weight gain. Early detection and treatment of VOD may help to limit the liver damage and is best attained with careful fluid charting alongside twice-daily weight and (premarked) girth measurements so that staff are alerted to any rapid increases.

19.2.1.2 Diagnostic Tests

Doppler ultrasound may demonstrate a reversal in hepatic portal venous flow. This is the preferred radiological technique as it is noninvasive. A transvenous liver biopsy or liver biopsy may be performed, though this is used infrequently as the child may have clotting abnormalities and is likely to be thrombocytopenic. Hepatic venous pressure gradient (HVPG) may be measured if bleeding risk is high (a balloon-tip catheter can be used).

19.2.1.3 Etiology

Though the actual cause of VOD is unknown, there are some risk factors:

- Conditioning agents, especially in high doses (e.g. busulphan)
- Drugs such as 6-thioguanine and Myelotarg have been implicated and may be exacerbated by concurrent use of other hepatotoxic drugs, particularly the azoles

- Total body irradiation (TBI)
- Preexisting hepatitis (one of the most predictive)
- Elevated liver function tests
- Fever or infection invading the liver immediately pretransplant
- Female gender
- Refractory leukaemia
- Age >15 years
- Underlying metastatic liver tumour
- Positive serological cytomegalovirus status
- Mismatched or unrelated allogeneic transplants
- Second transplant

19.2.1.4 Treatment

The management of the child with VOD mainly consists of supportive care. There is little consensus among clinicians about when to start specific treatments (Reiss et al., 2002). Symptomatic ascites is treated with diuretics (such as furosemide and spironolactone); however, albumin may need to be given concurrently in order to maintain intravascular volume.

If the child has gross ascites that is not responding to the above, it may be necessary to remove some of the peritoneal fluid via paracentesis with intravascular colloid replacement. This may improve the child's respiratory function and comfort.

In severe and deteriorating VOD, nonrandomised studies have shown that in a number of cases, treatment with recombinant tissue plasminogen activator (rt-PA) has been successful (Baglin et al., 1990; Vogelsang, 2002). However, as rt-PA can cause overwhelming bleeding, during such treatment the child requires careful observation and monitoring. Defibrotide is now increasingly being used with promising results, its advantage being, unlike rt-PA, it causes no systemic anticoagulant effect (Richardson et al., 1998).

Adequate pain relief (subcutaneous or IV morphine if necessary) is important. The child should be observed for petechiae, bleeding, and respiratory function. Platelets, albumin, and fresh frozen plasma should be given as required, and the platelet level should be kept above 20×10^9 if possible.

The child's fluid volumes and sodium content must be restricted, and an accurate fluid balance chart is essential, with recognised local agreement between inclusion or exclusion of blood products within the balance. Some centres restrict fluids to 75 % of maintenance (using minimum drug dilutions and flushes) and maximise calorific intake, e.g. parenteral nutrition. Fluid balance charts should be totalled frequently, e.g. every 2 hours. If a positive fluid balance is present, the child's weight, respirations, and blood pressure should be monitored and medical staff informed. Twice-daily weights and girths should continue to be charted.

Blood pressure should be monitored at least every 4 hours. Daily clotting and liver function tests (LFT) should be monitored as requested, and support and explanations for the child and family should be provided.

19.2.1.5 Prevention

Lower total doses of total body irradiation (TBI) or shielding of the liver during TBI[3] and the use of T-cell depleted marrow may reduce VOD toxicity. There are conflicting reports regarding the usefulness of heparin prophylaxis, and this once-common practice is now infrequently used.

Oral ursodeoxycholic acid (ursodiol) has been reported to reduce the incidence of nonfatal VOD in both randomised and historical control studies (Vogelsang et al., 2002). Many centres start ursodiol at a dose around 300 mg/m²/day in two or three divided doses, during conditioning and continuing until between days 28 and 80, depending on disease and regimen.

All compatible IV drugs should be administered with 5 % dextrose rather than 0.9 % sodium chloride to reduce the child's sodium load. Some centres test urinary sodium daily as an early warning sign. Scrupulous attention is required regarding the fluid balance chart; this charting, alongside twice-daily

---

3 In the setting of BMT for leukaemia, this is difficult.

weight and girth charting, is the most useful method of early detection of the rapid weight gain indicative of VOD.

19.2.1.6 Prognosis

The outcome from VOD ranges from full recovery to hepatic failure and death. Differing classification of VOD has led to a great disparity in reported outcomes. In some studies, death rates of up to 47% have been reported (Reiss et al., 2002).

The severity of pathological change in the liver directly correlates with the severity of clinical symptoms the child presents. Classification of severity has sometimes been made retrospectively. Death before day 100 with ongoing VOD or persistent VOD after day 100 is classified as severe and all other cases as mild/moderate (McDonald et al., cited in Reiss et al., 2002).

Despite enhanced knowledge of the pathogenesis of VOD, overall incidence remains similar and the consequences severe. Research continues with regard to etiology, pathogenesis, prevention, and cure of this complication.

19.2.2 Pulmonary Veno-occlusive Disease

Pulmonary veno-occlusive disease (PVOD) mainly affects children and young adults. It causes pulmonary hypertension resembling the clinical picture of right-sided heart failure and pulmonary arterial hypertension. Fibrosis and thrombi narrow the pulmonary venules and veins, leading to alveolar oedema and hypertrophy of pulmonary arteries.

19.2.2.1 Incidence

PVOD is rare; the literature reports it accounting for less than 10% of the 1–2 per million cases of primary pulmonary hypertension. A recent rise in incidence may be due in part to an increased awareness of the disease.

19.2.2.2 Etiology

Most cases are idiopathic. Several theories of etiology have been proposed, with viral infection being thought to be important and correlations reported with HIV. The use of appetite-suppressant drugs and some herbal preparations such as bush tea has been discussed.

PVOD has been reported in 40 oncology patients from 1983 to the present (Trobaugh-Lotrario et al., 2003), with a possible link to hepatic VOD and BMT.

19.2.2.3 Treatment

There is no definitive treatment for PVOD. Anticoagulation therapy, azathioprine, nifedipine, steroids, and treatment of infection have all been used with limited success. Lung transplantation may offer some hope, but patients do not tend to survive the waiting period.

19.2.2.4 Diagnosis

It is difficult to diagnose PVOD ante mortem. A chest x-ray would commonly show signs of cardiac failure, including cardiomegaly, dilated pulmonary arteries, pleural effusions, and Kerley B lines. Dyspnoea is usual. PVOD can be diagnosed by lung biopsy. There are no conclusive blood tests, though the patient should be tested for HIV.

19.2.2.5 Prognosis

Most patients with PVOD die within 2 years of diagnosis. In the 40 reported cases in oncology patients, there were four survivors (Trobaugh-Lotrario, 2003).

References

Baglin T, Harper P, Marcus R, (1990) Veno-occlusive disease of the liver complicating ABMT successfully treated with recombinant tissue plasminogen activator (rtPA). Bone Marrow Transplantation 5(3):439–441

Bearman SI, Appelbaum FR, Buckner CD, Petersen FB Fisher LD, Clift RA, Thomas ED (1988) Regimen-related toxicity in patients undergoing bone marrow transplantation. Journal of Clinical Oncology 6(10):1562–1568

Bu Lock FA, Mott MG, Oajhill A, Martin RP (1996) Early identification of anthracycline cardiomyopathy: possibilities and implications. Archives of Disease in Childhood 75(5): 416–422

Cancer Therapy Evaluation Program (2003) Common Terminology Criteria for Adverse Events, Version 3.0. DCTD, NCI, NIH, DHHS March 31, 2003. http://ctep.cancer.gov June 10

Grenier MA, Lipshultz SE (1998) Epidemiology of anthracycline cardiotoxicity in children and adults. Seminars in Oncology 25(4 Supp 10):72–85

Hrstkova H, Brazdova Z, Novotny J, Bajer M (2001) Nutrition and exercise in the lifestyle of long-term survivors of childhood cancer. Scripta Medica Facultatis Medicae Universitatis Bruensis Masarykianae 74(6):379–390

Iarussi D, Indolfi P, Galderisi M, Bossone E (2000) Cardiac toxicity after anthracycline chemotherapy in childhood. Herz 25(7):676–688

Jensen BV, Neilson SL, Skovsgaard T (1996) Treatment with angiotensin-converting-enzyme inhibitor for epirubicin-induced dilated cardiomyopathy. Lancet 347(8997):297–299

Kremer LC, van der Pal HJ, Offringa M, van Dalen EC, Voute PA (2002) Frequency and risk factors of subclinical cardiotoxicity after anthracycline therapy in children: a systemic review. Annals of Oncology 13(6):819–829

Langebrake C, Reinhardt D, Ritter J (2002) Minimising the long-term adverse effects of childhood leukaemia therapy. Drug Safety 25(15):1057–1077

Lanzarini L, Bossi G, Laudisa ML, Klersy C, Arico M (2000) Lack of clinically significant cardiac dysfunction during intermediate dobutamine doses in long-term childhood cancer survivors exposed to anthracyclines. American Heart Journal 140(2):315–323

Lanzkowsky, P (1999) Manual of Pediatric Hematology, 3rd edn. London, Academic Press

Levitt G, Bunch K, Rogers CA, Whitehead B (1996) Cardiac transplantation in childhood cancer survivors in Great Britain. European Journal of Cancer 32A(5):826–830

Lipshultz SE, Giantris AL, Lipshultz SR, Kimball Dalton V, Asselin BL, Barr RD, et al. (2002) Doxorubicin administration by continuous infusion is not cardioprotective: the Dana-Farber 91-01 acute lymphoblastic leukemia protocol. Journal of Clinical Oncology 20(6):1677–82

Lopez M (1999) Dexrazoxane. Current status and prospectives of cardiotoxicity of chemotherapy. Clinica Terapeutica 150(1):37–49

Oeffinger KC, Buchanan GR, Eshelman DA, Denke MA, Andrews C, Germak JA, Tomlinson GE, Snell LE, Foster BM (2001) Cardiovascular risk factors in young adult survivors of childhood acute lymphoblastic leukemia. Journal of Pediatric Hematology/Oncology 23(7):424–430

Ortega JA, Donaldson SS, Ivy SP, Pappo A, Maurer HM (1997) Venoocclusive disease of the liver after chemotherapy with vincristine, actinomycin D and cyclophosphamide for the treatment of rhabdomyosarcoma. A report of the Intergroup Rhabdomyosarcoma Study Group, Children's Cancer Group, the Pediatric Oncology Group, and the Pediatric Intergroup Statistical Centre Cancer 70(12):2435–2439

Reiss U, Cowan M, McMillan A & Horn B, (2002) Hepatic venoocclusive disease in blood and bone marrow transplantation in children and young adults: incidence, risk factors and outcome in a cohort of 241 patients. Journal of Pediatric Hematology and Oncology 24(9):746–750

Richardson PG, Elias AD, Krishnan A, Wheeler C, Nath R, Hoppensteadt D, Kinchla NM, Neuberg D, Waller EK, Antin JH, Soiffer R, Vredenburgh J. Lill M. Woolfrey AE, Bearman SI, Iacobelli M, Fareed J, Guinan EC (1998) Treatment of severe veno-occlusive disease with defibrotide: compassionate use results in response without significant toxicity in high-risk population. Blood 92(3):737–744

Speyer J, Wasserheit C (1998) Strategies for reduction of anthracycline cardiac toxicity. Seminars in Oncology 25(5): 525–537

Trobaugh-Lotrarion A, Greffe B, Deterding R, Deutsch G, Quinones R (2003) Pulmonary veno-occlusive disease after autologous bone marrow transplant in a child with stage iv neuroblastoma: case report and literature review. Journal of Pediatric Hematology and Oncology 25(5):405–409

Vogelsang G B, Dalal J (2002) Hepatic venoocclusive disease in blood and bone marrow transplantation in children: incidence, risk factors and outcome. Journal of Pediatric Hematology and Oncology 24(9):706–709

Bibliography

Evans M, Gibson F (1999) Paediatric Oncology: Acute Nursing Care. London, Whurr

Lilleyman J, Hann I, Blanchette V, (2000) Pediatric Hematology, 2nd edn. Edinburgh, Churchill Livingston

Central Nervous System

Jane Belmore · Deborah Tomlinson

20.1 Spinal Cord Compression

20.1.1 Incidence

Spinal cord compression (SCC) is uncommon in children, occurring in 2.7–5% of children with cancer and 4% of children at diagnosis of cancer (Kelly and Lange, 1997).

SCC is most common in terminal stages of metastatic cancer, but 25–35% of cases occur as a presenting complaint, usually due to extension of a paravertebral neuroblastoma, Ewing's sarcoma, non-Hodgkin's lymphoma (NHL), or Hodgkin's disease through one or more intravertebral foramina – known as the "dumb-bell tumor" (Nicolin, 2002). SCC can also present as a manifestation of tumour recurrence that is most commonly seen in children with rhabdomyosarcoma or osteosarcoma.

20.1.2 Etiology

SCC occurs when extension of a primary tumour causes compression of the vertebral venous plexus, leading to

- Vasogenic oedema
- Venous haemorrhage
- Demyelination
- Ischaemic cell death

Presenting features of SCC in children include

1. Back pain
   - Localised or radicular
2. Weakness
   - Ambulatory
   - Nonambulatory
   - Paraplegic

3. Localised spine tenderness
4. Sphincter disturbances – usually urinary retention or constipation
5. Sensory disturbances (difficult to ascertain in children)
6. Gait disturbances

(Nicolin, 2002; Kelly and Lange, 1997)

Back pain is unusual in children and should be investigated promptly. Pain may be aggravated by movement, neck flexion, or a recumbent position.

Magnetic resonance imaging (MRI) is the current initial investigation required because radiographs are abnormal in only one-third of cases (Parisi et al., 1999; Nicolin, 2002). MRI gives high-quality images of the spinal cord, epidural space, and paravertebral areas.

If possible, lumbar puncture (LP) should not be performed when SCC is suspected, due to the risk of impaction of the cord (spinal coning). If LP is necessary, close neurological monitoring is essential.

20.1.3 Treatment

The goal of emergency treatment is to restore neurological function and avoid irreversible damage. Intravenous dexamethasone 1 mg/kg infused over 30 minutes should be administered. Cases without neurological deficits may be given a lower dose of dexamethasone, 0.25–0.5 mg/kg orally every 6 hours. *Doses are empiric, and large doses of dexamethasone are not justified* (Kelly and Lange, 1997).

Surgical debulking of the tumour may be necessary through laminectomy (removal of the posterior arch of the spinal canal) (Acquaviva et al., 2003). These procedures often lead to later problems, with further reconstructive spinal treatments required. Osteoplastic laminotomies, followed by bracing for 6–8 weeks, are now the preference of some surgeons. Long-term incidence of deformities with this procedure has not yet been established.

If there is a known diagnosis, radiotherapy can be used in radiosensitive tumours (Nguyen et al., 2000). Low-dose radiotherapy is recommended because spinal radiation >2,000 cGy can cause late scoliosis and kyphosis, particularly in young children.

Chemotherapy is also effective in relieving pressure on the spinal cord from chemosensitive tumours, such as neuroblastoma, NHL, Hodgkin's disease, and Ewing's sarcoma. Chemotherapy has the advantages of avoiding long-term deformities and gaining control of the cancer at the primary or metastatic sites.

20.1.4 Prognosis

The ultimate outcome for these children depends on

- The extent of cancer at diagnosis
- The response to treatment

Quality of life, however, depends on neurological recovery, which is related to the degree of disability at diagnosis. In turn, this is associated with the duration of symptoms and time to diagnosis. Patients who are ambulatory at diagnosis generally remain ambulatory, and about half of the children who are nonambulatory at diagnosis regain ability (Kelly and Lange, 1997). Immediate treatment is essential.

20.2 Fatigue

A study carried out at two major cancer centres in the southern United States arrived at a definition for fatigue from focus group sessions: *Fatigue is a profound sense of being tired or having difficulty with movement, such as using arms and legs or opening eyes, and is influenced by environmental, personal/social, and treatment-related factors and can result in difficulties with play, concentration, and negative emotions, most typically anger and sadness* (Hockenberry-Eaton et al., 1999). The profound sense of tiredness can be acute, episodic, or chronic, and is relieved by rest and distraction.

20.2.1 Incidence

Fatigue during treatment for cancer in childhood and adolescence is now accepted as being a near-universal experience that adversely affects the quality of life of patients and their families. Fatigue is reported by clinicians to be particularly common in children and adolescents with leukaemia. Healthy people seldom regard fatigue as a serious problem because it is usually a temporary phenomenon; however, for those with cancer, it is a chronic and frequently relentless symptom.

The actual incidence of fatigue in children or adolescents treated for cancer is unreported, although Bottomley et al. (1995) found that over 50% of school-age children (n=75) with cancer reported being tired and playing less than they did before the illness. It is acknowledged that fatigue is probably underrecognised and undertreated despite its being a prevalent problem in the paediatric population (White, 2001).

20.2.2 Etiology

The etiology of this type of fatigue is complex. There can be many contributing factors in the cause of this type of fatigue:

1. Physiological
   Physiological causes include anaemia, nutritional status, and biochemical changes secondary to disease and treatment. Fatigue may be attributed to bone marrow transplantation, surgery, radiation, or/and chemotherapy. Treatment for childhood cancer is aggressive, with every effort made to administer maximum doses of therapy when possible. Unlike adult regimens, dose-limiting parameters do not include fatigue as a side effect.
   Young children may be unaware of changes in their physical stamina and activities of daily living, while parents and older children/adolescents may simply accept their fatigue and lack of energy as a consequence of having cancer.
2. Psychological
   Anxiety and depression can lead to fatigue (Langeveld et al., 2000). These are complex issues because fatigue may be due to a depressed mood, or people may become depressed if they perceive that they are constantly fatigued (Langeveld et al., 2000). Additionally, depression and fatigue may co-occur in cancer patients, as they can both originate from the same pathology (Visser and Smets, 1998).

Table 20.1. Causes of fatigue identified by children (Hockenberry-Eaton et al., 1999)

Cause of fatigue	Contributing factors
Treatment	Chemotherapy, radiation, surgery
	Fatigue associated with being sick
Being active	Easily tired after play and activities
Pain	Being tired when experiencing discomfort such as pain
Hospital environment	Noises, frequent interruptions, location of bed. Trouble falling asleep
Sleep changes	Sleep patterns change making it hard to get to sleep or sleep all night
Low counts	Feeling tired when experiencing myelosuppression

3. Situational
   Sleep patterns are very frequently changed, especially during stays in hospital, which again can be a contributing factor to feelings of general lethargy and tiredness.

The causes of fatigue and their contributing factors identified by children are listed in Table 20.1. Adolescents recognised the following as reasons for fatigue:

- Noise
- Inability to sleep
- Feeling upset
- Fear
- Effects of treatment
- Boredom

(Hockenberry-Eaton et al., 1999)
Parents, however, stated the following factors:

- Hospital sounds
- Interruptions
- Waiting
- Needing to interact with too many other individuals

A study by Davies et al. (2002) found that children with cancer may experience three subjectively distinct types of tiredness: typical tiredness, treatment fatigue, and shutdown fatigue.

20.2.3 Treatment

Because fatigue is commonly unrecognised in this patient population, interventions need to begin with an educational component that provides patients, parents, and staff with critical information about diagnosing fatigue and describing the type of fatigue experienced. It is only once the type of fatigue is identified that interventions can then be suggested. Precursors to fatigue identified in various studies have included physical, environmental, mental, and psychological causes that have implications for clinical care (Davies et al., 2002).

Cancer and cancer treatment can place an increasing and extraordinary demand on the child's energy. Fatigue may also be an issue related to mental health for paediatric oncology patients. Some of the common symptoms of fatigue may be misinterpreted as indications of depression. After careful nursing assessment for signs of fatigue versus depression, the child/adolescent may need to be referred to the mental health team. The relationship between nutrition and fatigue is also a concern because inadequate nutrition and anorexia can affect the child's energy levels. Efforts to optimise nutritional status can help support children through the potential for fatigue.

An improved understanding of the contributing and alleviating factors associated with fatigue in this patient population will provide children with greater comfort during treatment. Within the plethora of information the families receive during treatment of their child's cancer, it is important for the nurse to discuss fatigue as a symptom both during and after treatment. Awareness of interventions that will decrease fatigue can also be discussed, both for the hospital and for the home. In the study by Hockenberry-Eaton et al. (1998), children and adolescents reported factors that may help overcome fatigue (see Table 20.2).

The realisation that the hospital environment can be a major contributor to fatigue in children and ado-

Table 20.2. Children and adolescents description of what helps overcome fatigue (Hockenberry-Eaton et al., 1999)

Reported methods of help to overcome fatigue	Explanation
Naps/sleep	Resting during the day and night
Visitors	Someone coming to visit may help
Fun/activities	Going to the movies/listening to music/reading a book
Blood transfusion	Can give back some energy
Protected rest time	Not getting interrupted during rest times
Going outside	Outside to enjoy the day and get some fresh air
Having fun	Doing something they like in hospital and at home

lescents is important. Awareness that fatigue during hospitalisation occurs because of disrupted sleep due to noises, frequent interruptions, and even the location of the room can stimulate thoughts and ideas on how to make the hospital setting more conducive to rest and sleep.

Table 20.3 gives examples of nursing interventions that can relate to fatigue-alleviating factors as described by Hinds and Hockenberry-Eaton (2001).

20.2.4 Prognosis

Any effort to define, measure, and intervene with fatigue needs to take into consideration the major components of these children and adolescents' treatment context. Fatigue is a problem for many long-term survivors of childhood cancer and may be multifactorial in nature. Fatigue in these patients may be associated with certain late effects of chemotherapy, including irreversible cardiac and pulmonary toxicities. Efforts should focus on educating survivors to avoid factors that may contribute to fatigue, including those behaviours that may potentiate organ toxicity, such as tobacco and alcohol use (Hollen and Hobbie, 1993).

Table 20.3. Nursing interventions in the alleviation of fatigue (Hinds and Hockenberry-Eaton, 2001)

Factor	Interventions
Hospital environment	Decrease unit noise levels Group nursing activities together Implement protected rest times Maintain quiet hours at the nurses' station
Personal/behavioural	Establish a routine/schedule in the hospital setting Offer choices in relation to care where possible Provide activities to prevent boredom in the hospital setting Encourage participation of care in a positive manner
Treatment-related	Assess the need for blood transfusion Consider physical exercise as part of the daily hospital schedule Support nutritional needs Manage other side effects that may enhance fatigue
Cultural/family/other	Educate families on the symptom of fatigue Inform parents that children/adolescents receive cues from their behaviour Promote visits by family and friends Encourage quiet activities that expend minimal energy

Most young children seem to recover their energy levels fairly quickly even between pulses of chemotherapy, whereas adolescents seem to take much longer. Those who seem at risk of trying to fight off fatigue in the long term are those adolescents who have had some form of megatherapy. Follow-up treatment for these patients can be lengthy, requiring many outpatient visits, which in turn can lead to psychological and physical distress that may manifest itself as increasing fatigue.

As future work is carried out in the whole area of fatigue in paediatric oncology patients, we should improve our understanding of the individuals' experiences and ultimately provide them with a greater sense of understanding and comfort during treatment for their cancer.

20.3 Cognitive Deficits

20.3.1 Incidence

It is now generally accepted that central nervous system (CNS) treatments for childhood cancer can result in significant cognitive impairment, most commonly in the areas of attention/concentration.

Kingma et al. (2000) found that magnetic resonance imaging (MRI) of the brain revealed abnormalities in 63% of cases of children treated for acute lymphoblastic leukaemia (ALL) who received cranial irradiation and intrathecal methotrexate. The resultant cognitive impairment is commonly manifested as lower intelligence (IQ) and memory capacity and poorer academic achievement and visual-motor functioning. It remains unclear whether these deficits stabilise or diminish with time since treatment or if there may be an ongoing decline in abilities.

Altered mental status is frequently observed in children being actively treated for systemic cancer. However, the majority of these patients suffer from iatrogenically-induced encephalopathy, predominantly opioid-related.

Children treated at or before 5 years of age are considered to be at high risk with respect to neurobehavioral impairment, as researchers believe that the developing central nervous system may be particularly vulnerable to toxic agents during this time. The nature of the deficits suggests that children treated with cranial radiotherapy and chemotherapy are able to learn but do so more slowly than other children.

Table 20.4. Risk factors for cognitive effects following treatment for ALL

Precedent factor	Risk
Treatment modality	CNS radiation, TBI, intrathecal cytotoxics, high-dose systemic methotrexate
Age at time of initial CNS treatment	Increased risk if <3 years of age
Concomitant therapy	Combination of treatment modalities
Dosage of irradiation	18 Gy or greater of whole brain irradiation for one or more treatments
Gender	Girls appear to be more vulnerable than boys

A large study carried out in Great Ormond Street Hospital in London concerning cranial radiotherapy in leukaemia reemphasised the significant contribution of treatment at an early age to cognitive impairment and also confirmed that girls are more vulnerable than boys (Christie et al., 1995).

20.3.2 Etiology

There is well-documented evidence that children who have received cranial irradiation for treatment of ALL are likely to have resulting cognitive deficits (Moore et al., 2000; Precourt et al., 2002).

Neuroradiological signs in ALL survivors include brain abnormalities such as calcification, white matter changes, and parenchymal atrophy. The underlying cerebral pathology includes necrotising leucoencephalopathy and mineralising microangiopathy.

Organicity in behavioural sequelae for survivors, documented as lack of initiative, loss of motivation, increased distractibility, flat affect, and irritability, has been described as similar to that of patients with frontal lobe abnormalities.

The most important antecedent factors precipitating cognitive late effects in long-term survivors of childhood cancer are listed in Table 20.4.

20.3.3 Treatment

Cranial irradiation has been eliminated from most treatment protocols. However, patients with meningeal leukaemia or those receiving bone marrow transplantation may be confronted with academic limitations. Initial studies have also shown that dexamethasone therapy (compared with predniso-

lone) may increase the risk for neurocognitive effects in children treated for ALL (Waber et al., 2000).

A study done in the United States found that cancer-surviving adolescents may require intervention to improve their decision-making skills (Hollen et al., 1997). Poor-quality decision making was also clearly linked to adolescents who exhibited more risk behaviours.

Particular attention should therefore be paid to the development of concentration, attention, short-term memory, and abstract reasoning ability in all children, with the development of verbal processing skills needing greater attention in girls. Deficits in abstract reasoning, problem solving, and planning ability have also been found in survivors of childhood cancer.

Time missed from school is likely to be correlated with the degree of illness and medical complications, making periods of absence unavoidable. But when children are well, parents should be encouraged to send them to school as often as possible.

20.3.4 Prognosis

As the number of children surviving cancer for extended periods of time continues to increase, the phenomenon of symptoms that persist following completion of treatment is being recognised. Some children may benefit from special educational assistance to improve their educational outcomes. This is important in order to improve the quality of life of survivors and to help them achieve their maximum potential, initially at school and ultimately in the workforce.

20.4 Diabetes Insipidus

20.4.1 Incidence

Diabetes insipidus (DI) is found postoperatively in patients with craniopharyngioma. It is also the most common clinical presentation of patients with CNS disease in Langerhans cell histiocytosis (LCH). The clinical features of polyuria and polydipsia are usually dramatic. However, formal confirmation of the diagnosis by a water deprivation test is recommended because of occasional confusion with psychogenic polydipsia. DI may also be a late sequela of LCH, as found in one study in which 25% of patients followed up more than 3 years after diagnosis were on treatment (Broadbent and Pritchard, 1997). DI may also be one of the presenting features in intracranial germ cell tumours (Tarng and Huang, 1995).

20.4.2 Etiology

DI is characterised by polyuria and polydipsia, due to a disorder of antidiuretic hormone (ADH) availability. There are two types:-

1. Central or neurogenic DI: a defect in the synthesis or release of ADH
2. Nephrogenic DI: failure of the kidneys to respond to ADH

An abnormal growth hormone response has been correlated with the presence of DI in some studies. The diagnosis of DI is based on the results of a water deprivation test with measurement of urinary arginine vasopressin (AVP). The DI may be termed as "complete" or "partial."

20.4.3 Treatment

The aim of treatment is to treat any underlying disorder and supply the body with pharmacologic preparations that contain the missing hormone. These preparations cannot be given orally because the gastrointestinal tract destroys them; they must be administered parenterally or nasally. The preferred drug for treating chronic DI is 1-desamino-8-D arginine vasopressin (DDAVP). This can be given by in-

tranasal spray and has a duration of action of 8–20 hours.

20.4.4 Prognosis

The most appropriate treatment for reversing DI-complicating LCH is yet to be determined (Broadbent and Pritchard, 1997). The reports of one study that looked at the endocrine sequelae of childhood craniopharyngioma found that most children developed DI postoperatively (Bin-Abbas et al., 2001). Patients with an initial diagnosis of idiopathic DI require vigilant medical follow-up including repeated neuroimaging studies, particularly when there is evidence of evolving pituitary hormone deficiencies.

References

Acquaviva A, Marconcini S, Municchi G, Vallone I, Palma L (2003) Non-Hodgkin lymphoma in a child presenting with acute paraplegia: a case report. Pediatric Hematology and Oncology 20(3):245–251

Bin-Abbas B, Mawlawi H, Sakati N, Khafaja Y, Chaudhary MA, Al-Ashwal A (2001) Endocrine sequelae of childhood craniopharyngioma. Journal of Paediatric Endocrinology and Metabolism 14(7):869–874

Broadbent V, Pritchard J (1997) Diabetes insipidus associated with Langerhans cell histiocytosis. Medical and Paediatric Oncology 28(4):289–293

Christie D, Leiper A, Chessells J, Vargha-Khaden F (1995) Intellectual performance after presymptomatic cranial radiotherapy for leukaemia: effects of age and sex. Archives of Disease in Childhood 73:136–140

Davies B, Whitsett SF, Bruce A, McCarthy P (2002) A typology of fatigue in children with cancer. Journal of Pediatric Oncology Nursing 1(1):12–21

Hinds P, Hockenberry-Eaton M (2001) Developing a research program on fatigue in children and adolescents diagnosed with cancer. Journal of Paediatric Oncology Nursing 18(2):3–12

Hockenberry-Eaton M, Hinds P, O'Neill J, Alcoser P, Bottomley S, Kline N, Euell K, Howard V, Gattuso J (1999) Developing a conceptual model for fatigue in children. European Journal of Oncology Nursing 3(1):5–11

Hockenberry-Eaton M, Hinds P, Alcoser P, O'Neill J, Euell K, Howard V, Gattuso J, Taylor J (1998) Fatigue in children and adolescents with cancer. Journal of Paediatric Oncology Nursing 15(3):172–182

Hollen P, Hobbie WL (1993) Risk taking and decision making of adolescent long-term survivors of cancer. Oncology Nursing Forum 20:769–776

Hollen P, Hobbie W, Finley S (1997) Cognitive late effect factors related to decision making and risk behaviors of cancer-surviving adolescents. Cancer Nursing 20(5):305–314

Kelly KM, Lange B (1997) Pediatric Oncology: Oncologic emergencies. Pediatric Clinics of North America 44(4):809–830

Kingma A, Rammeloo LA, van Der Does-van den Berg A, Rekers-Mombarg L, Postma A. (2000) Academic career after treatment for acute lymphoblastic leukaemia. Archives of Disease in Childhood 82(5):353–7

Langeveld N, Ubbink M, Smets E on behalf of the Dutch Late Effects Study Group (2000) "I don't have any energy": The experience of fatigue in young adult survivors of childhood cancer. European Journal of Oncology Nursing 4(1):20–28

Moore IM, Espy KA, Kaufmann P, Kramer J, Kaemingk K, Miketova P, Mollova N, Kaspar M, Pasvogel A, Schram K, Wara W, Hutter J, Matthay K (2000) Cognitive consequences and central nervous system injury following treatment for childhood leukemia. Seminars in Oncology Nursing 16(4):279–290

Nguyen NP, Sallah S, Ludin A, Salehpour MR, Karlsson U, Files B, Strandjord S (2000) Neuroblastoma producing spinal cord compression: rapid relief with low dose of radiation. Anticancer Research 20(6C):4687–4690

Nicolin G (2002) Emergencies and their management. European Journal of Cancer 38(10):1365–1377

Parisi MT, Fahmy JL, Kaminsky CK, Malogolowkin MH (1999) Complications of cancer therapy in children: a radiologist's guide. Radiographics 19(2):283–297

Precourt S, Robaey P, Lamothe I, Lassonde M, Sauerwein HC, Moghrabi A. (2002) Verbal cognitive functioning and learning in girls treated for acute lymphoblastic leukemia by chemotherapy with or without cranial irradiation. Developmental Neuropsychology 21(2):173–195

Tarng DC, Huang TP (1995) Diabetes insipidus as an early sign of pineal tumor. American Journal of Nephrology 15(2):161–165

Visser MRM, Smets EMA (1998) Fatigue, depression and quality of life in cancer patients: how are they related? Supportive Care in Cancer 6:101–108

Waber DP, Carpentieri SC, Klar N, Silverman LB, Schwenn M, Hurwitz CA, Mullenix PJ, Tarbell NJ, Sallan SE (2000) Cognitive sequelae in children treated for acute lymphoblastic leukemia with dexamethasone or prednisone. Journal of Pediatric Hematology and Oncology 22(3):206–213

White AM (2001) Clinical applications of research on fatigue in children with cancer. Journal of Pediatric Oncology Nursing 18(2 Suppl 1):1720

Chapter 21

Musculoskeletal System

Chris M. Senter · Deborah Tomlinson

Contents

The two predominant primary bone tumors in children are osteosarcoma (60%) and Ewing's sarcoma (34%). (Solid tumors are detailed in Chapter 2.) Combined, these are the most predominant causes of bone tumors in the lower extremities (Nagarajan et al., 2002). Upper- and lower-extremity bone tumors are effectively treated with multimodal treatment that often involves local control by one of two surgical options:

- Limb-sparing resection
- Amputation

21.1 Limb Salvage Procedures

21.1.1 Incidence

Limb-salvage procedures are feasible in approximately 80% of childhood sarcomas (Kumta et al., 2002).

21.1.2 Procedure

The decision to proceed with limb-salvage surgery must consider the following:

- Aggressiveness of the underlying tumor and its stage
- Need to achieve a satisfactorily wide excision of the tumor
- Ability of the reconstructed extremity to be at least as functional as an ablative procedure and prosthesis
- Response to neo-adjuvant therapy

(Kumta et al., 2002; Nagarajan et al., 2002)

Table 21.1. Types of limb-sparing reconstruction and amputation (Nagarajan et al., 2002)

Type of reconstruction	Brief description of procedure	Joint or bone commonly affected	Advantages	Disadvantages	Complications
Arthrodesis	Involved resection of the tumor and adjacent joint. Joint is then fixated using plating and autogenous bone or allografts	Knee, shoulder (occasionally wrist and ankle)	Extremely stable and functional reconstruction for a young adult	Physical limitations – inability to bend knee. Not sufficient for children with large growth potential	Infection (particularly with allograft bone) Delayed union or nonunion Fracture
Allograft bone	Allograft bones from deceased donors (removed with ligaments, x-rayed for sizing, and frozen). Before use, allograft is cultured, placed in antibiotic solution, and thawed. Autogenous bone (hip or fibula) may also be used. Grafted bone is incorporated over time with native bone	Any without joint involvement. Large segment defects usually require allografts over autogenous grafts	Overall allograft survival is good (60–80%) despite complications. Can be stable for prolonged time period	May need protracted periods of non-weightbearing. Bracing or casting may be necessary to achieve bone healing. High incidence of complications	Nonunion – absence of osseous healing Infection – may require removal of allograft and prolonged use of antibiotics. Fracture – usually treated by internal fixation
Endoprosthetic implants	Resection of entire segment of bone involving tumor and replacement with metallic implant used to replace bone and joint. Implant has four components: – Metallic stem that anchors prosthesis to remaining femur – Metallic distal femur that fills the defect created by resection – Prosthetic replacement of proximal tibial articular surface – Rotating hinge knee joint	Distal femur	Postoperative rehabilitation. Stable joint. Immediate weightbearing. Rapid functional use of extremity	Survival of prosthesis progressively decreases over time	Infection Aseptic loosening, i.e, loosening of stem within the bone (tibia or femur) Bone resorption. Loosening
Composite endoprosthetic allografts	Attachment of articulating prosthesis to allograft bone that serves as site of attachment to remaining native bone	Proximal femur Proximal tibia Proximal humeral	Stable joint, incorporation of additional bone, and allows for attachment of major musculotendinous units	Protracted periods of non-weight-bearing	– As for endo-prostheses and allografts

Table 21.1. (Continued)

Type of reconstruction	Brief description of procedure	Joint or bone commonly affected	Advantages	Disadvantages	Complications
Expanding endoprosthetic implants	Implants inserted as endoprosthetic knee joint. Implant has a mechanism for "active growth" achieved by several interventions from turning of a key within implant to replacement of spacers that increase in size or number as the child grows	Lower extremities	For children with growth potential >4–5 cm (bone age of 12 in boys, 10 in girls). Lengthens and provides growth of supporting structures of affected limb while providing ambulation for child. Replace when adult height has been reached	Multiple surgeries may be required – Limb lengthening[a] – Prosthesis revision – Replacement for prosthesis failure – Larger prosthesis – Aseptic loosening – Infections	Aseptic loosening Infection
Amputation	Wide excision of tumor is impossible without complete amputation Four main types: – Transtibial (below-the-knee) – Knee disarticulation – Transfemoral amputation (above-knee) – Hip disarticulation	Majority are transfemoral due to high incidence of bone tumors in distal femur	Provides wide resection for tumors when limb salvage is not possible	May delay chemotherapy Possible greater psychosocial issues	Stump-prostheses problems Stump pain Phantom limb pain Bone overgrowth Infection
Rotationplasty	Tumor and soft tissues removed from the back of the thigh, leaving neurovascular bundle and the distal end of tibia and foot. The leg is rotated 180 degrees and tibia is reattached to the femur with blood vessels reconnected. The ankle is now at the level of the knee, and the foot that is now pointing backwards acts as the stump which can be fitted with an artificial limb at the level of a below-knee amputation	Majority for tumors of the distal femur (Van Nes rotationplasty)	Impressive functionally, stable reconstruction, useful knee movement, less energy consumption. Potentially fewer surgeries. No phantom limb pain (Kotz, 1997)	Appearance of the limb following reconstruction is less well accepted	Infection Delayed wound healing Disturbances in circulation (particularly thromboses)

[a] An extendable prosthesis is now beginning to be replaced by a noninvasive lengthening device. The extendable prosthesis, which contains a small internal magnet, is activated by an external power source. This enables the affected limb to be placed in a box, which stimulates a mechanism within the prosthesis to extend approximately 1 mm every 20 minutes, without the need for further surgical intervention

Various options are available for skeletal reconstruction, and the type used usually depends on the following:

1. Site of the tumor
2. Patient's age
3. Patient's prognosis
4. Orthopedic surgeon's expertise

Table 21.1 provides a general outline of the types of limb-sparing reconstructions that are available. However, bones such as ribs, clavicles, digits, scapulae, and fibulae can be removed with adequate margins and with no effect on function.

21.1.2.1 Management

Management is complicated for these patients who face life-threatening illness exacerbated by life-changing surgery. Heightened awareness should be made to psychosocial care. Nursing care encompasses meeting important physical and psychosocial needs. Patients receiving limb-sparing surgery of this nature will often be adolescents, and any change in body image may be detrimental to their psychological well-being. The nursing challenge is to help adolescents balance the limits of their illness and recovery with normal developmental needs (Dealy et al., 1995).

Table 21.2. Limb-sparing postoperative nursing care guidelines for dressing changes (from Gilger et al., 2002)

Dressing changes
First dressing change is done by surgical staff 5–7 days following surgery
After this time, dressing is changed about every 3 days
Frequency of dressing changes is very dependent on healing

Postoperative management regarding dressing changes and rehabilitation of a patient following limb-sparing surgery is briefly highlighted in Tables 21.2 and 21.3, respectively. Rehabilitation can take 2 years, by which time the patient should have a functioning limb.

21.2 Amputation

21.2.1 Incidence

Before the 1980s, amputation was the main surgical option for malignant bone tumors. Currently performed in less than 15% of patients, amputation is reserved for patients with widespread local disease where it is necessary to achieve wide excision. However, the procedure includes the premise that the resultant limb reconstruction be as functional as possible.

Table 21.3. Guidelines for limb-sparing postoperative rehabilitation (from Gilger et al., 2002)

Recovery	Day 1	Day 2	Day 3	Outpatient follow-up
Initiate use of continuous passive motion (CPM). Early mobility – Decreases risk of contractures – Facilitates early ambulation – May decrease pain	Encourage sitting in bed as much as possible to decrease chances of orthostatic hypotension during transfers. Physiotherapy referral Encourage open discussion regarding pain. For transfer and while sitting, use orthosis to maintain extension to avoid knee flexion contractures	Continue CPM when in bed	Ambulate with crutches	Check patient notes and protocol for information regarding use of brace, assistance with ambulation, use of CPM, etc.

21.2.2 Procedure

Amputation in children raises several issues because of the following important considerations:

- The etiology of childhood limb deficiencies
- Expected skeletal growth
- Functional demand on the locomotor system and prosthesis
- Appositional bone stump overgrowth
- Psychological challenges

(Krajbich, 1998)

Despite the increased use of limb-sparing procedures, amputation remains a valuable procedure. A tumor that extends into an adjacent joint involving blood vessels and nerves would be impossible to remove without contaminating the surgical margins, increasing the risk of local recurrence. The limb's function and movement are important, and inadequate surgical intervention may risk long-term survival. Amputation and an artificial limb may offer the best surgical option and function (see Table 21.1).

It is important to decide the level of local bone resection to ensure adequate tumor clearance and sufficient tissue availability to ensure skin closure. A measurement of 13 cm above the radiological visible tumor has been reported as the appropriate level; however, a more distal level of amputation offers the best functional level.

In the lower extremities, above-knee amputation is the most common level of amputation due to the frequent presentation around the knee joint, and below-knee amputation is done for tumors of the distal tibia. In the upper limb, tumors tend to present more commonly at the proximal humerus. If limb salvage is not possible due to the extent of disease, then disarticulation and forequarter amputation of the shoulder maybe required. This level is very disabling, and artificial limbs are often for cosmetic purposes only.

In children, if the aim is to restore function to the limb, it is crucial to consider how much potential skeletal growth they still have before undertaking surgery. The distal epiphyseal plates provide 70% of the potential longitudinal growth of the femur (Nagarajan et al,. 2002). Initially, if this plate is lost in surgery, the amputated limb is functional. But as growth

Table 21.4. Amputation postoperative nursing care guidelines for dressing changes

Dressing changes
Casts generally applied during surgery
First cast change within 10 days after surgery
Number of changes depends on extent of edema, infection, and muscle involvement

occurs, the stump becomes shorter, function becomes limited, and further surgery may be necessary. It is also recognized that in children under the age of 12 years, further bone growth may occur at the ends of long bones, which would also necessitate further surgical intervention.

21.2.3 Rotationplasty

Rotationplasty is a surgical procedure that is considered a method of amputation because it involves total removal of the tumor and surrounding tissue without reconstruction. A brief outline of the procedure is included in Table 21.1. This surgical option is always discussed in relation to treatment because of its functional outcomes. However, in the United Kingdom, it is a choice rarely made by patients and parents.

21.2.3.1 Management

Postoperative management regarding dressing changes and rehabilitation of a patient following amputation surgery is briefly highlighted in Tables 21.4 and 21.5, respectively. Phantom limb pain can be a particular problem (described in Chapter 28), and appropriate aggressive pain management is required immediately post amputation in an attempt to avoid chronic phantom limb pain.

When limb preservation is not possible, patients often view amputation as failure and begin grieving not only the potential loss of the limb but also the belief that life will never be normal again. Restoring individual belief in acquiring some form of normal activity with realistic goals is paramount. Depending

Table 21.5. Guidelines for amputation postoperative rehabilitation (from Gilger et al., 2002)

Day 1	Day 2	Day 3	Outpatient follow-up
Encourage sitting in bed as much as possible to decrease chances of orthostatic hypotension during transfers. Physiotherapy referral Encourage discussion about phantom (neuropathic) pain/sensation. Do not remove cast – provides protection and controls edema. Do not elevate limb after first 24 hours unless instructed by physician – prolonged hip flexion can lead to contractures		Ambulate on crutches	Check patient notes and protocol for information regarding use of brace, assistance with ambulation, use of CPM, etc.

on the child's age, preamputation assessment and preparation are offered. The involvement of a play specialist can be beneficial to help prepare children and explain what will happen. The opportunity to visit a local artificial limb center prior to admission has been shown to be not only beneficial preoperatively but appears to help the individual cope better following surgery. Meeting someone who has had an amputation at the same level can be inspiring and create a role model as to what can be achieved.

For children who are admitted for amputation, the stay in hospital is quite short. Once over the initial surgery and with adequate pain management, discharge follows soon after the individual is able to transfer and mobilize safely. Function, movement, balance, and safety are part of the physiotherapist's rehabilitation program for working on daily activities. The occupational therapist helps promote independence by providing equipment; advice, and referrals to local services to help patients and their families achieve realistic goals. Ideally seen in hospital initially by the limb rehabilitation team, the patient will be referred back to his or her local artificial limb center for prosthetic rehabilitation.

Younger children may lack or have only limited understanding and will need to be constantly monitored to reinforce the need to exercise to maintain movement. If exercises are not maintained, then more problems will develop.

21.2.3.2 Comparison of Limb Salvage and Amputation

Many studies have investigated the comparisons between limb salvage and amputation with regard to

- Duration of survival
- Immediate and ultimate morbidity
- Function
- Quality of life

Duration of Survival

Survival rates and local recurrence rates have been comparable in both groups (Sluga, 1999; Weiss, 1999; Bacci et al., 2003).

Immediate and Ultimate Morbidity

Complications following limb-sparing procedures occur more frequently than in amputation procedures (Nagarajan et al., 2002). These complications can directly impact future function and quality of life.

Function

Functional outcome is complex and based on more than physical ability (Nagarajan et al., 2002). A commonly used assessment of function is the Musculoskeletal Tumor Society scoring system. This is a physician assessment based on the patient's overall pain, level of activity restriction, emotional acceptance, use of supports, walking, and gait. Another assessment is the self-administered questionnaire of the Toronto Extremity Salvage Score (TESS), which divides functional outcome into

1. Disability, referring to inability or restriction in performing normal activities
2. Handicap, referring to the inability to assume, or limitation in assuming, a role that is normal for that person (depending on age, gender, social, and cultural factors) (Davis et al., 1996).

The difficulty in determining whether functional differences are notable is the lack of consistency in measurements of function. Generally it would appear that any functional differences are small (Nagarajan et al., 2003; Davis et al., 1999), but reports have also indicated significant improved function with limb-saving surgery when compared with ablative surgery (Renard et al., 2000). More consistently, however, reports state that functional outcome following rotationplasty is superior to that of amputation (Heeg and Torode, 1998; Hillman et al., 2000; Fuchs et al., 2003).

Quality of Life

Definitions of quality of life have varied; therefore, comparison between studies on quality of life has been difficult, and reports on differences in quality of life between these patients have varied in their conclusions. Certainly, it would appear that there is little difference (Refaat et al., 2002; Lane et al., 2001; Postma, 1992), despite predictions that the quality of life of patients undergoing limb-salvage procedures would be superior to that of patients undergoing amputation. There are little data available regarding quality of life measurements in children following limb-salvage or amputation procedures.

Despite the higher complication rate and equivocal improved quality of life, limb-sparing surgery remains current practice at most centers (Nagarajan et al., 2002). This may be due to a perception that "saving" the limb is of utmost importance.

The management of these patients includes an individualized surgical plan and an awareness of their psychosocial needs after surgery.

21.3 Altered Bone Density and Increased Risk of Fracture

21.3.1 Incidence

Children with malignancy are at risk of developing osteopenia. Van der Sluis et al. (2002) have reported a fracture risk six times higher in children with acute lymphoblastic leukemia (ALL) compared with healthy controls. The risk of fractures increases considerably during treatment and for a period after treatment.

21.3.2 Etiology

In childhood ALL, skeletal changes are often detected at diagnosis, including osteolysis, sclerosis, osteoporosis, and, occasionally, pathological fractures (Arikoski et al., 1999). These changes are probably caused by the disease process and alterations in mineral homeostasis and bone mass.

In addition, methotrexate, radiotherapy, and corticosteroids are some of the adjuvant antineoplastic treatments currently used and have been described as hindering normal development of bone mass (Nysom et al., 2001). (Some molecular mechanisms are outlined in Table 21.6.) In the older age group, the bone mass is calculated on the degree of bone loss and the maximum bone mass acquired in the 2nd and 3rd decades of life. If the normal acquisition of bone mass is disrupted during childhood and adolescence, survivors of childhood cancer may develop osteopenia, osteoporosis, and pathological fractures in later life (Azcona et al., 2003). Chemotherapy drugs such as ifosfamide and cisplatinum used in the treatment of bone tumors may interfere with the process of renal calcium and vitamin D metabolism. During treatment for ALL, persistent low levels of bone alkaline phosphatase have indicated a potential flaw in osteoblast differentiation. Azcona et al. (2003) further suggest that many other factors may affect bone mineralization in children with malignancy, including long periods of bed rest, poor diet, growth hormone deficiency (see Chapter 23), and variations in vitamin D metabolism. Diagnoses of these anomalies are often made by radiological imaging. However, it is im-

Table 21.6. Molecular mechanisms accounting for loss of bone mass (Cohen, 2003)

Treatment	Mechanism in bone loss
Methotrexate	Appears to increase bone resorption and excretion
Glucocorticoids	Prevent 1-alpha-hydroxylation of vitamin D in the kidneys to form the active metabolite 1,25-dihydroxy-vitamin D; this leads to impaired intestinal absorption of calcium. Inhibit the expression of vitamin D receptor in bone. Inhibit production of osteocalcin (principle bone matrix protein). Decrease local production of cytokines, which inhibit bone resorption
Bone marrow transplant	Increase in bone marrow interleukin-6, which may stimulate bone resorption Differentiation of bone marrow stromal cells into osteoblasts is impaired

portant to be able to recognize potential changes within the skeleton and to be able to differentiate from metastatic disease and recurrence (Roebuck, 1999).

21.3.3 Treatment

Bone marrow density (BMD) can be assessed using dual-energy x-ray absorptiometry (DEXA). Established osteoporosis may necessitate treatment with bisphosphonates; e.g., intravenous pamidronate. Future studies may lead to prophylactic treatment with bisphosphonates.

21.3.4 Prognosis

Bone marrow density does tend to improve, but children have been reported as having low BMD 1 year following cessation of treatment. Follow-up for patients with malignancy should include assessment for osteoporosis.

References

Arikoski P, Komulainen J, Riikonen P, Jurvelin JS, Voutilainen R, Kröger H (1999) Reduced bone mineral density at completion of chemotherapy for a malignancy. Archives of Disease in Childhood 80:143–148

Azcona C, Burghard E, Ruza E, Gimeno J, Sierrasesumaga L (2003) Reduced bone mineralization in adolescent survivors of malignant bone tumors: comparison of quantitative ultrasound and dual-energy x-ray absorptiometry. Journal of Paediatric Haematology/Oncology 25(4):297–301

Bacci C, Ferrari S, Longhi A, Donati D, Manfrini M, Giacoma S, Briccoli A, Forni C, Galletti S (2003) Nonmetastatic osteosarcoma of the extremity with pathological fracture at presentation: local and systemic control by amputation or limb salvage after preoperative chemotherapy. Acta Orthopaedic Scandinavia 74(4):449–459

Cohen LE (2003) Endocrine late effects of cancer treatment. Current Opinion in Pediatrics 15:3–9

Dealy MF, Pazola K, Heislein DM (1995) Care of the adolescent undergoing an allograft procedure. Cancer Nursing 18(2):130–137

Davis AM, Devlin M, Griffin AM, Wunder JS, Bell RS (1999) Functional outcome in amputation versus limb sparing of patients with lower extremity sarcoma: a matched case-control study. Archives of Physical Medical Rehabilitation 80(6):615–618

Davis AM, Wright JG, Williams JI, Bombardier C, Griffin A, Bell RS (1996) Development of a measure of physical function for patients with bone and soft tissue sarcoma. Quality of Life Research 5(5):508–516

Fuchs B, Kotajaravi BR, Kaufman KR, Sim FH (2003) Functional outcome of patients with rotationplasty about the knee. Clinical Orthopedics 415:52–58

Gilger EA, Groben VJ, Hinds PS (2002) Osteosarcoma nursing care guidelines: a tool to enhance the nursing care of children and adolescents enrolled on a medical research protocol. Journal of Pediatric Oncology Nursing 19(5):172–181

Heeg M, Torode IP (1998) Rotationplasty of the lower limb for childhood osteosarcoma of the femur. Australia and New Zealand Journal of Surgery 68(9):643–646

Hillman A, Gosheger G, Hoffman C, Ozaki T, Winkelmann W (2000) Rotationplasty: surgical treatment modality after failed limb salvage procedure. Archives in Orthopedic Trauma Surgery 120(10): 55–558

Kotz R (1997) Rotationplasty. Seminars in Surgical Oncology 13(1):34–40

Krajbich JI (1998) Lower-limb deficiencies and amputations in children. Journal of American Academy of Orthopedic Surgery 6(6):358–367

Kumta SM, Cheng JC, Li CK, Griffith JF, Chow LT, Quintos AD (2002) Scope and limitations of limb-sparing surgery in childhood sarcomas. Journal of Pediatric Orthopedics 22(2):244–248

Lane JM, Christ GH, Khan SN, Backus SI (2001) Rehabilitation for limb salvage patients: kinesiological parameters and psychological assessment. Cancer 92(4):1013–1019

Nagarajan R, Neglia JP, Clohisy DR, Robison LL (2002) Limb salvage and amputation in survivors of paediatric lower-extremity bone tumors: what are the long term implications? Journal of Clinical Oncology 20(20):4493–4501

Nagarajan R, Neglia JP, Clohisy DR, Yasui Y, Greenberg M, Hudson M, Zevon MA, Tersak JM, Ablin A, Robison LL (2003) Education, employment, insurance, and marital status among 694 survivors of pediatric lower extremity bone tumors: a report from the childhood cancer survivor study. Cancer 97(10):2554–2564

Nysom K, Holm K, Hertz H, Muller J, Fleischer Michaelsen K, Molgaard C (2001) Bone mass after treatment for acute lymphoblastic leukaemia in childhood. Journal of Clinical Oncology19 (11):2970–2971

Postma A, Kingma A, Ruiter JH Schraffordt Koops H, Veth RP, Goeken LN, Kamps WA (1992) Quality of life in bone tumor patients comparing limb salvage and amputation of the lower extremity. Journal of Surgical Oncology 51(1):47–51

Refaat Y, Gunnoe J, Hornicek FJ, Mankin HJ (2002) Comparison of quality of life after amputation or limb salvage. Clinical Orthopedics 397:298–305

Renard AJ, Veth RP, Schreuder HW, van Loon CJ, Koops HS, van Horn JR (2000) Function and complications after ablative and limb-salvage therapy in lower extremity sarcoma of the bone. Journal of Surgical Oncology 73(4):198–205

Roebuck DJ (1999) Skeletal complications in paediatric oncology patient. Radiographics. 19:873–885

Sluga M, Windhager R, Lang S, Heinzl H, Bielack S, Kotz R (1999) Local and systemic control after ablative and limb sparing surgery in patients with osteosarcoma. Clinical Orthopedics 358:120–127

van der Sluis IM, van den Heuvel-Eibrink MM, Hahlen K, Krenning EP, de Muinck Keizer-Schrama SM (2002) Altered bone mineral density and body composition, and increased fracture risk in childhood acute lymphoblastic leukemia. Journal of Pediatrics 141(2):204–210

Weis LD (1999) The success of limb-salvage surgery in the adolescent patient with osteogenic sarcoma. Adolescent Medicine 10(3):451–458, xii

Skin
Cutaneous Toxicities

Deborah Tomlinson · Nan D. McIntosh

Contents

22.1 Alopecia

22.1.1 Incidence

Alopecia is one of the most common dermatological side effects of cancer therapy. It can vary in degree from sporadic thinning to complete baldness (Batchelor, 2001). The majority of chemotherapy protocols, particularly those with mitotic inhibitors, and any radiation involving the scalp (including total body irradiation) will affect the rapidly dividing cells in the hair follicles. Chou et al. (1996) reported that approximately 50% of children receiving total body irradiation for bone marrow transplant displayed alopecia. The degree of hair loss was not described, though; the description of hair loss is frequently under-reported in the literature (Batchelor, 2001).

Table 22.1 describes cytotoxic drugs associated with alopecia in children. The severity of hair loss also depends on the route, dose, and schedule of the drugs and on the hair condition.

22.1.2 Etiology

The proliferating hair follicles are targeted by the treatment, which results in thin, weak hair or complete loss of the hair shaft formation (Alley et al., 2002). Up to 90% of all hair follicles are in a phase of rapid growth. The hair follicles of skin areas with the most rapid growth, such as the scalp, are affected more than the slower-growing eyebrows, eyelashes, and other body hair. However, repeated treatments with mitotic inhibitor agents can eventually lead to thinning and loss of hair in these areas as well (Alley et al., 2002). Alopecia of this nature is reversible, but the hair that grows back may be different in color or

Table 22.1. Cytotoxic agents that cause hair loss in children (adapted from Batchelor 2001)

Mild hair loss	Moderate hair loss	Severe hair loss
Bleomycin	Busulphan	Cyclophosphamide
5-Flurouracil	Methotrexate	Daunorubicin
Hydroxyurea	Mitomycin	Doxorubicin (Adriamycin)
Melphalan	Teniposide	Ifosfamide
Cisplatin	Actinomycin	Etoposide
Cytarabine arabinoside	Vincristine	High-dose vincristine
Thioguanine	Vinblastine	
Chlorambucil		
L-asparaginase		
Thiotepa		
Mercaptopurine (6-mp)		

texture. The pathobiology of the response of hair follicles to cytotoxic treatment is largely unknown (Botchkarev 2003). Research by Botchkarev and colleagues (2000) has indicated an essential role of the p53 gene in the process of chemotherapy-induced hair loss.

22.1.3 Treatment

Methods to reduce the incidence of chemotherapy-induced alopecia have been studied since the 1970s, with varying evidence for the efficacy of the measures taken. Recent devices have included gel cool caps (Macduff et al., 2003), digitized scalp-cooling systems (Ridderheim et al., 2003), and Penguin Cold Cap systems (Katsimbri et al., 2000). Marginal benefits in preventing alopecia in adult cancer patients were reported; these devices are time-consuming and usually present some discomfort.

Patient reactions to hair loss vary and may be related to the individual's perception of the importance of hair. Hair can have religious connotations; reflect trends of personal expression; and characterize beauty, age, and one's gender (Batchelor, 2001). In the pediatric population, adolescents (particularly girls) are generally more likely to be affected by the resulting change in body image caused by hair loss (Wu and Chin, 2003). In a study on quality of life among childhood leukemia patients, Hicks et al. (2003) found that hair loss was one of five emergent themes. Ten of the 13 children (5–9 years old) in this study mentioned hair loss; however, only one was distressed when it occurred (Hicks et al., 2003). Parents may be more distressed than their child about the hair loss, as it confirms the harsh reality of initial treatment (McGrath, 2002).

Nurses can play an important role in assisting children, adolescents, and parents to cope with alopecia. Nurses can help prepare for alopecia by providing information on the process and strategies for protecting the skin and eyes following hair loss (Batchelor, 2001). Adolescents may warrant more attention related to how they perceive their appearance and how to help them develop a positive body image (Wu and Chin, 2003). Shaving the head once hair loss becomes apparent is relatively common and can help with scalp irritation as well as avoiding prolonged hair loss, which may be uncomfortable for the patient. Wearing caps, scarves, and wigs can help the individual cope with alopecia (Alley et al., 2002).

22.1.4 Prognosis

Alopecia does not present a medical threat to children or adolescents with cancer; however, it may be psychologically devastating, particularly to the adolescent.

Table 22.2. Stages of radiation skin damage (Boot-Vickers and Eaton, 1999; Hopkins et al., 1999)

Stage	Reaction	Cause	Treatment
Erythema	Reddening of skin within 1 week of beginning therapy. Hot, irritable rash	Dilation of capillaries in response to the damage	Water-based moisturizing cream/aqueous cream. A topical steroid (usually 1% hydrocortisone) to reduce irritation, itching and soreness. *This treatment should be prescribed and used sparingly as it can inhibit healing due to its anti-inflammatory properties*
Dry desquamation	Dry, flaky skin usually 2–4 weeks after onset of therapy. Peeling skin Irritation Often occurring in skin folds	Cell death in the upper layers of skin. Decreased ability of epidermal basal cells to replace surface cells. Sweat and sebaceous glands are damaged. Friction increases damage	As for erythema. If damage is due to friction, a self-adhesive, thin, aerated dressing may be applied and left intact until treatment is complete. If used, this dressing needs to be kept dry
Moist desquamation	Skin peeling or denuding with exudate; often white or yellow in color	Damage to the epidermis that exposes the dermis and allows leakage of serous fluid from the tissues. Area is at risk from infection and fluid loss. *A break in therapy may be necessary to allow repair of tissue*	Wound-healing principles (institutions may vary in treatment policies). Hydrogel dressing covered with gauze and secured *without* the use of adhesive tape. *Dressing must be removed during radiotherapy treatment as it could alter the dimensions for the penetration of the radiation*
Necrosis	Darkened tissue that eventually turns black	Therapy has exceeded the tolerance dose and causes basal cell death, leading to ulceration and necrosis	Surgery with debridement ± grafting

22.2 Altered Skin Integrity Associated with Radiation Therapy

22.2.1 Incidence

It has been reported that 95% of patients treated with radiation therapy experience a skin reaction (Porock et al., 1999). It is unclear whether this incidence includes children, and the severity of the reaction is unreported, but it does include radiation-recall skin reactions.

Advanced planning and delivery techniques of radiotherapy help decrease its effect on the skin, but the radiation invariably affects some of the skin cells.

22.2.2 Etiology

The radiotherapy acts on the proliferating cells of the epidermis at the point of entry (or exit) of the radiation. Cells in the epidermis have a life cycle of 2–3 weeks, and skin reactions often begin around this time.

Table 22.2 lists four recognized stages of radiation skin reaction.

22.2.3 Prevention

Preventative measures must be instigated from the day radiotherapy begins. The skin condition of children receiving radiotherapy should be assessed daily.

Radiation skin reactions may not be preventable, but general principles of skin care included in skin-care policies may help decrease the severity of reactions (Campbell and Lane, 1996; Boot-Vickers and Eaton, 1999). Principles include the following:

1. Ensuring good skin hygiene to prevent increased irritation of the epithelium and to prevent bacteria build-up. Advice should include the need to use mild soap and warm water, pat skin dry, and preserve treatment marks
2. Washing hair gently, if the head area is treated, avoiding scrubbing; drying hair on a low setting if a hair dryer if necessary
3. Avoiding deodorants and perfumes at the radiation site
4. Preventing dehydration of the skin by applying moisturizing cream or aqueous cream, which helps to retain water and lubricates to reduce friction
5. Protecting skin from the sun during treatment and for 8 weeks following treatment. High-factor sunscreen should be used for at least 1 year post-treatment (and preferably for life)
6. Avoiding hot water bottles and ice packs
7. Swimming may be allowed, but the irradiated area should be showered gently afterwards and an aqueous cream applied
8. Choosing loose-fitting clothing that will not cause friction or trauma to the treatment site

22.2.4 Treatment

Treatment options are included in Table 22.2.

22.2.5 Prognosis

Good assessment and proper skin care should prevent permanent skin damage from radiation therapy. Nurses have a role to instigate skin assessment and deal with concerns about altered skin integrity for these children and adolescents

Table 22.3. Cytotoxic drugs commonly associated with radiation interactions (adapted from Alley et al., 2002)

Radiation interaction	Drug
Radiation sensitization and recall	Bleomycin
	Dactinomycin
	Daunorubicin
	Etoposide
	5-Fluorouracil
	Hydroxyurea
	Melphalan
	Methotrexate
	Vinblastine
Photosensitivity	5-Fluorouracil
	Methotrexate
	Vinblastine

22.3 Radiation Sensitivity and Recall

22.3.1 Incidence

Some cytotoxic drugs can sensitize the skin to radiation (Alley, 2002). Radiation recall dermatitis is the occurrence of an acute inflammatory toxicity in a previously radiated field following subsequent administration of cytotoxic therapy (Yeo and Johnson, 2000). The incidence in the pediatric population is unreported, but drugs that are particularly associated with radiation sensitization and recall are listed in Table 22.3. The radiation dermatitis develops days to weeks (and sometimes years) after radiation therapy with subsequent administration of chemotherapy.

Ataxia telangiectasia gene mutation and protein kinase deficiency have been associated with an increased susceptibility to severe radiation-induced skin toxicity (Yeo and Johnson, 2000).

22.3.2 Etiology

The mechanisms of radiation-recall sensitivity are undefined. Possibilities include the following:

— Depletion in tissue stem cells within the irradiated field caused by the radiation therapy and subsequent chemotherapy exposure causes a "remembered" reaction by the remaining cells (Yeo and Johnson, 2000).

- Radiation induces heritable mutations within surviving cells, producing a group of defective stem cells that are unable to tolerate a second insult with systemic chemotherapy (Indinnimeo et al., 2003).

Skin reactions can range from a mild rash to severe skin necrosis with manifestations that include maculopapular eruptions with erythema, vesicle formation, and desquamation of the affected skin areas (Alley et al., 2002).

22.3.3 Treatment

There is no specific treatment for this dermatitis, but topical steroids are often used. Other anti-inflammatory agents may also be prescribed, and supportive therapy is necessary. On rare occasions the cytotoxic therapy may be discontinued.

22.3.4 Prognosis

Most of the lesions will heal with supportive therapy. A decision to continue with the chemotherapeutic agent is usually determined by the severity of the reaction and the chemoresponsiveness of the tumor to that particular drug (Yeo and Johnson, 2000).

22.4 Photosensitivity

There is no reported incidence of photosensitivity in children; however, it is established that ultraviolet radiation (sunlight) can produce effects on the skin of patients previously treated with cytotoxic therapy similar to those seen in radiation-recall. Table 22.3 lists the main drugs used in pediatrics that are likely to cause photosensitivity.

It has also been reported that children previously treated for malignancy have an increased number of benign melanocytic nevi (moles), which may increase their risk of developing melanoma (Hughes et al., 1989).

Children and caregivers should be educated on the need for adequate sun protection: using sunscreen, seeking shade, wearing sun hats. Interestingly, studies show that the use of sunscreen can often increase the number of sunburn incidences (Davis et al., 2002; Horsley et al., 2003). This finding emphasizes a need for education regarding the proper use of these products and an increased need for protective measures for the entire population.

22.5 Cutaneous Reactions Associated with High-dose Cytosine Arabinoside

22.5.1 Incidence

The incidence of cutaneous toxicity associated with high-dose cytosine arabinoside (HDAC) has been stated to range from 3% to 72% (Richards and Wujick, 1992). A study by Cetkovska et al. (2002) reported the overall incidence of cutaneous reaction to be 53% in 172 patients aged 16–71 treated with HDAC. Whitlock and colleagues (1997) found that 22% (4 of 18) of children developed cutaneous reactions with HDAC.

22.5.2 Etiology

The etiology of toxicity associated with HDAC is unclear. This toxicity can range from erythema to painful swelling, bullae formation, and desquamation. The severity of the reaction appears to be related to the dose and the number of consecutive doses. Erythema of this nature that begins on the palms and soles is known as hand-foot syndrome, or palmarplantar erythrodysesthesia, and was originally described in patients receiving HDAC (Alley et al., 2002). However, other drugs have been associated with this toxicity, including 5-fluorouracil, doxorubicin, and methotrexate (Alley et al., 2002).

22.5.3 Prevention and Treatment

No therapy has been shown to prevent this condition, but most skin changes clear spontaneously (Cetkovska et al., 2002). Although this side effect is considered manageable, nurses must explore measures that could minimize these complications and reduce their impact on the patient's quality of life.

22.6 Nail Dystrophies

Although nail changes in patients receiving chemotherapy are reportedly fairly common (Alley et al., 2002), they are unreported as a problem for children. However, transverse ridges may occur, reflecting cyclic damage to the nail matrix. Nurses should be aware that nail changes are a possibility.

22.7 Graft Versus Host Disease

22.7.1 Incidence and Etiology

Graft versus host disease (GvHD) occurs when transplanted donor cells recognize and react to recipient histoincompatible cells, causing tissue damage (Fig. 1). It remains a major complication after allogeneic hematopoietic stem cell transplantation, especially with the increased use of stem cells from unrelated and mismatched donors. GvHD is classified as acute and chronic, although the distinction between them is not simply chronological. They both result from activation of donor T-cells against host antigens, but they have a different pathogenesis.

The acute form of GvHD usually develops up to 100 days after allogeneic SCT and is graded according to severity (Table 22.4).

Clinically relevant grades II to IV occur in approximately 20–50% of patients who receive stem cells from a human leukocyte antigen (HLA) identical sibling donor and in 50–80% whose donor is an HLA-

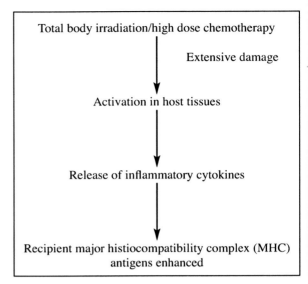

Figure 22.1

Mechanisms involved in phase 1 of GvHD

mismatched sibling or HLA-identical unrelated donor (Tabbara et al., 2002).

The classically recognized target organs affected by acute GvHD are the skin, liver, and gastrointestinal tract, but other organs may be affected.

Chronic GvHD is a result of a later phase of alloreactivity. It occurs in approximately 30% of patients, usually after the first 100 days but up to years after transplantation. It can follow acute GvHD (progressive); can occur after the resolution of acute GvHD

Table 22.4. Clinical grading of acute GvHD

Grade	Skin	Liver	Gastrointestinal
0	No rash	Bilirubin <2 mg/dl	<500 ml diarrhea/24 hours
I	Rash on <25% of body surface	Bilirubin 2–3 mg/d	>500 ml diarrhea/24 hours
II	Rash on 25–50% of body surface	Bilirubin 3–6 mg/d	>1,000 ml diarrhea/24 hours
III	Generalized erythroderma	Bilirubin 6–15 mg/dl	>1,500 ml diarrhea/24 hours
IV	Desquamation and bullae	Bilirubin >15 mg/dl	Severe abdominal pain ± ileus

Table 22.5. Classification of chronic GvHD

Limited chronic GvHD	Extensive chronic GvHD
Either or both:	Either generalized skin involvement or localized skin involvement
Localized skin involvement	with or without hepatic dysfunction
Hepatic dysfunction	or eye involvement or oral mucosa involvement or any other target organ involvement

(quiescent); or be de novo, in which case there was no acute GvHD. Clinical manifestations of chronic GvHD are similar to autoimmune collagen vascular diseases. It appears to be a syndrome of immune dysregulation resulting in autoimmunity and immunodeficiency (Shere and Shoenfield, 1998). It may involve various organs including the skin, liver, mouth, and eyes. Chronic GvHD is classified as either limited or extensive (Table 22.5) in an attempt to determine which patients need treatment.

Patients who receive an allogeneic bone marrow transplant fulfill the criteria necessary for the development of GvHD (Billingham, 1966):

— Administration of adequate numbers of immunocompetent cells
— Donor and recipient histocompatibility
— Inability of the recipient to destroy the donor cells

Table 22.6 shows a three-phase model that elucidates the major processes that lead to GvHD (Ferrara et al., 1999).

22.7.2 Treatment

The skin is the most commonly affected system of acute GvHD. It is typically characterized by the following signs and symptoms, but these may also be a consequence of chemotherapy, radiation, or other drugs and are therefore not diagnostic of acute GvHD (Goker et al., 2001).

— A pruritic maculopapular rash involving the face, trunk, palms, and soles of the feet usually marks the onset (see Fig. 22.2)
— The rash usually occurs at or near the time of engraftment
— The rash may look like a sunburn
— In severe cases, the rash develops into generalized erythroderma, bullous lesions, and desquamation, and may progress to epidermal necrosis

GvHD may also affect the liver, with derangement of hepatic function resulting in increased bilirubin, alkaline phosphatase, and aminotransferase levels. In the post-transplant setting, these abnormalities may occur secondary to drug-induced liver toxicity, venoocclusive disease, or hepatitis. Abdominal cramping and profuse diarrhea are characteristic manifestations of acute GvHD of the gastrointestinal tract. Other symptoms may include anorexia and weight loss.

Table 22.6. Processes leading to GvHD (Goker et al., 2001)

Phase	Processes
Phase 1 (conditioning) Afferent phase	Recipient conditioning resulting in damage to the tissues that starts before the infusion of the graft; see Fig. 22.1
Phase 2 (induction and expansion) Afferent phase	Recognition of the foreign host antigens by donor T-cells and activation, stimulation, and proliferation of T-cells
Phase 3 Effector phase (the cytokine storm)	Direct and indirect damage to host cells

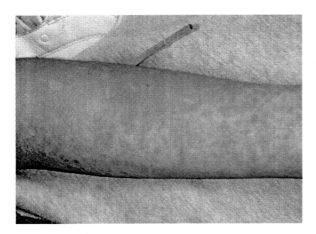

For diagnostic purposes, skin, rectal, and colonic biopsies may be performed. Liver biopsies are usually only performed when isolated GvHD is suspected. Histologically, the diagnosis is confirmed by lymphocyte infiltration characterized by Woodruff "satellite cell necrosis."

22.7.3 Prevention

The first approach for GvHD prevention is to reduce the risk factors if possible. The incidence of GvHD without prophylaxis can reach 100% (Sullivan et al., 1986). The most effective approaches to GvHD prevention involve removing T-cells from the graft by lymphocyte depletion. However, these methods increase the risk of graft failure or rejection and relapse as a consequence of a loss of the graft-versus-leukemia (GvL) effect, which is the attack of immunocompetent cells in the graft against any remaining disease cells in the patient after transplantation. Pharmacologic GvHD prophylaxis using immunosuppressive drugs is the preferred approach to disrupt the three phases of the GvHD cascade and prevent GvHD. It is aimed at removing or attenuating the activity of donor T-lymphocytes, reducing the risk of graft failure and attempts to maximize the GvL effect (Peters et al., 2000). Immunosuppression with combined drugs is more effective (Sullivan et al., 1986); the most commonly used drugs are cyclosporin and methotrexate.

There are no pharmacologic drugs to prevent chronic GvHD.

22.7.4 Treatment

Acute GvHD (grades II–IV) is treated by continuing immunosuppression and adding methylprednisolone at 2–2.5 mg/kg/day, with starting doses ranging from 1 to >20 mg/kg/day (Jacobsohn and Vogelsang, 2002). Steroids are tapered based on the patient's response rather than a fixed schedule. Bacterial, fungal, and viral infections may complicate acute GvHD and are the most common cause of death in these patients.

Immunosuppressive drugs such as steroids, cyclosporin, and tacrolimus are used to treat patients classified as having extensive chronic GvHD. Chronic GvHD may cause significant morbidity, and when mortality occurs it is most often due to infection.

Clinical trials have evaluated various monoclonal antibodies as treatment for GvHD in various settings, with different reported success rates. Future studies will aim to develop agents that will use stem cell transplantation with GvL effect devoid of GvHD.

22.7.5 Prognosis

Although significant improvements have been made in allogeneic stem cell transplantation, GvHD remains a major complication that can lead to significant morbidity and mortality. The more recent and less damaging approaches to allogeneic stem cell transplantation may help to reduce GvHD by decreasing the intense conditioning regimen, which

1. reduces early transplant-related mortality
2. plays an important role in the development of GvHD

Supportive measures such as symptomatic control, parenteral nutrition, infection prophylaxis, skin care, psychological support, and physical rehabilitation are equally important to minimize further complications and improve quality of life.

References

Alley E, Green R, Schuchter L (2002) Cutaneous toxicities of cancer therapy. Current Opinions in Oncology 14:212–216

Batchelor D (2001) Hair and cancer chemotherapy: consequence and nursing care- a literature study. European Journal of Cancer Care10 (3):147–163

Billingham RE (1966) The biology of graft-vs-host reactions. In: The Harvey Lectures. New York: Academic Press, 62:21

Boot-Vickers M, Eaton K (1999) Skin care for patients receiving radiotherapy. Professional Nurse 14(10):706–708

Botchkarev VA (2003) Molecular mechanisms of chemotherapy-induced hair loss. Journal of Investigative Dermatology Symposium Proceedings 8(1):72–75

Botchkarev VA, Komarova EA, Siebenhaar F, Botchkarev NV, Kmarov PG, Maurer M, Gilchrest BA, Gudkov AV (2000) p53 is essential for chemotherapy-induced hair loss. Cancer Research 60(18):5002–5006

Campbell J, Lane C (1996) Developing a skin-care protocol in radiotherapy. Professional Nurse 12(2):105-8

Cetkovska P, Pizinger K, Cetkovsky P (2002) High-dose cytosine arabinoside-induced cutaneous reactions. Journal of the European Academy of Dermatology and Venerology 16(5):481–485

Chou RH, Wong GB, Kramer JH, Wara DW, Matthay KK, Crittenden MR, Swift PS, Cowan MJ, Wara WM (1996) Toxicities of total-body irradiation for pediatric bone marrow transplantation. International Journal of radiation Oncology, Biology and Physics 34(4):843–851

Davis KJ, Cokkinides VE, Weinstock MA, O'Connell MC, Wingo PA (2002) Summer sunburn and sun exposure among US youths ages 11 to 18: national prevalence and associated factors. Pediatrics 110 (1 part 1):27–35

Ferrara JL, Levy R, Chao NJ (1999) Pathophysiologic mechanisms of acute graft-vs-host disease. Biology of Blood and Marrow Transplant 5(6):347–356

Goker H, Ibrahim CH, Chao NJ (2001) Acute graft-vs-host disease: pathophysiology and management. Experimental Hematology 29(3):259–277

Hicks J, Bartholomew J, Ward-Smith P, Hutto CJ (2003) Quality of life among childhood cancer patients. Journal of Pediatric Oncology Nursing 20(4):192–200

Hopkins M, Pownall J, Scott L (1999) Acute and subacute side effects of radiotherapy. In Gibson F, Evans M (eds) Paediatric Oncology: Acute Nursing care. London: Whurr

Horsley L, Charlton A, Waterman C (2003) Reducing skin cancer mortality by 2010: lessons from children's sunburn. British Journal of Dermatology 148(3):607

Hughes BR, Cunliffe WJ, Bailey CC (1989) Excess benign melanocytic naevi after chemotherapy for malignancy in childhood. British Medical Journal 299(6691):88–91

Indinnimeo M, Cicchini C, Kanakaki S, Larcinese A, Mingazzini PL (2003) Chemotherapy-induced radiation recall myositis. Oncology Reports 10(5):1401–1403

Jacobsohn DA, Vogelsang GB (2002) Novel Pharmacotherapeutic Approaches to Prevention and Treatment of GVHD. Drugs 62(6):879–889.

Katsimbri P, Bamias A, Pavlidis N (2000) Prevention of chemotherapy-induced alopecia using an effective scalp cooling system. European Journal of Cancer 36(6):766–771

Macduff C, Mackenzie T, Hutcheson A, Melville L, Archibald H (2003) The effectiveness of scalp cooling in preventing alopecia for patients receiving epirubicin and docetaxel. European Journal of Cancer Care 12(2):154–161

McGrath P (2002) Beginning treatment for childhood acute lymphoblastic: insights from the parents' perspective. Oncology Nurses Forum 29(6):988–996

Peters C, Minkov M, Gadner H, Klingebiel T, Vossen J, Locatelli F, Cornish J, Ortega J, Bekasi A, Souillet G, Stary J, Niethammer D; European Group for Blood and Marrow Transplantation (EBMT) Working Party Paediatric Diseases; International BFM Study Group–Subcommittee Bone Marrow Transplantation (IBFM-SG) (2000) Statement of current majority practices in graft-versus-host disease prophylaxis and treatment in children. Bone Marrow Transplant 26(4):405–411

Porock D, Nikoletti S, Kristjanson L (1999) Management of radiation skin reactions: literature review and clinical application. Plastic Surgery Nursing 19(4):185–192

Richards C, Wujcik D (1992) Cutaneous toxicity associated with high-dose cytosine arabinoside. Oncology Nurses Forum 19(8):1191–1195.

Ridderheim M, Bjurberg M, Gustavsson A (2003) Scalp hypothermia to prevent chemotherapy-induced alopecia is effective and safe: a pilot study of a new digitized scalp-cooling system used in 74 patients. Support Care Cancer 11(6):371–377

Shere Y, Shoenfield Y (1998) Autoimmune diseases and autoimmunity post-bone marrow transplantation. Bone Marrow Transplant 22(9):873–881

Sullivan KM, Deeg HJ, Sanders J, Klosterman A, Amos D, Shulman H, Sale G, Martin P, Witherspoon R, Appelbaum F, et al. (1986) Hyperacute graft-versus-host disease in patients not given immunosuppression after allogeneic marrow transplantation. Blood 67(4):1172–1175

Tabbara IA, Zimmerman K, Morgan C, Nahleh Z. Allogeneic hematopoietic stem cell transplantation (2002) Allogeneic Hematopoietic Stem Cell Transplantation: complications and results. Archives of Internal Medicine 162 (14):1558–1566

Whitlock JA, Wells RJ, Hord JD, Janco RL, Greer JP, Gay JC, Edwards JR, McCurley TL, Lukens JN (1997) High-dose cytosine arabinoside and etoposide: an effective regimen without anthracyclines for refractory childhood acute non-lymphocytic leukemia. Leukemia 11(2):185–189

Wu LM, Chin CC (2003) Factors related to satisfaction with body image in children undergoing chemotherapy. Kaohsiung Journal of Medical Science 19(5):217–224

Yeo W, Johnson PJ (2000) Radiation-recall skin disorders associated with the use of antineoplastic drugs: pathogenesis, prevalence, and management. American Journal of Clinical Dermatology 1(2):113–116

Endocrine System

Deborah Tomlinson · Ethel McNeill

Contents

Sklar (1999) suggests that approximately 40 % of cancer patients present with at least one endocrine abnormality at follow-up. Endocrine disturbances are attributed to location of disease, the type and dosage of chemotherapy, and the amount and schedule of radiotherapy (Cohen, 2003).

23.1 Hypothalamic-Pituitary Dysfunction

Table 23.1 summarises the physiology of hypothalamic-pituitary function.

23.1.1 Incidence and Etiology

The hypothalamic-pituitary axis is central to the control of the endocrine system (Brougham et al., 2002). Pituitary hormone deficiencies can occur as a result of

- Radiation therapy for central nervous system, orbital, facial, or nasopharyngeal tumours
- Radiation therapy for acute lymphoblastic leukaemia (ALL)
- Total body irradiation pre-bone marrow (stem cell) transplant (Cohen, 2003)

The resultant hormone deficiency depends on several factors, as shown in Table 23.2.

Table 23.1. Hypothalamic releasing hormones and the pituitary trophic hormones (Drury, 1990)

Hypothalamic hormones	Pituitary hormones	Peripheral hormones
Gonadotrophin-releasing hormone (GnRH, LHRH)	Luteinising hormone (LH) Follicle stimulating hormone (FSH)	Oestrogens/androgens
Prolactin inhibiting factor (PIF)	Prolactin	–
Growth hormone-releasing factor (GHRH) Somatostatin (GHRIH)	Growth hormone (GH)	Somatomedin C (insulin-like growth factor) and others
Thyrotropin-releasing hormone (TRH)	Thyroid-stimulating hormone (TSH)	Thyroxine (T_4), triiodothyronine (T_3) Both are present as free and bound forms
Corticotrophin-releasing factor (CRF)	Adrenocorticotrophic hormone	Cortisol
Vasopressin, antidiuretic hormone (ADH)	–	–
Oxytocin	–	–

Table 23.2. Factors related to pituitary hormone deficiencies in paediatric oncology (Cohen, 2003, Brougham et al., 2002)

Dependent factor	Effect on hypothalamic-pituitary dysfunction
Radiation dose received	Directly related. Growth hormone is the most radiosensitive, caused by doses as low as 18 Gy. Increasing radiation doses cause deficiencies in gonadotrophin, corticotrophin, and thyrotropin secretion
Fractionation schedule	Inversely related, i.e. therapy administered over more fractions will reduce the degree of dysfunction
Interval since completion of therapy	Dysfunction becomes progressively more severe with time since radiation treatment, possibly due to delayed effects of radiotherapy on the axis or to pituitary dysfunction secondary to earlier damage to the hypothalamus. Evidence indicates that the hypothalamus is more sensitive to radiotherapy than the pituitary
Age at treatment	Younger children are more sensitive to radiation-induced damage of the hypothalamic-pituitary axis compared with older children and adults.

23.2 Growth Hormone Deficiency

Growth hormone (GH) deficiency is the most common endocrine abnormality following cranial radiation. The main presentation of GH deficiency in children is short stature; however, the causes for short stature are not dependent on GH alone. Other treatments that inhibit growth include spinal irradiation, glucocorticoids, and chemotherapeutic agents, as well as altered nutrition/inadequate caloric intake. Incidence rates of the deficiency vary because of these confounding factors.

GH deficiency has also been associated with reduced lean body mass and increased fat mass, metabolic abnormalities (including glucose intolerance), a reduction in bone mineral density, and consequent impaired quality of life.

Growth can be divided into three stages:

1. Infancy – from birth to 2 years, growth is influenced by adequate nutrition and is at least partly independent from GH
2. Childhood – GH is the dominant factor and along with adequate nutrition will influence growth

3. Puberty – the sex hormones along with GH and nutrition influence growth until epiphyseal fusion is complete and growth is finished

Consequently, children treated for cancer at an early age are less likely to achieve their expected stature unless they receive GH replacement.

23.2.1 Treatment

23.2.1.1 Investigation

Statural growth should be monitored for 6 months before the fusion of growth plates. If there is any decline in growth velocity, formal testing of GH reserve should be performed (Oberfield and Sklar, 2002). Before establishing any hormone treatment, the following assessment should be made:

1. Accurate measurement of supine length (if under 2 years), standing height, sitting height, and weight
2. Measurement of parents
3. Calculation of decimal age
4. Plotting of growth measurements on appropriate chart
5. Calculation of mid-parental height and target range
6. Calculation of height velocity
7. Pubertal staging
8. Bone age

A GH stimulation test is performed once there is a suspicion of GH deficiency. Numerous tests can be performed, including clonidine, arginine, and insulin tolerance tests. The gold standard test is the insulin tolerance test, which is a safe and reliable test provided that a strict procedure is followed (Galloway et al., 2002). Pituitary function tests used to diagnose GH deficiency rely on these pharmacological provocation tests. However, although peak responses to these tests may remain normal, the physiologic secretion of pituitary hormones is often impaired (neurosecretory dysfunction). The assessment of physiological secretion is difficult, which emphasises the importance of continued long-term follow-up.

The insulin test should only be performed in paediatric endocrine units and in children over 5 years of age.

23.2.1.2 Growth Hormone Replacement Therapy

Once it is confirmed that the child is GH-deficient and is 2 years post-cancer treatment, replacement with recombinant GH therapy can be advocated.

Somatropin (synthetic human growth hormone) is given in the form of daily subcutaneous injections. The recommended dose is 5 mg/m^2/week.

GH replacement therapy is normally discontinued once the patient's final height has been achieved. However, consideration needs to be given to the continuation of GH replacement beyond this time in order to avoid the other adverse consequences associated with GH deficiency mentioned previously (Gleeson et al., 2002). Therefore, replacement therapy may continue, at a reduced dose, into adulthood (Brougham et al., 2002).

23.2.2 Prognosis

Growth hormone is potentially mitogenic, and there have been numerous clinical studies investigating any evidence of recurrence of disease in the children treated with GH. There has been no evidence found to support that there is a significant risk. It is therefore thought that GH treatment benefits most GH-deficient children. Oberfield and Sklar (2002) observe the importance of tracking adults who have survived childhood cancers and who are now starting to receive GH as part of the newly suggested lower-dose GH replacement regimens for adults.

23.3 Hypothalamic-Pituitary-Gonadal Axis

23.3.1 Gonadotrophin Deficiency

Higher doses of cranial irradiation (>35 Gy) can damage the hypothalamic-pituitary axis, with a result in gonadotrophin secretion deficiency (Cohen, 2003). Patients have demonstrated deficiencies in the secretion of

- Follicle stimulating hormone (FSH)
- Luteinising hormone (LH)

Clinically, gonadotrophin deficiency can exhibit a broad spectrum of severity, from subclinical abnormalities, which are detectable by gonadotrophin releasing hormone (GnRH) testing, to a significant reduction in circulating sex hormone levels and delayed puberty (Brougham et al., 2002). The etiology of hypogonadism following cranial irradiation is often hypothalamic GnRH deficiency. Exogenous GnRH replacement therapy may possibly restore gonadal function and fertility.

23.3.2 Early or Precocious Puberty

In contrast, lower doses of cranial irradiation can cause premature activation of the hypothalamic-pituitary-gonadal axis. This can lead to early or precocious puberty. True central precocious puberty occurs before the age of 8 years in girls and before 9 years in boys. Early puberty is defined as onset between ages 8 and 10 in girls (with the development of pubic hair) and between 9 and 11 in boys (using testicular enlargement). The etiology of radiation-induced early puberty is thought to be through the disinhibition of cortical influences on the hypothalamus (Brougham et al., 2002). The incidence of radiation-induced early puberty is dependent on dose. The dose threshold is then gender-specific; low doses of cranial radiation, 18–24 Gy (used in ALL treatment), may cause early puberty predominately in girls, but higher doses of 25–47 Gy (used to treat brain tumours) affects both genders equally (Cohen, 2002). Additionally, a patient may enter puberty early but subsequently develop gonadotrophin deficiency, suggesting the differential effects of radiotherapy with time (Brougham et al., 2002).

Entering puberty early causes a premature growth spurt that is followed by early epiphyseal fusion with a consequential reduction in final height. Puberty is usually of normal duration, but early puberty is often combined with GH deficiency, which further reduces the final height potential.

23.3.2.1 Treatment

These patients also require clinical assessment with regard to their growth and puberty. This assessment includes

- Pubertal status
- Auxological assessment, including standing and sitting heights
- Biochemical assessment of growth hormone and gonadotrophin secretion
- Radiological assessment of bone age

It is advantageous to suppress puberty by using a GnRH analogue, e.g. Zoladex LA 10.8 mg every 10–12 weeks. In this situation, combined treatment of GH with GnRH analogue will improve the height potential. To achieve improved auxological outcome, Gleeson et al. (2003) recommend

1. The use of standardised GH schedules and better dosing regimens
2. A reduction in the time interval between finishing radiotherapy and starting GH replacement
3. The use of GnRH analogue in addition to GH replacement in carefully selected patients

23.3.2.2 Prognosis

Despite treatment, final height obtained is generally lower than the target height. Also, growth is often disproportionate due to a reduction in sitting height. This is due to disruption to spinal growth caused by

- Early onset of puberty and GH deficiency (spinal growth is significant in the latter part of the pubertal growth spurt)
- Spinal irradiation

23.4 Thyroid Disorders

Thyroid disorders can occur following treatment for childhood cancer due to

- Disruption of the hypothalamic-pituitary-thyroid axis
- Direct damage to the thyroid gland

The thyroid gland is radiosensitive and can be affected by craniospinal radiation and total body irradiation, as well as treatments with iodine radiolabeled monoclonal antibodies, such as I^{131}-MIBG for neuroblastoma.

Disorders manifest as

- Dysfunction of the thyroid gland – Hypothyroidism is the most common abnormality following direct thyroid damage. Radiation-induced thyroid stimulating hormone (TSH) deficiency is dose-dependent and uncommon with doses less than 40 Gy in children. Hyperthyroidism is less common but can occur, particularly when patients receive higher doses.
- Thyroid nodules – Gleeson et al. (2002) report a varying incidence of thyroid nodules, 2–65%, in children and adolescents treated for Hodgkin's disease.
- Slight risk of secondary thyroid function – Papillary carcinoma is the most common thyroid cancer that develops secondary to irradiation (Brougham et al., 2002).

Direct damage to the thyroid is usually secondary to radiotherapy in which the radiation field includes the neck. Chemotherapy has been reported to potentiate this damage; however, van Santen and colleagues (2003) have concluded that chemotherapy does not contribute to damage on the thyroid axis.

23.4.1 Treatment

Biochemical diagnosis of central hypothyroidism relies on measurement of TSH and thyroid hormone as free T_4. Primary hypothyroidism results in an elevated TSH and a low free T_4; compensated hypothyroidism is indicated by an elevated TSH and a normal free T_4. However, TSH and free T_4 may both fall within normal range, but more detailed investigation of TSH dynamics, including thyrotrophin secretion, can suggest significant central hypothyroidism. This detail may be important when deciding thresholds for treatment with thyroxine supplements and may be particularly important in paediatric patients because reduced thyroid function may affect growth (Brougham et al., 2002).

It is advisable that thyroid function be assessed at least twice a year following treatment. The greatest risk of hypothyroidism occurs during the first 5 years after treatment, but new cases continue to emerge more than 20 years after irradiation (Gleeson et al., 2002). If treatment is necessary, thyroxin is prescribed orally in a dose of 100 mcg/m^2 to fully suppress and replace endogenous thyroid function.

23.5 Hypothalamic-Pituitary-Adrenal Axis

The hypothalamic-pituitary-adrenal axis appears to be relatively radio-resistant, and adrenal insufficiency due to radiotherapy or cranial tumour is rare. Treatment doses of glucocorticoids may suppress the hypothalamic-pituitary-adrenal axis. Dexamethasone at a dosage of 6 mg/m^2/day for 28–42 days can mildly suppress the axis for up to 4–8 weeks (Cohen, 2002; Peterson et al., 2003). However, clinical manifestation of adrenal insufficiency in these cases is rare.

Deficiency in adrenocorticotrophic hormone (ACTH) can develop in patients treated with radiation doses in excess of 50 Gy and in patients treated for pituitary tumours (Brougham et al., 2002). Excessive tiredness in patients treated with cranial radiation warrants testing of the hypothalamic-pituitary-adrenal axis. Aldosterone is usually unaffected because secretion depends more on angiotensin II than on ACTH.

Diagnosis is difficult, and the insulin tolerance test is usually the assessment of choice, as with GH secretion. Treatments of high-dose glucocorticoids should be tapered. Hydrocortisone replacement may be necessary, and increased doses are required during periods of illness and surgery (Brougham et al., 2002).

23.6 Other Pituitary Hormones

Prolactin secretion is inhibited by dopamine from the hypothalamus. High-dose cranial radiation, especially >50 Gy, can disrupt this inhibitory control and result in hyperprolactinemia (Cohen, 2002; Brougham et al., 2002). However, this is unusual in children.

Antidiuretic hormone (ADH) deficiency causing central diabetes insipidus has not been attributed to cranial irradiation. However, central diabetes insipidus has been associated with intracranial tumours involving the pituitary gland following cranial surgery or secondary to leukemic infiltration. The deficiency in these cases usually persists despite treatment of the underlying malignancy (Brougham et al., 2002) and may require treatment with exogenous vasopressin.

The syndrome of inappropriate ADH secretion (SIADH) with water retention and secondary hyponatremia has been associated with malignancy and its treatment. The associated malignancies are those more commonly seen in adults, including gastrointestinal tumours, breast and prostatic cancers, and primary brain tumours. However, treatments used for adults and children that can cause SIADH include the vinca alkaloids, cisplatin, cyclophosphamide, and melphalan. Other aspects of treatment associated with SIADH include intrathoracic infection and artificial ventilation. Fortunately, SIADH is only a problem for the short term and is rarely a long-term complication (Brougham et al., 2002).

23.6.1 Fertility

Radiotherapy involving the pelvic area or systemic chemotherapy can cause direct damage to gonadal tissue (testes and ovaries). This damage can result in subfertility or infertility in both males and females.

23.6.1.1 Testicular Failure

The adult male testes has two functions:

- Steroidogenesis
- Spermatogenesis

Table 23.3 outlines the physiology of the testes and the effects of radiotherapy and chemotherapy on their function. The mechanism that makes the testes susceptible to the toxic effects of radiation and chemotherapy appears to involve the combination of destruction of the germ cell pool and, when the germ cells survive, inhibition of further differentiation (Thomson et al., 2002).

23.6.1.2 Ovarian Failure

Ovarian function is very complex. Table 23.4 outlines the main functions and the consequential effects of radiotherapy and chemotherapy.

Additionally, radiotherapy involving the uterus in childhood is associated with

- Increased incidence of nulliparity
- Spontaneous miscarriage
- Intrauterine growth retardation with decreased uterine volume and decreased elasticity

Obstetricians must be aware of potential problems.

26.6.2 Treatment

23.6.2.1 Assessment of Gonadal Function

Table 23.5 summarises the patient history and investigations necessary when assessing gonadal function in males and females.

23.6.2.2 Treatment for Gonadal Dysfunction

Oestrogen replacement in girls starts at a small dose of ethinyl oestradiol 2 mcg, increasing in small increments over 2 years until full establishment of puberty. A combined pill of oestrogen and progesterone can then be given, e.g. Loestrin 30.

Table 23.3. Outline of the function of the testes and the associated effects of radiotherapy and chemotherapy (Drury,1990; Cohen, 2002; Brougham et al., 2002)

Function	Associated hormones	Target cells	Action	Effects of radiotherapy	Effects of chemotherapy
Steroido-genesis	GnRH released from hypothala-mus stimulates luteinising hor-mone (LH) from the pituitary	Leydig's cells of somatic cells of testes to produce testosterone	Testosterone acts systemically to produce male secondary sexual characteristics, anabolism, and the maintenance of libido (Testosterone feeds back on hypo-thalamus/pituitary to inhibit GnRH secretion)	Leydig's cells are more resistant to damage. Damage occurs at doses of 20 Gy in pre-pubertal boys and up to 30 Gy in sexually mature males. Second-ary sexual characteris-tics may develop despite impaired sper-matogenesis	Similar to radiotherapy effects. Leydig's cells are less sensitive and may be unaffected. Higher doses may cause Leydig cell dys-function
Spermato-genesis	GnRH released from hypothala-mus stimulates follicle stimu-lating hormone (FSH)	Sertoli's cells in germinal epithelium of the seminiferous tubules	Produces mature sperm (and feedback hormone inhibin that appears to feed back on pituitary to decrease FSH secre-tion.) Testosterone also acts locally to aid spermatogenesis	Damage depends on field of treatment, total dose, and frac-tionation schedule. Doses as low as 0.1 Gy can affect sper-matogenesis, with temporary azoospermia and oligospermia. Doses over 4 Gy may have a permanent effect	Extent of damage depends on agent administered and dose received.[a] Gonado-toxic chemotherapy can cause oligosper-mia or azoospermia

[a] Gonadotoxic agents include cisplatin, procarbazine, cytarabine, vinblastine and alkylating agents such as cyclophosphamide, melphalan, chlorambucil

Boys will start with 100 mg Sustanon every 6 weeks increasing to every 4 weeks until puberty is es-tablished.

26.6.3 Prognosis

Concerns that the offspring of patients successfully treated for cancer might have an increased risk of congenital abnormality and childhood cancer have not been substantiated (Thomson et al., 2002).

Techniques in preserving fertility continue to be developed. Established options include cryop-reservation of spermatozoa and collection of mature oocytes with fertilisation and subsequent cryop-reservation of embryos in the female with a partner. Options are limited in children. Experimental strate-gies are focusing on the harvesting and storage of go-nadal tissue, cryopreservation of immature sper-matogenic cells or oocytes, gonadotrophin suppres-sion, and inhibition of follicle apoptosis (Thomson et al., 2002). Following cure, stored tissue could possibly be autotransplanted or stored tissue could be matured in vitro until sufficiently mature for fertili-sation with assisted reproductive techniques (Broug-ham et al., 2002). Human primordial follicles survive cryopreservation, and the return of ovarian hormon-al activity has been achieved after reimplantation; however, no pregnancies have been reported (Thom-son et al., 2002). The potential developments raise many ethical and legal issues that must be addressed to ensure adequate regulation. Children with cancer must be ensured realistic, safe prospects for fertility in the future, and patients at risk of subfertility re-quire appropriate counselling as part of their routine care.

Table 23.4. Outline of the function of the ovaries and the associated effects of radiotherapy and chemotherapy (Drury, 1990; Cohen, 2002; Brougham et al., 2002)

Function	Associated hormones	Target cells	Action	Effects of radiotherapy	Effects of chemotherapy
Oestrogen and progesterone production	Pulses of GnRH stimulate release of pituitary LH and FSH	LH stimulates ovarian androgen production (mid-cycle LH surge induces ovulation).\n\nFSH stimulates follicular development and aromatase activity (Follicle differentiates into corpus luteum and secretes progesterone and oestradiol during 2nd half of cycle; aromatase is an enzyme required to convert ovarian androgens to oestrogen).\n\nFSH stimulates inhibin from ovarian stromal cells (feedback of inhibin inhibits FSH release)	Oestrogen initially, then progesterone, cause uterine endometrial proliferation in preparation for possible implantation; if implantation does not occur, corpus luteum regresses, progesterone secretion falls, and menstruation occurs. (Pregnancy causes human chorionic gonadotrophin production from corpus luteum until 10–12 weeks. Placenta then makes sufficient oestrogen and progesterone).\n\nOestrogens induce secondary sexual characteristics	Ovaries may be in the field of pelvic, abdominal or spinal radiation. Degree of impairment depends on dose, fractionation schedule, and age at time of treatment.\n\nThe human oocyte is highly sensitive to radiation, with 50% death of oocytes at a dose of 4 Gy. The younger the girl at the time of radiotherapy, the larger the oocyte pool and hence the later onset of premature menopause. Premature menopause can occur in women >40 years of age following treatment dose of 6 Gy. (Early menopause has implications for fertility, but also other medical complications including osteoporosis). Doses >20 Gy can cause complete ovarian failure.	Prepubertal ovaries appear to be more resistant to cytotoxic agents than postpubertal, possibly because they have more follicles. Ovarian function is often retained or recovered with standard doses of chemotherapy. High doses of alkylating agents or myeloablative therapy for bone marrow transplant are likely to result in permanent ovarian failure

Table 23.5. Assessment of gonadal function

Females – ovarian function	Males – testicular function
Pubertal staging	Pubertal staging
Menstrual history	Testicular volume using Prader orchidometer
Basal LH and FSH	Basal LH, FSH, and inhibin B
Basal oestradiol	Basal testosterone
Pelvic ultrasound	Semen analysis

References

Brougham MFH, Kelnar CJH, Wallace WHB (2002) The late endocrine effects of childhood cancer. Pediatric Rehabilitation 5(4): 191–201

Cohen LE (2003) Endocrine late effects of cancer treatment. Current Opinion in Pediatrics 15: 3–9.

Drury PL (1990) Endocrinology. In Kumar PJ, Clark ML Clinical Medicine, 2nd edn. Balliere Tindall, London

Galloway PJ, McNeill E, Paterson WF, Donaldson (2002) Safety of the insulin tolerance test. Archives of Disease in Childhood 87(4): 354–356

Gleeson HK, Darzy K, Shalet SM (2002) Late endocrine, metabolic and skeletal sequelae following treatment of childhood cancer. Best Practice and Research Clinical Endocrinology and Metabolism 16(2): 335–348

Gleeson HK, Stoeter R, Ogilvy-Stuart AL, Gattamaneni HR, Brennan BM, Shalet SM (2003) Improvements in final height over 25 years in growth hormone (GH)-deficient childhood survivors of brain tumors receiving GH replacement. Journal of Clinical Endocrinology and Metabolism 88(8): 3682–3689

Oberfield SE, Sklar CA (2002) Endocrine sequelae in survivors of childhood cancer. Adolescent Medicine 13(1): 161–169

Petersen KB, Muller J, Rasmussen M, Schmiegelow K (2003) Impaired adrenal function after glucocorticoid therapy in children with acute lymphoblastic leukemia. Medical Pediatric Oncology 41(2): 110–114

Sklar CA (1999) Overview of the effects of cancer therapies: the nature, scale and breadth of the problem. Acta Paediatrica (supplement) 88: 1–4

Thomson AB, Critchley HOD, Kelnar CJH, Wallace WHB (2002) Late reproductive sequelae following treatment of childhood cancer and options for fertility preservation. Best Practice and Research Clinical Endocrinology and Metabolism 16(2):311–334

Van Santen HM, Vulsma T, Dijkgraaf MG, Blumer RM, Heinen R, Jaspers Mw, Geenen MM, Offringa MO, de Vijlder JJ, van den Bos C (2003) No damaging effect of chemotherapy in addition to radiotherapy on the thyroid axis in young adult survivors of childhood cancer. Journal of Clinical Endocrinology Metabolism 88(8): 3657–3663

Ototoxicity

Colleen Nixon

Contents

Higher doses of chemotherapy and radiation increase the occurrence of side effects, especially sensorineural hearing loss (SNHL) (Huang et al., 2002). SNHL results from damage to the inner ear or auditory nerve. At some point during most children's cancer treatment, they will receive an agent or a combination of agents that will put them at risk of developing ototoxicity (Landier, 1998). Hearing loss affects a child's total quality of life; high-frequency hearing loss can result in difficulties with communication, including acquisition and development of speech and language, as well as emotional and social difficulties (Schweitzer, 1993).

24.1 Incidence

Ototoxic agents used for pediatric oncology patients include platinum-based chemotherapeutic agents, radiation therapy, aminoglycosides, and loop diuretics (Brookhouser, 2002).

Cisplatin and carboplatin are platinum-based chemotherapeutic agents. In one study, Brookhouser (2002) cites an 84–100% incidence of cisplatin-induced ototoxicity in the pediatric population. Cisplatin produces a high-frequency SNHL (i.e., 6000–8000-Hertz [Hz] range) (Michaud et al., 2002). This generally irreversible hearing loss is caused by damage to the inner ear, specifically to hair cells of the organ of Corti, and possibly by damage to the stria vascularis (Michaud et al., 2002). Less common is vestibular toxicity with ataxia, vertigo, and nystagmus (Meyer, 2001). Damage to the inner ear hair cells should be considered permanent, as hair cells do not regenerate (Landier, 1998). The hearing loss may first be noticed 3–4 days after the initial dose of cisplatin. Ototoxicity caused by cisplatin is dose-related, cumulative, and inversely related to age (Schweitzer, 1993). The dose of cisplatin at which SNHL occurs is around 400 mg/m² (Brookhouser, 2002). Continued exposure to cisplatin will ultimately affect the lower frequencies used in speech (i.e., 1,000–2,000 Hz) (Huang, 2002). Ototoxicity remains an irreversible, dose-limiting side effect of cisplatin, despite vigorous prehydration and in combination with mannitol diuresis (Schweitzer, 1993). Carboplatin, an analog of cisplatin, introduced in the early 1980s, can also cause a high-frequency hearing loss but without the loss of hair cells (Michaud et al., 2002).

Hearing loss is not typically associated with cranial irradiation alone (Halperin et al., 1999). Ototoxicity becomes increasingly of concern when radiotherapy is used in combination with cisplatin. The administration of cisplatin after cranial radiation appears to enhance the ototoxic effects of cisplatin (Halperin et al., 1999).

Aminoglycoside antibiotics are used mainly to treat infections caused by aerobic gram-negative bacteria. Ototoxicity, a known side effect of these drugs, is often irreversible. Aminoglycosides initially injure outer hair cell membranes, followed by inner hair cell destruction, with damage most often occurring during prolonged elevated serum trough levels (Matz, 1993).

A synergism exists between aminoglycosides and loop diuretics (frusemide). Studies have shown that giving a loop diuretic and then an aminoglycoside antibiotic does not affect hearing more than giving either drug alone. But when the aminoglycoside is given first, and then the loop diuretic, the organ of Corti is damaged, causing synergistic hearing loss (Brookhouser, 2002). Ototoxicity caused by a loop diuretic is often due to fluid changes within the inner ear, resulting in problems with nerve transmission. This type of hearing loss typically develops quickly and is reversible (Brookhouser, 2002). Ototoxicity most often occurs after rapid intravenous infusion of frusemide (Landier, 1998).

The incidence of ototoxicity in the pediatric oncology population is well documented in the literature (Table 24.1). Many factors are associated with the development of hearing loss in this group: age (3 years or younger), platinum-based chemotherapy or other ototoxic agents, rapid infusion of ototoxic medications, cranial irradiation, presence of a central nervous system tumor, surgery involving the 8th cranial nerve, excessive noise exposure, and prior ototoxic therapy (Schell et al., 1989). Patients with poor renal function, associated with chemotherapeutic drugs, are at increased risk of hearing loss (Landier, 1998). Berg et al. (1999) noted studies that suggest that other factors such as nutrition, iris color, and skin pigmentation play a role in the development of cisplatin ototoxicity.

Despite known toxicities, many of the ototoxic drugs play a critical role in the treatment of the child with cancer. Often, when early hearing loss develops after treatment initiation, treatment protocols – particularly ones containing platinum-based agents – may be altered (Landier, 1998).

Other children at high risk for hearing loss include those who had perinatal anoxia or hypoxia, low Apgar scores (<1 at 5 minutes), hyperbilirubinemia requiring an exchange transfusion, or mechanical ventilation for more than 10 days. Children with a history of bacterial meningitis, birth weight <1500 g, maternal infection (e.g., toxoplasmosis, rubella, cytomegalovirus, or herpes) while in utero, recurrent or persistent otitis media with effusion for at least 3 months, prior treatment with ototoxic drugs, or a family history of SNHL (presumably congenital) are also at risk (Cunningham & Cox, 2003). Clinical manifestations during infancy and early toddlerhood that may signify a hearing deficit include lack of a startle, failure to be awakened by loud environmental noises, absence of well-formed syllables ("da," "na," "ya") by 11 months, and monotone and difficult to understand speech (Kline and Bloom, 2003).

The three main types of hearing loss, conductive, sensorineural, and mixed, are described according to the site of damage (Fig. 24.1). A conductive hearing loss occurs in the outer or middle ear and results in the prevention of sound waves progressing to the inner ear. This is often temporary, due to fluid in the middle ear or to otitis media, and reversible. Sensorineural loss results from damage to the inner ear or auditory nerve. For a child with SNHL, sounds are

Table 24.1. Studies of ototoxic agents in pediatric oncology

Author	Ototoxic agent	Results	Recommendations
Berg et al. (1999)	Cisplatin 60–120 mg/m²/ course treatment	26% of children developed bilateral symmetrical high-frequency sensori-neural hearing loss	Audiologic assessment should be incorporated into regular medical examination because the onset of hearing loss can be delayed. Hearing aids may be useful for patients with hearing loss affecting low or middle frequencies. Assessment, evaluation, and intervention by a speech pathologist to address possible communication issues.
Schell, et al. (1983)	Cisplatin, medium cumulative dose 360 mg/m²	>50% of patients had substantial hearing loss (50 dB or greater) at higher frequencies (4,000–8,000 Hz), and 11% had hearing loss at speech frequency level (500–3,000 Hz). Hearing loss was related to cumulative dose of cisplatin	Obtain audiogram at least 3 weeks after cisplatin to monitor for delayed appearance of hearing loss. Serial audiograms for younger patients, patients receiving cranial irradiation, patients with CNS neoplasm, and any patient receiving cisplatin >360 mg/m²
Huang et al. (2002)	Comparing ototoxicity in patients with medulloblastoma receiving conventional radiotherapy vs. intensity-modulated radiation therapy (IMRT)	Compared with conventional radiotherapy, IMRT delivered 68% of the radiation dose to the auditory apparatus (cochlea and 8th cranial nerve) while still delivering full doses to the desired target volume; 13% of the IMRT group had a Grade 3 or 4 hearing loss vs. 64% of the conventional RT group	Larger sample size Further studies Longer follow-ups
Parsons et al. (1998)	Carboplatin, high-dose, 2 g/m²	82% of children with neuroblastoma treated with autologous bone marrow transplant developed speech frequency hearing loss requiring hearing aids	Continued efforts to monitor and evaluate hearing loss in patients treated with platinum-based agents as well as other ototoxic agents. Prepare patients and parents for this difficult side effect of treatment

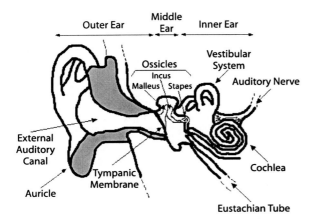

Figure 24.1

Sound waves are funneled through the external auditory canal and hit the tympanic membrane (eardrum). The sound waves hitting the tympanic membrane cause the ossicles of the middle ear to vibrate, setting the oval window (beginning point of the inner ear) in motion. The organ of Corti, located inside the fluid-filled cochlea, is the sensory receptor, which holds the hair cells, or the nerve receptors for hearing. The vibration of the ossicles causes fluid in the cochlea to move, stimulating the hair cells. Specific hair cells react to specific sound frequencies (pitch). Depending on the pitch, specific hair cells are stimulated. Signals from the cochlear hair cells are transmitted into nerve impulses and sent to the brain via the acoustic nerve (Children's Oncology Group, 2003)

indistinct, and it is often difficult to perceive speech accurately. A mixed conductive-sensorineural hearing loss results from disruption of the transmission of sound along the auditory nerve (Kline and Bloom, 2003).

24.2 Prevention and Treatment

Early detection, with possible prevention, of hearing loss is an important consideration for a patient's primary care team. Baseline audiologic testing is recommended before a patient receives any platinum-based therapy or other potential ototoxic agents (Schweitzer, 1993). Serial audiologic testing should continue throughout the entire treatment course, with close attention paid to the delayed effects of cisplatin ototoxicity. The testing is typically done before starting each cycle of cisplatin therapy (Landier, 1998).

Multiple audiologic tests exist for infants and children (Table 24.2). The method for evaluation can vary depending on the child's age, state of health, and ability to cooperate (Parsons et al., 1998).

Pure tone audiometry remains the standard as well as the most common test for hearing evaluation (Cunningham and Cox, 2003). This test includes air and bone conduction testing to establish hearing sensitivity. Tones heard through earphones are presented at different frequencies (pitch) ranging from 125–8,000 Hz. Hearing impairment or sensitivity is measured in decibels (dB), a measurement of loudness or intensity (Fig. 24.2) (Landier, 1998).

Normal hearing is considered to be in the 0–20 dB range for all frequencies tested in the 125–8,000 Hz (Fig. 24.3). A mild hearing loss for a child (20–40 dB) results in the inability to hear soft sounds or a whispered conversation in a quiet room. The child with a moderate hearing loss (40–60 dB) will have great difficulty understanding a typical conversation even in a quiet room. A child with a severe hearing loss (60–90 dB) will be able to have a conversation only if the speaker is within 6–12 inches of the child. A child with a profound loss of 90 dB or more may hear only loud sounds and will typically experience sound as a vibration (Landier, 1998)

Children's ability to accurately understand what is being spoken is crucial. Many of the consonants are high-frequency sounds, such as "s," "sh," "f," and "th." Most of the consonants are pitched higher than vowels and are more difficult to identify, especially in a noisy environment (Berg et al., 1999). As the pediatric cancer survival rates continue to climb; the effect of hearing loss on a child's life must be closely evaluated. New promising treatments may help with the incidence of ototoxicity. Eloxatin (oxaliplatin) is a cell-cycle nonspecific platinum-based chemotherapeutic agent; its main side effects are nausea, neuropathy, and dyspnea, without the ototoxicity of cisplatin. As of this writing, Eloxatin has not been approved for the pediatric population but has shown promise in

Table 24.2. Audiologic tests for infants and children (Cunningham and Cox, 2003)

Developmental age of child	Auditory test	Type of measurement	Test procedures	What the test reveals
Birth to 9 months	Brainstem auditory evoked response (BAER). 15-minute test	Electrophysiologic measurement that evaluates function in auditory nerve pathways	Placement of electrodes on child's head that record electrical responses to sound stimuli. The child must be asleep or sedated	Patient's hearing is evaluated by studying the size of the peaks and the time to form them
9 months to 2.5 years	Visual reinforcement audiogram (VRA). 30-minute test	Behavioral test obtained in a sound-treated room. The child is seated on the parent's lap between two speakers or wearing earphones. When a sound is presented at a specific frequency, the infant's head-turn response is reinforced with a lighted toy	Requires a sound-treated room. Condition the child to associate speech or specific sound with a reinforcement stimulus	Assesses hearing of better ear (if earphones not worn). Used to evaluate frequencies in the 500–4000 Hz range
2.5–4 years	Play audiometry. 30-minute test	Behavioral test assessing auditory thresholds in response to speech and specific tones delivered through earphones	Child is instructed to perform a repetitive task, such as placing a peg in a pegboard, each time the child hears a sound. If the child refuses to wear the earphones, the test can be administered in a sound field	Ear-specific results if the child does not wear earphones. Assess auditory perception of the child
All ages	Evokes otoacoustic emissions (OAE). 10-minute test	Physiologic test measuring cochlear response to an auditory stimulus	Small microphone placed in ear canal; signals are generated by the cochlear hair cells in response	Otoacoustic emissions cannot be picked up with >40 dB hearing loss
Extended high-frequency audiometry (Landier, 1998)			Measures frequencies in the 8,000–20,000 Hz range	Important in monitoring early hearing loss

the adult population (National Cancer Institute). Amifostine has been approved to prevent neurotoxicity from alkylating agents, platinum analogues, and radiation therapy while preserving the antineoplastic effect on tumors. It has shown efficacy in decreasing cisplatin neurotoxicity; however, its otoprotective effect is uncertain. One study showed a 7% incidence of ototoxicity with amifostine and chemotherapy compared with 22% with chemotherapy alone (Meyer, 2001). In another study using cisplatin and amifostine, neither a tumor-protective effect nor reduced toxicity was noted (Gradishar et al., 2001). The latest technology in radiotherapy is intensity-modulated radiotherapy (IMRT). IMRT is a complex type of three-dimensional conformal radiotherapy. The benefit of IMRT is its capability to deliver radiation to the intended site while avoiding surrounding tissues, such as the cochlea and auditory apparatus. This allows for less irradiation of normal tissue and decreased side effects (Huang et al., 2002).

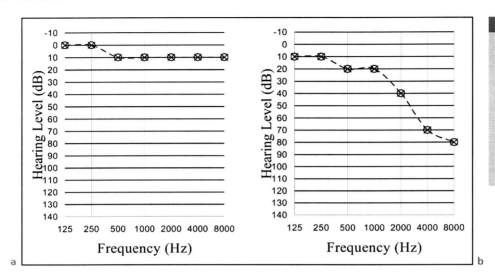

Figure 24.2

a Illustration of normal audiogram (air conduction, right ear)
b Illustration of audiogram showing sensorineural hearing loss (air conduction, right ear)

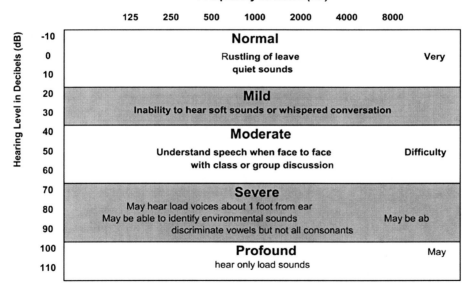

Figure 24.3

Degree of hearing loss and effect on speech and language (Kline and Bloom, 2003)

Primary prevention and early detection are important in the care and management of the child with a sensorineural hearing loss. Studies show that the incidence of hearing loss due to ototoxic agents ranges from minimal loss to greater than 80%. A multidisciplinary team needs to be involved to manage the acute and long-term needs of the child with a hearing loss. Serial monitoring is recommended so that if ototoxicity develops, treatments can be changed or services added. The onset of ototoxicity cannot be predicted or delayed, making regular audiology exams of the utmost importance (Berg et al., 1999). The Children's Oncology Group has developed guidelines for monitoring hearing loss (Children's Oncology Group, 2003). Any child who received any dose of carboplatin or cisplatin should be tested at least once 2 years post-treatment, and if problems develop, then yearly until stable. Any child who received any dose of aminoglycoside or loop diuretics should be tested once post-treatment and if any other problems arise. A child receiving doses of 30 Gy (3,000 cGy) or higher to the ear, brain, or nasopharyngeal or infratemporal area should be screened yearly for 5 years after completion of treatment and then every 5 years as long as no problems arise.

Hearing loss affects a child's total quality of life. Strategies to reach dose intensification and to maximize antineoplastic effects require interventions to minimize the associated side effects. This is particularly important as higher doses of cisplatin and carboplatin continue to be used in attempt for cure. The future holds new developments of chemotherapeutic agents, chemoprotectants, and radiologic technology. It is hoped that these new innovative treatments will greatly decrease the incidence of ototoxicity associated with childhood cancer.

References

American Cancer Society. http://www.cancer.org/docroot/CRI. Retrieved 12/30/03

Berg A.L., Spitzer J.B., Garvin J.H. (1999) Ototoxic impact of cisplatin in pediatric oncology patients. Laryngoscope 109(11):1806–1814

Brookhouser P.E. (2002) Diseases of the inner ear and sensorineural hearing. In: Bluestone C.D., Casselbrant M.L., Stool S.E., Dohar J.E., Alper C.M., Arjmand E.M., Yellon R.F. (eds) Pediatric Otolaryngology, 4th edn. Philadelphia: Saunders, pp. 798–800

Children's Oncology Group. Healthy living after treatment for childhood cancer. http://www.childrensoncologygroup.org. Retrieved 1/5/04

Cunningham M., Cox E.O. (2003) Hearing assessment in infants and children: Recommendation beyond neonatal screening. Pediatrics 111(2):436–440

Gradishar W.J., Stephenson P., Glover D.J., Neuber D.S., Moore M.R., Windschiti H.E., et al. (2001) A phase II trial of cisplatin plus WR-2721 (amifostine) for metastatic breast carcinoma: An eastern cooperative oncology study (E8188). Cancer 92(10):2517–2522

Halperin E.C., Constine L.S., Tarbell N.J., Kun L.E. (eds) (1999) Late effects of cancer treatment. In: Pediatric Oncology, 3rd edn. Philadelphia: Lippincott Williams & Wilkins, pp. 515–517

Huang E., Teh B.S., Strother D.R., Davis Q.G., Chiu, J.K., Lu H.H. (2002) Intensity-modulated radiation therapy for pediatric medulloblastoma: Early report on the reduction of ototoxicity. International Journal of Radiation Oncology, Biology, Physics 52(3):599

Kline N. E., Bloom D (2003) The child with cognitive, sensory, or communication impairment. In: Hockenberry M.J., Wilson D., Winkelstein M., Kline N.E. (eds.) Wong's Nursing Care of Infants and Children, 7th edn. St. Louis: Mosby, pp. 994–997

Landier W. (1998) Hearing loss related to ototoxicity in children with cancer. Journal of Pediatric Oncology 15(4): 195–207

Matz G. (1993) Aminoglycoside cochlear ototoxicity. Otolaryngologic Clinics of North America 26(5):705–711

Meyer M.A. (2001) Neurotoxicity of chemotherapy agents. In: Perry M.C. (ed) The Chemotherapy Source Book. Philadelphia: Lippincott Williams & Wilkins, pp. 504–509

National Cancer Institute. Late effects of childhood cancer. http://seer.cnacer.gov/publications/childhoo/forward.html Retrieved 12/30/03

Michaud L.J., Ried S.R., McMahon M.A. (2002) Rehabilitation of the child with cancer. In: Pizzo P.A., Poplak D.G. (eds) Principles and Practice of Pediatric Oncology. Philadelphia: Lippincott Williams & Wilkins, p. 1356

Parsons S.K, Neault M.W., Lehmann L.E., Brennan L.L., Eickhoff C.E., Kretschmar C.S., Diller L.R. (1998) Severe ototoxicity following carboplatin-containing conditioning regimen for autologous marrow transplantation for neuroblastoma. Bone Marrow Transplantation 22:669–674

Schell M. J., McHaney V.A, Green A.A., Kun L.E., Hayes A., Horowitz M., et al. (1989) Hearing loss in children and young adults receiving cisplatin with or without prior cranial irradiation. Journal of Clinical Oncology, 7(6):754–760

Schweitzer V.G. (1993) Ototoxicity of chemotherapeutic agents. Otolaryngologic Clinics of North America 26(5):759–779

Eyes – Ocular complications

Deborah Tomlinson

Contents

25.1 Ocular Toxicity Associated with High-dose Cytarabine Arabinoside

25.1.1 Incidence and Etiology

Keratoconjunctivitis is a known side effect of systemic high-dose cytarabine arabinoside (HDAC). HDAC may be given as doses of 4–6 g/m^2/day twice a day for usually 2–4 days (Barrios et al. 1987). Corneal toxicity associated with HDAC is a function of tear concentration that causes an inhibition of corneal epithelial DNA synthesis (Ritch et al. 1983). Symptoms include photophobia, foreign body sensation, and excessive tearing (Higa et al. 1991).

The incidence appears to be related to the duration of cytarabine arabinoside (also referred to as cytosine or ara-c) therapy, the intraocular fluid concentration of the drug, the cerebrospinal fluid (CSF) pharmacokinetics, and the use of corticosteroid eye drops (Higa et al. 1991):

- Extended periods of administration of HDAC (6–8 days) appear to increase the likelihood of eye problems.
- High levels of cytarabine arabinoside have been found in the CSF, tears, and aqueous humor of patients treated with HDAC. Conventional doses of cytarabine arabinoside (100 mg/m^2/day) also cross the blood-brain barrier but cause a low concentration in the CSF, accounting for the absence of ocular reactions. Any reaction that does occur in conventional dose therapy may be attributed to allergic reaction.
- Cytarabine arabinoside undergoes slower inactivation in the CSF.

— Compared with no therapy, the use of eye drops can decrease the incidence of ocular symptoms from about 40% to 20% or less (Itoh et al. 1999; Higa et al. 1991; Barrios et al. 1987).

25.1.2 Prevention

Generally, all treatment schedules that include HDAC also incorporate the administration of corticosteroid eye drops as routine prophylaxis against ocular toxic reactions. The frequency of administration of eye drops (prednisolone 1%) varies from every 2 hours to every 8 hours (Gococo et al. 1991; Higa et al. 1991). Eye-drop administration begins before the first dose of HDAC and usually extends to 48 hours following the last dose. Results regarding the optimum frequency of eye-drop administration are inconclusive, and even 5 minutes of drug exposure to the corneal epithelium has been associated with cell injury (Gococo et al. 1991).

Research involving the use of eye drops for ocular toxicity associated with HDAC is always subject to small numbers of patients. Higa et al. (1991) compared the efficacy of corticosteroid eye drops and artificial tears. They suggested that eye drops decrease ocular toxicity by diluting intraocular concentrations of cytarabine arabinoside and concluded that artificial tears appeared to be as effective as corticosteroid eye drops if a rigorous administration schedule is employed. However, although glucocorticoid eye drops should not be used indiscriminately, they are safe and efficacious given over short periods of time (Gococo et al. 1991). A study by Itoh and colleagues (1999) suggested that the incidence could be reduced further with additional eye washing with 0.9% saline and monitoring for proper technique of eye-drop administration (including eye closure and nasolacrimal occlusion). These procedures were performed on 34 patients, and no ocular toxicity was observed in these cases. It is important to remember that these procedures may be more difficult to adhere to in a young pediatric population.

25.1.3 Treatment

Ocular toxicity that occurs despite prophylaxis will usually continue to be treated with corticosteroid eye drops. More severe reactions may require referral to an ophthalmologist. Very rarely would the treatment need to be discontinued.

25.1.4 Prognosis

The associated conjunctivitis usually resolves in affected patients within 7 days of discontinuation of HDAC (Barrios et al. 1987). Glucocorticoid eye drops will probably remain the prophylactic choice against HDAC-induced keratoconjunctivitis. However, rigorous administration of artificial tears may also decrease the incidence of ocular reaction (Higa 1991).

25.2 Cataracts

25.2.1 Incidence

The incidence of cataracts in children who receive a conditioning treatment of total body irradiation (TBI) prior to bone marrow transplant (BMT) has been reported to be 95% (20 of 21 children) to 100% (21 children) (Holmstrom et al. 2002; Frisk et al. 2002). Busulfan has also been related to cataract development, with Holmstrom et al. (2002) reporting an incidence of 21% (five of 24 children).

25.2.2 Etiology

Opacity of the crystalline lens is referred to as a cataract. Several cataractogenic factors involved in cytotoxic therapy include ionizing radiation, corticosteroid treatment, and chemotherapeutic agents. Further factors related to radiation include the total dose, fractionation scheme, and dose rate (van Kempen-Harteveld et al. 2002). Autologous BMT patients appear to have a slower progression of cataracts than allogenic BMT patients (Frisk et al. 200). This may be due to less need for corticosteroids after autologous BMT (Aristei et al. 2002; van Kempen-Harteveld 2002).

25.2.3 Prevention

To minimize the risk of cataracts with TBI, it would appear that steroid therapy should be minimized and that TBI regimens should include appropriate biologic effective doses (van Kempen-Harteveld et al. 2002). Eyes are not shielded during TBI because the orbit and the central nervous system are potential sites for residual disease.

25.2.4 Treatment

Surgical repair of cataracts is the treatment of choice, including extracapsular cataract extraction and intraocular lens implantation.

25.2.5 Prognosis

Therapy-induced cataracts are not considered a severe complication because visual acuity can be restored by surgical treatment without significant complications. However, early diagnosis of cataracts in children is important in order to prevent the development of amblyopia (Holmstrom et al. 2002). Long-term follow-up should assess those children at risk for developing cataracts.

References

Aristei C, Alessandro M, Santucci A, Aversa F, Tabillo A, Carotti A, Latini RA, Cagini C, Latini P (2002) Cataracts in patients receiving stem cell transplantation after conditioning with total body irradiation. Bone Marrow Transplant 29(6): 503–507

Barrios NJ, Tebbi CK, Freeman AI, Brecher ML (1987) Toxicity of high-dose ara-c in children and adolescents. Cancer 60: 165–167

Frisk P, Hagberg H, Mandahl A, Soderberg P, Lonnerholm G (2000) Cataracts after autologous bone marrow transplantation in children. Acta Paediatrica 89(7): 814–819

Gococo KO, Lazarus HM, Lass JH (1991) The use of prophylactic eye drops during high-dose cytosine arabinoside therapy. Cancer 69(11): 2866–2867

Higa GM (1991) Reply to Gococo et al. Cancer 69(11): 2867

Higa GM, Gockerman JP, Hunt AL, Jones MR, Horne BJ (1991) The use of prophylactic eye drops during high-dose cytosine arabinoside therapy. Cancer 68: 1691–1693

Holstrom G, Borstrom B, Calissendorff B (2002) Cataract in children after bone marrow transplantation: relation to conditioning regimen. Acta Opthalmology Scandinavia 80(2):211–215

Itoh M, Aoyama T, Yamamura Y, Nakajima K, Nakamura K, Kotaki H, Matsuyama T, Saitoh T, Kami M, Chiba S, Hirai H, Yazaki Y, Iga T (1999) Effects of the rational use of corticosteroids eye drops for the prevention of ocular toxicity in high-dose cytosine arabinoside therapy. Yakugaku Zasshi 119(3): 229–235

Ritch PS, Hansen RM, Hener DK (1983) Ocular toxicity from high dose cytosine arabinoside. Cancer 51: 430–32

Van Kempen-Harteveld ML, Belkacemi Y, Kal HB, Labopin M, Frassoni F (2002) Dose-effect relationship for cataract induction after single-dose total body irradiation and bone marrow transplantation for acute leukemia. International Journal of Radiation Oncology, Biology and Physics 52(5): 1367–1374

PART V

Nutrition and Hydration in Children with Cancer

Elizabeth Kassner

Contents

26.1 Introduction

Cachexia is a well-known form of malnutrition that results from malignant tumors, therapy, and associated side effects. Children are at a higher risk of developing cachexia due to limited nutritional reserves and increased demands already required for normal growth and development. Weight loss in children with cancer is attributed to a phenomenon called anorexia-cachexia syndrome and differs greatly from the weight loss seen with starvation (Inui, 2002).

Factors contributing to the development of cachexia in children with cancer include tumor effects, therapy-related effects, and host response. Tumor site, histology, and rate of growth affect normal nutrient metabolism and homeostasis. Tumor production of cytokines (tumor necrosis factor alpha [TNF-a], IL-6, IL-1 and interferon-gamma) is proposed to promote cachexia by altering the leptin feedback signal, mimicking a hypothalamic effect. Altered protein, carbohydrate, and lipid metabolism contributes to cancer cachexia. Protein stores are depleted during cachexia in place of fat typically used during starvation. The demand for amino acids is met in the form of nitrogen depletion, leading to skeletal muscle breakdown and eventual lactic acidosis. Additionally, cytokine release by tumors affects the muscle repair process. Carbohydrate metabolism is altered, promoting glucose intolerance and mimicking insulin resistance. Abnormal lipid metabolism includes depletion of lipid stores; increased oxidation of fatty acids, causing hyperlipidemia; and decreased activity of lipoprotein lipase. Lipoprotein lipase production is also inhibited by cytokines. Tumors may block areas of the gastrointestinal (GI) tract, causing altered absorption.

Common side effects of cancer therapy may interfere with the child's ability to ingest, digest, and absorb food. Nausea, vomiting, anorexia, diarrhea, early satiety, altered taste perception, disruption of mucous membranes, xerostomia, colitis, and enteritis contribute to decreased intake or absorption. Administration of high-dose steroids for some treatment protocols may cause steroid-induced diabetes, further affecting carbohydrate metabolism. Children can experience anticipatory vomiting, depression, anxiety, and learned food aversion behaviors, contributing to decreased caloric intake.

Symptoms of cachexia vary depending on tumor location, size, and rate of growth; treatment plan; and developmental stage. Common symptoms include wasting, weakness, anorexia, anemia, hypoglycemia, lactic acidosis, hypoalbuminemia, hyperlipidemia, glucose intolerance, skeletal muscle atrophy, anergy, impaired liver function, and tissue depletion.

26.2 Principles of Treatment

26.2.1 Nutritional Assessment

A registered dietician should be consulted once a diagnosis of cancer has been determined and a therapy regimen selected. The dietician can assist the treatment team to determine nutritional requirements for the child related to diagnosis and GI function. They may also discuss and provide written materials for managing treatment toxicities (e.g., nausea, vomiting, diarrhea, anorexia, stomatitis, mucositis, mouth dryness, dysphagia, constipation, and altered taste and sense of smell) with the family and patient. A complete nutritional assessment should include assessment of the family's and patient's capabilities and compliance, available resources (e.g., insurance, home health), financial issues, and potential cultural or ethical issues relative to nutritional support. Nutritional assessment begins by determining the existence and extent of cachexia (Table 26.1).

A complete biochemical assessment would include evaluation of sodium, potassium, chloride, bicarbonate, glucose, creatinine, blood urea nitrogen (BUN), calcium, phosphorus, magnesium, total protein, albumin, triglycerides, cholesterol, alkaline phosphatase,

Table 26.1. Measurements of developing cachexia

Intake <80% estimated needs
Growth charts demonstrate decrease of 2 percentile channels
>5% weight loss from prediagnosis
>5% weight loss over 1 month   Weight loss percentage should be calculated based on the previous highest weight; not allowing for weight gains related to large tumors, edema, pulmonary congestion, or the administration of large volumes of fluids
<5th percentile for height and or weight
<5% percentile weight for age
<90% ideal body weight for height

alkaline aminotransferase, γ-glutamyltransferase, total bilirubin, serum albumin (<3.2 mg/dl indicates decreased protein stores), serum prealbumin (increases with impaired renal function and decreases with altered hepatic function), and transferase. Clinical findings during physical exam may include abnormal core temperature (normothermic, febrile, or hypothermic); cheilosis; glossitis; sunken cheeks; prominent zygomatic arches; bulging appearance of eyeballs; dry, scaly, shiny, flaky, atrophic skin; muscle wasting or atrophy; and peripheral edema.

Measurements of nutritional status and energy requirements should be ongoing during therapy. Serial anthropometric studies (e.g., weight, weight/height ratio, calf circumference, midarm circumference) provide easy and quick monitoring of weight loss or body mass changes. The degree of malnutrition may be determined by dividing the patient's actual weight by the ideal body weight for height. Body mass index (BMI) is a measurement used to assess nutritional changes based on the child's weight in relation to height (Table 26.2). Basal metabolic rate (BMR) is used to calculate energy needs for acute or chronically ill individuals and expresses BMR in kcal/24 hours. Resting energy expenditure (REE) represents the number of calories the body requires in a 24-hour nonactive period (Table 26.2). Estimated REE increases during normal activity and with psychological and physiological stressors. The human body at-

Table 26.2. Calculating body mass index and resting energy expenditure (*W* weight in kg, *H* height in cm, *A* age in years, *BMR* basal metabolic rate; adapted from Apovian et al., 1998)

$$BMI = \frac{kg}{m^2}$$

Harris-Benedict equation: (expresses BMR in kcal/24 hours)

Male BMR = 66.5 + (13.7W) + (5H) × (6.8A)

Female BMR = 65.5 + (9.6W) + (1.8H) × (4.7A)

tempts to maintain homeostasis by regulating REE in accordance with calorie consumption. Children often experience imbalance because of continued growth and development requirements. One of the more frequently used formulas to predict energy expenditure is the Harris-Benedict equation, which takes into account gender, age, height, and weight.

Goals for optimal nutrition include preventing or correcting malnutrition, muscle, and organ wasting; maintaining or promoting strength, energy, and immune functioning; and promoting the tolerance of cancer treatment and its associated side effects. Nutritional therapy options include medications to stimulate appetite, supplemental high-caloric solutions, enteral feedings, and total parenteral nutrition (intravenous hyperalimentation). Commonly administered appetite stimulants include the following:

- Megestrol acetate (Megace)
  Progestational agent
  10 mg/kg PO given in one or two doses
  (maximum dose 800 mg/day)
- Dronabinol (Marinol TCH)
  15 mg/m²/day
- Metoclopramide hydrochloride or cisapride
  Prokinetic agent with additional dyspeptic symptom relief benefit
  Metoclopramide: 1–2 mg/kg/dose
  Cisapride: 0.15–0.3 mg/kg/dose
  (maximum dose 10 mg)

26.3 Method of Delivery

26.3.1 Oral and Enteral Replacement Strategies

Oral replacement is the nutritional treatment of choice, if tolerated. Some children may require enteral tube feedings, which allow for the maintenance of GI flora immune status and prevention of mucosal atrophy. Assessment to determine physical safety for tube placement includes oral mucosa status; function of the GI tract; tolerance of feedings without acute side effects; presence of nausea, vomiting, or diarrhea; and an adequate platelet count. Nasogastric (NG) tube placement is warranted when short-term requirement is anticipated. In general, a small bore (i.e., 6–12 French) silicone tube is placed and requires replacement every 4–6 weeks.

When long-term use is anticipated, or in children prone to dislodging an oral tube, percutaneous placement may be indicated. Gastrostomy tubes are placed via a surgical opening through the abdominal wall directly into the stomach. The stomach retains the ability to dilute hyperosmolar solutions. There is less incidence of diarrhea with gastrostomy tubes than with jejunostomy tubes. Jejunostomy tubes are surgically placed through the abdominal wall directly into the jejunum. This method is recommended if the child has known upper GI dysfunction, insufficient gastric motility, high aspiration risk, obstruction, or fistulas. Jejunostomy tubes have fewer problems with stomal leakage and skin erosion, nausea, vomiting, or bloating than gastrostomy tubes do, but have an increased risk of diarrhea.

26.3.2 Selection of Supplemental Enteral Nutritional Solutions

Standard polymeric (full digestion) options contain whole proteins, triglycerides, and long-chain carbohydrates, with an average caloric density of 1–2 calories/ml. These supplemental solutions require an intact GI tract capable of digestion, absorption, and excretion. Examples include blenderized food, Carnation Instant Breakfast, Pediasure, Osmolite, Isocal, Sustacal, and Nutren Junior.

Table 26.3. Initiation and progression of feedings

NPO <3 days
Continuous   Start with full-strength formula at 0.5–2 ml/kg/hr   Increase 1–2 ml/kg/hr q8–24h as tolerated
Bolus   Start with full-strength formula at 1–5 ml/kg/hr
Advance as tolerated   <12 months   10–30 ml/feeding   1–6 years   30–45 ml/feeding   >7 years   60–90 ml/feeding

NPO >3 days or with GI problems
Continuous   Start with half-strength formula at 0.5–2 ml/kg/hr   Increase to full-strength formula in 12–24 hours   Increase 1–2 ml/kg/hr q8–24h as tolerated
Bolus   Start with half-strength formula at 1–5 ml/kg/hr   Increase to full-strength formula in 24 hours
Advance as tolerated   <12 months   10–30 ml/feeding   1–6 years   30–45 ml/feeding   >7 years   60–90 ml/feeding
May require water in addition to supplemental feedings

Chemically defined or specifically formulated (partial digestion) options require little or no digestive capability, allowing for easy absorption. These products contain protein in the form of essential and nonessential amino acids and low fat percentages.

Partial digestion solutions are recommended for patients with malabsorption, maldigestion, or rapid GI transit. Examples include high-calorie Nutren, Magnacal, Resource Plus, Ensure Plus, High Nitrogen-Osmolite HN, Isocal HN, Replete, Ensure HN, Vital High Nitrogen, Predigested- Peptamen, Vivonex, products, and Neocare.

Supplemental solutions may be delivered by a feeding pump or by gravity flow. Feeding schedules can be adjusted to meet the individual child's requirements, activity levels, and family administration requirements. Some children benefit from continuous nocturnal feeding that delivers one-half the estimated calorie and energy needs, followed by daytime feedings that provide the other half of the calorie requirements. Bolus feeding schedules mimic normal feeding routines and may be divided into two or three boluses. Continuous infusions may be better tolerated in children who have a high incidence of nausea.

The child's individual tolerance and the duration of time the child has been without oral intake determine initiation and progression of tube feedings (Table 26.3). Monitoring for all children receiving enteral feedings includes daily weight, fluid intake and output, assessment of GI function, daily confirmation of tube placement, and assessment for residual feeding. Monitoring of biochemical laboratory values (i.e., glucose, BUN/urea, electrolytes, calcium, phosphorus, magnesium) is recommended daily until stabilized, and then every 3–7 days.

26.4 Special Considerations

26.4.1 Common Complications of Oral/Enteral Nutritional Supplementation

- Refeeding syndrome develops within 1–2 weeks after initiation of nutritional supplementation in children with chronic nutritional deficits. Symptoms include metabolic complications, severe fluid shifts, hypophosphatemia, and hypokalemia. Treatment is achieved through slow replacement of nutrients during initiation of refeeding. Strict monitoring of sodium, magnesium, potassium, chloride, bicarbonate, BUN/urea, creatinine, calcium, and phosphorus is required.
- High gastric residual volume is caused by delayed gastric emptying, and confirmation of correct tube placement is needed. Treatment options include holding the feedings if the residual volume is determined less than 2 hours of the feeding and reassessing for residual volume every hour until the volume is absorbed. Administration of prokinetic medications (cisapride or metoclopramide) and elevating the head of the bed at least 30° during and after feeding may decrease the incidence of recurrent gastric residual.
- Aspiration pneumonia may occur from incorrect placement or movement of an NG tube. Symptoms

include cough, congestion, rales, rhonchi, wheezing, and respiratory distress. Appropriate placement of the NG tube should be assessed before any bolus feeding and when placement is in question. Elevating the head of the bed at least 30° during feedings decreases the risk of aspiration.

- Skin irritation and excoriation may occur at the site of NG, gastrostomy, or jejunostomy tubes. Local infection and cellulitis can be treated with strict skin care and antibiotics as needed.

- Tube obstruction can occur when the tube is not flushed adequately between fluid boluses or medication administration. All tubes should be flushed with water at least every 4 hours during continuous feedings and after all boluses and medication administration. The use of medication in liquid elixir formulations is recommended. Many institutions recommend once-daily maintenance flushes using one of the following: water and 1 tablespoon meat tenderizer or water and 1 tablespoon seltzer mixed with 1/8 teaspoon baking soda or cola beverage.

- Vomiting, bloating, or diarrhea may occur if the rate is too fast for the child's absorption capabilities or if the child has lactose intolerance. Treatment options include slowing the infusion rate and doing frequent residual assessments. Additionally, administering lactose-free supplements, formulas with a lower fat content, and room-temperature formulas may decrease GI side effects.

- Hyperglycemia is treated by reducing the infusion rate, using formula with less carbohydrate and sugar, or administering insulin as needed.

26.4.2 Total Parental Nutrition (TPN)/ Hyperalimentation

Total parental nutrition (TPN) is required when oral and enteral feedings are unable to provide adequate calories and nutrients; components of TPN are listed in Table 26.4. There is no clear evidence that initiation of TPN is helpful or detrimental to treatment tolerance, response rates, or survival. Therapeutic goals of TPN include restoring the child's normal body weight, reversing malnutrition, promoting growth, improving immunologic status, potentially accelerating marrow recovery, and generally supporting activity and energy expenditure.

Peripheral venous catheter administration of TPN is appropriate for short-term therapy. Central venous catheter administration is indicated if TPN is anticipated to be required for several weeks or months. The initiation of TPN should be coordinated with a pharmacist, dietician, and physician or nurse practitioner.

Guidelines for formulation are frequently institution-specific. Patient-specific energy needs should be calculated based on the degree of malnutrition, diagnosis, and individual treatment plan. A basic approach for initiating TPN includes the following steps:

1. Assess protein and energy requirements of child
2. Protein g/day = (g/kg/day) × weight (kg)
3. Energy/day = (kcal/kg/day) × weight (kg)
4. Calculate maintenance fluid requirements
   - 1,500 ml for the first 20 kg, then 20–30 ml/kg for each additional kg of body weight
5. Determine fat, dextrose, and amino acid energy requirements
   - (30 % fat, 70 % dextrose)
6. Determine lipid requirements
7. Select amino acid, electrolyte, mineral, and vitamin concentration
   - Typically institution-dependent
8. Determine volume based on calculations
9. Compare maintenance fluids, calculate with total fluids, and adjust as needed

Table 26.4. Components of total parenteral nutrition

Component	Contents
Protein	Amino acids
Fat	Lipids
Carbohydrate	Glucose
Electrolytes	Sodium, potassium, chloride, calcium, phosphate, magnesium
Trace elements	Copper, zinc, manganese, chromium, selenium
Vitamins	A, C, D, E, K, thiamine, riboflavin, niacin, pantothenic acid, pyridoxine, B12, choline, biotin, folic acid

Table 26.5. Electrolyte requirements by patient weight

Electrolyte	25 kg (mEq/kg)	25–45 kg (mEq/kg)	>45 kg
Sodium	2–6	2–6	60–150 mEq
Potassium	2–5	2–5	60–150 mEq
Calcium	1–2	1	0.2–0.3 mEq
Magnesium	0.5	0.5	0.35–0.45 mEq
Phosphate	0.5–1 mmol	0.5–1 mmol	7–10 mmol/1,000 cal
Chloride	2–3 mEq/kg/day		2–3 mEq/kg/day

Table 26.6. Energy and protein requirement recommendations

Age in years	Resting energy expenditure kcal/kg/day	Total energy kcal/kg/day	Protein requirement g/kg/day (total g/day)
0–1	55	90–120	1.6–3.2 (16–18)
1–3	50	70–100	1.2–3 (19–22)
4–10	40–45	50–70	1–3 (25–39)
11–14	30		1–2.5 (51–74)
Males		60–70	
Females		50–60	
>15	25		0.9–2.5 (66–80)
Males		45–55	
Females		35–45	

Electrolyte needs and protein and energy requirements are listed in Tables 26.5 and 26.6, respectively.

Peripheral and central TPN concentrations will differ in composition, primary calorie source, rate of administration, and associated risks. Peripheral administration of TPN limits dextrose concentrations to 10%, protein (amino acids) concentrations to 1.5–2%, and lipid solutions to either 20%, providing 2 kcal/ml, or 10%, providing 1.1 kcal/ml. Administration of TPN via central venous access allows delivery of greater volumes and greater caloric replacement. Dextrose concentrations may range from 10–12.5%, providing 3.4 kcal/g, with rates of administration ranging from 3–4 mg/kg/hour. Dextrose may be advanced by 2.5–5% every 24 hours as tolerated until the preferred caloric level of 20–25% dextrose concentration is attained. Infusion rates should not exceed 5 mg/kg/min. Protein (standard amino acids) concentrations of 10% will deliver 4 kcal/g and may be administered at 1 g/kg/day. Protein levels may be advanced by 0.5–1 g/kg/day until the maximum goal of 1.5–3 g/kg/day is achieved. Lipid concentrations of 20%, administered at 1–2 g/kg/day, are advanced by 0.5–1 g/kg/day until a total of 1–3 g/kg/day are attained as tolerated. Lipid concentrations should not exceed 4 g/kg/day or 60% of the total calories in order to prevent essential fatty acid deficiency.

Recommended monitoring during TPN administration includes daily weights and intake and output measurements. Urine glucose should be monitored initially with each void and may be decreased to daily monitoring if normal. Electrolyte and BUN evaluation is recommended two to three times a week until the TPN dose is stabilized, and then monitoring may be decreased to weekly. Calcium, phosphorus, and magnesium serum levels should be obtained weekly until the TPN rate is stable, and then monitoring may be decreased to every other week. A baseline albumin should be obtained and then repeated every 3 weeks. Prealbumin levels are recommended weekly, and triglyceride levels should be obtained 4 hours after the initiation of TPN and 4 hours after each rate increase.

26.4.3 Complications of TPN/Hyperalimentation

- Hypoglycemia is a common side effect and is easily prevented by avoiding rapid discontinuation of TPN and by tapering the administration rate when an infusion is being discontinued.
- Hyperglycemia can be managed by decreasing dextrose concentrations or by adding insulin.
- Hepatic dysfunction may include fatty liver symptoms or cholestatic jaundice. Treatment strategies include avoiding excessive infusion of carbohydrates; maintaining a balance of dextrose, protein and lipids; and converting to enteral feeding as soon as therapeutically possible.
- Hyponatremia, fluid overload, and infection are all possible complications of TPN; they can be prevented or treated with strict monitoring and early interventions.
- Mechanical difficulty may include catheter tip migration, obstruction, or thrombosis. Evaluation of proper line functioning is essential and is determined by adequate blood return. Radiologic evaluation is warranted if displacement or obstruction is suspected.

26.4.4 Glutamine

Glutamine is a nonessential amino acid that is an important fuel source for proliferating cells. During periods of physiological stress (i.e., injury, illness), the body's demand for plasma glutamine increases. Preliminary investigational use of supplemental glutamine suggests that it may promote improved muscle protein and facilitate muscle repair and excessive catabolism. Additional studies have shown that glutamine supplements may improve a suppressed immune system by supporting lymphocytes and macrophages. Research is still indicated to determine safety data, appropriate replacement dose levels, and long-term effects. Large doses of glutamine have been associated with abdominal pain and diarrhea (Bechard et al., 2002).

26.4.5 Intravenous Fluid and Electrolyte Requirements

The hydration status of a child receiving treatment for cancer is another important area to continually assess. Early intervention may prevent severe electrolyte imbalance and even prevent hospitalizations. Most hydration imbalances result from therapy and its associated side effects. Children receiving chemotherapy and blood products are at increased risk of fluid overload, and side effects of chemotherapy and radiotherapy that affect gastric functioning and the perception of taste and smell predispose the child to dehydration.

Weight is the single most accurate variable for assessing hydration status. Additional measurements of hydration include vital sign monitoring to assess vascular volume and 24-hour input and output monitoring to provide data regarding hydration imbalances. Serum electrolytes, serum osmolality, blood sugar, BUN, creatinine, and urine electrolytes and osmolality can provide additional information regarding the child's hydration status. Common findings observed on physical exam are listed in Table 26.7.

Fluid requirements for a healthy child with a routine activity level may be based on body surface area ($1500\ ml/m^2/day$) or more often by weight (Table 26.8). Intravenous replacement options include isotonic or hypotonic fluids or colloids. The most common form of dehydration is isotonic dehydration, which is corrected using isotonic fluids. Examples of isotonic fluids include normal saline (NS), lactated Ringer's (LR), and $D_5 1/2NS$. Hypotonic fluids such as 1/2NS or D_5W have a lower degree of osmotic pressure than individual cells. The administration of hypotonic fluids causes migration of fluid into the cells and could cause cellular rupture. Hypertonic solutions such as D_5NS or D_5LR cause the flow of intra-

Table 26.7. Physical exam findings associated with dehydration

Sign	Symptom
Weight loss	5–15% of body weight
Behavior	irritable to lethargic
Thirst	slight to intense
Mucous membranes	dry
Tears	absent
Anterior fontanel	flat or sunken
Skin turgor	decreased, dry, warm
Urine output	decreased, concentrated, increased urine specific gravity
Cardiac	Pulse increased, weak
Laboratory	increased hematocrit, BUN/urea

Table 26.8. Weight-based fluid requirements

Weight	Volume
<10 kg	100 ml/kg/day
11–20 kg	1,000 ml + (50 ml for each kg >10)kg/day
20–30 kg	1,500 ml + (20 ml for each kg >20)kg/day
>30 kg	35 ml/kg/day

Table 26.9. Volume replacement guide for dehydration

Degree of dehydration	Volume
Mild	50 ml/kg within 4 hours
Moderate	100 ml/kg within 4 hours
Severe	IVF for stabilization, then 100 ml/kg
Hypovolemic shock	20 ml/kg in two aliquots of 10 ml/kg

cellular fluids into extracellular space, causing blood volume to expand and blood pressure to increase. Small volume replacement over a short time period is recommended. Colloids exert an oncotic pressure, pulling fluid from other spaces into vascular compartments. Examples are 5% albumin, fresh frozen plasma, and dextran 4% and 6%.

Oral replacement of fluids for children with mild and moderate levels of dehydration is preferred. Patients requiring rehydration and electrolyte replacement may benefit from products such as Ricelyte, Pedialyte, and Rehydrate. Children exhibiting signs and symptoms of hypovolemic shock require rapid intravenous replacement (Table 26.9).

Children with malignancy can develop electrolyte imbalances due to the disease process itself or to the associated treatment. Routine laboratory evaluations are necessary at the time of diagnosis and before and during therapy (Table 26.10).

26.4.6 Specific Nutritional Concerns During Palliative Care

Children receiving palliative care for unresponsive or progressive oncologic diseases have different nutritional concerns than children receiving aggressive therapy. The primary focus of all interventions during this time is on the child's quality of life. Families frequently need education and support to understand that reduced nutrient intake will not alter the occurring pathologic process or shorten the child's life. The child's loss of interest in food and a decreased appetite are normal near death and indicate that the body can no longer manage caloric intake. As adequate metabolization is declining, forcing the child to consume foods will only tire the child and cause discomfort in the form of diarrhea, nausea, vomiting, choking, or pneumonia. Family members should be encouraged to give permission for child to refuse intake. Children who remain interested in eating may benefit from smaller, more frequent meals of soft, easily digested foods and by avoiding strong smells.

Fluid requirements during palliative care are also decreased. Thirst is rare during the final days of life. Again, there are no data to suggest that withholding fluids, orally or intravenously, in the final stages of life is detrimental. Children may be supported with minimal intravenous fluid (IVF) administration if intravenous access is not a problem and it is the wish of the child or family. Advantages of IVF administration

Table 26.10. Common electrolyte imbalances in pediatric cancer patients

Condition	Serum levels	Causes	Symptoms	Treatment
Hypercalcemia	>10.5 mg/dl	Bone malignancies and metastases, excessive concentrations in TPN, poor dietary intake of phosphorus, renal absorption or excretion, diuretics	Weakness, irritability, lethargy, seizures, coma, abdominal cramping, anorexia, nausea, vomiting, ECG changes	Hydration, hemodialysis, steroids
Hypocalcemia	<8 mg/dl	Decreased intake; vitamin D deficiency, intake, or malabsorption; hypoparathyroidism, pancreatitis	Neuromuscular irritability, weakness, cramping, fatigue, change in level of consciousness, seizures, ECG changes	IV or oral replacement, correct underlying cause
Hyperkalemia	6–7 mEq/l	Renal failure, cellular breakdown, leukocytosis, metabolic acidosis	ECG changes	Kayexalate, insulin, $NaHCO_3$, calcium gluconate
Hypokalemia	<3.5 mEq/l	Decreased intake, increased renal excretion, therapy-induced renal tubular defects, diarrhea, vomiting	Skeletal muscle weakness, dysrhythmias: prolonged Q-T interval, flattened T-waves	Replace with potassium acetate or gluconate
Hyponatremia	<130 mEq/l	Syndrome of inappropriate secretion of antidiuretic hormone (SIADH); ectopic secretion of antidiuretic hormone; renal, adrenal cortical, or cardiac insufficiency; excessive loss secondary to vomiting, diarrhea, or salt-losing nephropathy; neurotoxic effect of cyclophosphamide and vinca alkaloids	Convulsions, shock, lethargy	Fluid restriction, replace losses, treat underlying cause
Hypomagnesemia	<1 mEq/l	Nephrotoxic agents, decreased intake, diarrhea, vomiting, urinary loss	Tetany, seizures, tremors, anorexia, nausea, cardiac abnormalities, weakness, clonus	IV or oral magnesium sulfate, oxide, or gluconate
Hypermagnesemia	>5 mg/dl	Renal dysfunction	Hyporeflexia, respiratory depression, confusion, coma	IV administration of calcium, diuresis
Hypophosphatemia	<3 mg/dl	Poor dietary intake, malabsorption, excessive renal excretion, vitamin D deficiency	Usually not until severe (<1 mg/dl); irritability, paresthesias	IV or oral potassium-phosphate or sodium-phosphate
Hyperphosphatemia	>6 mg/dl	Chemotherapeutic agents, renal insufficiency: glomerular filtration rate <25% normal	Symptoms relative to resulting from hypocalcemia	Restrict intake, phosphorus binders: calcium carbonate, aluminum hydroxide

include possible improved oral comfort and bowel function, less delirium, and a more productive cough due to thinning of secretions. Administration of minimal IVF allows family members to feel as if they are doing "everything possible." Disadvantages include increased oral, respiratory, and GI secretions and urine output, which predisposes the child to an increased chance of choking, cough, pulmonary congestion, edema (peripheral and pulmonary), vomiting, and urinary incontinence.

References

Apovian CM, Still CD, Blackburn GL (1998). Nutrition support. In Berger, Portenoy & Weissman's Principles and Practice of Supportive Oncology, pp 571–588. Lippincott-Raven, Philadelphia

Bechard LJ, Adiv OE, Jaksic T, Duggan C (2002). Nutritional supportive care. In Poplack & Pizzo's Principles and Practice of Pediatric Oncology, 4th edn, pp1285–1300. Lippincott Williams & Wilkins, Philadelphia.

Inui A (2002) Cancer anorexia-cachexia syndrome: current issues in research and management. CA: A Cancer Journal for Clinicians 52(2):72-91

Bibliography

Sacks N, Meek RS (1997). Nutritional support. In Ablin's Supportive Care of Children with Cancer: Current Therapy and Guidelines from the Children's Cancer Group, pp 193–209. The Johns Hopkins University Press, Baltimore

Sacks N, Meek RS (1998). Nutritional support of the child with cancer. In Hockenberry-Eaton's Essentials of Pediatric Oncology Nursing: A Core Curriculum, pp 164–168. Association of Oncology Nursing, Glenview, IL

Waller A, Caroline NL (2000). Nutrition and hydration. In Waller & Caroline's Handbook of Palliative Care in Cancer: 2nd edn, pp 61 – 74. Butterworth-Heinemann: Woburn, MA

Pain in Children with Cancer

Debbie Rembert

Contents

27.1 Introduction

Pain is an unpleasant sensory and emotional experience with actual or potential tissue damage, or described in terms of such damage. It is always subjective and interpreted by the individual. Unrelieved pain in children can lead to mistrust of the medical staff, create fear, and increase anxiety and pain in future procedures. Children may also experience night terrors, flashbacks, sleep disturbances, and eating problems. Long-lasting effects of childhood pain can include post-traumatic stress syndrome, phobic reactions, and depression (World Health Organization, 1998).

Uncontrolled or chronic pain in children can lead them to victimized, depressed, isolated, and lonely. It can also affect their ability to cope with the cancer. The effects of uncontrolled chronic or acute pain are extended to the family and healthcare providers. Parents may experience guilt, anger and depression. Healthcare providers may have decreased ability to show compassion, may experience feelings of guilt, and may deny that children are, in fact, suffering (World Health Organization, 1998). Nurses and other healthcare providers must realize that children feel pain just as adults do (Table 27.1) and that their pain must be treated appropriately.

Table 27.1. Myths and misconceptions about pain control in children

Myths and misconceptions about pain control in children	
Myth: Infants cannot feel pain because their nervous systems are immature.	**Fact supported by evidence:** Pain pathways are formed before birth. Neonates and infants can remember pain.
Myth: Some health providers and parents believe that opioids should be administered only as a last resort to avoid drug addiction.	**Consequences:** Children do not always receive the strong analgesic required to relieve severe pain. Opioid side effects may not be treated as aggressively as they should.
Misconception: The pharmacology of opioid analgesics, especially their pharmacodynamics and pharmacokinetics, is poorly understood.	**Consequence:** Health professionals do not select the most appropriate drug, dose, or route of administration for children in pain.
Misconception: Health professionals do not know how to assess a child's pain level or factors that intensify the pain.	**Consequence:** Health professional cannot evaluate if changes in drug therapy are effective.
Misconception: Some health professionals do not know that simple nondrug therapies are effective and can lessen a child's pain.	**Consequence:** Children and patients are not taught how to use practical cognitive, physical, and behavioral strategies to reduce pain and distress.

Adapted from McGrath PA. Pain in children: Nature, Assessment and Treatment. New York: Guilford Publications, 1990. In World Health Organization (2003) Pain control in pediatric palliative care. Cancer Pain Release 16 (3,4): http://www.whocancerpain.wisc.edu/eng/16_3-4/myths.html

27.2 Causes of Pain in Childhood Cancer

Almost all children diagnosed with cancer will experience pain at some point in their treatment. The most common causes of pain can be directly related to the disease itself, to the treatment, or to procedures (Table 27.2). Children often do not convey that they are in pain, but turn inward and become quiet to cope with it.

In addition, children who undergo limb amputation may develop phantom limb pain, phantom limb sensations, or stump pain. The precise cause of phantom limb pain is unknown. Injury to the nerves during amputation causes changes in the way the central nervous system conducts impulses. The parts of the brain that control the missing limb stay active, causing the illusion of the missing limb even though the amputee knows that the limb is gone.

Phantom limb pain refers to pain felt in an absent limb that was removed because of disease, and it usu-

ally comes in bursts. Very few children have constant pain. The attacks can come frequently or only occasionally. Phantom pain is often described as shooting, stabbing, or burning. The pain is felt at the "end" of the limb, in phantom fingers or toes. In contrast, phantom limb sensations, which are also felt in the absent limb, are not painful. Stump pain is only felt in the stump of the amputated limb. Phantom limb pain is treated with medications (see Table 27.3), stimulation therapy, prosthesis use, and rehabilitation.

27.3 Assessment

Children learn to adapt and may not show visible signs of pain. But it is the health professional's ethical obligation to ask them if they are in pain. Pain assessment is an essential component of the process of pain management in children and is often referred to as the "fifth vital sign."

Table 27.2. Causes of pain in childhood cancer

Type	Clinical presentation	Causes
Bone – Skull – Vertebrae – Pelvis/femur	Aching to sharp, severe pain generally more pronounced with movement. Point tenderness common Skul – headaches, blurred vision Spine – tenderness over spinous process Arms/extremities – pain associated with movement or lifting Pelvis/femur – associated with movement; pain with weight bearing and walking	Infiltration of bone Skeletal metastases – irritation and stretching of pain receptors in the periosteum and endosteum. Prostaglandins released from bone destruction.
Neuropathic – Peripheral – Plexus – Epidural – Cord compression	Complaints of pain without any detectable tissue damage Abnormal or unpleasant sensations, generally described as tingling, burning, or stabbing Often a delay in onset Brief, shooting pain Increased intensity of pain with receptive stimuli	Nerve injury caused by tumor infiltration; can also be caused by injury from treatment (i.e., vincristine toxicity) Infiltration or compression of peripheral nerves Surgical interruption of nerves (phantom pain post-amputation)
Visceral – Soft tissue – Tumors of the bowel – Retroperitoneum	Poorly localized Varies in intensity Pressure, deep or aching	Obstruction – bowel, urinary tract, biliary tract Mucosal ulceration Metabolic alteration Nociceptor activation, generally from distension or inflammation of visceral organs
Treatment-related – Mucositis – Infection – Post-lumbar puncture headaches – Radiation dermatitis – Postsurgical	Difficulty swallowing, pain from lesions in the oropharynx. May extend throughout the entire GI tract. Infection may be localized pain from a focused infection or generalized (i.e., tissue infection versus septicemia). Severe headache following lumbar puncture. Skin inflammation causing redness and breakdown Pain related to tissue trauma secondary to surgery	Direct side-effects of Treatment for cancer – Chemotherapy – Radiation – Surgery

From Hockenberry-Eaton M., Barrera P., Brown M., Bottomley S., O'Neill J. (1999) Pain Management in Children with Cancer Handbook. Austin, TX: Texas Cancer Council. Reprinted with permission.

Healthcare providers should specifically assess the presence, severity, location, quality, and intensity of pain in a manner appropriate for the child's cognitive ability. One method is the QUESTT method (Hockenberry et al., 2003):

Question the child
Use pain rating scales
Evaluate behavior

Secure parents' involvement
Take cause of pain into account
Take action and evaluate results

Because pain is subjective, self-reporting is preferred. However, behavioral observations can complement self-reporting or may be used along with physical findings for the preverbal or nonverbal child.

Table 27.3. Co-analgesic agents

Category/Drug	Dosage	Indication	Comments
Antidepressants			
Amitriptyline	0.2–0.5 mg/kg PO hs Titrate upward by 0.25 mg/kg every 5–7 days as needed Available in 10 mg and 25 mg tablets Usual starting dose is 10–25 mg	Continuous neuropathic pain with burning, aching, dysthesia with insomnia	Provides analgesia by blocking re-uptake of serotonin and norepinephrine possibly slowing transmissions of pain signals. Helps with pain related to insomnia and depression (use nortriptyline if patient is over-sedated) Analgesic effects seen earlier than antidepressant effects Side effects include dry mouth, constipation, urinary retention
Nortriptyline	0.2–1.0 mg/kg PO a.m. or bid Titrate up by 0.5 mg q 5–7 days max: 25 mg/dose	Neuropathic pain as above without insomnia	
Anticonvulsants			
Gabapentin	5 mg/kg PO at bedtime Increase to bid on day 2, tid on day 3 max: 300 mg/day	Neuropathic pain	Mechanism of action unknown Side effects include sedation, ataxia, nystagmus, dizziness
Carbamazepine	*<6 years* 2.5–5 mg/kg PO bid initially Increase 20 mg/kg/24 hr Divide bid q week prn; max: 100 mg bid *6–12 years* 5 mg/kg PO bid initially Increase 10 mg/kg/24 hr divide q week Prn to usual max: 100 mg/dose bid *>12 years* 200 mg PO bid initially Increase 200 mg/24 hr divide bid q week Prn to max: 1.6–2.4 g/24 hr	Sharp, lancinating neuropathic pain Peripheral Neuropathies Phantom limb pain	Similar analgesic effect as amitriptyline Monitor blood levels for toxicity only Side effects include decreased blood counts, ataxia, and GI irritation
Anxiolytics			
Lorazepam	0.03–0.1 mg/kg q4–6h PO/IV; max: 2 mg/dose	Muscle spasm Anxiety	May increase sedation in combination with opioids Can cause depression with prolonged use
Diazepam	0.1–0.3 mg/kg q4–6h PO/IV; max:10 mg/dose		

Table 27.3. (Continued)

Category/Drug	Dosage	Indication	Comments
Corticosteroids			
Dexamethasone	Dose dependent on clinical situation Higher bolus doses in cord compression then lower daily dose. Try to wean to NSAIDs if pain allows Cerebral edema: 1–2 mg/kg load then 1–1.5 mg/kg/day divided q6h; max: 4 mg/dose	Pain from increased intracranial pressure Bony metastasis Spinal/nerve compression	Side effects include edema, gastrointestinal irritation, increased weight, acne Use gastroprotectants such as H_2 blockers (ranitidine) or proton pump inhibitors such as omeprazole for long-term administration of steroids or NSAIDs in end-stage cancer with bony pain
	Anti-inflammatory: 0.08–0.3 mg/kg/day divided q6–12h		
Others			
Clonidine	2–4 mcg/kg PO q4–6h May also use a 100 mcg transdermal patch q 7 days for patients >40kg	Neuropathic pain. Lancinating, sharp, electrical, shooting pain. Phantom limb pain	Alpha 2 adrenoreceptor agonist modulates ascending pain sensations Routes of administration include oral, transdermal, and spinal Management of withdrawal symptoms Monitor for orthostatic hypertension, bradycardia Sedation common
Mexiletine	2–3 mg/kg/dose PO tid may titrate 0.5 mg/kg q2–3 weeks as needed max: 300 mg/dose	Neuropathic pain. Lancinating, sharp, electrical, shooting pain Phantom limb pain	Similar to lidocaine, longer acting Stabilizes sodium conduction in nerve cells, reduces neuronal firing Can enhance action of opioids, antidepressants, anticonvulsants Side effects include dizziness, ataxia, nausea, vomiting May measure blood levels for toxicity

From Hockenberry-Eaton M., Barrera P., Brown M., Bottomley S., O'Neill J. (1999) Pain Management in Children with Cancer Handbook. Austin, TX: Texas Cancer Council. Reprinted with permission.

A variety of tools are available to assess pediatric pain. The FACES pain rating scale is a well studied and commonly used method to assess children's pain (Fig. 27.1). Children as young as 3 years old are able to appropriately use this scale. It has been translated into seven different languages and can be correlated with a scale of 0–5 or of 0–10. The numeric scale is also a common tool used to assess a child's pain and can be used with children 5 years of age or older; however, it does assume that they have some concept of numbers and their value. It is represented by a line with equal increments from 0 to 5 or 10, with "0" representing no pain and "5" or "10" representing the worst pain imaginable. This tool may be used vertically or horizontally.

When assessing pain in children, it is important to consider that the lack of reporting pain does not equate to the lack of pain itself (Twycross et al., 1998). Behaviors such as watching television, talking on the phone, playing, and sleeping are often distraction methods used to cope with pain but are often misinterpreted by healthcare professionals, (Hockenberry-

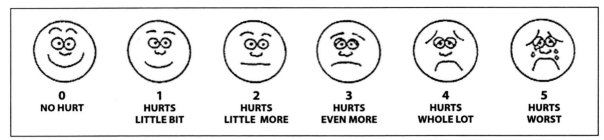

Figure 27.1

FACES pain rating scale (from Wong et al., 2001) Original instructions: Explain to the person that each face is for a person who feels happy because he has no pain (hurt) or sad because he has some or a lot of pain. Face 0 is very happy because he doesn't hurt at all. Face 1 hurts just a little bit. Face 2 hurts a little more. Face 3 hurts even more. Face 4 hurts a whole lot. Face 5 hurts as much as you can imagine, although you don't have to be crying to feel this bad. Ask the person to choose the face that best describes how he is feeling. Brief word instructions: Point to each face using the words to describe the pain intensity. Ask the child to choose the face that best describes own pain and record the appropriate number. Copyright Mosby, Inc.; reprinted by permission

Eaton et al., 1999). Due to the nature of childhood cancer diagnosis and treatment it is reasonable to expect that all children will need some type of pain management plan, and certainly all children should be assessed for the presence of pain. Physiologic responses to pain from sympathetic involvement include diaphoresis, flushing, pallor, hypertension, tachycardia, tachypnea, and hypoxia. These measures are more commonly observed during acute pain and may dissipate if the pain becomes more chronic in nature.

Manifestations of pain in children differ according to developmental stage (Table 27.4). There are some distinct differences between how infants communicate and react to pain and how children communicate and react to pain. The infant or preverbal child is especially vulnerable to untreated or undertreated pain. Therefore, specific measures have been taken to identify consistent behaviors in infants undergoing painful procedures to quantify cry, oxygen requirements, vital sign parameters, facial expression and sleep pattern.

27.4 Cultural Issues

The World Health Organization (1998) states that family and cultural factors greatly affect pain and suffering. Some of these factors (e.g., a child's response to pain) may be misinterpreted by the health care provider. Stoic children may not report or show expected signs of pain. In some cultures and religions, pain and suffering are seen as punishment or even as a necessity for reaching an individual's spiritual destination or status. Language differences can also impact pain assessment and treatment. Using an appropriate interpreter in combination with behavioral and physiologic measures can help to more accurately assess pain. After an assessment is made, the healthcare provider should establish a pain management plan that incorporates the patient's and family's cultural or religious practices that are compatible with medical treatment.

Table 27.4. Developmental differences in pain expression

Developmental group	Expressions of pain
Infants	May Exhibit body rigidity or thrashing, may include arching Exhibit facial expression of pain (brows lowered and drawn together, eyes tightly closed, mouth open and squarish) Cry intensely/loudly Be inconsolable Draw knees to chest Exhibit hypersensitivity or irritability Have poor oral intake Be unable to sleep
Toddlers	May Be verbally aggressive, cry intensely Exhibit regressive behavior or withdraw Exhibit physical resistance by pushing painful stimulus away after it is applied Guard painful area of body Be unable to sleep
Preschoolers/young children	May Verbalize intensity of pain See pain as punishment Exhibit thrashing of arms and legs Attempt to push stimulus away before it is applied Be uncooperative Need physical restraint Cling to parent, nurse, or significant other Request emotional support (e.g., hugs, kisses) Understand that there can be secondary gains associated with pain Be unable to sleep
School-age children	May Verbalize pain Use an objective measurement of pain Be influenced by cultural beliefs Experience nightmares related to pain Exhibit stalling behaviors (e.g., "Wait a minute" or "I'm not ready") Have muscular rigidity such as clenched fists, white knuckles, gritted teeth, contracted limbs, body stiffness, closed eyes, or wrinkled forehead Include behaviors of preschoolers/young children Be unable to sleep
Adolescents	May Localize and verbalize pain Deny pain in presence of peers Have changes in sleep patterns or appetite Be influenced by cultural beliefs Exhibit muscle tension and body control Display regressive behavior in presence of family Be unable to sleep

From Hockenberry-Eaton M., Barrera P., Brown M., Bottomley S., O'Neill J. (1999) Pain Management in Children with Cancer Handbook. Austin, TX: Texas Cancer Council. Reprinted with permission.

27.5 Principles of Treatment

Because of the nature of childhood cancer pain, it is optimal to have a multidisciplinary approach with the advanced practice nurse the coordinator of various disciplines that may need to be consulted. In so doing, it is feasible to address all the variables mentioned earlier (i.e., physical, emotional, and social issues). Prevention of pain or early intervention is always best.

Unfortunately, some providers still inadequately medicate pain in children because of fear of side effects or addiction. Painkillers are *not* addictive in therapeutic doses. Overdoses are rare and in most cases reversible. Practitioners need to understand the difference between tolerance, physical dependence, and addiction. Definitions recognized by the American Pain Society and the American Society of Addiction Medicine (2001) include the following:

— Tolerance: "a state of adaptation in which exposure to a drug induces changes that result in a diminution of one or more of the drug's effects"
— Physical dependence: "a state of adaptation that is manifested by a drug-class-specific withdrawal syndrome that can be produced by abrupt cessation, rapid dose reduction, decreasing blood level of the drug, and/or administration of an antagonist"
— Addiction: "a primary chronic, neurobiological disease with genetic and environmental influencing factors characterized by behaviors that include one or more of the following: impaired control over drug use, compulsive use, continued use despite harm, and craving"

27.6 Treatment

27.6.1 By the Ladder

The World Health Organization has put forth recommendations for a sequential, stepwise approach to the pharmacologic management of pain in children (Fig. 27.2). It is important to note that the primary "step" is based on the level of the child's pain and that

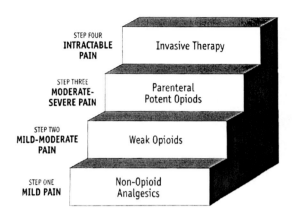

Figure 27.2

Therapeutic ladder for pain management (World Health Organization, http://www.who.int/cancer/palliative/painladder/en/)

not all children will start on step one. If upon assessment the pain is severe, then the appropriate initial step for that child would be step three, which indicates the use of opioids such as morphine for moderate to severe pain. This child may also benefit from the use of a nonopioid and/or the addition of an adjuvant drug. There should be no delay or hesitation in moving up to the next step if the pain does not respond to the current treatment.

27.6.1.1 Step I: Mild Pain

Step one in controlling mild pain is the use of a nonopioid analgesic.

This includes paracetamol/acetaminophen and other non steroidal anti-inflammatory drugs (NSAIDs). Additionally, they are limited by the "ceiling" effect; higher doses cause increased risk of toxicity, not more analgesia. However, NSAIDs are very effective in controlling pain associated with bony metastasis, although they must be used with caution in pediatric cancer patients because of their possible effect on platelet aggregation (Table 27.5).

Table 27.5. Nonsteroidal anti-inflammatory drugs used for cancer pain

Drug type	Typical starting dose
Paracetamol/acetaminophen	10–15 mg/kg/dose q4hr PO to a max of 650 mg/dose
Aspirin	10–15 mg/kg/dose q6–8hr PO to a max of 650 mg/dose
Ibuprofen	10 mg/kg/dose to a max single dose of 800 mg q6–8hr PO
Choline magnesium trisalicylate	7.5–25 mg/kg/dose bid-tid; max single close of 1,500 mg PO
Diclofenac sodium	1–1.5 mg/kg/dose to a max single does of 75 mg q8–12hr PO
Naproxen	5–7.5 mg/kg/dose to a max of 500 mg/dose q12hr PO
Naproxen sodium	Same as naproxen
Ketorolac	0.5–1 mg/kg as single dose IM to a max of 60 mg, followed by 0.5 mg/kg IV q6hr to a max single dose of 30 mg. Max duration is 5 days (useful in short-term pain management). Limited data on use of oral ketorolac
Celecoxib (Cox-2inhibitor)	100–200 mg PO q day for patients >18 years. No information in patients<18 years
Rofecoxib (Cox-2 inhibitor)	12.5 PO q day for patients >18 years, max of 25 mg/day. No information for patients <18 years

From Hockenberry-Eaton M., Barrera P., Brown M., Bottomley S., O'Neill J. (1999) Pain Management in Children with Cancer Handbook. Austin, TX: Texas Cancer Council. Reprinted with permission.

27.6.1.2 Step II: Mild to Moderate Pain

If pain persists or is not relieved, an opioid for mild to moderate pain should be prescribed (Table 27.6). The child should continue to receive the nonopioid analgesic, if appropriate, to provide supplemental analgesia. If a nonopioid and opioid combined fail to provide adequate analgesia, then step III should be taken.

27.6.1.3 Step III: Moderate to Severe Pain

To provide pain relief, an opioid for moderate to severe pain should be used, and the dose should be increased until pain is relieved or toxicities occur. If side effects occur, supportive management can be provided (Table 27.7). If appropriate, the nonopioid can be continued. Morphine is the drug of choice. In general, only one medication from each group should be used at the same time.

27.6.1.4 Step IV: Intractable Pain

Extreme pain unresolved by the previous steps may require more aggressive treatment. Some children with bone metastasis or nerve involvement may be candidates for this step. Invasive therapy or procedures may include opioids via epidural catheter, therapeutic nerve block, or cordotomy. These techniques are used as a last resort, with the risk and discomfort of the procedure weighed heavily against the benefit of pain relief. It is also important to note that there is no guarantee these procedures will provide total or permanent pain relief. If the invasive technique is successful, then one should proceed cautiously when discontinuing previously used opioids, instituting the weaning guidelines as appropriate (Table 27.8).

Table 27.6. Starting doses for commonly prescribed opioids

Drug	Oral starting doses	Dosage forms	Starting doses IV	IV to PO
Codeine	0.5 1 mg/kg q4 6 hr; max: 60 mg/dose	Tablet, as sulfate: 30 mg Liquid: 3 mg/ml	N/A	N/A
Paracetamol/ acetaminophen w/codeine	0.5 1.0 mg/kg/dose of codeine q4 6 hr; max: 2 tablets/dose; 15 ml/dose	Elixir: Paracetamol/acetaminophen 24 mg and codeine 2.4 mg/ml with alcohol 7% Suspension: acetaminophen 24 mg and codeine 2.4 mg/ml alcohol free Tablet: #3: Paracetamol/acetamino- phen 300 mg and codeine 30 mg	N/A	N/A
Hydrocodone and Paracetamol/ acetaminophen	3–6 years: 5 ml 3–4 times/day 7–12 years: 10 ml 3–4 times/day >12 years: 1–2 tablets q4–6 hr; max 8 tablets/day	Tablet: hydrocodone 5 mg and acetaminophen 500 mg Oral solution at: 0.5 mg hydro codone and 33.4 mg/ml Paracetamol/acetaminophen	N/A	N/A
Oxycodone	Instant release: 0.05–0.15 mg/kg/dose up to 5 mg/dose q4–6hr Sustained release: for patients taking >20 mg/day of oxycodone can administer 10 mg q12hr	Instant release: 5 mg Sustained release: 10 mg, 20 mg, 40 mg, 80 mg	N/A	N/A
Morphine	0.3–0.6 mg/kg/dose every 12 hr for sustained release 0.2 to 0.5 mg/kg/dose q4–6hr prn for solution of instant release tablets	Injection: 2 mg/ml, 5 mg/ml Injection, preservative-free: 1 mg/ml Solution: 2 mg/ml Tablet: 15 mg (instant release) Tablet, controlled release: 15 mg, 30 mg, 60 mg, 100 mg, 200 mg	0.1 mg/kg/dose 0.1–0.2 mg/kg/dose q1–4hr; max 15 mg/dose	10 mg IV = 30–60 mg PO
Fentanyl	Lozenge: <15 kg: contraindicated >2 years (15–40 kg): 5–15 mcg/kg; max dose 400 mcg >40 kg: 5 mcg/kg; max dose of 400 mcg Transdermal	Lozenge: 100 mcg, 200 mcg, 300 mcg, 400 mcg Patch: 25 mcg/hr, 50 mcg/hr, 75 mcg/hr, 100 mcg/hr Injection: 50 mcg/ml	1–2 mcg/kg/dose; max: 50 mcg/dose Continuous IV infusion	N/A
Hydromorphone	0.03–0.08 mg/kg/dose PO q4–6 hr; max: 5 mg/dose	Injection: 1, 2, 3 and 4 mg/ml Tablet: 2 mg, 4 mg Syrup: hydromorphone 1 mg and guaifenesin 100 mg/5 ml Suppository: 3 mg	15 mcg/kg IV q4–6 hr; max: 2 mg/dose	1.5 mg IV = 7.5 mg PO
Methadone	0.1–0.2 mg/kg q4–12 hr; max: 10 mg/dose	Tablet: 5 mg, 10 mg Solution: 1 mg/ml Concentrate: 10 mg/ml	0.1 mg/kg IV q 4 to 12 hr; max: 10 mg	10 mg IV = 20 mg PO

From Hockenberry-Eaton M., Barrera P., Brown M., Bottomley S., O'Neill J. (1999) Pain Management in Children with Cancer Hand-book. Austin, TX: Texas Cancer Council. Reprinted with permission.

Table 27.7. Management of opioid side effects

Side effect	Adjuvant drugs	Nonpharmacologic techniques
Constipation	Senna and docusate sodium: Tablet: 2–6 yearst: 1/2 tablet once a day; max: 1 tablet twice a day 6–12 years: 1 tablet once a day; max: 2 tablets twice a day >12 years: Start 2 tablets once a day; max: 4 tablets twice a day Liquid: 1 month to 1 year: 1.25–5 ml q hs 1–5 years = 2.5 ml q hs 5–15 years = 5–10 ml q hs >15 years = 10–25 ml q hs Casanthranol and docusate sodium Liquid: 5–15 ml q hs Capsules: 1 cap PO q hs Bisacodyl: PO or PR 3–12 years 5 mg/dose/day >12 years 10 to 15 mg/dose/day Lactulose: 7.5 ml/day after breakfast Adult: 15 to 30 ml PO q day Mineral oil: 1–2 tsp PO/day Magnesium citrate: >6 years = 2–4 ml/kg PO once 6–12 years = 100–150 ml PO once >12 years = 150–300 ml PO once Milk of magnesia (MOM) <2 years = 0.5 ml/kg/dose PO once 2–5 years = 5–15 ml PO q day 6–12 years = 15–30 ml PO once >12 years = 30–60 ml PO once	Increase water intake, prune juice, bran cereal, vegetables
Sedation	Caffeine: single dose of 1–1.5 mg PO Dextroamphetamine: 2.5–5 mg PO in a.m. and early afternoon Methylphenidate: 2.5–5 mg PO in a.m. and early afternoon Consider opioid switch if sedation is persistent	Caffeinated drinks (i.e., Mountain Dew, cola drinks)
Nausea/vomiting	Promethazine: 0.5 mg/kg q4–6hr; max: 25 mg/dose Ondansetron: 0.1–0.15 mg/kg IV or PO q 4 hr; max: 8 mg/dose Granisetron: 10–40 mcg/kg q 2 to 4 hr; max: 1 mg/dose Droperidol: 0.05 to 0.06 mg/kg IV q4–6hr; can be very sedating	Imagery, relaxation Deep, slow breathing
Pruritus	Diphenhydramine: 1 mg/kg IV/PO q4–6hr prn; max: 25 mg/dose Hydroxyzine: 0.6 mg/kg dose PO q6hr; max: 50 mg/dose Naloxone: 0.5 mcg/kg/hr continuous infusion(diluted in a solution of 0.1 mg of naloxone per 10 ml of saline) Butorphanol: 0.3–0.5 mg/kg IV (use cautiously in opioid tolerant children, may cause withdrawal symptoms); max: 2 mg/dose because mixed agonist/antagonist	Oatmeal baths, good hygiene Exclude other causes of itching Change opioids

Table 27.7. (Continued)

Side effect	Adjuvant drugs	Nonpharmacologic techniques
Respiratory depression: Mild-moderate	Hold dose of opioid Reduce subsequent doses by 25%	Arouse gently, give O₂, encourage to deep breath
Respiratory depression: Severe	Naloxone: During disease pain management: 0.5 mcg/kg in 2-minute increments until breathing improves Reduce opioid dose if possible Consider opioid switch During sedation for procedures: 5 to 10 mcg/kg until breathing improves Reduce opioid dose if possible Consider opioid switch	O₂ bag and mask if indicated
Dysphoria/confusion/ Hallucinations	Evaluate medications, eliminate adjuvant medications with CNS effects as symptoms allow Consider opioid switch if possible Haloperidol (Haldol): 0.05–0.15 mg/kg/day divided in 2–3 doses; max: 2–4 mg/day	Rule out other physiologic causes
Urinary retention	Evaluate medications, eliminate adjuvant medications with anticholinergic effects; i.e., antihistamines, tricyclic antidepressants Occurs with spinal analgesia more frequently than with systemic opioid use Oxybutynin: 1 year = 1 mg tid 1–2 years = 2 mg tid 2–3 years = 3 mg tid 4–5 years = 4 mg tid >5 years = 5 mg tid	Rule out other physiologic causes In/out or indwelling urinary catheter

From Hockenberry-Eaton M., Barrera P., Brown M., Bottomley S., O'Neill J. (1999) Pain Management in Children with Cancer Handbook. Austin, TX: Texas Cancer Council. Reprinted with permission.

Table 27.8. Opioid weaning guidelines

1. Give 1/2 of previous daily dose for 2 days

2. Reduce dose by 25% every 2 days

3. Continue until daily dose equals 0.6 mg/kg/day
   for child <50 kg
   30 mg/day for a child >50 kg
   (of morphine or equivalent)

4. After 2 days at this dose (0.6 mg/kg/day), discontinue opioid

*Oral methadone may be used to wean as follows

Use 1/4 of the equianalgesic dose as initial wean dose, then proceed as stated above

From World Health Organization (1998) Cancer pain relief and palliative care in children. Geneva: WHO

27.6.2 By the Route

Medications should be administered by the simplest, most effective, least painful route. Oral analgesics are usually available in tablets or elixirs. Intravenous, subcutaneous, and transdermal are also appropriate routes. Intramuscular injections should be avoided because they are painful and may alter the patient's report of pain in order to avoid more pain. Factors that influence the selection of administration route include severity of pain, type of pain, potency of the analgesic, and the required dosing interval.

27.6.3 By the Clock

When using pharmacologic agents, scheduled or by-the-clock dosing is recommended over "as needed" or prn dosing. Rescue dosing for intermittent or breakthrough pain is also suggested. The dosing interval is determined by the severity of the pain and the duration of the medication used (World Health Organization, 1998).

27.6.4 Opioids

There are many considerations when implementing opioid analgesia. First, there is no standard dose. The appropriate dose of an opioid is the dose that provides effective pain relief. Addiction in children with cancer is rare; however, tolerance is common in long-term use and will affect the dose required to maintain analgesia. Tolerance to side effects is also common and beneficial when titrating the dose to achieve desired analgesia. Common side effects include constipation, sedation, pruritus, nausea, and urinary retention (Table 27.7). Physical dependence may occur with prolonged use (longer than 7 days) and is more common than addiction, and opioid weaning is strongly recommended (Table 27.8). Signs and symptoms of withdrawal or physical dependence include diaphoresis, rhinorrhea, lacrimation, irritability, tremors, anorexia, dilated pupils, and goose bumps.

The most common opioid used in treating childhood cancer pain is morphine. Demerol is not recommended due to its short duration of action and toxic metabolite normeperidine, which has been associated with seizures in children. The risk of respiratory depression is still a common barrier to the appropriate dosing of morphine, especially intravenous morphine. This is a rare side effect that is reversible with the administration of naloxone. It occurs more frequently in patients with little or no prior opioid exposure, and is antagonized by pain.

27.6.5 Equianalgesia

Because there are a variety of routes by which to administer opioids, and because patients may need to be switched from one opioid to another, one must

Table 27.9. Common procedures in childhood cancer

Procedure	Suggested analgesia
Intravenous catheter insertion venipuncture	Ice pack, topical lidocaine preparations (e.g., EMLA, ELA-Max)
Implanted catheter access	Ethyl chloride coolant spray
Lumbar puncture	Conscious sedation with midazolam, morphine, and/or fentanyl (see Table 27.6)
Bone marrow aspirate or biopsy	Buffered lidocaine (use in addition to EMLA, ELA-Max, or ethyl chloride coolant spray)

consider the equianalgesic conversion factor. For example, when going from an intravenous dose of morphine to an oral dose, the oral dose may need to be larger in order to achieve the same analgesic effect. This is due largely to the first-pass effect that oral medications undergo in the liver before entering the systemic circulation. Likewise, when switching from one opioid to another, even if it is the same route, the equianalgesia factor still exists. For example, 1 mg of oral hydromorphone is equal to 4 mg of oral morphine. Equianalgesia doses are listed with the opioid doses in Table 27.6.

27.6.6 Procedure-related Pain

For procedure-related pain, premedication with the appropriate analgesic is warranted (Table 27.9). Non-pharmacologic methods in conjunction with the appropriate analgesia, such as distraction, guided imagery, and relaxation, can be used to successfully relieve this type of pain.

For more invasive procedures, sedation is widely accepted as standard of care in many centers (Table 27.10). Because of the potential for severe side effects, it is necessary to have appropriately trained staff administer the analgesia and the reversal drug if indicated, monitor the patient at regular intervals, and ensure recovery to baseline neurological and res-

Table 27.10. Conscious sedation protocol example

Agent	Dose	Reversal
Midazolam	0.1 mg/kg IV × 3 doses prn	Flumazenil 0.01 mg/kg, max. dose 0.2 mg Then 0.005–0.01 mg/kg max dose 0.2 mg Given q 1 min. Total cumulative dose = 1 mg Doses may be repeated in 20 minutes up to a maximum of 3 mg in 1 hour
Fentanyl	1 mcg/kg IV × 3 doses prn	Naloxone <20 kg: 0.1 mg/kg/dose q2–3min >20 kg or >5 yrs: 2 mg/dose q2–3min

piratory status upon completion of the process. Most centers have instituted protocols to ensure continuity and safety while providing a higher level of analgesia. Included in the protocols are recommendations for NPO status, type and dose of analgesic agents, and their reversals.

27.6.7 Patient-controlled Analgesia (PCA)

For extended pain control in children with cancer, administration of intravenous morphine and other appropriate opioids is often delivered by continuous infusion via a patient-controlled device. Although the opioid of choice is morphine, hydromorphone and fentanyl have also been used. This type of medication delivery is most effective when the parent, caregiver, or child has the ability to understand and implement it. Children who are able to understand and correlate pain relief with pushing the button are appropriate candidates. This method also has the advantage of putting the child in control and prevents the delays that often occur when waiting on a medication to be administered by personnel.

Medications can be delivered in several ways with this method: intermittent boluses, nurse- or parent-administered boluses, and continuous infusion. The delivery device usually has a mechanism for collecting and storing data so that a team member can look at how much medication the patient is receiving, or trying to receive, and correlate that with the level of pain relief. The device also provides the ability to set a maximum amount to be delivered in a given time frame to avoid overdosing. The ability to deliver a constant background infusion helps to achieve and maintain a more steady state of the drug and provide a more constant level of analgesia.

27.6.8 Adjuvant Medications

Medications that are used to provide additional analgesia are known as adjuvant drugs or co-analgesics (Table 27.3). They can aid in providing pain relief by enhancing mood, decreasing anxiety, or by directly providing additional analgesia. They may also be used to treat the side effects of the primary analgesic (Table 27.7).

Adjuvant medications are not routinely prescribed, but are instituted on a per case basis. Ongoing assessment and evaluation of their efficacy is indicated to guide their continued use in the overall plan. It is important to consider that most adjuvant medications also have possible side effects.

27.6.9 Nonpharmacologic Treatment

Nonpharmacologic treatment is indicated as an adjuvant to, not a replacement of, pharmacologic treatment. These treatments are indicated for procedure-related pain as well as for chronic pain.

Cognitive methods are directed at influencing the child's thoughts and/or images. This is also known as distraction and can be very successful with young children because they can be engaged in an activity that interests them, such as music, toys, games, or story telling (Table 27.11). If appropriate, children can be allowed to pick their preferred method.

Table 27.11. Distraction techniques by age

Age	Methods
0–2 years	Touching, stroking, patting, rocking, music, mobile over crib
2–4 years	Puppet play, storytelling, reading books, blowing bubbles
4–6 years	Breathing, storytelling, puppet play, television, activities
6–11 years	Music, breathing, counting, eye fixation, television, humor

From Hockenberry-Eaton M., Barrera P., Brown M., Bottomley S., O'Neill J. (1999) Pain Management in Children with Cancer Handbook. Austin, TX: Texas Cancer Council. Reprinted with permission.

Table 27.12. Favorite imagery scenes for children

Visual imagery

Favorite places

Animals

Flower gardens

TV or movies

Favorite room

Favorite sport

Auditory imagery

Conversations with significant others

Favorite song

Playing a musical instrument

Listening to music

Environmental sound (waves, etc)

Movement imagery

Flying

Swimming

Skating

Amusement rides

Any activity

From Hockenberry-Eaton M., Barrera P., Brown M., Bottomley S., O'Neill J. (1999) Pain Management in Children with Cancer Handbook. Austin, TX: Texas Cancer Council. Reprinted with permission.

Imagery is also used to focus the child on a pleasant event, place, or experience that engages all of the senses: sight, sound, taste, smell, touch (Table 27.12). True hypnosis requires specialized training and good cooperation from the child.

Other nonpharmacologic methods include deep breathing, relaxation, cold or warm compresses and transcutaneous electrical nerve stimulation (TENS). These nonpharmacological methods may be used individually or in combination to enhance the overall pain management plan. Choosing a nonpharmacological technique may depend on the child's age and cognitive ability and the type, severity, and nature of the pain. It may also require the support and participation of the family.

27.7 Summary

Pain in children with cancer can be caused by a number of factors. The cancer mass itself can produce pain by tissue distention or infiltration. Inflammation due to infection, necrosis, or obstruction can also cause pain. Cancer treatment consisting of chemotherapy, radiation therapy, and surgery can cause pain. Nurses must accurately assess the child's pain and intervene appropriately; pain control is of paramount importance (Table 27.13).

Table 27.13. WHO clinical recommendations for pain control in childhood cancer

1	Severe pain in children with cancer is an emergency and should be dealt with expeditiously.
2	A multidisciplinary approach that offers comprehensive palliative care should be used.
3	Practical cognitive, behavioral, physical, and supportive therapies should be combined with appropriate drug treatment to relieve pain.
4	Pain and the efficacy of pain relief should be assessed at regular intervals throughout the course of treatment.
5	Where possible, the cause of the pain should be determined and treatment of the underlying cause initiated.
6	Procedure pain should be treated aggressively.
7	The WHO "analgesic ladder" should be used for selecting pain-relief drugs; that is, there should be a step-wise approach to pain management in which the severity of a child's pain determines the type and dose of analgesics.
8	Oral administration of analgesics should be used whenever possible.
9	Misperceptions regarding opioid addiction and drug abuse should be corrected. Fear of addiction in patients receiving opioids for pain relief is a problem that must be addressed.
10	The appropriate dose of an opioid is the dose that effectively relieves pain.
11	Adequate analgesic doses should be given "by the clock", i.e. at regular times, not on an "as-required" basis.
12	A sufficient analgesic dose should be given to allow children to sleep throughout the night.
13	Side-effects should be anticipated and treated aggressively, and the effects of treatment should be regularly assessed.
14	When opioids are to be reduced or stopped, doses should be tapered gradually to avoid causing severe pain flare or withdrawal symptoms.
15	Palliative care for children dying of cancer should be part of a comprehensive approach that addresses their physical symptoms, and their psychological, cultural and spiritual needs. It should be possible to provide such care in children's own homes, should they so wish.

From World Health Organization (1998) Cancer pain relief and palliative care in children. Geneva: WHO

References

American Pain Society and the American Society of Addiction Medicine (2001) Definitions related to the use of opioids for the treatment of pain: a consensus document. www.ampainsoc.org

Hockenberry-Eaton M., Barrera P., Brown M., Bottomley S., O'Neill J. (1999) Pain Management in Children with Cancer Handbook. Austin, TX: Texas Cancer Council

Hockenberry M., Wilson D., Winklestein M., Kline N. (2003) Family centered care of the child during hospitalization and illness. In Wong's Nursing Care of Infants and Children, 7th edn, pp. 1031–1100. St. Louis: Mosby

McGrath P.A. (1990) Pain in children: Nature, Assessment and Treatment. New York: Guilford Publications

Twycross A., Moriarty A., Betts T. (1998) Paediatric Pain Management: A Multidisciplinary Approach. Oxon, UK: Radcliffe Medical Press

Wong D.L., Hockenberry-Eaton M., Wilson D., Winkelstein M.L., Schwartz P. (2001) FACES pain rating scale. In Wong's Essentials of Pediatric Nursing, 6th edn, p. 1301. St. Louis: Mosby

World Health Organization (1998) Cancer pain relief and palliative care in children. Geneva: WHO

World Health Organization (2003) Pain control in pediatric palliative care. Cancer Pain Release 16 (3,4): http://www.whocancerpain.wisc.edu/eng/16_3-4/myths.html

World Health Organization. WHO's pain relief ladder. Retrieved January 23, 2004, from http://www.who.int/cancer/palliative/painladder/en/

Bibliography

American Academy of Pediatrics, American Pain Society (2001) The assessment and management of acute pain in infants, children and adolescents. Pediatrics 108:793–797

American Academy of Pain Medicine, the American Pain Society, and the American Society of Addiction Medicine (1996) The use of opioids for the treatment of chronic pain: a consensus statement. www.ampainsoc.org/advocacy/opioids.htm

McMarthy A., Cool V., Hanrahan K. (1998) Cognitive behavioral interventions for children during painful procedures: research challenges and program development. Journal of Pediatric Nursing 13(1):55–63

Tavier-Sojo J. (2002) Analgesia and sedation. In Gunn V., Nechyba C. (eds) The Harriet Lane Handbook: A Manual For Pediatric House Officers, 16th edn, pp. 891–905. Philadelphia: Mosby

Blood Transfusion Therapy

Elizabeth Kassner

Contents

28.1 Introduction

Blood transfusion is an essential part of modern health care. Used correctly, it can save life and improve health. However, as with any therapeutic intervention, it may result in acute or delayed complications and carries the risk of transmission of infectious agents, such as human immunodeficiency virus (HIV), hepatitis viruses, syphilis, and Chagas disease. It is also expensive and uses a scarce human resource.

The decision to transfuse blood or blood products must be based on a careful assessment of clinical and laboratory indications that a transfusion is necessary to save the individual's life or prevent significant morbidity (Tables 28.1, 28.2, 28.3).

Children with malignancy or who are undergoing immunosuppressive treatment often experience myelosuppression that requires the necessary, and sometimes emergent, transfusion of blood products.

28.2 Blood Screening Guidelines

The differences in human blood are due to the presence or absence of certain protein molecules called antigens and antibodies. The antigens are located on the surface of the red blood cells (RBCs), and the antibodies are in the blood plasma. Individuals have different types and combinations of these molecules. There are more than 20 genetically-determined blood group systems known today, but the AB0 and Rh systems are the most important ones used for blood transfusions. Not all blood groups are compatible with each other. Mixing incompatible blood groups leads to blood clumping or agglutination, which is dangerous for blood recipients.

For a blood transfusion to be successful, AB0 and Rh blood groups must be compatible between the donor blood and the patient blood (Table 28.4). If they are not, the RBCs from the donated blood will agglutinate. The agglutinated red cells can clog blood vessels and stop the circulation of the blood to various parts of the body. The agglutinated RBCs also hemolyze.

Table 28.1. Age-appropriate blood volumes (adapted from Lanzkowsky, 1999)

Age	Total blood volume (ml/kg)
Newborn	82–86
1–3 years	74–81
4–6 years	80–85
7–9 years	86–88
10–15 years	83–88
16–18 years	90

Table 28.2. Disease and treatment transfusion guidelines based on hemoglobin (Rogers et al., 2002; Norville and Bryant, 2002)

Indication	Hemoglobin
Prior to a course of chemotherapy[a]	<8 g/l
Receiving radiation therapy[b]	<10 g/l
Recovering from therapy-induced bone marrow suppression	<7–8 g/l and low reticulocyte count
Signs and symptoms of anemia	<10 g/l
Active bleeding	<8 g/l or acute blood loss of >10% total blood volume

If child is asymptomatic, hold transfusion during known chemotherapy or radiation therapy-induced myelosuppression

[a] Unless child is beginning an intensive course of therapy with an existing low hemoglobin (8–10 g/dl), even if asymptomatic

[b] During radiation therapy, hemoglobin should be maintained above 6–7 g/dl for optimal oxygen-carrying capacity

Table 28.3. Disease/treatment specific transfusion guidelines (Norville and Bryant, 2002; Rogers et al., 2002)

Disease/treatment	Platelet count
Leukemia	10,000–20,000/mm³
Brain tumor	<30,000/mm³
Requiring lumbar puncture	<20,000/mm³
Requiring bone marrow aspirate/biopsy	<5,000 /mm³
Requiring surgery	>50,000/mm³
	>100,00/mm³ for surgery of eye or brain
Requiring intramuscular injection	>20,000/mm³
Presence of bleeding	60,000/mm³ (with normal prothrombin, partial thromboplastin, and fibrinogen level)
Child on therapy, with platelet recovery anticipated to be >1–2 days	Platelet count <5,000/ul
Febrile patient with acute illness	<20,000/mm³

Table 28.4. Blood type compatibility

Blood group	Antigens	Antibodies	Can give blood to	Can receive blood from
AB	A and B	None	AB	AB, A, B, 0
A	A	B	A and AB	A and 0
B	B	A	B and AB	B and 0
0	None	A and B	AB, A, B, 0	0

Type and screen requested when likelihood of transfusion is low
Includes ABO, Rh crossmatching and antibody screen
Good for 72 hours; may use sample for type and crossmatch

Type and crossmatch: Required for every PRBC transfusion
Includes ABO and Rh typing and antibody screen
Antibody identification performed for positive antibody screen

28.2.1 Blood Product Processing

Processing of blood products may include:
- Addition of:
  1. Citrate-phosphate dextrose adenine (CPDA-1) Anticoagulant: binds to calcium, inhibiting coagulation pathways
  2. ADSOL (dextrose, adenine, mannitol, sodium chloride)
  Enhances red cell survival

Each unit contains approximately 350–380 ml, with a hematocrit of 75–80% if preserved with CPDA-1 and 55–60% if preserved with ADSOL (Kulkarnis and Gera, 1999; Norville and Bryant, 2002; Rogers et al., 2002)

- Washed cells: uses normal saline to remove white blood cells (WBCs), platelets, and plasma proteins
- Leukocyte depletion (leukopore filtration): allows for greater percentage of leukocyte removal than washed or frozen platelets (99.5% versus 90%, respectively). This will prevent alloimmunization to human leukocyte antigens (HLA), cytomegalovirus (CMV) transmission, immune suppression, and nonhemolytic febrile reactions, and will possibly decrease the incidence of graft versus host (GvHD) disease. The recommended Food

Table 28.5. Indications for irradiated blood products in pediatric hematology/oncology patients

Generally accepted indications
  Bone marrow transplant recipients
  Patients with Hodgkin's disease or
  non-Hodgkin's lymphoma
  Patients with certain solid tumors including
  neuroblastoma and glioblastoma
  Patients receiving HLA-matched components
  or components from biological relatives
Indications under review
  Patients with certain hematologic malignancies
  such as acute leukemia
  Patients receiving crossmatched compatible platelets
No established indications
  Most patients receiving chemotherapy
  Patients with aplastic anemia not receiving
  immunosuppressive therapy

and Drug Administration guidelines allow 5×10^6 leukocytes per unit of blood or platelets (Rogers et al., 2002) Indications for leukocyte-reduced blood products include chronic transfusions, patients receiving chemotherapy, and bone marrow transplant candidates.

- Irradiation of blood products: This causes depletion of lymphocytes. Graft versus host disease (GVHD) occurs when donor lymphocytes engraft in a susceptible recipient. These donor lymphocytes proliferate and damage target organs, especially the bone marrow, skin, liver, and gastrointestinal tract, which ultimately can be fatal. The disease initially was recognized as a complication of intrauterine transfusion and transfusion to recipients of allogeneic marrow transplant in patients who had received total body irradiation. If irradiated blood products are recommended, (Table 28.5), the irradiation dose is 1,500–2,500 cGy to the midplane with at least 1,500 cGy in the field without resultant cellular damage (Kulkarnis and Gera, 1999; Rogers et al., 2002; Wuest, 1996). Irradiation of red blood cells decreases the storage time to 28 days.

28.3 Transfusion Complications

28.3.1 Hemolytic Reactions

Hemolytic transfusion reactions (HTR) typically occur when immunologic incompatibility between transfused donor RBCs and recipient alloantibodies produces accelerated destruction of transfused cells. Transfusion of ABO-incompatible RBCs to a recipient with the corresponding preformed antibodies is the most common etiology. Complement-mediated intravascular hemolysis is associated with acute hemolytic transfusion reactions (AHTR) and extravascular RBC destruction with delayed hemolytic transfusion reactions (DHTR). AHTR are the most severe and are a medical emergency requiring rapid identification of the event, discontinuation of the transfusion, hydration, and intensive patient monitoring.

The risk of hemolytic reactions from transfusions is approximately 1:25,000, with the risk of fatal hemolytic reactions approximately 1:160,000. AHTR are most often caused by ABO incompatibility between patient and donor during red cell transfusion.

The signs and symptoms of ATHR will usually appear within the first 5–15 minutes after the transfusion is started, but can happen at any time during the transfusion. They generally consist of

- Temperature increase >1 °C or 2 °F
- Hemoglobinuria
- Chills
- Hypotension
- Severe low back pain or chest pain
- Anuria
- Nausea and vomiting
- Dyspnea, wheezing
- Anxiety, impending sense of doom
- Diaphoresis
- Generalized bleeding
- Disseminated intravascular coagulation (DIC)

Laboratory findings include hemoglobinemia, hemoglobinuria, and decreased haptoglobin.

Treatment consists of the following:

- Stop transfusion
- Administer diphenhydramine (1 mg/kg PO or IV; maximum 50 mg/dose) and Paracetamol/acetaminophen (15 mg/kg PO; maximum 1,000 mg/dose)

In contrast to RBC transfusion – in which ABO incompatibility has potentially lethal implications – ABO matching has historically been considered less critical for platelet transfusion. Nonetheless, platelets bear ABO blood group antigens, and the plasma contained in platelet concentrates results in passive transfer of anti-A or anti-B antibodies (Heal et al., 1989)

28.3.2 Nonhemolytic Reactions

Nonhemolytic reactions are certainly more common than hemolytic reactions (30% rate of occurrence – 10% PRBC, 20% platelets) (Norville and Bryant, 2002) These reactions occur more often in children receiving frequent transfusions and begin shortly after the transfusion is started. They result from alloantibodies in the patient's plasma that react to HLA or other antigens on leukocytes or tumor necrosis factor, interleukin-1, -6, -8, and other cytokines.

Symptoms include:

- Chills
- Fever (rise of 1 °C in 24-hour period)
- Urticaria
- Rigors
- Headache
- Nausea

Treatment consists of the following:

- Stop transfusion
- Administer diphenhydramine (1 mg/kg PO or IV; maximum 50 mg/dose) and acetaminophen (15 mg/kg PO; maximum 1,000 mg/dose)
- Consider premedicating future transfusion with diphenhydramine (0.5–1mg/kg; maximum 50 mg PO or IV) and acetaminophen (10–15 mg/kg PO); Solu-Cortef 1–2 mg/kg IVP may also be given prior to transfusion in children with repeated transfusion reactions)

- Platelet transfusion may be restarted. However, if patient has a second reaction, the transfusion must be discontinued

28.3.3 Allergic Reactions

Allergens found in plasma may cause allergic transfusion reactions. If the recipient is sensitive to these, antibodies will be produced.

Clinical signs include:

- Skin erythema
- Pruritis
- Swollen lips
- Vomiting
- Hypotension
- Wheezing
- Laryngeal edema
- Anxiety
- Irritability
- Progression to anaphylaxis

Management aims to stop the allergic process. Antihistamine can be administered. In the absence of fever the infusion can continue/restart. Recurrent allergic reactions indicate the routine use of antihistamine with the possible addition of a steroid. However, if bronchospasm or life-threatening symptoms occur the infusion must be discontinued and the reaction treated.

28.3.4 Graft Versus Host Disease (GvHD)

GvHD occurs when transfused lymphocytes are not recognized by the immunocompromised patient, resulting in engraftment of transfused cells that mount an attack against the host. Blood-relative donors with similar HLA haplotypes may increase the risk of occurrence.

Symptoms may occur up to 30 days after transfusion and include

- Erythematous maculopapular dermatitis
- High fever
- Liver dysfunction
- Severe gastrointestinal symptoms (anorexia, diarrhea, vomiting)
- Pancytopenia

Prevention should be attempted and includes the following:

— Avoid donations from blood relatives
— Administer only irradiated blood components

28.3.5 Fluid Overload

Fluid overload may occur during blood product transfusion if the transfusion is administered too rapidly or the wrong volume is infused.
Symptoms include:

— Dyspnea
— Cough
— Tachycardia
— Hypertension
— Edema
— Headache

Treatment consists of the following:

— Stop transfusion
— Administer oxygen
— Diuretics (furosemide 1–2 mg/kg dose IV)

28.3.6 Transfusion-acquired Infections

28.3.6.1 Bacterial Infections

Transfusion-transmitted bacterial reaction has been identified as the most common and severe infectious complication associated with transfusion. Approximately 57% of all transfusion-transmitted infections and 16% of transfusion-related deaths have been associated with bacterial contamination. It has been estimated that 1 in 38,500 units of red cells, 1 in 3,300 units of random donor platelets, and 1 in 2,000 units of apheresis platelets are contaminated with bacteria (Blajchman, 1999).

Blood components may be contaminated with bacteria throughout many stages of preparation, including blood collection, processing, pooling, and transfusion. Bacteria may enter into blood components through several sources: donors' bacteremia, exposure to donor skin bacteria by venipuncture, and contaminated bags and environment in blood banks or hospitals.

The bacteria implicated in bacterial reactions associated with red cells are typically Gram-negative bacilli such as *Yersinia enterocolitica* and *Pseudomonas fluorescens*. In contrast, bacteria implicated in reactions associated with platelets are mostly Gram-positive species such as *Staphylococcus* and *Streptococcus*. The clinical severity of transfusion-transmitted bacterial reactions depends largely on the type and load of bacteria involved as well as the recipient's condition. Gram-negative agents usually produce endotoxins and cause severe reactions, whereas Gram-positive agents often cause minor reactions. The load of bacteria is determined by the storage time. Platelet units that are stored over 3 days and red cell units that are stored over 21 days are strongly associated with an increased risk of bacterial reactions. In addition, age and underlying diseases in recipients may also play an important role in determining the severity of a bacterial reaction.
Symptoms include:

— Fever
— Chills, rigors
— Hypotension

Treatment consists of the following:

— Obtain cultures and treat with antibiotics as appropriate
— Treat with acetaminophen (15 mg/kg PO; maximum dose 1,000 mg) and meperidine (0.5–1 mg/kg) for rigors
— Consider pre-medicating future transfusion with diphenhydramine (0.5–1mg/kg, maximum 50 mg, PO or IV) and acetaminophen (10–15 mg/kg PO)
— Prestorage filtration may decrease febrile reactions

28.3.6.2 Cytomegalovirus (CMV)
(See section 16.4.3 in chapter 16)

Infection with cytomegalovirus (CMV) is common and often lasts for a lifetime. The prevalence of CMV antibodies increases with age, and approximately 50–80% of the adult population are infected with the virus. The acute infection is usually asymptomatic, particularly in immunocompetent individuals. How-

Table 28.6. Normal hematocrit, hemoglobin, and reticulocyte values for age (Lankowsky, 1999; Schwartz, 2000)

Age	Hematocrit (%)[a]	Hemoglobin (g/dl)	Reticulocyte
Cord blood	51–55	13.5–20	3.2–5
2 weeks	50–51	12.5–20	0.5–1
3 months	35–36	9.5–14.5	0.7–1
6 months–6 years	36–37	10.5–14	1
7–12 years	38–40	11–16	1
Adult male	43–47	13–18	1
Adult female	41–42	12–16	1

[a] Hematocrit is defined as the percentage of blood volume that is specifically comprised of RBCs; can be influenced by hydration status

Table 28.7. Age-appropriate iron, ferritin, bilirubin values (adapted from Choukair, 2000)

Age	Iron	Ferritin	Total bilirubin
Newborn infant	100–250 mcg/dl	25–200 ng/ml	<1 mg/dl
1 month	40–100 mcg/dl	200–600 ng/ml	<1 mg/dl
2–5 months	40–100 mcg/dl	50–200 ng/ml	<1 mg/dl
6 months–15 years	50–120 mcg/dl	7–140 ng/ml	<1 mg/dl
Adult male	65–170 mcg/dl	15–200 ng/ml	0.1–0.2 mg/dl
Adult female	50–170 mcg/dl	12–150 ng/ml	0.1–0.2 mg/dl

ever, CMV infection may result in severe outcomes in immunocompromised or immunodeficient individuals, including those receiving bone marrow or solid organ transplants.

The prevalence of CMV antibodies among blood donors is 35–50%. Prevention of transfusion-transmitted CMV infection in high-risk recipients is critical.

- Use CMV-seronegative blood products for CMV-negative patients
- Use leukocyte-depleting filters capable of >3 log removal of white blood cells if only CMV-positive blood products are available

28.4 Erythrocyte Transfusion

Erythrocytes originate from pluripotent stem cells, which undergo proliferation, differentiation, and maturation. Iron and chemical growth factors stimulate the process of erythropoiesis. Erythrocyte values vary with age until 12 years,, and thereafter according to gender (Table 28.6). Iron, ferritin, and bilirubin values vary until age 15 years, and thereafter according to gender (Table 28.7). The lifespan of erythrocytes in serum is approximately 90–120 days; therefore, signs or symptoms of treatment-associated anemia may not be observed for 4–6 weeks after the myelosuppressive therapy has been administered.

Table 28.8. Hemoglobin-specific dosing recommendations (Kulkarnis and Gera, 1999; Norville and Bryant, 2002; Rogers et al., 2002)

Hemoglobin value	Transfusion dose
<8 g/l	10–15 ml/kg over 3–4 hours
<5 g/l	PRBC volume = (ml/kg = Hgb value) over 4 hours; e.g., 10 kg child with Hgb of 5 would receive 50 ml PRBC safely over 4 hours

10 ml/kg yields increase in hemoglobin of 2–4/dl

28.4.1 Erythrocyte Transfusion Options

- Whole blood
  - Used when massive blood loss has occurred
  - Contains RBCs, WBCs, platelets, and plasma
  - Requires crossmatching within 72 hours; must be ABO-identical and Rh-compatible
  - 8 cc/kg increases hemoglobin (Hgb) 1 g/dl
- PRBCs (Packed red blood cells)
  - Treatment choice (Table 28.8)
  - Does not significantly increase volume
  - Preparation includes removing plasma from whole blood; sediment and erythrocytes are centrifuged from 1 unit of whole blood
  - Shelf life 42 days; lifespan after transfusion 30 days
  - Requires crossmatching within 72 hours; must be ABO-identical and Rh compatible
  - Transfuse over 3–4 hours (must be completed in 4 hours)
  - Filter with 40-micron microaggregate (leukopore) filter
- Directed donor
  - Donation and screening takes approximately 2 days
  - Donate whole blood every 8 weeks
  - Check local blood bank specific guidelines regarding use of expiring products

28.4.2 Special Transfusion Considerations

28.4.2.1 Partial Exchange Transfusion

- Preferred to single or frequent PRBC transfusions
- Requires two large IV catheters
- Process involves withdrawing patient's blood and administering PRBCs in small increments of 10–50 ml, determined by the patient's weight
- Allows for rapid correction of severe anemia with less risk of pulmonary congestion. Recommended for newly diagnosed children with hyperleukocytosis (>100,000/mm^3) with associated hyperuricemia or tumor lysis syndrome

28.4.2.2 Specific Risks of Erythrocyte Transfusion

- Electrolyte imbalances (potassium and calcium), hypothermia, arrhythmias, post-transfusion purpura, hemolytic transfusion reactions, pulmonary edema with rapid or repeated transfusions

28.5 Platelet Transfusion Options

- Single donor (apheresis)
  - 6–8 units equivalent to random donor unit
  - Collected by apheresis
  - Volume ~200–300 ml; adjust per child's weight in kg
  - Reduces patient risk of alloimmunization because of limited donor exposures
  - Standard apheresis unit
  - 3.5×10^{11} platelet content and $<50\times10^6$ WBCs
  - Standard apheresis unit leukocyte-reduced
  - 3.5×10^{11} platelet content and $<5\times10^6$ WBCs
  - Facilitates matched or type-specific platelets
  - Can obtain partially or fully HLA-matched platelets from family members
- Random donor
  - Obtained from whole blood
  - 6 units typically considered pooled concentrate
  - 6 units = 4.8×10^{11} platelet content and 600×10^6 WBCs
  - 6 units leukocyte-reduced = 3.8×10^{11} platelet content and $<5\times10^6$ WBCs

28.5.1 Procurement and Storage

- Single units of whole blood are processed and platelet-rich plasma is removed; platelets are then separated from plasma by centrifugation
- May be stored for up to 5 days when processed in 50–60 ml anticoagulant and gently agitated to prevent clumping
- Require plastic bags that permit entry of oxygen, which enhances aerobic metabolism and prevents accumulation of lactic acid

28.5.2 Transfusion Guidelines

- Specific guidelines for platelet transfusion continue to vary and be disputed widely
- Platelet counts between 5,000–10,000/mm^3 are considered safe in a stable pediatric oncology patient
- Platelet count, clinical manifestations, and the child's diagnosis and therapy schedule should guide the decision to transfuse for treatment and/or prophylaxis

28.5.3 Dosing Recommendations

- 1 unit/m^2 or 1 unit/7.5 kg
  (each unit = 5.5–10^{10} platelets)
- Transfusion response may be assessed in 1 and 24 hours
- 60 minutes post-transfusion standard dose increases platelet count 10,000–12,000/mm^3 (Rogers et al., 2002). Note: Platelet increase/recovery also depends on variables such as infection, prior alloimmunization, and injury of platelets during procurement, storage, or transfusion

28.5.4 Infusion Guidelines

- ABO compatibility is recommended
- ABO incompatibility may contribute to a poor post-transfusion increase and a shorter survival time of transfused platelets
- Rh antigens are not expressed on platelets
- Females who are Rh-negative should ideally not receive Rh-positive transfusions

- Infuse rapidly (20–60 minutes) through 170-mm-diameter filter

28.5.5 Platelet-specific Transfusion Risks

- Nonhemolytic reactions
  – 20–30% occurrence (Norville and Bryant, 2002)

28.5.6 Platelet Alloimmunization

- Children receiving multiple transfusions may develop antibodies against HLA-A and B antigens, which destroy platelets expressing the HLA-A or B antigens
- Platelet refractoriness is defined as post-transfusion increment of <5,000/ul measured 60 minutes post-transfusion and recurring on two sequential occasions

28.5.7 Treatment Options

- Platelets stored <24 hours
- Antibody testing
- If antibodies are not detected, consider nonimmune causes
- HLA-matched single-donor platelets
- Crossmatching compatible platelets
- Intravenous immunoglobulin 400 mg/kg/day before the platelet transfusion for up to 9 days
- Massive transfusion with random-donor platelets
- Vinblastine-loaded platelets

28.6 Granulocyte Transfusion

- Granulocytopenia: absolute granulocyte count <200/l
- Obtained by leukopheresis, which is labor-intensive and expensive
- Granulocytes have a half-life of 6–10 hours, serum survival 12–14 hours, tissue survival 5 days
- ABO/Rh-compatible, HLA-matched preferred

28.6.1 Indications

— Absolute neutrophil count (ANC) <100 with systemic bacterial or fungal infection, culture-positive and unresponsive to antibiotic or antifungal coverage for 24–48 hour-period
— ANC <500 with expected recovery more than several days *and* prolonged survival is anticipated if the infection is controlled
— Agranulocytosis or granulocyte dysfunction

28.6.2 Dosing Guidelines

— $1-2\times10^9$ WBC/kg infused over 2–4 hours daily until infection clears or ANC increases to 500 (Kulkarnis and Gera, 1999; Norville and Bryant, 2002)
— Maintain at room temperature until transfusion
— Administer through a standard blood set 170-micron filter
— Do not administer with a leukocyte-depleting filter
— Irradiation is questionable – possible compromise of cell integrity

28.6.3 Specific Risks

— CMV infection
— GvHD
— Granulocyte preparations contain viable lymphocytes
— Alloimmunization
— Hemolytic reactions
— Respiratory distress with pulmonary infiltration

28.7 Albumin

— Protein component of plasma; requires separation from blood plasma by centrifuge
— Crossmatching not required
— Indications include hypovolemia, hypoproteinemia, ascites, pleural effusion

28.7.1 Volume

— 1 g/kg=20 ml/kg of 5%
— 1 g/kg=4 ml/kg of 25%

28.7.2 Transfusion

— 5% solution: 1–10 ml/minute; increase rate for patients in shock
— 25% solution: 0.2–0.4 ml/minute

28.8 Fresh Frozen Plasma (FFP)

— FFP contains plasma proteins, fibrinogen (1–2 mg/ml), factor IX, factor V, and factor VIII (approximately 1 unit/ml of each coagulation factor)
— Plasma portion remaining after RBCs are removed from whole blood
— Frozen at 18 °C within 8 hours of processing

28.8.1 Indications

— Replace coagulation factors
— Massive blood loss
— Active bleeding and abnormal PT/PTT
— Antithrombin III (AT-III) deficiency, protein C or S deficiency requiring surgery
— Thrombocytic thrombocytopenia purpura (TTP)
— Crossmatching not required, but donor and recipient must be ABO-identical and Rh-compatible

28.8.2 Volume

— 10–15 ml/kg

28.8.3 Transfusion

— Over 2–4 hours, infused within 6 hours of thaw time

28.9 Cryoprecipitate

- Precipitated product when FFP is thawed; rich in clotting factors
- Not virally inactivated
- 10–15 ml (1 unit) contains
  - 80–100 units factor VIII
  - 150–250 mg fibrinogen/10–15 ml
  - 40–70% vWF activity
  - 20–30% factor XIII activity
- Crossmatching not required

28.9.1 Indications

- Replace fibrinogen deficiencies

28.9.2 Volume

Varies related to diagnosis and condition

28.9.3 Transfusion

1–2 hours, within 4 hours of thaw time
  Repeat every 8–12 hours until bleeding is stopped or factor VIII level is normalized

28.10 Intravenous Immunoglobulin (IVIG)

28.10.1 Indications

- Antibiotic deficiency, immunoregulatory disorder
- Crossmatching not required

28.10.2 Volume

- 200–400 mg/kg every 3–4 weeks, infuse over 2–4 hours

28.10.3 Side Effects

- Fever, chills, tachycardia, headache, flushing

28.11 Recombinant Human (rHu) Erythropoietin Alpha

- Erythropoietin (EPO) is a glycoprotein that increases the number of stem cells committed to the red cell line
- 90% produced in kidneys, 10% in liver
- Production and maturation of RBCs may be expedited with administration of EPO
- Therapeutic experience in children is limited
- May be indicated in specific patient populations; e.g., Jehovah Witnesses
- Agents expensive, require additional injections, and side-effect profile unknown for children

28.12 Palliative Care Issues for Transfusion Therapy

In general, blood component therapy is deferred unless it is clear that the child would receive immediate and direct benefit from transfusion therapy

28.12.1 Erythrocyte Transfusion

- Temporarily improve physical and psychological functioning and respiratory status

28.12.2 Platelet Transfusion

- Decrease active bleeding
- Prevent spontaneous intracranial hemorrhaging

References

Blajchman MA (1999). Reducing the risk of bacterial contamination of cellular blood components. Advances in Transfusion Safety, 102: 183–193

Choukair, MK (2000). Blood chemistries/body fluids. In Siberry, Iannone (eds) The Harriet Lane Handbook, 15th edn, pp 199–130. Mosby, St Louis

Heal JM, Mullin A, Blumberg N (1989). The importance of ABH antigens in platelet crossmatching. Transfusion, 29: 514–20

Kulkarnis, R, Gera, R (1999). Pediatric transfusion therapy: Practical considerations. Indian Journal of Pediatrics 66: 307–317

Lanzkowsky, P (1999). Supportive care and management of oncologic emergencies. Manual of Pediatric Hematology and Oncology, 3rd edn, pp 669–717. Academic Press, San Diego

Norville, R, Bryant, R (2002). Blood component therapy. In Baggott, Kelly, Fochtman, Foley (eds.) Nursing Care of Children and Adolescents with Cancer, 3rd edn, pp 347–364. WB Saunders, Philadelphia

Rogers, ZR, Aquino, VM, Buchanan, GR (2002). Hematologic supportive care and hematopoietic cytokines. In Pizzo and Poplack (eds) Principles and Practice of Pediatric Oncology, 4th edition, pp 1205–1238. Lippincott-Raven Publishers, Philadelphia

Schwartz, E (2000). The Anemias. Behrman, Kliegman, Jensen's Nelson's Textbook of Pediatrics, 16th edn, pp 1461–1462. WB Saunders, Philadelphia

Wuest, DL (1996). Transfusion and stem cell support in cancer treatment. Hematology Oncology Clinics of North America, 10(2): 397–429

Bibliography

Blood transfusions. www.bloodsafety.com/complications.asp

Loney, J, Chernecky, C (2000). Anemia. Oncology Nursing Forum, 27: 951–964

Growth Factors

Nancy E. Kline

Contents

29.1 Principles of Treatment

Growth factors are proteins that bind to receptors on the cell surface, with the primary result of activating cellular proliferation and/or differentiation. Many growth factors are quite versatile, stimulating cellular division in numerous different cell types, whereas others are specific to a particular cell type. The lists in the following tables as well as the descriptions of several factors are intended neither to be comprehensive nor complete, but rather a look at some of the more commonly known factors and their principal activities.

Cytokines are a unique family of growth factors. Secreted primarily from leukocytes, cytokines stimulate both the humoral and cellular immune responses as well as the activation of phagocytic cells. Cytokines that are secreted from lymphocytes are termed lymphokines, whereas those secreted by monocytes or macrophages are termed monokines. A large family of cytokines is produced by various cells of the body. Many of the lymphokines are also known as interleukins (ILs) because they are not only secreted by leukocytes but are also able to affect the cellular responses of leukocytes. Specifically, interleukins are growth factors targeted to cells of hematopoietic origin (Table 29.1). The list of identified interleukins grows continuously, with the total number of individual activities now at 22.

Placebo-controlled clinical trials of recombinant human interleukin-11 (rhIL-11, also known as oprelvekin [Neumega, Wyeth]) in patients with non-myeloid malignancies have demonstrated significant efficacy in preventing post-chemotherapy platelet nadirs ≤20,000/ml, and reducing the need for platelet

Table 29.1. Source and activity of selected interleukins and interferons

Interleukins	Primary source	Primary activity
IL1-α and -β	Monocytes	Activation of natural killer cells, hematopoiesis
	Macrophages	Activation of natural killer cells, hematopoiesis
IL-3	Activated T-cells	Growth and differentiation of hematopoietic progenitor cells
IL-6	Monocytes	Acute phase response, B-cell proliferation, thrombopoiesis, cell differentiation
	Macrophages	Acute phase response, B-cell proliferation, thrombopoiesis, cell differentiation
	Stromal cells	Acute phase response, B-cell proliferation, thrombopoiesis, cell differentiation
IL-9	T-cells	Hematopoietic and thymopoietic effects
IL-11	Stromal cells	Synergistic hematopoietic and thrombopoietic effects
IL-12	B-cells, macrophages	Activates and induces a proliferation of cytotoxic T-cells and natural killer (NK) cells
INF-α and -β	Macrophages, neutrophils and some somatic cells	Antiviral effects, induction of class I MHC on all somatic cells, activation of NK cells and macrophages
INF-γ	Activated TH$_1$ and NK cells	Activates macrophages, neutrophils, NK cells, promotes cell-mediated immunity, antiviral effects

transfusions while chemotherapy can continue without dose reductions. The recommended pediatric dose of rhIL-11 is 75 mcg/kg subcutaneously(SQ) once daily, beginning 6–24 hours after the administration of chemotherapy until a post-nadir platelet count ≥50,000/microL is reached (Reynolds, 2000). Laboratory studies including a complete blood count (CBC) should be done twice or three times weekly while the child is receiving IL-11.

Erythropoietin (Epo) is synthesized by the kidney in response to the amount of oxygen available to the tissues and renal cells and is the primary regulator of erythropoiesis. It was the first hematopoietic growth factor to be identified as an important regulatory factor in erythropoiesis. Epo stimulates the proliferation and differentiation of immature erythrocytes; it also stimulates the growth of erythroid progenitor cells (e. g., erythrocyte burst-forming and colony-forming units) and induces the differentiation of erythrocyte colony-forming units into proerythroblasts. When patients suffering from anemia due to kidney failure are given Epo, the result is a rapid and significant increase in red blood cell count. It can be given to people with cancer who have anemia either because of the disease or the chemotherapy treatment (Table 29.2).

Colony-stimulating factors (CSFs) are cytokines that stimulate the proliferation of specific pluripotent stem cells of the bone marrow in adults. Granulocyte-CSF (G-CSF) is specific for proliferative effects on cells of the granulocyte lineage. G-CSF also increases the activity of erythropoietin. G-CSF has been used to treat myelosuppression since the early 1990s.

Granulocyte-macrophage-CSF (GM-CSF) has proliferative effects on both classes of lymphoid cells. Epo is also considered a CSF as well as a growth factor because it stimulates the proliferation of erythrocyte colony-forming units. IL-3 (secreted primarily from T-cells) is also known as multi-CSF because it stimulates stem cells to produce all forms of hematopoietic cells.

Myeloid growth factors are widely used in both pediatric and adult oncology. Although the literature supporting the use of growth factors in pediatric on-

Table 29.2. Colony stimulating factors

Factor	Commercial product	Principle source	Indication	Primary activity
Erythropoietin	Epoetin-alpha (Epogen, Amgen); (Procrit, Ortho-Biotech)	Kidney	Anemia related to chronic renal failure, zidovudine-treated HIV infection, cancer chemotherapy	Promotes proliferation and differentiation of erythrocytes
G-CSF	Filgrastim (Neupogen, Amgen)	Monocytes Macrophages	Neutropenia related to cancer chemotherapy; mobilize stem cells prior to PBSC transplant	Promotes growth of granulocytes, primarily neutrophils
GM-CSF	Sargramostim (Leukine, Immunex)	T-cells Epithelial cells Fibroblasts		
Thrombopoietin		E. coli	Thrombocytopenia (not approved by FDA for use)	Stimulates the production and maturation of megakaryocytes

cology is less extensive than the adult-related literature, some uses are clearly established. Both granulocyte colony-stimulating factor and granulocyte-macrophage colony-stimulating factor shorten the duration of febrile neutropenia after myelosuppressive chemotherapy, effectively mobilize hematopoietic stem cells for transplantation, and enhance neutrophil engraftment after hematopoietic stem cell transplantation (Levine and Boxer, 2002).

Thrombopoietin (TPO) is a colony-stimulating factor that stimulates the production of blood cells, especially platelets, during chemotherapy. It is a cytokine that belongs to the family of drugs called hematopoietic (blood-forming) agents. In clinical trials, TPO has proven useful in shortening the time for platelet recovery after chemotherapy, but it is not currently approved for routine use (Table 29.2). It is quite clear, however, that TPO does not regulate the release of platelets by megakaryocytes. This final step in platelet formation seems to be regulated by a separate process. Most people with thrombocytopenia have a normal or high TPO level in their blood. It is not clear whether additional doses of this investigational drug would improve platelet production (Wolff et al., 2001).

29.2 Method of Delivery

Erythropoietin is generally given as an injection under the skin (SQ), although it can be given intravenously (IV). It usually needs to be given three times a week. Recombinant human erythropoietin is generally well tolerated and may offer the benefit of reducing the need for blood transfusions in pediatric patients. G-CSF and GM-CSF are also well tolerated but need to be given daily, either SQ or IV. Laboratory monitoring is needed to determine when therapy can be discontinued (Table 29.3).

Approval of thrombopoietin for clinical use has been delayed because studies showed less impressive platelet recovery after chemotherapy than expected, and because a small percentage of recipients developed an immune reaction to the drug (Table 29.4).

Table 29.3. Doses of selected growth factors

Factor	Dose	Laboratory monitoring
Erythropoietin	Cancer chemotherapy: 150 units/kg IV or SQ three times weekly Chronic renal failure: 50 units/kg IV or SQ three times weekly Zidovudine -treated HIV infection: 100 units/kg SQ three times weekly	CBC and reticulocyte count at least weekly; check iron level and endogenous serum erythropoietin levels at baseline
G-CSF	Neutropenia: 5–10 mcg/kg/dose SQ or IV daily until post-nadir ANC ≥10,000 cells/mm^3. First dose administered 24 hours after last dose of chemotherapy PBSC mobilization: 10 mcg/kg/day SQ for at least 4 days prior to leukopheresis	CBC two to three times per week
GM-CSF	Neutropenia: 250 mcg/m^2/day for 3 weeks or until post-nadir ANC ≥1,500 cells/mm^3 for 3 consecutive days PBSC mobilization: 250 mcg/m^2/day IV over 24 hours, or SQ daily	Neutropenia related to cancer chemo- therapy; mobilize stem cells prior to PBSC transplant

Table 29.4. Potential side effects

Factor	Reported side effects
Erythropoietin	High blood pressure, skin rash, headaches, flu-like symptoms, bone pain, seizures
G-CSF	Headache, fever, chills, nausea, vomiting, diarrhea, fatigue, weakness, decreased appetite, thrombosis, flushing, muscle and bone pain, local reactions at site of injection, rashes, decreased kidney or liver function
GM-CSF	Redness at the injection site, low-grade fever, muscle aches, fatigue, rash, headache, nausea, dizziness
Thrombopoietin	Thrombocytosis, thrombosis, marrow fibrosis, veno-occlusive disease, interactions with other growth factors

29.3 Future Perspectives

Pegfilgrastim (SC/01), a long-acting pegylated G-CSF preparation, is being studied as a one-time dose per cycle given 24 hours after the completion of chemotherapy to prevent prolonged neutropenia following cancer chemotherapy. Initial studies suggest that the one-time dose per cycle is as effective as daily doses of G-CSF (Holmes et al., 2002). If this is found to be the case, it would certainly have a positive effect on quality of life.

IL-3 is capable of stimulating multipotential hematopoietic stem cells to differentiate. It has been tested in adult patients with bone marrow failure, but its role in the treatment of children with cancer is not certain. It does not seem to be superior to G-CSF and is less well tolerated (Maslak and Nimer, 1998).

Recombinant human TPO remains in active clinical development. Unquestionably, the need to develop a more effective platelet growth factor remains for the treatment of treatment-related thrombocytopenia, especially in myelodysplasia, idiopathic thrombocytopenic purpura (ITP), and lymphoproliferative disorders. This type of growth factor would also improve the yield of platelet donations, thus perhaps decreasing the number of donors needed.

References

Holmes, F. A., O'Shaughnessy, J. A., Vukelja, S., Jones, S. E., Shogan, J., Savin, M., Glaspy, J., Moore, M., Meza, L., Wiznitzer, I., Neumann, T. A., Hill, L. R., Liang, B. C. (2002) Blinded, randomized, multicenter study to evaluate single administration pegfilgrastim once per cycle versus daily filgrastim as an adjunct to chemotherapy in patients with high-risk stage I or stage III/VI breast cancer. Journal of Clinical Oncology, 20:727–731

Levine, J.E., Boxer, L.A. (2002) Clinical applications of hematopoietic growth factors in pediatric oncology. Current Opinions in Hematology, 9:222–227

Maslak, P., Nimer, S. D. (1998). The efficacy of IL-3, SCF, IL-6 and IL-11 in treating thrombocytopenia. Seminars in Hematology, 35:253–260

Reynolds, C.H. (2000). Clinical efficacy of rhIL-11. Oncology 14(9 Suppl 8):32–40

Wolff, S. N., Herzig, R., Lynch, J., Ericson, S. G., Greer, J.P., Stein, R., Goodman, S., Benyunes, M. C., Ashby, M., Jones, D. V., Fay, J. (2001) Recombinant human thrombopoietin (rhTPO) after autologous bone marrow transplantation: A phase I pharmacokinetic and pharmacodynamic study. Bone Marrow Transplantation 27:261–268

Care of the Dying Child and the Family

Angela M. Ethier

30.1   Children's Understanding of Death

Understanding death is a never-ending process that begins in childhood. An individual's concept of death matures as he or she ages (Grollman, 1990). Children's concepts of death are influenced by their personal experiences with death and by explanations and attitudes of those around them (Table 30.1). When children's questions about dying and death are avoided, their fears are magnified. Nurses can assist parents in their children's age-specific understanding of death (Ethier, in press).

30.1.1   Infants and Toddlers (0–36 Months)

It is unknown how preverbal children view death, but it is believed that they have no concept of it. Some toddlers perceive death as temporary. Infants and toddlers are affected by their parents' emotional and physical state and respond to the emotions of those around them. They react to separation from caregivers and to alterations in routine and surroundings. Behavioral responses can include crying, fussiness, clinging, biting, hitting, turning away, withdrawal, regression in speech or toileting or both, and changes in eating patterns (Ethier, in press).

30.1.2   Preschool Children (3–5 Years)

Preschoolers have a limited understanding of death. They perceive death as a state of being less alive, comparable to the state of someone who is sleeping or who goes away on a trip. They view death as reversible and temporary. Preschoolers' magical thinking can lead them to believe that their misdeeds or

Table 30.1. Children's understanding of death and characteristic behaviors

Understanding of death	Characteristic behaviors
Age 0–3 Does not comprehend death Aware of constant activity in the house Aware of Mom and Dad looking sad Aware that someone in the home is missing	Altered sleeping patterns Irritable Clings to others
Age 3–5 Sees death as temporary and reversible; continually asks if person will return May feel ambivalent Through magical thinking, may assume responsibility for the death	Concerned about own well-being Feels confused and guilty May use imaginative play Withdraws Irritable Regresses
Age 6–9 Begins to understand concept of death Feels it happens to others May be superstitious about death May be uncomfortable in expressing feelings Worries that other important people will die	May seem outwardly uncaring, inwardly upset May use denial to cope May attempt to "parent" May act out in school or home May play death games
Age 10–12 Accepts death as final Has personal fear of death May be morbidly interested in skeletons, gruesome details of violent deaths Concerned with practical matters about child's lifestyle	May appear tough or funny May express and demonstrate anger or sadness May act like adult, but regress to earlier stage of emotional response
Adolescents Has adult concept of death, but ability to deal with loss is based on experience and developmental factors Experiences thrill of recklessness Focuses on present Develops strong philosophical view Questions existence of an afterlife	Allow for informed participation Encourage peer support Suggest individualized and group expressions of grief Recommend creative outlets (e.g., writing, art, and music)

From Hellsten MB, Hockenberry-Eaton M, Lamb D, Kline N, Bottomley S (2000) End-of-life care for children. Texas Cancer Council, Austin, TX, pp. 68–69. Copyright 2000 by the Texas Cancer Council. Reprinted with permission

thoughts have caused their illness or the illness of family members. As a result, they might feel guilty and responsible for having caused someone's illness or death. Preschoolers hear the literal meaning of words (Ethier, in press). Therefore, euphemisms regarding death (e.g., "pass away," "lost") should not be used (Grollman, 1990). Children at this age who hear death as "gone to sleep" may fear going to sleep for fear of dying. Their greatest fear about death is being separated from their parents. Children of this age often hear, see, and understand more than adults are aware that they can. Their ideas and feelings of death are strongly influenced by their parents' reactions. Because of their limited coping strategies for dealing with loss, they may appear to be indifferent, being unable to tolerate feelings of grief for long. Playing can provide them with relief and an alternative method of coping. Behavioral responses among preschoolers can include asking repeated questions, complaining about physical symptoms (stomachaches, headaches), showing signs of regression, displaying intensification of their normal fears, having emotional outbursts, displaying irritability, and undergoing disturbances in their eating and sleeping patterns (Ethier, in press).

30.1.3 School-age Children (6–12 Years)

School-age children have a deeper understanding of death, although 6–9-year-olds may continue to believe that their own thoughts or misdeeds can cause death and may feel guilt and responsibility for death. They frequently personify death as someone who comes in the night, dressed in black. By the age of 9–10 years, they typically understand death in realistic concepts and view it as final and universal. School-age children ask more questions about life and death than younger children do. They tend to ask questions about what happens to the body after it is dead. They are aware that they can die, and they fear death. Dying is viewed as a threat to the school-age child's security. Their behavioral responses can include asking repeated questions, experiencing eating and sleeping disturbances, complaining about physical symptoms (stomach aches, headaches), displaying intensification of normal fears, having emotional outbursts and exhibiting irritability, and showing signs of regression (Ethier, in press).

30.1.4 Adolescents (13–20 Years)

Adolescents understand death much as adults do. They ask about dying and death and search for the spiritual meaning of what follows it. Their immediate concerns may relate to their physical appearance and to being different from their peers. Isolation from their peers and increased dependence on their families are difficult for adolescents. They often display intense emotional reactions towards dying and death, and their behavioral responses can include anger, withdrawal, an intensified fear of death, and risk-taking behaviors, such as reckless driving, drug use, and sexual activity (Ethier, in press).

30.2 Explaining Death to Children

Approach the discussion of death with a child gently. "*What* is said is significant, but *how* you say it will have a greater bearing on whether youngsters develop morbid fears or will be able to accept, within their capacity, the reality of death" (Grollman, 1990, p. 1). Grollman (1990) advises beginning the discussion of death with a child by using a nonthreatening example such as trees and leaves and how long they live. Speak on the child's developmental level, providing basic information slowly, directly, and honestly (Fochtman, 2002). Allow the child's questions to guide the discussion, avoiding unnecessary or unwarranted information. Avoid the use of euphemisms ("pass away," "lost"), and use words such as "die" and "dead." Allow the child to express his or her feelings, while accepting whatever emotions the child expresses. Provide warmth and support during the discussion, and speak with a calm and reassuring voice. Ask the child to repeat what has been discussed in order to clarify any misconceptions (Hellsten et al., 2000). Books or movies can be used to encourage discussion (Fochtman, 2002). Play, art, and music can facilitate the child's expression of feelings. Encourage family members to discuss the child's impending death openly and honestly with the child and other family members, including siblings (Ethier, in press).

30.3 Pediatric Palliative Care

30.3.1 Principles

Pediatric palliative care is family-centered, encompassing the child and the child's family members (Fig. 30.1) (Fochtman, 2002). The goal of palliative care is to attain the best quality of life for the dying child. Care is transitioned from curative to palliative, with a focus on managing symptoms to promote comfort (Ferrell and Coyle, 2002). A model of pediatric palliative care, Fig. 30.1, depicts the child and family as the center of care that addresses their physical, psychological, spiritual, cultural, and social needs. An interdisciplinary team is utilized to build systems and mechanisms of support. It involves con-

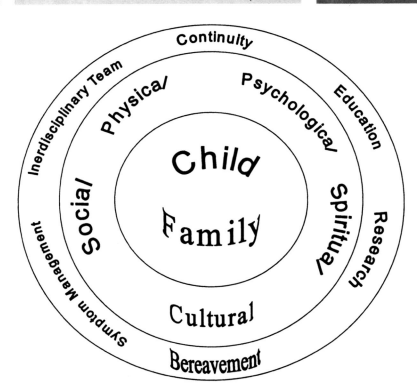

Figure 30.1

Model of pediatric palliative care

tinuity of team members and shared decision making consisting of open communication and respect for the goals, preferences, and choices of the child and family to guide the child's medical care (Last Acts, 2003). Palliative care affirms life and views death as a normal process. It does not hasten or postpone death. Bereavement care is provided to family members following the child's death (Fochtman, 2002).

30.3.2 Location of Care

It is important to determine the child's and family's preference for the location of palliative care. Pediatric palliative care can be provided in the hospital or home, or sometimes in the hospice setting. Often, the child and families will move among the various settings. Care in the hospital can be provided amongst familiar staff and surroundings, with consistent interdisciplinary team members providing care. The hospital setting affords immediate access to medications for pain and symptom management. Home care

provides the necessary supplies, medications, and periodic nursing visits to allow the child to receive care at home, and hospice provides supportive care to the dying child and family members in the child's home (Ferrell and Coyle, 2002). An interdisciplinary team, trained in the care of dying individuals and their families, provides the care. Bereavement care is provided to the family members following the child's death. Respite care is sometimes available in an inpatient hospital or hospice setting. Unfortunately, only a limited number of hospices in the United States provide care for children.

30.4 Grief

30.4.1 Principles

Grief is the emotional reaction to anticipated or actual loss and is exhibited by both children and adults (Table 30.2). Buckman (1996) describes grieving as a continuous process that usually follows three stages.

Table 30.2. Normal grief symptoms

Physical/behavioral*	Guilt feelings
Accident proneness	Indecisiveness
Allergies/asthma	Irritability
Appetite changes	Jealousy
Constipation/diarrhea	Lack of initiative
Dizziness/dry mouth	Loss of interest in living
Heartache	Moodiness
High blood pressure	Nightmares
Hives/rashes/itching	Rumination
Indigestion	Sadness
Insomnia/oversleeping	Suspiciousness
Loss of appetite/overeating	Thoughts of own death
Low energy	Withdrawal from relationships
Low resistance to infection	
Migraine headaches	**Intellectual**
Muscle tightness	Confusion
Pounding, rapid heartbeat	Difficulty concentrating
Recurrent nausea	Disbelief/denial
Restlessness	Errors in language usage
Sexual disinterest or difficulty	Forgetfulness
Stomachache	Inattention
Tearfulness	Lack of attention to detail
Weakness in legs	Lack of awareness of external events
	Loss of creativity
Emotional/social	Loss of productivity
Agitation	Memory loss
Anger	Overachievement
Angry outbursts	Past-oriented
Anxiousness	
Complacency	**Spiritual**
Critical of self	Anger at God
Difficulty in relationships	Feelings of abandonment
Exaggerated positive behaviors	"Why" questions
Fear of groups or crowds	

From Hellsten MB, Hockenberry-Eaton M, Lamb D, Kline N, Bottomley S (2000) End-of-life care for children. Texas Cancer Council, Austin, TX, p. 69. Copyright 2000 by the Texas Cancer Council. Reprinted with permission
* Any recurrent physical reaction should be evaluated by a physician to rule out the existence of a condition that may require medical treatment

The initial stage of grief involves shock and deep sadness. Physical symptoms (e.g., nausea, pain in the chest or throat, general aches and pains) during this initial phase are common. The middle phase involves realizing that the living individual's life will go on. Anger and resentment towards those who have not lost a child or sibling can occur. The final phase involves the resolution of grief, being able to remember the person who has died without acute pain and distress. Most individuals never completely resolve their grief, but rather achieve a degree of resolution (Buckman, 1996). Children and adolescents rework their loss and grief as they mature and achieve developmental milestones (Ethier, in press). Children work through grief through play, art activities, conversation, introspection, and written expressions (Ethier, in press). Adults work through grief through verbal, written, physical, and creative expressions. Sharing grief is often therapeutic (Hellsten et al., 2000).

Table 30.3. Warning signs of complicated grief

Absence of grief

Persistent blame or guilt

Aggressive, antisocial, or destructive acts

Suicidal thoughts or actions

Unwillingness to speak about the deceased
or expression of only positive or only negative feelings
about the deceased

Prolonged dysfunction in school/work

Exhibiting proneness to accidents

Engaging in addictive behaviors (e.g., drugs, food)

Adapted from N Kline (ed) (in press) Essentials of pediatric oncology nursing: a core curriculum, 2nd edn. Association of Pediatric Oncology Nurses, Glenview, IL. Copyright by the Association of Pediatric Oncology Nurses

Complicated grief is defined as the intensity and duration of behaviors, as shown in Table 30.3, persisting over several months (Field and Behrman, 2003). There are four types of complicated grief: chronic grief, delayed grief, exaggerated grief, and masked grief (American Association of Colleges of Nursing and City of Hope National Medical Center, 2003). Chronic grief reactions continue over long periods of time. Delayed grief reactions are suppressed, and the individual consciously or unconsciously avoids the pain of the loved one's death. Exaggerated grief involves the individual's resorting to destructive behaviors, including suicide. Masked grief manifests itself when individuals are unaware that their behaviors are interfering with normal functioning as a result of their loss (American Association of Colleges of Nursing and City of Hope National Medical Center, 2003). Complicated grief symptoms may necessitate referral to a mental healthcare provider (Table 30.3). Suicidal thoughts or actions and expressions to inflict hurt on another require immediate professional care (Hellsten et al., 2000).

30.4.2 Assessment of Child and Family

A grief assessment should include the child; the family members, including siblings; and significant others. Assessment begins at diagnosis and is ongoing throughout the child's care and following death during the bereavement period (American Association of Colleges of Nursing and City of Hope National Medical Center, 2003). Cultural and spiritual beliefs should be considered for each individual because these may affect the grief process.

30.4.3 Interventions

Interventions for the child (Table 30.4) and family (Table 30.5) should include educating them about the grief process; encouraging mutual participation among family members, including siblings, in caring for the child; providing the child and family with a safe and nonjudgmental environment in which to express their grief while supporting them with expressions of acceptance, patience, and respect; facilitating honest, open communication among the child, parents, siblings, and the healthcare team; avoiding euphemisms and trite expressions; assisting the child and siblings to express their feelings through the use of play and creative activities (e.g., providing art supplies, musical instruments, puppets, toy figures); educating the family about their child's age-specific understanding of death; answering all questions, avoiding unnecessary or unwarranted information; and sharing personal feelings of grief, which demonstrates that sadness, tears, anger, disbelief, and guilt are acceptable (Ethier, in press). Comfort care measures are provided to enhance the child's sense of security and include distraction techniques (such as music, video games, movies, books), pets, familiar toys, therapeutic touch or massage, and visits from friends and family members.

Table 30.4. Grief interventions for children

Age 0–3	**Maintain routines but allow for flexibility**
	Choose familiar and supportive caregivers
	Assign a support person for each child during funeral, burial, and other rituals
	Acknowledge all feelings of child and adult by naming feelings and giving permission to express anger and sadness in developmentally appropriate ways
	Give hugs when needed to help child feel secure
Age 3–5	**Reinforce that when people are sad, they cry; crying is natural**
	Read stories
	Provide materials for child to draw pictures
	Encourage dialogue among family meetings
	Expect misbehavior as child struggles with confusing feelings
	Offer play with themes of death while providing supportive guidance
	Preschool and school-age kids may benefit from knowing that the person is no longer breathing, unable to talk or other physical indicators that person is not alive
Age 6–9	**Listen to determine what information the child is seeking**
	Increase physical activity while role-modeling stress-reducing behaviors
	Work on identifying more sophisticated feelings (i.e., frustration, confusion)
	Encourage creative outlets for feelings (i.e., drawing, painting, clay, blank books)
	Preschool and school-age kids may benefit from knowing that the person is no longer breathing, unable to talk, or other physical indicators that person is not alive
Age 10–12	**Encourage creative expressions of feelings**
	Explore support group/peer-to-peer connection
	Establish family traditions and memorials
	Incorporate children into rituals, not just at time of death, but at important anniversaries (e.g., taking balloons to the cemetery; creating a special Christmas tree ornament which is always hung first; having birthday dinners and memory nights)
Adolescents	**Allow for informed participation**
	Encourage peer support
	Suggest individualized and group expressions of grief
	Recommend creative outlets, (i.e., writing, art, and music)

From Hellsten MB, Hockenberry-Eaton M, Lamb D, Kline N, Bottomley S (2000) End-of-life care for children. Texas Cancer Council, Austin, TX, pp. 68–69. Copyright 2000 by the Texas Cancer Council. Reprinted with permission

Table 30.5. Grief interventions for parents and siblings

Parents should be	Siblings should be
Encouraged to spend time with all of their children	Informed about dying sibling's situation
Encouraged to maintain normal activities	Allowed to talk and ask questions
Encouraged to take time for themselves	Comforted and supported regardless of expressions
Encouraged to share their feelings with spouse/significant other	Involved in activities with dying sibling
Encouraged to seek respite care as needed	Encouraged to see and say good-bye after sibling dies
	Encouraged to attend funeral or memorial services

30.5 Cultural and Spiritual Care

30.5.1 Principles

Culture is a system of socially-acquired beliefs, values, and rules of conduct for a particular group (Hellsten et al., 2000). Race is only one aspect of an individual's culture. Culture is multifaceted (Table 30.6), frequently changes, and is often transmitted unconsciously (American Association of Colleges of Nursing and City of Hope National Medical Center, 2003).

Spirituality involves finding the meaning of one's life, connecting with a higher power or others, and developing the ability to live with uncertainty (Mazanec and Tyler, 2003). Spirituality may or may not involve participation in organized religion.

30.5.2 Assessment of Child and Family

Components of cultural and spiritual assessment (Table 30.7) include identifying the child and family's beliefs, concerns, wishes related to their culture, and wishes related to their religious, spiritual, or existential issues.

30.5.3 Interventions

Providing culturally competent care includes being flexible, displaying empathy, portraying a nonjudgmental approach, and facilitating communication (American Association of Colleges of Nursing and City of Hope National Medical Center, 2003). Cultural sensitivity involves knowledge, attitudes, attributes, and skills (American Association of Colleges of Nursing and City of Hope National Medical Center, 2003).

Communication with the child and family who speak a different language from the nurse should involve an interpreter (Table 30.8). If possible, family members should not be used as translators for the child. Conversational style, personal space, eye contact, touch, time orientation, view of healthcare providers, and auditory versus visual learning styles should be considered when communicating with the child and family (American Association of Colleges of Nursing and City of Hope National Medical Center, 2003). Respect should be shown for the child and family's cultural and spiritual beliefs and traditions.

Table 30.6. Components within culture

Ethnic identity
Gender
Age
Differing abilities
Sexual orientation
Religion and spirituality
Financial status
Place of residency
Child's role
Educational level

Adapted from American Association of Colleges of Nursing and City of Hope National Medical Center (2003) ELNEC/End-of-Life Nursing Education Consortium/Pediatric Palliative Care Faculty Guide, pp. M5-5–M5-7. Copyright 2003 by the American Association of Colleges of Nursing and City of Hope National Medical Center

Table 30.7. Components of cultural and religious assessment

How does the child identify him/herself?
Where were the child and family/caregivers born?
If immigrants, how long have they lived in this country?
How old were they when they came to this country?
Where were their grandparents born?

What is the child and family's ethnic affiliation and how strong is the ethnic identity?

Who are the child's and family's major support people: family members, friends? Does the patient live in an ethnic community?

How does the child and family's culture affect decisions regarding their medical treatment? Who makes decisions? What are the gender issues in the child's culture and in their family structure? Is the decision-making a shared responsibility?

What are the primary and secondary languages, speaking and reading ability, and educational level?

How would you characterize the nonverbal communication styles of the child and family?

What is their religion, its importance in daily life, and current practices? Is religion an important source of support and comfort? What are other aspects of spirituality?

What are the food preferences and prohibitions?

What is the economic situation, and is the income adequate to meet the needs of the child and family? What healthcare coverage is available?

What are the health and illness beliefs and practices?

What are the customs and beliefs around the transitions of illness and death? What are their past experiences regarding death and bereavement? How much do the child and family wish to know about the disease and prognosis? What are their beliefs about the afterlife and miracles? What are their beliefs about hope? What are their beliefs about pain and suffering?

Adapted from American Association of Colleges of Nursing and City of Hope National Medical Center (2003) ELNEC/End-of-Life Nursing Education Consortium/Pediatric Palliative Care Faculty Guide, pp. M5-8–M5-9. Copyright 2003 by the American Association of Colleges of Nursing and City of Hope National Medical Center

Table 30.8. Communicating with the use of translators

Assess the translator's comfort with the topic to be discussed before the conversation

Explain the purpose of the meeting to the translator

Ask the translator to meet with the child and family before the discussion to establish trust

Speak to the child and family, not the interpreter, using simple language and avoiding medical jargon, pausing between sentences to allow the interpreter to translate every word

Ask the child and family to repeat what you've discussed to verify comprehension

Encourage the same translator to continue working with the same family throughout care

Adapted from American Association of Colleges of Nursing and City of Hope National Medical Center (2003) ELNEC/End-of-Life Nursing Education Consortium/Pediatric Palliative Care Faculty Guide, p. M5-10. Copyright 2003 by the American Association of Colleges of Nursing and City of Hope National Medical Center

30.6 Bereavement

30.6.1 Principles

Bereavement is the state of having suffered a loss. The death of a child is frequently viewed as out of the normal order. Experiencing the death of a child is one of the most difficult losses (Field and Behrman, 2003), and it affects the entire family. The stages of bereavement include shock and disbelief, experience of grief, disorganization and despair, and reorganization (Ethier, in press). The tasks of bereavement include acknowledging and accepting the loss, experiencing pain, and adjusting to life without the child (Ethier, in press). The nurse's role includes facilitating the grieving process (Table 30.9).

Table 30.9. Facilitating bereavement

Allow children and adults who are grieving to complete process, which includes these steps:
1. Tell story of their loved one
2. Identify and express emotion
3. Find meaning from experience and loss
4. Make transition from their relationship with the physical presence of the deceased child/sibling to development of a relationship based on the history, memories, and the notion of who the child/sibling would have been

Adapted from Hockenberry-Eaton MJ (ed) (1998) Essentials of pediatric oncology nursing: a core curriculum. Association of Pediatric Oncology Nurses, Glenview, IL, p. 230. Copyright 1998 by the Association of Pediatric Oncology Nurses

30.6.2 Assessment of Child and Family

The grief assessment (Tables 30.2 and 30.3) should include the family members and significant others and should take place several times during the bereavement period (American Association of Colleges of Nursing and City of Hope National Medical Center, 2003). Cultural and spiritual beliefs should be considered for each individual because these may affect the grief process.

30.6.3 Interventions

Interventions at the time of death include allowing the parents and siblings to participate, if desired, in preparing the child's body; supporting the family's cultural and spiritual preferences; and assisting with notification of the child's death and with any funeral or memorial arrangements, if requested (Hellsten et al., 2000). Facilitating bereavement (Table 30.9) assists family members through the grief process. Helping the family to find healthy ways to remember the child may include storytelling, developing rituals, and creating a memory book. Family members should be referred to other healthcare providers (social workers, psychologists, psychiatrists, counselors, marriage and family therapists, pastoral counselors, and school-based guidance counselors) as indicated. Complicated grief symptoms may necessitate referral

to a mental healthcare provider. Suicidal thoughts or actions and expressions to inflict hurt on another require immediate professional care (Hellsten et al., 2000). Many believe that the process of grieving is never fully completed (American Association of Colleges of Nursing and City of Hope National Medical Center, 2003).

30.7 Resources

30.7.1 Resources for Children

Preschool to age 8

Baumgart Klaus (2000) Laura's Star. Little Tiger Press, London.

Hickman M (1984) Last week my brother Anthony died. Abingdon Press, Nashville, TN

Lawrence M (1987) For everyone I love. Children's Hospice International, Alexandria, VA

Mellonie B, Ingpen R (1983) Lifetimes. Bantam Books, New York

Smith Joy (2004) The Day Great grandma moved house: a story explaining death and bereavement to young children. Kevin Mayhew.

Stickney D (2002) Waterbugs and Dragonflies. Continuum International Publishing Group, Academi.

Varley Susan (1997) Badger's parting gifts. HarperCollins, London.

Williams M (1971) The velveteen rabbit. Doubleday, Garden City, NY

Ages 8 to 11

Buck P (1947) The big wave. John Day, New York

Buscaglia L (1982) The fall of Freddie the leaf. Holt, Rinehart and Winston, New York

Center for Attitudinal Healing (1979) There is a rainbow behind every dark cloud. Celestial Arts, Berkeley, CA

Coutant H (1974) First snow. Knopf, New York

Krasny Brown L & Brown M (1996) When dinosaurs die: a guide to understanding death. Time Warner Trade Publishing, New York.

Varley Susan (1997) Badger's parting gifts. HarperCollins, London.
(Or younger age group).

White EB (1952) Charlotte's web. Harper & Row, New York

Ages 12 and Up

Agee J (1959) A death in the family. Avon, New York

Coerr E (1977) Sadako and the thousand paper cranes. Putnam, New York

Craven M (1973) I heard the owl call my name. Doubleday, Garden City, NY

Grollman S (1988) Shira: a legacy of courage. Doubleday, New York

Klein N (1974) Sunshine. Avon, New York

Rofes E (1985) The kids' book about death and dying. Little, Brown, Boston

30.7.2 Resources for Adults

Books

Buckman R (1996) "I don't know what to say...": how to help and support someone who is dying, 2nd edn. Key Porter Books, Toronto

Farrant A (1998) Sibling Bereavement: Helping children cope with loss. Continuum International Publishing Group, Academi.

Fitzgerald H (1992) The grieving child: a parent's guide. Simon & Schuster, New York

Grollman EA (1990) Talking about death to children: a dialogue between parent and child. Beacon Press, Boston

Kübler-Ross E (1983) On children and death: how children and their parents can and do cope with death. Simon & Schuster, New York

Phillips Kerstin (1996) What do we tell the children?: Books to use with children affected by illness and bereavement. Barnardo's, London.

Organizations

Center for Loss and Grief Therapy, 10400 Connecticut Avenue, Suite 514, Kensington, MD 20985, USA (+1-301-942-6440)

Children's Hospice International, 2202 Mt. Vernon Avenue, Suite 3C, Alexandria, VA 22301, USA (+1-800-703-684-0300; www.chionline.org)

Christian Lewis Trust, Cancer Care for Children Tel.: (01792) 480500 Fax (01792) 480700 (http://www.childrens-cancer-care.org.uk/)

CLIC (Cancer and Leukaemia in Childhood) Head office, Abbey Wood Business Park Filton, Bristol, BS34 7JU; Tel.: 0845 301 0031 Email: info@clic.org.uk (http://www.clic.uk.com/)

The Candelighter's Childhood Cancer Foundation, 7910 Woodmont Avenue, Suite 240, Bethesda, MD 20814, USA (+1-800-366-2223; www.candlelighters.org)

Web sites

Children's Cancer Web: http://www.cancerindex.org/ccw/

End-of-Life Care for Children: www.childendoflifecare.org

Last Acts: www.lastacts.org

Macmillan Cancer Relief: http://www.cancerlink.org

References

American Association of Colleges of Nursing and City of Hope National Medical Center (2003) ELNEC/End-of-Life Nursing Education Consortium/Pediatric Palliative Care Faculty Guide

Buckman R (1996) "I don't know what to say...": how to help and support someone who is dying, 2nd edn. Key Porter Books, Toronto

Ethier AM (in press) Children and death. In N Kline (ed) Essentials of pediatric oncology nursing: a core curriculum, 2nd edn. Association of Pediatric Oncology Nurses, Glenview, IL

Ferrell BR, Coyle N (2002) An overview of palliative nursing care. American Journal of Nursing 102(5):26–31

Field MJ, Behrman RE (eds) (2003) When children die: improving palliative care for children and their families. National Academies Press, Washington, D.C.

Fochtman D (2002) Palliative care. In: Baggott CR, Kelly KP, Fochtman D, Foley GV (eds) Nursing care of children and adolescents with cancer, 3rd edn. Saunders, Philadelphia, pp. 400–425

Grollman EA (1990) Talking about death to children: a dialogue between parent and child. Beacon Press, Boston

Hellsten MB, Hockenberry-Eaton M, Lamb D, Kline N, Bottomley S (2000) End-of-life care for children. Texas Cancer Council, Austin, TX

Last Acts (2002) Precepts of palliative care for children/adolescents and their families. Retrieved November 30, 2002, from http://www.apon.org//files/public/last_acts_precepts.pdf

Mazanec P, Tyler MK (2003) Cultural considerations in end-of-life care. American Journal of Nursing 103(3):50–58

Bibliography

Bluebond-Langner M (1977) The private words of dying children. Princeton University Press, Princeton, NJ

Bluebond-Langner M (1996) In the shadow of illness: Parents and siblings of the chronically ill child. Princeton University Press, Princeton, NJ

Buckman R (1996) "I don't know what to say...": how to help and support someone who is dying, 2nd edn. Key Porter Books, Toronto

Ferrell BR, Coyle N (2002) An overview of palliative nursing care. American Journal of Nursing 102(5):26–31

Grollman EA (1990) Talking about death: a dialogue between parent and child, 3rd edn. Beacon Press, Boston

Hellsten MB, Hockenberry-Eaton M, Lamb D, Kline N, Bottomley S (2000) End-of-life care for children. Texas Cancer Council, Austin, TX

Hockenberry-Eaton MJ (ed) (1998) Essentials of pediatric oncology nursing: a core curriculum. Association of Pediatric Oncology Nurses, Glenview, IL

Kübler-Ross E (1983) On children and death: how children and their parents can and do cope with death. Simon & Schuster, New York

Mazanec P, Tyler MK (2003) Cultural considerations in end-of-life care. American Journal of Nursing 103(3):50–58

Pitorak EF (2003) Care at the time of death. American Journal of Nursing 103(7):42–52

Subject Index

Printed in the United States
118133LV00003B/3/P